NASPAG

*Essentials of Pediatric &
Adolescent Gynecology*

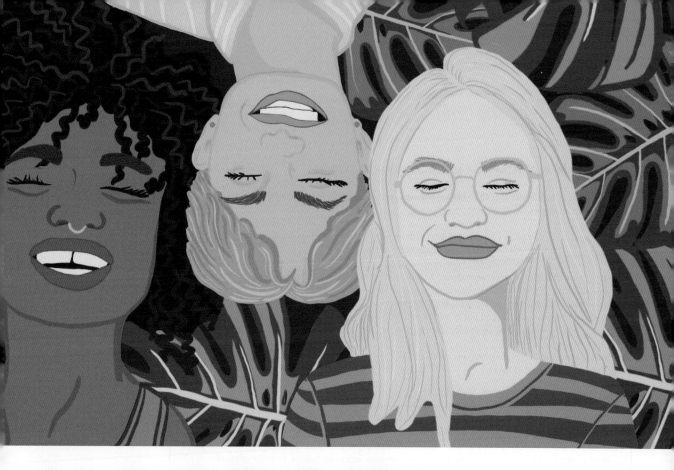

NASPAG

Essentials of Pediatric & Adolescent Gynecology

Nirupama K. DeSilva, MD
Professor
Division of Pediatric Adolescent Gynecology
Children's Medical Center
University of Texas Southwestern Medical Center
Dallas, Texas

Nichole Tyson, MD
Clinical Professor
Division of Pediatric Adolescent Gynecology
Stanford Medicine Children's Hospital
Stanford University
Palo Alto, California

ELSEVIER

Elsevier
1600 John F. Kennedy Blvd.
Ste 1800
Philadelphia, PA 19103-2899

NASPAG ESSENTIALS OF PEDIATRIC & ADOLESCENT GYNECOLOGY   ISBN: 978-0-443-10512-8

Senior Content Development Manager: Somodatta Roy Choudhury
Executive Content Strategist: Nancy Anastasi Duffy
Content Development Manager: Ranjana Sharma
Publishing Services Manager: Deepthi Unni
Project Manager: Nayagi Anandan
Senior Designer: Brian Salisbury
Cover Artist: Madelyn Frank

Printed in India

Last digit is the print number: 9 8 7 6 5 4 3 2 1

Working together
to grow libraries in
developing countries

www.elsevier.com • www.bookaid.org

CONTRIBUTORS

Oluyemisi Adeyemi-Fowode, MD, FACOG
Department of Obstetrics and Gynecology
Texas Pediatric and Adolescent Gynecology
Sugarland, Texas

Alexazandra Douglass Adler, MD
Resident Physician
Department of Obstetrics and Gynecology
University of Colorado
Aurora, Colorado

Elizabeth Alderman, MD
Professor of Pediatrics
Professor of Obstetrics and Gynecology and Women's
    Health
Department of Pediatrics, Division of Adolescent
    Medicine
Children's Hospital at Montefiore
Albert Einstein College of Medicine
Bronx, New York

Jennifer L. Bercaw-Pratt, MD
Associate Professor
Department of Obstetrics and Gynecology
Baylor College of Medicine
Houston, Texas

Elise D. Berlan, MD, MPH, FAAP, FSAHM
Professor
Department of Pediatrics, Division of Adolescent
    Medicine
Nationwide Children's Hospital
The Ohio State University College of Medicine
Columbus, Ohio

Valerie Bloomfield, MD, FRCSC
Assistant Professor
Department of Obstetrics and Gynecology
Hospital for Sick Children
Toronto, Ontario, Canada

Amy Boone, MD
Assistant Professor
Department of Obstetrics and Gynecology
University of Alabama at Birmingham
Birmingham, Alabama

Debra K. Braun-Courville, MD
Assistant Professor
Department of Pediatrics, Division of Adolescent and
    Young Adult Health
Vanderbilt University Medical Center
Nashville, Tennessee

Tania S. Burgert, MD
Associate Professor
Department of Pediatric Endocrinology
Children's Mercy Kansas City
Kansas City, Missouri

Hannah E. Canter, MD
Assistant Professor
Department of Pediatrics
Oregon Health and Science University
Portland, Oregon

Rachel Kastl Casey, MD
Department of Pediatric and Adolescent Gynecology
Inova Health System
Fairfax, Virginia

Emily Chi, MD
Resident Physician
Department of Pediatrics
University of Iowa Hospitals and Clinics
Iowa City, Iowa

Krista Childress, MD
Associate Professor
Department of Obstetrics and Gynecology
Department of Pediatric and Adolescent Gynecology
Primary Children's Hospital
University of Utah
Salt Lake City, Utah

Ana Luisa Cisneros-Camacho, MD
Assistant Professor
Department of Obstetrics and Gynecology
Baylor College of Medicine
Houston, Texas

Stephanie Marie Cizek, MD
Clinical Associate Professor
Department of Obstetrics and Gynecology
Stanford University School of Medicine
Stanford, California

Ellen Lancon Connor, MD
Professor
Department of Pediatrics
University of Wisconsin
Madison, Wisconsin

Courtney Crain, MD
Assistant Professor
Department of Obstetrics and Gynecology
Marshall Health
Huntington, West Virginia

Lauren Frances Damle, MD
Associate Professor
Department of Obstetrics and Gynecology,
Department of Pediatric and Adolescent Gynecology
Children's National Hospital
Georgetown University School of Medicine
Washington, District of Columbia

Shelby H. Davies, MD
Assistant Professor
Department of Pediatrics
Children's Hospital of Philadelphia
University of Pennsylvania School of Medicine
Philadelphia, Pennsylvania

Christina Davis-Kankanamge, MD, MS, FACOG
Assistant Professor
Department of Obstetrics and Gynecology
Baylor College of Medicine
Houston, Texas

Jennifer E. Dietrich, MD, MSc
Professor
Department of Obstetrics, Gynecology
    and Pediatrics
Texas Children's Hospital
Baylor College of Medicine
Houston, Texas

Tazim Dowlut-McElroy, MD, MS
Assistant Professor
Department of Obstetrics and Gynecology
Children's Mercy Hospital
University of Missouri-Kansas City School
    of Medicine
Kansas City, Missouri

Tania Dumont, MD, FRCSC
Associate Professor
Department of Obstetrics and Gynecology
Children's Hospital of Eastern Ontario
University of Ottawa
Ottawa, Ontario, Canada

Ashley Morgan Ebersole, MD, MS, FAAP
Assistant Professor
Department of Adolescent Medicine
Nationwide Children's Hospital
Columbus, Ohio

Amanda V. French, MD
Associate Professor
Department of Obstetrics and Gynecology and
    Pediatrics
Tufts Medical Center, Tufts Medical School
Boston, Massachusetts

Rachel Lynn Goldstein, MD
Clinical Associate Professor
Department of Pediatrics
Stanford University
Palo Alto, California

Frances Grimstad, MD, MS
Assistant Professor
Department of Obstetrics, Gynecology, and
    Reproductive Biology
Boston Children's Hospital
Harvard Medical School
Boston, Massachusetts

Megan E. Harrison, MD, FRCPC
Associate Professor
Department of Pediatrics, Division of Adolescent
    Health
Children's Hospital of Eastern Ontario
University of Ottawa
Ottawa, Ontario, Canada

Katherine G. Hayes, MD, FACOG
Assistant Professor (Clinical)
Department of Obstetrics and Gynecology
Department of Pediatric and Adolescent Gynecology
Intermountain Primary Children's Hospital
University of Utah
Salt Lake City, Utah

Cynthia Holland-Hall, MD, MPH
Professor
Department of Pediatrics, Division of Adolescent
    Medicine
Nationwide Children's Hospital
The Ohio State University
Columbus, Ohio

Laura Hollenbach, MD, FACOG
Associate Professor
Department of Pediatric and Adolescent Gynecology
University of Arkansas for Medical Sciences
Hot Springs, Arkansas

Kim Hoover, MD
Professor
Department of Obstetrics and Gynecology
University of Alabama Birmingham
Birmingham, Alabama

Patricia S. Huguelet, MD
Associate Professor
Department of Obstetrics and Gynecology, Division of
    Pediatric and Adolescent Gynecology
Children's Hospital Colorado
University of Colorado School of Medicine
Aurora, Colorado

Megan Jacobs, MD
Assistant Professor
Department of Pediatrics, Division of Adolescent
    Health
Oregon Health and Science University
Portland, Oregon

Jason Jarin, MD
Associate Professor
Department of Obstetrics and Gynecology, Division of
    Pediatric and Adolescent Gynecology
Children's Medical Center
UT Southwestern Medical Center
Dallas, Texas

Lauren A. Kanner, MD
Associate Clinical Professor
Department of Pediatrics, Division of Pediatric
    Endocrinology and Metabolism
University of Iowa Carver College of Medicine
Iowa City, Iowa

Rama D. Kastury, DO
Fellow
Department of Pediatric and Adolescent Gynecology
National Institutes of Health
Bethesda, Maryland

Olga Kciuk, MD, MSc
Fellow
Department of Obstetrics and Gynecology, Division of
　Pediatric and Adolescent Gynecology
Stanford Medicine Children's Health
Palo Alto, California

Sari Kives, MD, FRCSC, MSC
Associate Professor
Department of Gynecology
Hospital for Sick Children
Toronto, Ontario, Canada

Ashli Alyssa Lawson, MD
Assistant Professor
Department of Obstetrics and Gynecology
Children's Mercy Kansas City
University of Missouri-Kansas City
Kansas City, Missouri

Serena Margaret Liu, MD, FACOG
Assistant Professor
Department of Obstetrics and Gynecology
University of California San Francisco
San Francisco, California

Andrew Lupo, MD
Assistant Professor
Department of Obstetrics and Gynecology, Division of
　Pediatric and Adolescent Gynecology
Emory University
Atlanta, Georgia

Lauren Matera, DO
Department of Adolescent Medicine
Boston Children's Health Physicians
Valhalla, New York

Kate McCracken, MD, FACOG
Associate Professor
Department of Obstetrics and Gynecology
The University of Michigan
Ann Arbor, Michigan

Emily Paprocki, DO
Assistant Professor
Department of Pediatrics
Children's Mercy Kansas City
Kansas City, Missouri

Elisabeth H. Quint, MD
Emerita Clinical Professor
Department of Obstetrics and Gynecology
University of Michigan
Ann Arbor, Michigan

Mary E. Romano, MD, MPH
Associate Professor
Department of Pediatrics, Division of Adolescent
　Medicine/Young Adult Health
Monroe Carrell Jr. Children's Hospital at Vanderbilt
Nashville, Tennessee

Monica Woll Rosen, BA, MD
Assistant Professor
Department of Obstetrics and Gynecology
Michigan Medicine
Ann Arbor, Michigan

Amy Sass, MD, MPH
Associate Professor
Department of Pediatrics
University of Colorado
Aurora, Colorado

Nancy A. Sokkary, MD
Associate Professor
Department of Obstetrics and Gynecology
Children's Healthcare of Atlanta/Emory School of
　Medicine
Atlanta, Georgia

Shruthi Srinivas, MD
Resident Physician
Department of Pediatric Surgery
Nationwide Children's Hospital
Columbus, Ohio

Kathryn C. Stambough, MD
Assistant Professor
Department of Obstetrics and Gynecology
University of Arkansas for Medical Sciences
Little Rock, Arkansas

Clara Tang, MD
Obstetrics and Gynecology
SSM Health Medical Group
Oklahoma City, Oklahoma

Gylynthia E. Trotman, MD, MPH
Associate Professor
Department of Obstetrics, Gynecology and
    Reproductive Science and Department of Pediatrics
Mount Sinai Health System/Kravis Children's Hospital
Icahn School of Medicine at Mount Sinai
New York, New York

Nichole Tyson, MD
Clinical Professor
Division of Pediatric Adolescent Gynecology
Stanford Medicine Children's Hospital
Stanford University
Palo Alto, California

Alla Vash-Margita, MD
Associate Professor
Division of Pediatric and Adolescent Gynecology
Department of Obstetrics, Gynecology and
    Reproductive Sciences and Pediatrics
Yale University School of Medicine
New Haven, Connecticut

Jennie Yoost, MD, MSc
Associate Professor
Department of Obstetrics and Gynecology
Marshall University School of Medicine
Huntington, West Virginia

PREFACE

Pediatric and Adolescent Gynecology (PAG) is a unique speciality that focuses on the care of the youngest patients in the field of Gynecology. The North American Society of Pediatric and Adolescent Gynecology (NASPAG) was founded in 1986 in response to the growing need and development of this specialty. NASPAG has been dedicated to providing vital resources to support PAG providers in delivering the highest-quality, evidence-based care to our patients. Its mission is to provide multidisciplinary leadership in education, research, and gynecologic care to improve the reproductive health of youth.

PAG providers are experts in educating our young patients, as well as medical students, residents, and fellows. To date, training opportunities have expanded; there are now 20 PAG fellowships across the United States and Canada. Despite the significant growth of the specialty, the availability of PAG providers remains scarce both in the United States and globally, highlighting the continued need for more specialized care for PAG patients. Organizations such as International Federation of Pediatric and Adolescent Gynecology (FIGIJ) and European Association of Pediatric and Adolescent Gynecology (EUROPAG) unite PAG providers from all over the world to collaborate, train, optimize, and standardize PAG health care. This aligned mission is a goal and mandate for numerous global organizations, including Healthy People 2030 (Health.gov).

As our field has expanded, we have recognized the absence of a comprehensive collaborative text tailored to educate learners of today in the realm of PAG. Hence, our purpose in creating this book is to equip PAG learners with the knowledge necessary to address the entire range of gynecologic needs in young patients and to empower them to advocate for these patients effectively. The scope of diseases within our field is extensive, and our aim is to comprehensively educate learners on the entire spectrum. Therefore you will find chapters covering a wide array of topics, including müllerian anomalies, adnexal masses, prepubertal and postpubertal vaginal issues, sexually transmitted infections, contraception, fertility preservation, transgender patient care, and various other gynecologic issues relevant to young women. Additionally, we address common menstrual concerns, such as heavy vaginal bleeding, amenorrhea, and polycystic ovarian syndrome.

PAG providers have close partnerships across disciplines, including pediatricians, pediatric endocrinologists, adolescent medicine, pediatric and urologists and surgeons and reproductive endocrinologists to name a few. For example, young girls and teens with chronic illness such as transplants, cancer, and bleeding disorders will have routine gynecologic concerns. We strive to not only emphasize the essential aspects of health care maintenance but also shed light on frequently neglected gynecologic issues in medically complex young patients, including topics like human papilloma virus (HPV) vaccination, menstrual concerns, and contraception. PAG surgeons collaborate closely with pediatric surgeons, urologists, and colorectal surgeons to address conditions such as differences in sex development. With this goal in mind, all the authors contributing to this book are esteemed experts in their respective fields, representing various subspecialties within PAG. This diverse group ensures that learners gain a comprehensive understanding, benefitting from different perspectives across various service lines. The editors extend their profound gratitude to these authors for their invaluable expertise and unwavering commitment to educating in a manner tailored to resonate with today's learners.

In recognition of the modern learning styles embraced by today's learners, this book has been crafted to accommodate a diverse range of educational preferences. Alongside traditional text, each chapter features icons highlighting essential facts, key points, and thought-provoking questions. Furthermore, the electronic version of the book offers the convenience of hyperlinks to websites, videos, and PowerPoint presentations, allowing individuals to tailor their learning experience to their unique needs and preferences with ease and effectiveness.

Expertise in common PAG problems should be taught in all medical schools and residencies, and the ability to triage and refer to a PAG specialist is an essential skill for all providers who care for young patients. Although some of our learners who use this text may not become PAG providers, we hope that this book will be of service to all learners, so that whatever field of medicine you choose, you are able to recognize the complexities of the PAG field and triage or treat these patients effectively.

As a PAG specialist, the daily opportunity to effect meaningful changes in the lives of children and teenagers is profoundly rewarding. Within the realm of PAG, there exists an abundance of opportunities to advocate for and enact positive transformations at the community, national, and global levels. Our aspiration is for this book to equip you with the essential skills to seize these opportunities. This inaugural edition has been meticulously crafted to empower you in delivering the highest-quality care to the young women you encounter, as you play a pivotal role in enhancing the reproductive well-being of the world's youth.

Nichole Tyson, MD
Rupa DeSilva, MD

CONTENT

Visit eBooks.health.elsevier.com for videos.

Pediatric and Adolescent Well-Child Examination/Preventive Care

Amy Sass

INTRODUCTION

The American Academy of Pediatrics (AAP) developed the primary care medical home as a model of delivering primary care with the goal of addressing and integrating high-quality health promotion, acute care, and chronic condition management in a planned, coordinated, and family-centered manner. Children and adolescents may receive primary care by pediatric health care providers in a variety of settings, including hospital-based ambulatory clinics, neighborhood health centers, or school-based health centers, among other examples. It is important for pediatric and adolescent gynecology (PAG) providers to be familiar with components of well-care and preventive care for children and adolescents. Health services should be developmentally appropriate, inclusive, and culturally sensitive. Certified medical interpreters should be used to communicate clearly with the patient and/or parent/guardian in their preferred language if the provider is not already fluent in that language.

GUIDELINES FOR PREVENTIVE CARE

Bright Futures is a national health promotion and prevention initiative led by the AAP and supported, in part, by the U.S. Department of Health and Human Services, Health Resources and Service Administration, Maternal and Child Health Bureau.[1] The Bright Future Guidelines provide theory-based and evidence-driven guidance for preventive-care screenings and health supervision visits for newborns through age 21 years. The AAP/Bright Futures website (https://www.aap.org/brightfutures) has a compendium of useful resources for clinical practice, including a pictorial guide of specific screening recommendations by age, "Recommendations for Preventative Pediatric Health Care," which can be printed and displayed for reference in the clinical setting (https://downloads.aap.org/AAP/PDF/periodicity_schedule.pdf). These recommendations contain links for additional information, evidence-based guidelines, and validated screening and assessment tools.

For adolescents, the goals of these guidelines are to (1) deter adolescents from participating in behaviors that jeopardize health; (2) detect physical, emotional, and behavioral problems early and intervene promptly; (3) reinforce and encourage behaviors that promote healthful living; and (4) provide immunization against infectious diseases. The Guidelines recommend that adolescents between ages 11 and 21 years have annual routine health visits. Table 1.1 lists recommendations for universal screening and selective screening after risk factor assessments at these visits.

RELATING TO THE ADOLESCENT PATIENT

Adolescence is one of the physically healthiest periods in life. Providers who care for adolescents need to be aware of cognitive, emotional, and psychosocial changes that influence adolescents' health behaviors.[2] Each teenager is a unique individual; however, there are common developmental stages, feelings, and behaviors that many youth experience during adolescence. Adolescence is a dynamic time, and the brain continues to develop throughout adolescence into young adulthood, allowing youth to develop insight, judgement, and maturity as they navigate adolescence. See Table 1.2 for components of adolescent psychological development.

TABLE 1.1   Universal and Selective Health Screening During Health Supervision Visits

	Universal	Selective
Anemia	Screen all nonpregnant women every 5–10 y, starting in adolescence with HgB and/or HCT	Obtain HgB and/or HCT annually at minimum with ≥1 RF for anemia (diet low in iron-rich foods, history of iron deficiency anemia, excessive menstrual bleeding, poverty, food insecurities) annually
Depression	Screen youth ≥11 y annually with Patient Health Questionnaire-9 (PHQ9) tool: https://www.phqscreeners.com	
Dyslipidemia	Nonfasting lipid panel once between age 9 and 11 y and once between ages 11 and 17 y	Fasting lipid panel once ages 12–16 y if ≥1 RF in parent, grandparent, aunt/uncle, or sibling of myocardial infarction, angina, stroke, coronary artery bypass graft/stent/angioplasty, sudden cardiac death in males <55 y, females <65 y
Hypertension	Measure BP annually age ≥3 y for patients with normal BMI	Measure BP at every health care encounter for patients age ≥3 y if obese, have renal disease, a history of aortic arch obstruction or coarctation, or diabetes and/or take medication to manage high BP
Obesity	Screen BMI annually Plot BMI on CDC Clinical Growth Charts (https://www.cdc.gov/growthcharts/clinical_charts.htm) to assess sex- and age-specific BMI percentiles and identify BMI category: Underweight: <5th percentile Healthy weight: 5th percentile to <85th percentile Overweight: 85th percentile to <95th percentile Obese: ≥95th percentile	
Substance use	Screen youth ≥11 y annually with CRAFFT 2.1+N tool: https://crafft.org	
Tobacco use	Screen youth ≥11 y annually with CRAFFT 2.1+N tool: https://crafft.org	
Tuberculosis		Assess RF for TB infection annually with questionnaire: contact with people with confirmed or suspected contagious TB, radiographic or clinical findings suggesting TB, immigration (including international adoptees) from countries with endemic infection, history of significant travel to countries with endemic infection, current HIV infection; with ≥1 RF, administer TB skin test or interferon-gamma release assay

BMI, Body mass index; *BP,* blood pressure; *CDC,* Centers for Disease Control and Prevention; *HgB,* hemoglobin; *HCT,* hematocrit; *RF,* risk factor; *TB,* tuberculosis; *y,* year.
(Adapted from U.S. Department of Health and Human Services, Health Resources and Service Administration, Maternal and Child Health Bureau. Bright Futures. https://www.aap.org/brightfutures.)

TABLE 1.2	Components of Adolescent Psychological Development	
	Middle School and Early High School Years	**Late High School Years and Beyond**
Movement toward independence	Struggle with sense of identity Feeling awkward or strange about one's self and one's body Often an increased focus on self, alternating between high expectations and poor self-esteem Interests and clothing style influenced by peer group Moodiness Improved ability to use speech to express one's self Realization that parents are not perfect; identification of their faults Less overt affection shown to parents, with occasional rudeness Complaints that parents interfere with independence Learning to drive and share family automobiles Tendency to return to childish behavior, particularly when stressed Resistance to following their parents' belief system or cultural traditions, especially if these are different from what they see in their community	Increased independent functioning Firmer and more cohesive sense of identity Examination of inner experiences Ability to think ideas through Conflict with parents begins to decrease Increased ability for delayed gratification and compromise Increased emotional stability Increased concern for others Increased self-reliance Peer relationships remain important and take an appropriate place among other interests Firmer religious and cultural belief system, which may be different from their parents and family
Future interests and cognitive changes	Mostly interested in present, with limited thoughts of the future Intellectual interests expand and gain in importance Greater ability to do work (physical, mental, emotional)	Work habits become more defined Increased concern for the future and life beyond high school More importance is placed on one's role in life
Sexuality	Display shyness and modesty Increased interest in sex; this can be with the opposite sex, the same sex, or either Concerns regarding physical and sexual attractiveness to others Frequently changing relationships Worries about being normal	Feelings of love and passion Development of more serious relationships Firmer sense of sexual identity Increased capacity for tender and sensual love
Morals, values, and self-direction	Testing rules and limits Capacity for abstract thought; beginning to understand the potential consequences of future behaviors Development of ideals and selection of role models Experimentation with sex and drugs (cigarettes, alcohol, and marijuana)	Greater capacity for setting goals Capacity to use insight Increased emphasis on personal dignity and self-esteem Family, social, and cultural traditions regain some of their previous importance

(Adapted from the American Academy of Child & Adolescent Psychiatry. https://www.aacap.org/. *Facts for Families.*)

The majority of time during a routine health visit is devoted to screening and providing anticipatory guidance with a nonjudgmental, patient-centered focus. It can be helpful to have the patient complete a confidential health questionnaire before starting the visit. This can include questions about health concerns, updates of active health issues, medications, allergies, and changes in family history since the last routine health visit. The questionnaire may also include questions pertaining to risk behaviors and screening for depression (see later). There should be clear instructions for the young person to complete the questionnaire independently from an accompanying parent/guardian to ensure confidentiality about sensitive topics. There is evidence that youth may share health concerns and report risk behaviors more readily with a questionnaire format versus verbally to their provider. Care must be taken to ensure that electronic questionnaire data are protected in the electronic medical record for minors.

CONFIDENTIALITY

 Confidentiality is an essential component of health care for adolescents. For more than 25 years, national medical organizations have supported the need to provide confidential care for adolescents, including the AAP, the Society for Adolescent Health and Medicine (SAHM), the American Academy of Family Practice, the American College of Obstetricians and Gynecologists (ACOG), and the North American Society for Pediatric and Adolescent Gynecology.[3] Adolescents are more likely to disclose sensitive information, have positive perceptions of care, feel more actively involved in their own health care, and return for future care if providers assure confidentiality.

An important aspect of providing confidential health care for minor adolescents is having awareness of federal and state laws that govern a minor's ability to consent for medical treatment without consent from a parent or guardian. This is particularly relevant for PAG practices that provide sexual and reproductive health care for minors. The Guttmacher Institute is a leading research and policy organization committed to advancing sexual and reproductive health and rights (SRHR) worldwide (https://www.guttmacher.org).[4] It has a robust website detailing high-quality research and statistics, evidence-based advocacy, and regularly updated federal and state policies pertaining to SRHR topics, including an overview of individual state minor consent laws.

THE PATIENT INTERVIEW

Effective interviewing and counseling skills, characterized by respect, compassion, and a nonjudgmental attitude toward all patients, are essential to obtaining a thorough history and delivering effective prevention and health education messages. The AAP and SAHM recommend that providers have some time alone with their patients during visits starting in early adolescence to convey to the teenagers and their parents/guardians that this is a standard part of adolescent health care. This also provides an opportunity for the provider to develop an open and trusting relationship

with the young person and support the adolescent's individualization and developing autonomy. It is helpful to address confidentiality at the beginning of the clinical encounter and remind the adolescent that sensitive issues are discussed because they are important for health and to assure them that what you talk about is confidential, unless the behavior is life-threatening.

OBTAINING A PSYCHOSOCIAL HISTORY

The HEADSS Assessment

The major causes of morbidity and mortality for adolescents are associated with risk behaviors, including alcohol and substance use, violence, sexual activity, and the existence of undiagnosed and untreated behavioral health problems. In addition to using a questionnaire, health care providers who see adolescents must be able to take a developmentally appropriate psychosocial history. The HEADSS (Home, Education/employment, Activities, Drugs, Sexuality, and Suicide/depression) assessment acronym is useful for organizing this history (Table 1.3).[5] The sensitive aspects of the history should be obtained with the adolescent alone, and providers may need to be flexible with history taking to allow for this to happen after the parent/guardian leaves the examination room. Many questions can be asked in each area of the HEADSS assessment, and providers should determine which questions are most relevant to the patient population they care for. Providers in pediatric and gynecology clinics may consider using a tailored HEADSS assessment for their encounters. The adolescent's responses to the HEADSS questions may reveal what is going well in their life while also identifying risk behaviors that they may be engaged in. The provider can praise and encourage the positive behaviors and provide education, intervention, and/or treatment as needed for the unhealthy behaviors.

Depression Screening

Major depressive disorder is a common, debilitating mood disorder characterized by negative feelings, thoughts, and behaviors that causes significant impairment in social, occupational, and educational functioning and quality of life and is related to an increased risk of suicide and death. For youth ages 10 to 24 years, suicide is among the leading causes of death. Approximately 7 in 100,000 children aged 10 to 19 years died by

TABLE 1.3 The HEADSS Assessment Psychosocial History and Rationale

	Questions	Rationale
Home and environment	Where do you live, and who lives there with you? How do you get along with your parents/guardians, siblings? Is there anything you would like to change about your family?	Home life has an important impact on an adolescent's ability to succeed. It is important to know whether they live in a safe and supportive environment.
Education and employment	Are you in school? Where do you go to school? What grade are you in? What are you good at in school? What do you like about school? What is hard for you? What grades do you get? How much school did you miss last year? Why? Have you ever been suspended or expelled? Why? How do you get along with your teachers/peers? Have you been involved with bullying? What are your future plans/goals?	School is likely the primary social activity in the adolescent's life. Problems in school, academically or socially, can be an indicator of other issues. Future goals and plans can be important motivators in high-risk behavior change.
Activities	Tell me about your relationships with friends? What do you (or your friends) do for fun? Are you involved in any extracurricular activities or activities in your community? Do you have a job? How many hours a week do you work? Do you play sports or exercise? What activities do you do and how often? How many hours of screen time do you have per day?	Disengagement and withdrawal can be a sign of other problems.
Drugs	Many young people experiment with marijuana, drugs, smoking cigarettes, or drinking alcohol. Have you or your friends ever tried them? What did you try? How often do you use these things? Do you ever operate a vehicle under the influence of drugs or alcohol or ride with an impaired driver?	Positive answers can lead to diagnoses of nicotine and/or substance use disorders and need for intervention and treatment.
Sexuality/ relationships	Are you in a romantic relationship or have you been in one in the past? Tell me about your partner. Do you feel you have a healthy relationship? How do you define a healthy relationship? How do you identify your gender? How do you identify your sexuality? How do you define sex? Have you had sex? How do you feel about it? Have you ever been forced to have sex when you didn't want to?	It is important to normalize sexual feelings even in the absence of sexual activity. Teens not having sex can still have conversations about sexuality, including masturbation. It is also important to avoid assumptions about patients' sexual orientation and to be nonjudgmental about sexual practices.
Suicide/ depression	Have you had long periods where you felt down, depressed, or irritable? Have you ever thought about death, dying, or suicide?	Responses may reveal indicators of depression and/or suicidal ideation.

suicide in 2018 and 2019.[6] Recent data show that among adolescents aged 12 to 17 years, one in five (21%) had ever experienced a major depressive episode. Among high school students in 2019, more than one in three (37%) reported feeling sad or hopeless, and nearly one in five (19%) seriously considered attempting suicide. There are many risk factors for youth developing depression, including but not limited to previous history of mental health problems, family crisis, living in poverty and/or a violent household, lack of social or emotional support, being bullied, having a chronic illness, identifying as a member of the LGBTQIA+ (lesbian, gay, bisexual, transgender, queer, intersex, asexual, and more) community, and substance abuse. The AAP recommends screening youth ≥11 years for depression annually, at a minimum, at routine health care visits. The Patient Health Questionnaire-9 (PHQ-9) is a validated screening tool. The tool and instructions are available online at https://www.phqscreeners.com. If a patient expresses suicidal ideation during a clinical visit and/or if there are other serious safety concerns for the young person, they need urgent evaluation by a trained behavioral health provider, often in an emergency room to assess safety and provide an appropriate level of behavioral health care.

OBTAINING A MENSTRUAL HISTORY

A standard menstrual history includes age at menarche, frequency of menstrual periods, duration of periods, description of the volume of menstrual flow, and the types and numbers of menstrual hygiene products per day used to manage the flow. It is also helpful to inquire about any problems with periods (e.g., symptoms of dysmenorrhea, medication and supplements used to manage these symptoms, and whether the patient misses school or other activities because of these symptoms). Both the AAP and ACOG have recommended including an evaluation of the last menstrual period (LMP) as an additional or fifth vital sign.[7] By doing so, clinicians reinforce the importance of the LMP in assessing overall health status for both patients and parents. Just as abnormal blood pressure, heart rate, or respiratory rate may be key to the diagnosis of potentially serious health conditions, identification of abnormal menstrual patterns through adolescence may permit early identification of potential health concerns for adulthood.

Although menarche is an exciting event and may have significant cultural meaning for many teens, menstruation can also cause anxiety for teens and their parents/guardians, especially when there is concern that the teen's periods are abnormal. Furthermore, some patients may not inform their caretakers about heavy menstrual bleeding, prolonged periods, or missed menses, which subsequently often causes significant alarm for the caregiver when they do become aware. Teens may also seek information from peers or social media, which can lead to misinformation, incorrect self-diagnosis, and treatment seeking. It is also important to recognize that a teen may not provide accurate information about their periods during an evaluation when a parent/guardian is present, especially with concerns for pregnancy or sexually transmitted infection (STI). Providing an opportunity to meet with your patient alone allows you to discuss confidentiality again, clarify the history that was provided with the adult present, ask additional sensitive relevant questions, and offer the teen to ask any questions that they may have but were reluctant to ask with the adult present. This provides a unique opportunity to validate the teen's concerns, engage in shared decision making about the evaluation and management options, and provide education and reassurance. It is important to ask the teen for their permission regarding what specific information you can share with the parent/guardian, particularly in the context of protecting the teen's legal right to confidentiality about their reproductive health. Refer to Chapters 8 and 9 for discussion of normal and abnormal menstrual cycles.

OBTAINING A SEXUAL HISTORY

In addition to obtaining a menstrual history for patients who are female sex assigned at birth as part of the routine health care visit, health care providers should obtain sexual histories from all patients when relevant and address risk reduction. Primary prevention of STIs includes assessment of behavioral risk (e.g., assessing the sexual behaviors that can place persons at risk for infection) and biologic risk (e.g., testing for risk markers for STI and HIV acquisition or transmission). Discussions concerning sexual behavior should be tailored for the patient's developmental level and be aimed at identifying risk behaviors (e.g., multiple partners; oral, anal, or vaginal sex; or drug misuse behaviors). Careful,

Five P's	Dialogue With Patient
Partners	Are you currently having sex of any kind? If no, have you ever had sex of any kind with another person? In recent months, how many sex partners have you had? What is/are the gender(s) of your sex partner(s)? Do you or your partner(s) currently have other sex partners?
Practices	What kind of sexual contact do you have or have you had? Do you have vaginal sex, meaning penis in vagina sex? Do you have anal sex, meaning penis in rectum/anus sex? Do you have oral sex, meaning mouth on penis/vagina? Do you meet your partners online or through apps? Have you or any of your partners used drugs? Have you exchanged sex for your needs (e.g., money, housing, drugs)?
Protection from STIs	Do you and your partner(s) discuss STI and HIV prevention? Do you use condoms with your partner(s)? How often do you use condoms? Have you received HPV, hepatitis A, and/or hepatitis B vaccines? Are you aware of PrEP, a medicine that can prevent HIV? Have you considered using it?
Past history of STIs	Have you ever been tested for STIs and HIV? Would you like to get tested? Have you ever been diagnosed with an STI in the past? Did you get treatment? Did you complete treatment? Have any of your partners ever been diagnosed or treated for an STI? Do you know your partner's(s) HIV status? Have you or any of your partner(s) ever injected drugs?
Pregnancy intention	Do you desire to become pregnant? Do you think you would like to have (more) children in the future? How important is it to you to prevent pregnancy (until then)? Are you or your partner using contraception or practicing any form of birth control? Would you like to talk about ways to prevent pregnancy?

TABLE 1.4 Five P's Approach for Health Care Providers Obtaining Sexual Histories

HIV, Human immunodeficiency virus; *HPV,* human papilloma virus; *PrEP,* preexposure prophylaxis; *STI,* sexually transmitted infection. (Adapted from Centers for Disease Control and Prevention. Guide to Taking a Sexual History. https://www.cdc.gov/std/treatment/SexualHistory.htm.)

nonjudgmental, and thorough counseling is particularly vital for adolescents, who might not feel comfortable acknowledging their engagement in behaviors that make them more vulnerable to acquiring STIs. The Centers for Disease Control and Prevention (CDC) provides a "Guide to Taking a Sexual History" online (https://www.cdc.gov/std/treatment/SexualHistory.htm), which includes the "Five P's" approach (Table 1.4) to obtaining sexual histories: partners, practices, protection against STI, past history of STIs, and pregnancy intention.[8]

Sexually Transmitted Infections Screening

Twenty-six million new STIs were diagnosed in the United States in 2018, and almost half were among youth aged 15 to 24 years.[9] Table 1.5 lists STI screening recommendations from the CDC.[10] It is imperative that youth have access to confidential and free STI screening for early diagnosis and treatment of STIs, including HIV, to avoid developing morbidities of pelvic inflammatory disease, infertility, and immunodeficiency. Although STI screening is a recommended part of routine health care visits for sexually active youth, not all clinical settings provide confidential screening, which is a barrier for youth who are uncomfortable sharing or unable because of potential safety risks to share a history of sexual behaviors and need for STI screening. This may also be true in your pediatric and gynecology clinic setting. If confidential STI screening and testing are not available in your setting, providing a resource

TABLE 1.5 STI Screening Recommendations for Adolescents

Chlamydia	Screen all sexually active people AFAB <25 y at least annually. Use shared decision making to determine the frequency of screening and the sites to be tested (pharynx, vagina, urine, rectum) on the basis of sexual behavior and anatomic site of exposure.
Gonorrhea	Same as chlamydia.
HIV	Screen all sexually active AFAB people aged 13–64 y at least once in their lifetime. In addition, screen at least annually based on (1) personal risk factors: >1 sex partner since most recent HIV test, sex work, injection drug use and (2) sex partner(s) risk factors: injection drug use, HIV infection, MSM.
Syphilis	Screen sexually active AFAB people at increased risk of infection (current HIV or other STI infection, history of incarceration or sex work, MSM, living in area with higher rate of syphilis).

AFAB, Assigned female at birth; *HIV,* human immunodeficiency virus; *MCM,* men who have sex with men; *y,* year. (Adapted from Centers for Disease Control and Prevention. Sexually Transmitted Infections Treatment Guidelines, 2021, Detection of STIs in Special Populations, Adolescents. https://www.cdc.gov/std/treatment-guidelines/adolescents.htm; Adapted from American College of Obstetricians and Gynecologists. Routine human immunodeficiency virus screening. Committee opinion no. 596. *Obstet Gynecol.* 2014;123:1137-1139.)

list of locations in your local area for youth to access confidential and free STI testing is an alternative.

IMMUNIZATIONS

Providing appropriate vaccines at every routine health visit is a best-practice standard. The AAP and CDC have up-to-date information regarding recommended childhood and adolescent vaccines and schedules for individuals <18 years, including catch-up immunization schedules for children and adolescents (Table 1.6) who start late or who are more than 1 month behind. The schedules are available at the CDC website (https://www.cdc.gov/vaccines/schedules/ and include printable schedules for the office).[11] For the most up-to-date information on COVID vaccination,

TABLE 1.6 Vaccines Recommended for Adolescents Who Have Received Newborn and Pediatric Vaccines on Time

Age 11–12 y	Meningococcal disease (first dose MenACWY vaccine) Human papilloma virus (HPV) (two doses of nonavalent HPV vaccine, 6–12 mo apart) Tetanus, diphtheria, and pertussis (one dose Tdap vaccine) Influenza vaccine annually COVID-19 vaccinations
Age 13–15 y	HPV (two doses of nonavalent HPV vaccine, 6–12 mo apart; or three doses should be given over 6 mo if series started after 15th birthday Tetanus, diphtheria, and pertussis (one dose Tdap vaccine) if not given age 11–12 y Influenza vaccine annually COVID-19 vaccinations
Age 16–18 y	Meningococcal disease (second dose MenACWY vaccine) Influenza vaccine annually COVID-19 vaccinations

visit https://www.cdc.gov/coronavirus/2019-ncov/vaccines/stay-up-to-date.html#children.

PHYSICAL EXAMINATION

A complete physical examination is included as part of every routine health visit. Table 1.7 lists some of the components of a physical examination, with considerations that are unique to adolescents. Adolescents should be asked if they prefer their parent/guardian is in the room during the physical examination. Attempts should be made to keep the examination as discrete as possible by keeping any parts of the body that are not being examined covered by a gown, sheet, or clothing. Providers should start by asking the adolescent if they have any concerns about their bodies or the examination. The provider should explain the components of the examination as they move through the examination and ask the adolescent's permission before examining potentially sensitive parts of the body such as breasts and genitals. The patient may decline to have certain areas of their bodies examined, and those requests should be

TABLE 1.7 Physical Examination for Adolescents Assigned Female at Birth

Vital signs	Measure and plot height and weight on CDC clinical growth charts (http://www.cdc.gov/growthcharts/clinical_charts.htm). Calculate and plot BMI on CDC clinical growth charts. Measure BP and evaluate elevated BP by age and height percentiles to determine the degree of hypertension per the National Heart, Lung, and Blood Institute BP tables for children and adolescents (http://www.nhlbi.nih.gov/files/docs/guidelines/child_tbl.pdf). Record date of last menstrual period.
Skin	Inspect for acne, acanthosis nigricans, atypical nevi, tattoos, piercings, and signs of abuse or self-inflicted injury.
Spine	Examine back for scoliosis with Adam's forward bend test
Breasts	Visual inspection to assess SMR.[a] Conduct clinical breast examination for breast disorders if there is a reported concern.
Genitalia	Visual inspection of external genitalia to assess SMR,[a] anatomic and skin abnormalities, and signs of STIs (warts, vesicles, pathologic vaginal discharge).

[a]Refer to Chapter 5 on puberty progression for a table on SMR.
AFAB, Assigned female at birth; *BMI,* body mass index (height [cm]/weight [kg²]); *BP,* blood pressure; *CDC,* Centers for Disease Control and Prevention; *SMR,* sexual maturity rating; *STI,* sexually transmitted infection.

honored. Chaperones may be needed for breast and genital examinations depending on the patient's preference and office policies. Providers should explain any examination findings to the patient in sensitive and developmentally appropriate terms.

CONCLUSION

Although PAG providers may be more likely to see adolescents in a consultant role for reproductive health concerns, it is necessary for them to develop an understanding of the components of preventive health care and considerations that are unique to providing care to this age group (Table 1.8). Given that reproductive health is an integral part of overall health, the adolescent's developmental and psychosocial functioning directly affects reproductive health decision making. Developing communication skills to ask nonjudgmental, age and developmentally appropriate, sensitive questions, while respecting an adolescent's confidentiality, will make the adolescent feel heard and appreciated as a unique individual. Shared decision making is also a key component of patient-centered health care for an adolescent. When included in decision making and treatment planning, adolescents are more likely to be satisfied with the appointment, trust the provider, and be adherent with the treatment plan. When reviewing a treatment plan, it is important to recall minor consent laws, and providers should be cognizant of their local laws and avoid sharing confidential information (verbally, printed in an after-visit summary, or visible in the electronic health record) when appropriate.

TABLE 1.8 Summary of Health Care Considerations for Adolescents

Guidelines for preventive care	Bright Future Guidelines (AAP and HHS/MCHB) https://www.aap.org/brightfutures https://downloads.aap.org/AAP/PDF/periodicity_schedule.pdf).
Adolescent psychological development	Be familiar with assessing adolescent psychological developmental changes between middle school years and high school years in categories of movement toward independence; morals, values, and self-direction; future interests and cognitive changes; and sexuality. This will help promote developmentally appropriate discussion.
Confidentiality[a]	Allow for some time alone with your patient during the appointment to discuss confidential concerns. Be aware of state and federal policies pertaining to minor consent laws listed in the Guttmacher Institute (https://www.guttmacher.org).
Obtaining a psychosocial history[a]	Use the HEADSS Assessment to obtain a social history pertaining to the following areas: Home, Education/employment, Activities, Drugs, Sexuality, and Suicide/depression. Identify what is going well in an adolescent's life and risk behaviors that need to be addressed.

Continued

TABLE 1.8 **Summary of Health Care Considerations for Adolescents—cont'd**	
Depression screening[a]	The Patient Health Questionnaire-9 (PHQ-9; https://www.phqscreeners.com) is a validated tool to screen for depression and suicidality. Be aware of clinic resources (e.g., social work consultation for positive screens). Facilitate transport of patient to an emergency department for further evaluation of safety concerns such as suicidal ideations.
Obtaining a menstrual history[a]	Consider the LMP as a "fifth vital sign," and an indicator of reproductive health.
Obtaining a sexual history[a]	Use the "Guide to Taking a Sexual History" from the CDC, including the "Five Ps": partners, practices, protection for sexually transmitted infection, past history of sexually transmitted infections, and pregnancy intention (https://www.cdc.gov/std/treatment/SexualHistory.htm).
Immunizations	Use the adolescent vaccine schedule from the CDC (https://www.cdc.gov/vaccines/schedules/).

[a]Provide an opportunity to meet with your patient alone (separately from the accompanying parent/guardian) during the visit to discuss these topics.

AAP, American Academy of Pediatrics; *HHS/MCHB,* U.S. Department of Health and Human Services, Health Resources and Service Administration, Maternal and Child Health Bureau; *LMP,* last menstrual period.

KEY POINTS

- Annual health supervision visits are recommended during adolescence and should include universal health screening for anemia, depression, dyslipidemia, hypertension, obesity, tobacco and substance use, menstrual disorders, and provision of age-appropriate immunizations.
- Adolescence is a dynamic time of life characterized by physical, cognitive, emotional, and psychological developmental changes that influence teens' health behaviors. The major causes of morbidity and mortality for adolescents are associated with risk behaviors, including alcohol and substance use, violence, sexual activity, and the existence of undiagnosed and untreated behavioral health problems.
- Confidentiality is a necessary component of providing sexual and reproductive health care to adolescents. Providers should spend some time alone with the adolescent during an appointment when discussing sensitive topics such as sexual history, risk of pregnancy and STIs, and contraception. Providers must have awareness of federal and state laws that govern a minor's ability to consent for medical treatment without consent from a parent or guardian.
- Shared decision making is a helpful approach when caring for adolescents, as it engages them in their health care, they are more receptive to education and anticipatory guidance, and are more likely to be adherent with treatment recommendations.

REVIEW QUESTIONS

1. Which of the following is not considered part of recommended annual universal screening during a routine health care visit for an adolescent?
   a. Anemia
   b. Depression
   c. Hypertension
   d. Obesity
   e. Tobacco/substance use

2. Which of the following is not true about the human papilloma virus (HPV) vaccine?
   a. The second dose of HPV vaccine should be given at least 5 months after the first dose.
   b. The nonvalent HPV vaccine protects against nine HPV types.
   c. Patients must receive three doses of the HPV vaccine to complete the series.
   d. The HPV vaccine protects against HPV types that cause cervical cancers and anogenital warts.
   e. If the vaccination schedule is interrupted, vaccine doses do not need to be repeated.

3. The HEADSS acronym includes all of the following categories except:
   a. Home
   b. Education
   c. Activities
   d. Drugs
   e. Social media

REFERENCES

1. Hagan JF, Shaw JS, Duncan PM, eds. *Bright Futures: Guidelines for Health Supervision of Infants, Children and Adolescents*. 4th ed. American Academy of Pediatrics; 2017.
2. American Academy of Child & Adolescent Psychiatry. Facts for Families. Accessed January 5, 2023. https://www.aacap.org/
3. Maslyanskaya S, Alderman EM. Confidentiality and consent in the care of the adolescent patient. *Pediatr Rev*. 2019;40(10):508-516.
4. Guttmacher Institute. Accessed December 12, 2022. https://www.guttmacher.org/
5. Cohen E, Mackenzie RG, Yates GL. HEADSS, a psychosocial risk assessment instrument: implications for designing effective intervention programs for runaway youth. *J Adolesc Health*. 1991;12(7):539-544.
6. Bitsko RH, Claussen AH, Lichtstein J, et al. Surveillance of children's mental Health – United States, 2013–2019. *MMWR*. 2022;71(suppl 2):1-42.
7. American College of Obstetricians and Gynecologists. Committee opinion no. 651. Menstruation in girls and adolescents: using the menstrual cycle as a vital sign. *Obstet Gynecol*. 2015;126:e143-e146.
8. Centers for Disease Control and Prevention. Guide to Taking a Sexual History. Accessed December 12, 2022. https://www.cdc.gov/std/treatment/SexualHistory.htm
9. Kreisel KM, Spicknall IH, Gargano JW, et al. Sexually transmitted infections among US women and men: prevalence and incidence estimates, 2018. *Sex Transm Dis*. 2021;48(4):208-214.
10. Workowski KA, Bachmann LH, Chan PA, et al. Sexually transmitted infections treatment guidelines, 2021. *MMWR Recomm Rep*. 2021;70(4):1-187.
11. Centers for Disease Control and Prevention. Child and Adolescent Immunization Schedule, Recommendations for Ages 18 Years or Younger, United States, 2022. Accessed January 8, 2023. https://www.cdc.gov/vaccines/schedules/hcp/imz/child-adolescent.html

2

The Confidential Interview

Rachel Goldstein and Elizabeth Alderman

INTRODUCTION

Adolescence is a complex developmental phase with cognitive, physical, and psychosocial milestones (Table 2.1).[1] As a young person navigates this journey, they may engage in risk-taking behaviors as they explore their identity.[2] Studies have shown that adolescents are more likely to seek out appropriate health care when they are able to access confidential care as needed.[3] Screening for reproductive health, substance use, and mental health concerns in a developmentally appropriate way is key as you care for patients transitioning from early adolescence to young adulthood. The importance of giving adolescents the time and space to understand what kinds of health risk behaviors they are engaging in has become even more critical, as the top three causes of mortality among adolescents are firearm-related injuries, motor vehicle crashes, and drug overdose and poisoning.[4] Depression has also became more pervasive among youth, with recent data indicating nearly half of high school students report clinically significant hopelessness and sadness.[5] It should be noted, however, that the types of information that are considered confidential vary significantly across the United States.[6,7] Understanding the laws that apply locally is essential.

PART 1: SETTING THE STAGE

Setting expectations at the beginning of the visit is key in ensuring that both the adolescent and their family understand the limits of confidentiality, including the types of situations in which confidentiality must be breached.[8,9] This messaging is ideally delivered in a way that underscores the importance of "alone time" in a developmentally appropriate way, while acknowledging the supportive and positive relationships that parents and guardians can have in a young person's life.[10]

Part of setting the stage is also acknowledging any bias you may have as a provider.[11-13] It is essential to ask these questions of all teens and to not avoid asking these questions because of assumptions based on the patient's religious, socioeconomic, or cultural background.[14]

For adolescents with intellectual disability, it is important to gauge their level of independence and ability to consent for confidential care. It is key not to assume that patients with intellectual or physical disabilities are not engaging in the same risk-taking behaviors as their peers. If they have the capacity to consent to confidential services, they should be given the same time alone with their health care provider.[15] Additionally, as patients with intellectual and physical disability are at higher risk for experiencing sexual abuse,[16,17] these conversations are even more critical.

If interpreter services are needed, be sure to review confidentiality expectations for all persons involved in the interview.

As an example, stating:

"For today's visit, we'll all meet together and then I'll have you [parent/guardian] wait in the waiting room while I meet with [PATIENT'S NAME] alone. When you [PATIENT] and I meet alone, I'll be checking in with you about topics that affect teens, unless I have concerns about your safety, for instance, you hurting yourself, you hurting someone else, or someone else hurting you, then what we discuss will remain confidential. If any of those safety concerns come up, I will let you [parent/guardian] know. It is also up to you [PATIENT] who is in the room for your examination, which we can figure out later."

Rarely, there may be parents/guardians who are uncomfortable or apprehensive about leaving the room for

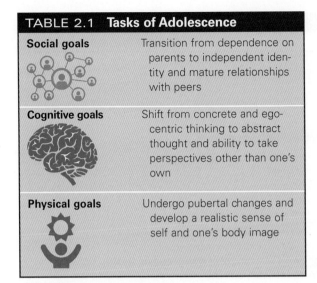

TABLE 2.1	Tasks of Adolescence
Social goals	Transition from dependence on parents to independent identity and mature relationships with peers
Cognitive goals	Shift from concrete and egocentric thinking to abstract thought and ability to take perspectives other than one's own
Physical goals	Undergo pubertal changes and develop a realistic sense of self and one's body image

the confidential interview. If this happens, you can begin by asking what their concerns are. Often, by reviewing the limits of confidentiality, many parents/guardians will be reassured that they will be informed if there are any significant concerns. For some, highlighting the importance of allowing their adolescent to practice speaking with a physician on their own as part of managing their health care, which will one day be their responsibility, can help to facilitate alone time with the teen.

For example, stating:

> "I hear your concerns and can understand this can be a difficult transition. Giving the space for your child to speak with the doctor alone allows them to practice having their own relationship with their health care provider and being responsible for their own health needs/health care. Also, in [YOUR STATE], adolescents have certain rights to confidential health care. I encourage you to have these conversations, as we both want your teen to be as healthy and safe as possible. Again, to reassure you, if I have any concerns about your child's safety, I will let you know."

The same conversation can be helpful for the adolescent who does not want their parent/guardian to leave. If ultimately, the parent/guardian remains in the room,

you can review the topics that would be addressed to see if the teen is willing to discuss any of them with their parent/guardian present and then document the context of how the history was obtained in your note.

For example:

> "Typically, I would check in with you [PATIENT] about substance use, things like birth control, and how your mood is. Are there any topics you'd like to discuss today?"

In this case, it is helpful to let the teen drive the conversations, as they can dictate the amount of information that is disclosed, and you can counsel about the health information topics relevant to them. As part of the discussion with the adolescent around confidential information sharing, it is important that they understand where their information goes within the electronic health record (EHR) and who has access to it.[18] For example, changing pronouns in the EHR to affirm their gender identity may be visible to any provider who opens their chart and could be inadvertently disclosed to their parents. Encouraging teens to have their own portal account can help them to take on more ownership of their health care and facilitates confidential communication with their health care team.[19] It is essential to educate yourself about what types of health information are shared within your EHR to patients and families so you can best counsel your patients and protect their confidentiality rights.

PART 2: HOW TO ASK THE QUESTIONS

Now that you have set the stage and are meeting with the adolescent by themselves, many providers wonder where to begin. The first step before obtaining this important information is ensuring you have accurate contact information for the teen in case you need to communicate with them directly after the visit. For many teens, if permitted within the EHR, messaging through the patient portal can be a convenient mode of communication.

Many frameworks exist to help you normalize what can be sensitive topics and structure the conversation (Fig. 2.1 and Table 2.2).

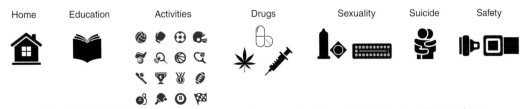

Fig. 2.1 HEADSSS[22] is a similar psychosocial screening tool but with the structure shown above.

TABLE 2.2 **Example of SHADESS Structure**[19]	
Domain	**Example Questions**
Strengths	What is your favorite part or quality about yourself? What would your best friend say they like best about you?
School	Where do you go to school? What grade are you in? How were your grades last year? What do you plan to do after you finish high school?
Home	Who all lives with you at home? How do you get along with folks at home? Do you feel safe at home?
Activities	What activities or hobbies are you into right now? What activities do you do in your free time?
Drugs	Any vaping, marijuana, alcohol, or other drug use? *If the patient answers yes, then you can ask the following questions:* How have you used _____? *(for example, with marijuana, it can be used in multiple different forms, e.g., vaping, smoking blunts, edibles)* How long have you been using _____? How often do you use _____? What do you like about using _____? Have you noticed any downsides to using _____?
Emotions/eating and depression	Do you have any concerns about body image or your eating habits? What is one word you would use to describe your mood? Have you ever felt really down or sad? If so, have you ever felt so down or sad that you had thoughts of hurting yourself? If so, have you ever hurt yourself?

Sexuality	Are you attracted to guys, girls, both or neither?[20]
	Have you ever had sex, which includes oral, anal, or vaginal sex?
	   If the patient answers yes, then you can ask the following questions:
	      How old were you when you first had sex?
	      How many sexual partners have you had in your whole life?
	      Have you ever been on birth control?
	      Have you ever had to take emergency contraception?
	      Have you ever been pregnant?
	      What do you use to protect yourself against sexually transmitted infections?
	   If the patient has been in a relationship, screening for intimate partner violence is important[21]*:*
	      Has anyone ever made you do something sexual that you were not comfortable with?
	      Have you ever felt afraid of your partner?

Safety	Do you feel safe at home? Do you feel safe in your neighborhood? Do you or anyone you know carry a weapon (e.g., gun, knife, etc.)? Have you ever been touched in a way that you did not want? Have you ever seen people at home hurt each other?

Of note, generally, we recommend confirming the adolescent's name and pronouns at the beginning of the visit. It can also be helpful tos inquire again during the confidential interview, as some teens may not feel comfortable sharing this information in front of parents/guardians or at the beginning of the visit. Typically, this question can be asked before sexuality.

PART 3: WHEN AND HOW TO BREAK CONFIDENTIALITY

There are certain situations where confidentiality must be breached because of concerns around safety. In those circumstances, it is best to remind the adolescent of the limits of confidentiality and that as their health care provider, you must disclose this confidential information to keep patients and others safe. It is important to assure the adolescent that you will let them know first about any disclosure before it is made. In the case of a patient with suicidal ideation, for instance, it may be helpful to inform the teen that you need to share the information with their family and describe in general terms the scope of the conversation.

For example, you can say:

"Thank you for sharing all of this with me today. As you may remember, before we began, I told you that if I had any concerns about your safety, I would need to let your family know. Based on what we have talked about today, I will let your family know that you have been struggling with depression and are having thoughts of hurting yourself. I'll speak with your family about ways that they can help to keep you safe."

For many adolescents, this can feel incredibly disempowering. To mitigate this, you can give them agency by allowing them to decide who is present for the disclosure. For example, you could offer to speak with the family separately or together with the teen. You can also offer to make the disclosure yourself or help the teen share the information with their family. Once the family has been informed, you would then connect with any other relevant resources (e.g., social work, mental health clinicians, law enforcement). Although these conversations can be quite challenging because the limits of confidentiality were described before beginning the confidential interview, breaking confidentiality is typically much more straightforward.

In contrast, there are other scenarios where the decision to break confidentiality is more nuanced. For instance, although in many states, gender identity may not be a legally protected topic for minors, many clinicians would not disclose gender dysphoria to a patient's family without their permission, given the potential risks for the teen in the event that their family is not supportive.[23] Substance use can be another gray area where adolescents may be engaging in harmful substance use, but it can be challenging to decide when the substance use crosses the line and confidentiality must be breached. If a health care provider feels that the safety of the patient or others is at risk because of their substance use, then they may decide to disclose this information to the patient's family—for example, if a patient shares that they consistently drive while under the influence of drugs or alcohol. Other topics that may pose challenges around confidentiality breaches include concerns for disordered eating and nonsuicidal self-injury. Ultimately, you need to use your professional judgment when determining whether breach of confidentiality is required. In the instance where you have determined that breach of confidentiality is not required and the teen does not feel they can speak only with their parent/guardian, it is important to encourage the teen to involve another trusted adult.

Finally, informing the adolescent about where information goes after the discussion ends, whether to other members of the health care team or within their health record, is essential. Part of being able to counsel patients about how information will be shared is understanding how confidential information is documented at your institution. This has become even more important after passage of the 21st Century Cures Act, which mandated the sharing of electronic health information to patients and their families. Implementation of this new law has presented notable challenges in terms of balancing information sharing and protection of confidentiality rights.[18] Having a separate note type to document confidential information can allow providers to share nonconfidential notes with patients and families. Understanding how other potentially confidential information like medications, laboratory tests/imaging, and diagnoses are handled within the EHR is also essential in caring for adolescents and young adults. Providers should be aware of how the patient portal is set up and who has access to it. Even when minors are allowed to have their own access, it is possible that a parent/guardian may have access because of the parents' email having been provided during portal setup.[19]

CONCLUSION

Although the teen may be seeing you specifically for gynecologic care, they may be engaging in other risk-taking behaviors that can affect their overall health. Therefore it is critical to take advantage of every encounter with an adolescent to screen for health risk behaviors. Regardless of which model you use to obtain the adolescent social history, it is important to pick one, practice asking the questions, and make it a consistent part of your visits with adolescent patients.

KEY POINTS

- Establishing rapport with the adolescent in a developmentally appropriate way is essential.
- Providing confidential care for certain types of health concerns such as reproductive health, mental health, and substance use, when allowable under the law, is the cornerstone of the provision of care for adolescents.
- Time with the adolescent alone is a necessary part of the visit. This should be explained to the teen and parent. There should be part of the visit with the teen and parent together, too, as well as offering the parent time alone, if they wish.
- Involving parents/guardians in the care of adolescents, if possible, should be encouraged.
- Explaining when confidentiality cannot be ensured is important.

REVIEW QUESTIONS

1. One of the instances in which confidentiality absolutely cannot be ensured in all states is:
   a. A 16-year-old discloses he is sexually active
   b. A 15-year-old discloses she needs treatment for chlamydia because her partner was diagnosed
   c. A 17-year-old wishes to obtain contraception without her parents' knowledge
   d. A 14-year-old discloses that a family member living with her family has "touched her in her privates"
2. One of the first steps in establishing rapport with a teen at a health care visit is:
   a. Asking if they wish their parent to be brought into the room
   b. Asking for their confidential contact information such as cell phone number
   c. Asking their preferred pronouns and name
   d. Asking the teen why they are seeking medical care
3. What potential activities associated with the teen's visit would not potentially compromise confidentiality and should be addressed with the teen, even those 18 years or older?
   a. Documentation in the medical record
   b. The questions you ask while obtaining a medical history
   c. Release of information in the patient portal
   d. Billing for the visit

REFERENCES

1. Neinstein LS, Katzman D, Callahan T, eds. *Neinstein's Adolescent and Young Adult Health Care: A Practical Guide*. 6th ed. Wolters Kluwer; 2016.
2. van Duijvenvoorde ACK, van Hoorn J, Blankenstein NE. Risks and rewards in adolescent decision-making. *Curr Opin Psychol*. 2022;48:101457. doi:10.1016/j.copsyc.2022.101457
3. Committee on Adolescence. Achieving quality health services for adolescents. *Pediatrics*. 2016;138(2):e20161347. doi:10.1542/peds.2016-1347
4. Goldstick JE, Cunningham RM, Carter PM. Current causes of death in children and adolescents in the United States. *N Engl J Med*. 2022;386(20):1955-1956. doi:10.1056/NEJMc2201761
5. Sharko M, Jameson R, Ancker JS, Krams L, Webber EC, Rosenbloom ST. State-by-state variability in adolescent privacy laws. *Pediatrics*. 2022;149(6):e2021053458. doi:10.1542/peds.2021-053458
6. An Overview of Consent to Reproductive Health Services by Young People. Guttmacher Institute. Accessed October 30, 2022. https://www.guttmacher.org/state-policy/explore/overview-minors-consent-law
7. English A, Ford CA. Adolescent health, confidentiality in healthcare, and communication with parents. *J Pediatr*. 2018;199:11-13. doi:10.1016/j.jpeds.2018.04.029
8. Maslyanskaya S, Alderman EM. Confidentiality and consent in the care of the adolescent patient. *Pediatr Rev*. 2019;40(10):508-516. doi:10.1542/pir.2018-0040
9. Centers for Disease Control and Prevention. Teen Health Services and One-on-One Time with a Healthcare Provider: An Infobrief for Parents. Accessed October 30, 2022. https://www.cdc.gov/healthyyouth/healthservices/pdf/oneononetime_factsheet.pdf
10. Goyal MK, Witt R, Hayes KL, Zaoutis TE, Gerber JS. Clinician adherence to recommendations for screening of

adolescents for sexual activity and sexually transmitted infection/human immunodeficiency virus. *J Pediatr.* 2014;165(2):343-347. doi:10.1016/j.jpeds.2014.04.009

11. Robertson C, Thomas A, Koyama A, et al. Missed opportunities for sexual history documentation and sexually transmitted infection testing in the pediatric emergency department. *J Adolesc Health.* 2022;70(3):429-434. doi:10.1016/j.jadohealth.2021.10.002

12. Sterling S, Kline-Simon AH, Wibbelsman C, Wong A, Weisner C. Screening for adolescent alcohol and drug use in pediatric health-care settings: predictors and implications for practice and policy. *Addict Sci Clin Pract.* 2012;7:13. doi:10.1186/1940-0640-7-13

13. American Academy of Pediatrics. Equitable Access to Sexual and Reproductive Health Care for All Youth. Published August 11, 2022. Accessed October 30, 2022. https://downloads.aap.org/AAP/PDF/FINAL_Equitable%20Youth%20Access%20to%20SRH%20Care.pdf?_ga=2.215149716.2043957043.1665925305-1044840319.1469394667

14. Houtrow A, Elias ER, Davis BE, Council on Children With Disabilities. Promoting healthy sexuality for children and adolescents with disabilities. *Pediatrics.* 2021;148(1):e2021052043. doi:10.1542/peds.2021-052043

15. Byrne G. Prevalence and psychological sequelae of sexual abuse among individuals with an intellectual disability: a review of the recent literature. *J Intellect Disabil.* 2018;22(3):294-310. doi:10.1177/1744629517698844

16. Alriksson-Schmidt AI, Armour BS, Thibadeau JK. Are adolescent girls with a physical disability at increased risk for sexual violence? *J Sch Health.* 2010;80(7):361-367. doi:10.1111/j.1746-1561.2010.00514.x

17. Carlson J, Goldstein R, Hoover K, Tyson N. NASPAG/SAHM statement: the 21st Century Cures Act and adolescent confidentiality. *J Pediatr Adolesc Gynecol.* 2021;34(1):3-5. doi:10.1016/j.jpag.2020.12.015

18. Lee JA, Holland-Hall C. Patient portals for the adolescent and young adult population: benefits, risks and guidance for use. *Curr Probl Pediatr Adolesc Health Care.* 2021;51(11):101101. doi:10.1016/j.cppeds.2021.101101

19. Ginsburg KR. The SSHADESS Screen: a strength-based psychosocial assessment. In: Ginsburg KR, Kinsman SB, eds. *Reaching Teens: Strength-Based Communication Strategies to Build Resilience and Support Healthy Adolescent Development.* American Academy of Pediatrics; 2014:225-228A. doi:10.1542/9781581108347-part04-ch18

20. Centers for Disease Control and Prevention. A Guide to Taking a Sexual History. Published January 14, 2022. Accessed October 30, 2022. https://www.cdc.gov/std/treatment/SexualHistory.htm

21. Rome ES, Miller E. Intimate partner violence in the adolescent. *Pediatr Rev.* 2020;41(2):73-80. doi:10.1542/pir.2018-0053

22. Klein D, Goldenring J, Adelman W. HEEADSSS 3.0: the psychosocial interview for adolescents updated for a new century fueled by media. *Contemp Pediatr.* 2014;31(1):16-28.

23. Rafferty J, Committee on Psychosocial Aspects of Child and Family Health, Committee on Adolescence, Section on Lesbian, Gay, Bisexual, and Transgender Health and Wellness. Ensuring comprehensive care and support for transgender and gender-diverse children and adolescents. *Pediatrics.* 2018;142(4):e20182162. doi:10.1542/peds.2018-2162

Care of the Transgender and Gender Diverse Adolescent

Jason Jarin and Frances Grimstad

INTRODUCTION

Transgender and gender diverse (TGD) adolescents are those whose gender identity differs from their sex assigned at birth (Table 3.1). Although the prevalence of gender diversity in the population is difficult to ascertain because of poor data collection at the national level, roughly 0.5% of adults are estimated to identify as transgender, with 1.3% of 18- to 24-year-olds and 1.4% of 13- to 17-year-olds.[1] As such, it is likely that all clinicians will provide care for TGD adolescents at some point in their career. Much of the specific medical and surgical care that TGD adolescents may seek is within the domain of pediatric and adolescent gynecology, including hormone therapy, fertility counseling, sexual health, and reproductive surgeries.[2-4] This chapter provides an overview of gender-affirming care as it relates to the field. Additional resources are provided in Table 3.2.

BOX 3.1 Complimentary Resources for Transgender Health Care

- World Professional Association for Transgender Health (WPATH) Standards of Care
- The Endocrine Society Guidelines on the Endocrine Treatment of Gender-Dysphoric/Gender-Incongruent Persons
- University of California San Francisco Guidelines for the Primary and Gender-Affirming Care of Transgender and Gender Nonbinary People.

See references 5 to 7.

BARRIERS TO CARE

TGD individuals face numerous systemic and specific health care barriers.[8] Many are grounded in the roots of inequities.[9] TGD individuals continue to face widespread societal discrimination, including in terms of education, housing, and employment discrimination; ostracization from families; and targeted exclusion from social spaces and activities as well as targeted violence.[8] These disparities are further heightened for those who are also persons of color.[10] In large part, as a result of these, TGD individuals have higher rates of mental health and chronic health disparities, being unable to obtain comprehensive insurance, experiencing homelessness, and living below the poverty line.[8,11] The 2015 US Transgender Survey found that one in four individuals experienced some degree of discrimination, violence, or refusal of necessary care because of being TGD, and one in three would delay or avoid engaging with health care because of fear of said concerns.[8] In reproductive health care settings, there are additional barriers and layers of discrimination. Many gynecologic spaces assume all individuals have the same sex traits and the same gender. Some gynecologists refuse to provide care to transgender men and transmasculine individuals who have anatomy and physiologic needs within gynecology but who are not women. Additionally, some gynecologists refuse to provide care for transgender women or transfeminine individuals who, although they identify as women, may have anatomy that differs from what gynecologists have training and familiarity with.[12] TGD individuals have documented concerns with the gendered nature of gynecology and seek

TABLE 3.1   Common Definitions

Sex: An assignment of male, female, or intersex at birth based on sex trait characteristics.
Gender: A person's inner sense of male, female, or something else. Gender is self-identified and may evolve over time.
Cisgender: An individual whose gender identity aligns with their sex assigned at birth.
Transgender: An individual whose gender identity differs from their sex assigned at birth.
Nonbinary: A person whose gender identity differs from their sex assigned at birth but is not fully encompassed by the terms male or female.
Gender diverse: A term used to encompass diverse, not entirely cisgenders. Alongside transgender, the phrases transgender and gender diverse are often used to encompass the umbrella of gender identities someone may espouse, including gender queer, gender nonbinary, gender fluid, agender, and many more.
Transgender man: A man who was assigned female sex at birth.
Transmasculine: An umbrella term used to encompass those who have masculine-of-center gender identities, including man, transgender man, nonbinary masculine, and others.
Transgender woman: A woman who was assigned male sex at birth.
Transfeminine: An umbrella term used to encompass those who have feminine-of-center gender identities, including woman, transgender woman, nonbinary feminine, and others.
Sexual orientation: Describes the general attraction of one individual toward others and is typically described in relation to gender, not sex.

From Hembree WC, Cohen-Kettenis PT, Gooren L, et al. Endocrine treatment of gender-dysphoric/gender-incongruent persons: an Endocrine Society clinical practice guideline. *J Clin Endocrinol Metab.* 2017;102(11):3869-3903.

competent and welcoming care.[13] Similarly, surveys of clinicians in obstetrics and gynecology find that few physicians feel prepared to care for TGD individuals.[14] Collectively, these chasms in care knowledge of the clinician, crossed with the experiences and preferences of TGD individuals, unite to support the call for more clinicians to be trained in culturally inclusive and competent care for TGD individuals.

Many clinicians see TGD individuals for the routine spectrum of care they provide for their cisgender patients, such as for menstrual suppression or vaginal discharge. As such, clinicians may not know a patient who is TGD is scheduled until they are seeing the patient. There are certain things that clinicians should employ universally to ensure that no assumptions are made about which of their patients are cisgender and which are TGD. All patients should be asked about their name in use and pronouns, and this information should be documented in a place that is universally accessible to all clinical staff. Clinics should review their environment to ensure it is reflective of the populations they serve, including diverse posters, magazines, and handouts.[15] Signage that specifically welcomes LGBTQIA+ (lesbian, gay, bisexual, transgender, queer, intersex, asexual, and more) individuals, such as rainbows or trans flags, can signal safety to TGD patients.[16] For patients who are presenting seeking gender-affirming hormone therapies or surgeries, the initial visit should

BOX 3.2   How to Take an Embodiment-Centered Approach to Gender Care

- Rather than asking which therapies or surgeries a patient is seeking, ask about the specific changes or goals they are seeking.
- Explore which, if any, therapies might help them best achieve these goals.

BOX 3.3   Key Topics When Addressing Therapies That May Affect Sexual and Reproductive Health[2,6]

- Fertility
- Family building
- Fertility preservation options
- Genital changes
- Sexual experience changes

additionally include discussions about gender identity, history of gender exploration, any social transition that has occurred (e.g., name change), and any gender-related goals (including any physical changes desired).[2,3] Patients should be asked about their desired timing for these changes and about their reasoning for timing so that clinicians can understand the patients' longitudinal plan.

Remove the assumption from clinicians that all TGD individuals of the same gender desire the same therapies and goals, and instead create a system where patients are offered therapies that best address their individual goals.[5]

Adolescence can also be a tumultuous time in life, and in accordance with general pediatric goals, all patients who are experiencing psychosocial concerns should be connected with mental health resources; TGD adolescents are no exception.[4] For those who are desiring hormonal or surgical therapies, mental health clinicians are recommended to be involved in care by national and international guidelines, and as such, clinicians should aid TGD patients in networking to find a TGD-inclusive mental health provider.[5,6]

PUBERTY SUPPRESSION

Puberty marks a particularly crucial time in the management of children and adolescents with gender dysphoria, as the unwanted physical changes that accompany puberty put them at the high risk of adverse mental health outcomes.[6] As previously stated, TGD youth are not only at a higher risk of suicide, substance abuse, and high-risk sexual behavior; they also comprise a disproportionate portion of the homeless population.[5] After the mental health provider has determined that the adolescent has met *Diagnostic and Statistical Manual of Mental Disorders, Fifth Edition* (DSM-5) criteria for gender dysphoria, the Endocrine Society guidelines support the use of puberty blockers starting when the youth reaches Tanner stage 2 of puberty.[6] This typically consists of breast budding in those assigned female at birth and reaching testicular volume of 4 cc in those assigned male. Initiating treatment to suppress these pubertal changes not only minimizes the mental distress brought about by puberty but also prevents the development of secondary sexual characteristics that may later be difficult to address, such as the sound of the voice, the Adam's apple, or large breasts.

Puberty suppression is typically achieved with the use of gonadotropin-releasing hormone (GnRH) analogues. This includes depot leuprolide acetate and the Histrelin implant. The suppression of pubertal changes allows the adolescents to engage with a mental health provider and explore their gender identity before engaging in gender-affirming medical and surgical interventions that have permanent effects.[17] Puberty suppression is reversible, and in the event that treatment is discontinued, endogenous puberty will ensue.

FOLLOW-UP AND MONITORING

Although puberty suppression is considered reversible, the effects of GnRH analogues on bone mineral density in adolescents are not completely known. Thus testing for bone mineral density annually is recommended by the Endocrine Society.[6] Calcium and vitamin D supplementation may be offered to adolescents undergoing pubertal suppression, and physical activity and weight-bearing exercise should be encouraged. The Endocrine Society also recommends evaluation of gonadotropins (luteinizing hormone/follicle-stimulating hormone [LH/FSH]) as well as testosterone or estradiol levels every 3 months, along with height and weight measurements and Tanner staging during each visit.[6]

SPECIAL CONSIDERATIONS

Transmasculine adolescents who start gender-affirming therapy at or beyond puberty may opt to forego pubertal suppression. Menstrual suppression may also be considered. Although cessation of menstruation can be expected within the first few months of testosterone use, those who are on neither puberty-suppressing nor testosterone treatment should be offered menstrual suppression should menses be a significant cause of distress.[18] Any agent that can be used to suppress periods in cisgender female adolescents can be considered; however, many transmasculine individuals may prefer methods without estrogen. Systemic progesterone—in the form of oral, depo, intrauterine, or an implant—can be considered in those wishing menstrual suppression without additional estrogen exposure. Progesterone-containing intrauterine devices specifically decrease menstrual flow or fully suppress periods.[15]

TGD adolescents should receive ongoing counseling regarding their options for fertility preservation throughout their gender-affirming care; however, this is especially true in adolescents seeking puberty suppression. GnRH analogue treatment results in cessation of germ cell maturation, and at this time there are no options for fertility preservation in children and adolescents who have not undergone puberty in their gender assigned at birth.[5] Providers should engage adolescents in discussions regarding their fertility and their options for fertility preservation before pubertal suppression and before the use of testosterone or estrogen (see Chapter 27). Menstrual Suppression Please refer to Appendix 3.1 for patient friendly handout reviewing all the options.

GENDER-AFFIRMING HORMONES

The Endocrine Society guidelines support the initiation of testosterone or estrogen around the age of 16, when adolescents are known to have the sufficient capacity to provide informed assent.[6] Although data surrounding the use of gender-affirming hormones before age 13.5 to 14 years are limited, special consideration can be given to adolescents before the age of 16 in cases where there is compelling support from both their medical and mental health providers.[6]

Written documentation from a dedicated mental health professional about the patient's eligibility and need for gender-affirming treatment was strongly recommended in the past by the prior World Professional Association for Transgender Health (WPATH) Standards of Care version 7; however, this presented a challenge to adolescents receiving gender-affirming care in a timely manner.[5] Although gender-affirming care is best undertaken in a multidisciplinary environment, not all TGD youth and their families have access to such care. In settings where multiple disciplines are available and accessible to patients, all relevant providers should be included in the provision of gender-affirming care to adolescents. Any written documentation recommending gender-affirming care should include assessments from both medical and mental health providers.[19] There are cases where parental consent is not required to receive gender-affirming care; however, obtaining consent is preferable, as parental support improves clinical outcomes during hormone therapy.[17]

Adolescents and their families should be made aware of the possible health effects of both masculinizing and feminizing therapy, and expectations should be set as to the timing and extent of the physical changes brought about by gender-affirming medications. Providers should be aware that although surgery can be an important component in the treatment of gender dysphoria, hormone therapy serves as the endpoint for many individuals, especially if surgery is not consistent with their goals toward their gender identity.[5]

Masculinizing Therapy

Testosterone is available as injectable esters for adolescents seeking masculinizing therapy. It can also be administered transdermally in the form of patches and gels and subcutaneously as pellets. Parenteral formulations, administered either subcutaneously or intramuscularly, are typically recommended during puberty induction because of the low cost and ease of self-administration.[20]

Puberty induction with testosterone in transmasculine adolescents typically starts at 25 mg every 7 to 14 days, increasing incrementally every 3 to 6 months to an adult maintenance dose of 50 to 100 mg every week.[6] After puberty induction, testosterone levels are typically maintained within physiologic levels for males (400–700 ng/dL), although it is unclear what the optimal ranges are in transmasculine patients.[5] Desired effects of testosterone include virilization of the body and development of male secondary sex characteristics, including growth of facial and body hair, lowering of the voice, and increase in muscle development.[21] Given the partially irreversible nature of these changes, the Endocrine Society recommends gradual and incremental dosing of testosterone regardless of whether or not puberty suppression was undertaken before starting androgen therapy.[6]

Clinical monitoring of their pubertal development as well as laboratory evaluation is also recommended every 3 to 6 months during treatment, including sex steroid hormone levels and complete blood counts.[6] This allows for close monitoring for adverse effects secondary to therapy (Table 3.2). Of particular concern is erythrocytosis secondary to testosterone, although hypertension and hyperlipidemia can occur with long-term use as well.[6] The decision regarding the frequency and breadth of surveillance should be individualized to each adolescent's comorbidities, lifestyle risks, and response to treatment. There is no evidence to suggest standardized testing intervals while undergoing treatment.[5]

TABLE 3.2 Physical Changes and Associated Risks With Testosterone Treatment

Physical Changes	Associated Risks
Deepening of voice	Erythrocytosis
Facial/body hair growth	Acne
Increased muscle mass and strength	Male-pattern hair loss
	Increased LDL cholesterol
Body fat redistribution	Decreased HDL cholesterol
Cessation of menstruation	Hypertension
Clitoral enlargement	Weight gain
Vaginal atrophy	

HDL, High-density lipoprotein; *LDL,* low-density lipoprotein. From Hembree WC, Cohen-Kettenis PT, Gooren L, et al. Endocrine treatment of gender-dysphoric/gender-incongruent persons: an Endocrine Society clinical practice guideline. *J Clin Endocrinol Metab.* 2017;102(11):3869-3903.

Feminizing Therapy

Feminizing therapy typically involves estrogen and anti-androgens, especially in patients who have not undergone puberty suppression. Estrogen alone has been shown to be insufficient in the suppression of testosterone when administered at physiologic doses, so adjunctive therapy is typically required to achieve testosterone levels in the female range.[6] Puberty induction with estrogen is typically initiated with oral formulations and transdermal estradiol, although parenteral formulations are also available for maintenance in older adolescents and adults. In adolescents undergoing puberty induction with oral formulations, estrogen treatment may begin with 1 mg daily dosing, incrementally increasing to typical adult maintenance doses of 4 to 6 mg daily every 3 to 4 months.[5] Similarly, puberty induction with transdermal estrogen may start with the 0.1 mg/day patch, which can then be incrementally increased to up to a 0.4 mg/day dose.[5] Serum estradiol levels are maintained at the level for premenopausal females (100–200 pg/mL), whereas testosterone levels are ideally suppressed below 50 ng/dL.[5] Physical changes secondary to feminizing therapy are typically evident within the first 3 to 12 months, including increased breast tissue growth, redistribution of fat mass to the hips and thighs, and decreased facial and body hair.[6] Similar to masculinizing therapy, these physical changes are partially irreversible; thus initiation of therapy is typically undertaken with a gradually increasing schedule.

Providers should be aware of a number of antiandrogen and progestin medications transfeminine adolescents may use as adjunctive therapy to estrogen. The most common antiandrogen is spironolactone, which works by blocking the action of testosterone at the level of the androgen receptors.[6] This results in a reduction in the rate of growth and thickness of male-pattern hair. The addition of antiandrogenic medications also allows for the reduction of testosterone levels toward the preferred physiologic levels as well as the reduction of the amount of estrogen needed to achieve the desired physical effects.[5] Spironolactone is a weak antihypertensive; thus providers should be aware of the potential for hypokalemia and reduced blood pressure. Current WPATH guidelines recommend regular assessment of renal function and potassium levels in conjunction with spironolactone use.[5] Alternative antiandrogens include finasteride, bicalutamide, and GnRH analogues. Some adolescents may also opt for progestin therapy in

TABLE 3.3 Physical Changes and Associated Risks With Estrogen Treatment

Physical Changes	Associated Risks
Breast growth	Venous thromboembolism
Redistribution of body fat	Decreased sperm
Decrease in muscle mass	production and
Softening of skin	testicular volume
Decreased sexual desire	Elevated prolactin
Decreased terminal hair	Liver dysfunction
growth	Hyperkalemia
Voice changes	Hypertriglyceridemia
	Weight gain

From Hembree WC, Cohen-Kettenis PT, Gooren L, et al. Endocrine treatment of gender-dysphoric/gender-incongruent persons: an Endocrine Society clinical practice guideline. *J Clin Endocrinol Metab*. 2017;102(11):3869-3903.

addition to estradiol in hopes of potentiating the breast growth brought about by estrogen; however, the evidence to support this practice is very limited.

As with masculinizing therapy, regular clinical and laboratory assessment is recommended every 3 to 6 months to prevent potential adverse events during treatment with estradiol (Table 3.3). Exogenous estrogen is known to increase the risk of venous thromboembolism, although this risk can be minimized by maintaining levels within the desired physiologic range and with the use of transdermal formulations.[5] There is also a risk of liver dysfunction, hypertension, and hyperprolactinemia, so appropriate monitoring should be undertaken, especially in adolescents at higher doses.[5]

GENDER-AFFIRMING SURGERIES

Although the majority of gender-affirming surgeries are performed after the age of majority (which is typically age 18 in the United States), some are performed before or shortly after the age of majority.[2] Some adolescents may express interest in, or are planning to undergo, gender-affirming surgeries. Nonsterilizing procedures are considered more acceptable to perform before the age of majority compared with sterilizing procedures. Surgical criteria are based on a number of elements, including WPATH Standards of Care, insurance company requirements, local regulations, and individual surgeon requirements (e.g., age, body mass index [BMI], and smoking).[5] All of these will be different depending on the surgery.

BOX 3.4 **The WPATH Standards of Care Readiness Standards for Gender-Affirming Surgery[5]**

- Diagnosis of gender incongruence by a qualified clinician
- Marked and sustained gender incongruence
- Capacity to consent (assent in the case of a minor)
- Understanding the effects of the specific surgery on reproductive health
- Management of mental health and physical comorbidities that can affect the outcomes of the surgery
- A minimum of 6 months on hormone therapy (12 months for adolescents) unless it is medically contraindicated or not desired

---

TABLE 3.4 **Common Masculinizing Procedures**

- **Chest masculinization (top surgery):** Reconstruction of chest tissue, removing most glandular tissue from the breasts to create a masculine contour. It also may involve free nipple grafts.
- **Hysterectomy:** When performed for the purposes of gender affirmation, it is typically done minimally invasively (laparoscopic or vaginal). Gender-affirming bilateral oophorectomy is an additional procedure that, although not required at the time of gender-affirming hysterectomy, is desired by some patients. Gender-affirming hysterectomies should be done with a risk-reducing bilateral salpingectomy.
- **Metoidioplasty and phalloplasty:** Metoidioplasty is a genital surgery to create a more prominent phallus using a hormonally enhanced clitoris. A phalloplasty uses the base of the metoidioplasty approach and adds a tube graft that expands the size. For those who also desire the ability to stand to urinate, the phallus can also have a neourethra grafted within. When this occurs, the surgery will also include a vaginectomy. Both phalloplasty and metoidioplasty may also include scrotoplasty and scrotal implants if desired. Metoidioplasties can become erect on their own, but phalloplasties will require an internal or external prosthesis.

From Coleman E, Radix AE, Bouman WP, et al. Standards of care for the health of transgender and gender diverse people, version 8. *Int J Transgend Health.* 2022;23(Supp 1):S1-S259.

Common gender-affirming surgeries for both transmasculine and transfeminine individuals are listed in Table 3.4 and Table 3.5.

TABLE 3.5 **Common Feminizing Procedures**

- **Breast augmentations:** Surgical expansion of breasts similar to other breast augmentation procedures.
- **Orchiectomies:** May be done as part of a vaginoplasty or in isolation (e.g., to remove the need for medical antiandrogen therapy or for scrotal dysphoria).
- **Vaginoplasty and vulvoplasty:** Vaginoplasty is the deconstruction of external genitalia (scrotum, phallus) and creation of a vaginal canal in the retro-prostatic space with a clitoris, shortened urethra, labia, and vestibule. The vaginal cavity is lined with a graft, which is often penoscrotal tissue but can also be peritoneal or other grafts. A vulvoplasty is a similar technique without the vaginal cavity.

From Coleman E, Radix AE, Bouman WP, et al. Standards of care for the health of transgender and gender diverse people, version 8. *Int J Transgend Health.* 2022;23(Supp 1):S1-S259.

HEALTH CONCERNS

Contraception

Some TGD individuals may have anatomy capable of, and may engage in sexual activity that can produce, a pregnancy.[22] For these individuals, if pregnancy is not desired, contraceptive counseling is recommended.[23,24] Neither testosterone, estrogen, nor GnRH agonists are Food and Drug Administration (FDA) approved for the purposes of contraception.

Some individuals may be on additional forms of menstrual suppression that are also forms of contraception.[25] There is no current evidence that any contraceptive method is contraindicated for those taking gender-affirming hormone therapy.[24] The decision as to which form of contraception TGD individuals would want to use is a personal one and comes with many considerations. Patient-centered counseling should address patient concerns such as whether or not the method contains estrogen, ease of discontinuation, concealability, risk of chest tenderness, and tolerance for breakthrough bleeding.[24] Clinicians should counsel on all options and ask patients what aspects of a method are most important to them to help guide selection. Emergency contraception is also available to TGD individuals, including those on gender-affirming hormones.[26]

Breakthrough Bleeding on Testosterone

Although the majority of individuals using testosterone will rapidly achieve amenorrhea (85%–100% at 1 year of use), up to a quarter may experience some degree of breakthrough bleeding.[27] Some individuals may experience breakthrough bleeding on testosterone alone, whereas others may experience it while on a concomitant menstrual suppression agent. The uterine linings of those who are on testosterone are mostly thin but can exhibit a range of endometrial activity, including atrophy, proliferative, and in some cases, secretory endometrium.[28] There does not appear to be an increased risk of precancerous or cancerous pathology in the uterus of younger individuals on testosterone.[28] As such, management of breakthrough bleeding is similar to those who are on other forms of menstrual suppression who experience breakthrough bleeding. This includes ensuring that other age- and activity-appropriate causes of genital and uterine bleeding are considered, including vulvovaginal atrophy (which can occur in individuals on testosterone), urethral and rectal bleeding, genital infections, thyroid dysfunction, uterine masses such as polyps and fibroids, and pregnancy. When other causes are ruled out, options for management of breakthrough bleeding include adjusting the testosterone dosage; initiation, discontinuation, or modification of a concomitant menstrual suppression agent; use of nonhormonal bleeding reduction methods; and consideration for surgical options.[27] The choice of method will depend on the patient's goals, contraceptive need, and desire for gender-affirming genital surgery. Hormonal options to help with breakthrough bleeding include progestin-only methods, estrogen and progestin combined methods, GnRH analogues, and danazol, a synthetic weak androgen with progestogenic activity. Patients who are on testosterone with testosterone levels in the cisgender male range can likely safely take GnRH analogues alongside testosterone long term.[27] All patients should be counseled that the rates of amenorrhea on any of these methods are based on individuals using those methods alone and not on concomitant testosterone. Additionally, aromatase inhibitors and selective estrogen receptor modulators have been proposed as methods of achieving amenorrhea with breakthrough bleeding but lack data on their efficacy.[27] Ulipristal acetate, a selective progestin receptor modulator, can also be considered, but clinical recommendations are only for short duration of use.[27] Nonhormonal methods to reduce bleeding include nonsteroidal antiinflammatory drugs (NSAIDs) and tranexamic acid.[29] Surgical options include ablation (generally avoided because of the low rates of long-term amenorrhea in younger individuals in cisgender populations[30]) and hysterectomy.

Fertility

Certain gender-affirming therapies can or may affect fertility.[6] Current guidelines recommend counseling about fertility implications of the specific gender-affirming hormone therapies and surgeries that a patient may be interested in before initiation of therapy or surgery.[5]

For those born with a uterus, current evidence suggests that hormone therapies do not adversely affect the fertility potential of the uterus. Individuals have discontinued testosterone and successfully carried pregnancies.[31] Those who desire a hysterectomy or a genital surgery that requires a preceding hysterectomy should be counseled that removal of the uterus renders a person unable to carry a pregnancy in the future.[2]

For those born with ovaries who initiate GnRH analogues at the onset of puberty, ovarian maturation arrests limiting the ability to retrieve oocytes.[6] As such, ovarian tissue cryopreservation is the only present option for fertility preservation; however, it remains experimental for this purpose, as the only current way to subsequently use the tissue is with auto-reimplantation. This may not be desired by TGD individuals.[32] For those who use testosterone, emerging data are countering previous concerns of infertility. A growing body of studies show individuals on testosterone have been able to discontinue testosterone and either carry a pregnancy or undergo oocyte retrieval.[33-36] These data, however, are limited, and more studies are needed to inform counseling. For those who desire to preserve their fertility after puberty and either before or while on testosterone, the standard fertility preservation option is oocyte cryopreservation.[6] Ovarian tissue cryopreservation was previously considered experimental but is now available for postpubertal transmasculine individuals. This option mitigates the need for oocyte stimulation and retrieval; however, the procedure remains costly, still presently requires intracorporeal replacement of tissue for oocyte maturation, and is offered only by a limited number of institutions.

For those born with testes who initiate GnRH analogues at the onset of puberty, it will cause arrest of testicular maturation.[6] Testicular tissue cryopreservation may be an experimental option for these patients to preserve testicular tissue.[37] For those born with testes, estrogen therapy has been shown to impair spermatogenesis with unclear future sperm viability should estrogen be later discontinued, and as such the recommendation is fertility preservation before initiation for those who desire to preserve gametes.[6]

Sexually Transmitted Infections

Just like cisgender individuals, TGD individuals engage in a variety of sexual behaviors that may necessitate sexually transmitted infection (STI) screening.[22,38] The risk of an individual TGD patient for STIs may be different depending on their anatomy (including history of genital surgeries), sexual activity, and risk-related behaviors (such as barrier method use or number of partners). When taking a sexual history, clinicians should ask about the patient's anatomy and the anatomies of their partners and the types of sex they are engaging in. As per Centers for Disease Control and Prevention guidelines, STI screening should be behavior specific.[39]

For those who have had genital surgery, STIs can still be acquired and transmitted even in grafted tissue.[40] Clinicians should take into consideration the graft donor site when counseling on transmissibility of different STIs (e.g., a split-thickness skin graft vagina may be more resistant to gonorrhea than mucosal graft); however, current guidelines recommend approaching patients who have undergone genital surgery the same as those who have similar natal anatomy with regard to counseling and screening.[7] Preexposure prophylaxis (PrEP) should be offered to all patients who meet criteria or who desire it.[41] Additionally, for those who have had vaginoplasty, clinicians currently recommend testing both the urethra and vagina during screening because of the possible resistance of the vaginal graft tissue to STIs.[40]

Cancer Screening in Adulthood

Cancer screening in TGD individuals follows similar recommendations to cisgender individuals. People should be screened for the anatomy present with consideration for risk factors, including presence and duration of hormonal exposure. The cancer screenings reviewed herein are those that have hormonal considerations.

For breast cancer screening in TGD individuals on testosterone, the guidelines are no different from cisgender women not on testosterone; however, the rates of breast cancer appear to be lower.[42] Those who have undergone masculinizing chest reconstruction may likely have most, but not all, of their breast tissue removed, and thus may still be at risk for future breast cancer development.[43] Mammography in these individuals will be less successful because of the lack of tissue, and as such, recommendations presently are to consider screening ultrasounds. In TGD individuals born with testes on estrogen therapy, breast cancer rates are higher than that of cisgender men; however, they are lower than that of cisgender women.[42] As such, guidelines have differed in screening frequency, but the general consensus is to begin mammograms at the age of 50 and to additionally consider not initiating them until a person has been on estrogen for at least 5 to 10 years.[7]

All individuals with a cervix should undergo cervical cancer screening. Some TGD individuals may undergo a hysterectomy, thus negating the need for this. The frequency of cervical cancer screening is the same for all individuals with a cervix, regardless of whether they are on testosterone. However, testosterone can cause decreased cervical cellularity, leading to a higher chance of inadequate Pap tests.[44] This may become less of a concern as cervical cancer screening continues to evolve away from reliance upon Pap tests and toward high-risk human papilloma virus (HPV) DNA primary screening (which is now approved for 25 years and older); however, it is still relevant to those undergoing cervical cancer screening before this age.[45] For those with inadequate Pap tests, some clinicians recommend pretreating with vaginal estrogen before the repeat Pap to improve cellularity. Current WPATH recommendations also include vaccination against HPV according to local guidelines, which currently includes individuals age 9 to 26.[5]

All TGD individuals born with a prostate should be counseled on screening. Prostates are not removed at the time of gender-affirming genital surgery.[40] However, the incidence of prostate cancer in TGD individuals on estrogen is lower than that of cisgender men, likely because estrogen causes prostatic atrophy.[46] There is presently no consensus on prostate cancer screening, as national guidelines are moving away from routine prostate specific antigen (PSA) or digital rectal examinations because of the lack of benefit in reducing mortality.[47] Additionally, PSA reference ranges for TGD individuals on estrogen have not yet been established. Finally, for those who have undergone a vaginoplasty, the prostate examination should be transvaginal, not transrectal, because of the prostate's anterior position to the vagina.[40] Current recommendations are to follow cisgender guidelines for prostate screening and to engage in shared decision making about the prostate cancer screening approach.

KEY POINTS

- TGD adolescents have gender identities that are incongruent from their sex assigned at birth. All clinicians will see TGD individuals in their practice and should be prepared to provide appropriate and sensitive medical care.
- TGD adolescents may be undergoing feminizing therapy with estrogen or masculinizing therapy with testosterone; there are other medical options available to them, including puberty suppression with GnRH agonists. Providers should be aware of all options that can be afforded to these patients in order to adequately provide care.
- Reproductive health concerns are of utmost importance among TGD adolescents, so they should be counseled regarding their options for fertility preservation, contraception, and optimizing their sexual health before and during treatment.
- There are limited data about screening for adult cancers specifically in TGD individuals. Current recommendations, such as HPV vaccines and cervical cancer screening, follow guidelines established for cisgender individuals.

REVIEW QUESTIONS

1. Which of the following statements is true regarding the care of transgender/gender diverse adolescents?
   a. In the United States, more adults identify as transgender and gender diverse than adolescents.
   b. Providers should ask all patients about their name and pronouns, and this information should not be disclosed to the staff to honor patient confidentiality.
   c. Gynecologists should not care for transgender women or transfeminine individuals, as they may have anatomy that gynecologists are not trained to care for.
   d. Clinicians caring for TGD patients should help patients find inclusive mental health providers, especially if they are desiring medical or surgical therapy.

2. An 18-year-old transgender male is under your care in urgent care with chest pain and dyspnea on exertion. He reports testosterone use for the past 2 years as provided by his endocrinologist. Which of the following is least likely to be found on examination and laboratory evaluation?
   a. A blood pressure of 129/80
   b. A hematocrit of 51.2%
   c. A prolactin of 30 μg/L
   d. A fasting LDL of 101 mg/dL

3. Which of the following contraceptive options is appropriate for use in healthy transmasculine individuals?
   a. Estrogen-containing hormonal contraception (such as oral contraceptive pills and the combined patch)
   b. Options with systemic progesterone, such as depo medroxyprogesterone acetate
   c. The levonorgestrel intrauterine device
   d. All options are appropriate and can be considered by the patient

---

REFERENCES

1. Herman JL, Flores AR, O'Neill KK. How Many Adults and Youth Identify as Transgender in the United States? UCLA School of Law; Published 2022. Accessed July 24, 2022. https://williamsinstitute.law.ucla.edu/publications/trans-adults-united-states/
2. Grimstad F, Boskey ER, Taghinia A, Ganor O. Gender-affirming surgeries in transgender and gender diverse adolescent and young adults: a pediatric and adolescent gynecology primer. *J Pediatr Adolesc Gynecol*. 2021;34(4):442-448.
3. Hodax JK, Wagner J, Sackett-Taylor AC, Rafferty J, Forcier M. Medical options for care of gender diverse and transgender youth. *J Pediatr Adolesc Gynecol*. 2020;33(1):3-9. doi:10.1016/j.jpag.2019.05.010
4. Wagner J, Sackett-Taylor AC, Hodax JK, Forcier M, Rafferty J. Psychosocial overview of gender-affirmative care. *J Pediatr Adolesc Gynecol*. 2019;32(6):567-573. doi:10.1016/j.jpag.2019.05.004
5. Coleman E, Radix AE, Bouman WP, et al. Standards of care for the health of transgender and gender diverse people, version 8. *Int J Transgend Health*. 2022;23(supp 1):S1-S259. doi:10.1080/26895269.2022.2100644
6. Hembree WC, Cohen-Kettenis PT, Gooren L, et al. Endocrine treatment of gender-dysphoric/gender-incongruent persons: an Endocrine Society clinical practice guideline. *J Clin Endocrinol Metab*. 2017;102(11):3869-3903.

7. Deutsch MB, ed. *Guidelines for the Primary and Gender-Affirming Care of Transgender and Gender Nonbinary People.* 2nd ed. 2016. transcare.ucsf.edu/guidelines

8. James SE, Herman JL, Keisling M, Mottet L, Anafi M. *The Report of the 2015 US Transgender Survey.* National Center for Transgender Equality; 2016.

9. White Hughto JM, Reisner SL, Pachankis JE. Transgender stigma and health: a critical review of stigma determinants, mechanisms, and interventions. *Soc Sci Med.* 2015;147:222-231. doi:10.1016/j.socscimed.2015.11.010

10. Howard SD, Lee KL, Nathan AG, Wenger HC, Chin MH, Cook SC. Healthcare experiences of transgender people of color. *J Gen Intern Med.* 2019;34(10):2068-2074. doi:10.1007/s11606-019-05179-0

11. ACOG Committee on Health Care for Underserved Women. Committee opinion no. 512: health care for transgender individuals. *Obstet Gynecol.* 2011;118(6):1454-1458.

12. Unger CA. Care of the transgender patient: the role of the gynecologist. *Am J Obstet Gynecol.* 2014;210(1):16-26.

13. Frecker H, Scheim A, Leonardi M, Yudin M. Experiences of transgender men in accessing care in gynecology clinics. *Obstet Gynecol.* 2018;131:81S. doi:10.1097/01. AOG.0000533374.66494.29

14. Unger CA. Care of the transgender patient: a survey of gynecologists' current knowledge and practice. *J Womens Health (Larchmt).* 2015;24(2):114-118.

15. American College of Obstetricians and Gynecologists' Committee on Gynecologic Practice, American College of Obstetricians and Gynecologists' Committee on Health Care for Underserved Women. Health care for transgender and gender diverse individuals: ACOG committee opinion, no. 823. *Obstet Gynecol.* 2021;137(3): e75-e88. doi:10.1097/AOG.0000000000004294

16. Stroumsa D, Wu JP. Welcoming transgender and nonbinary patients: expanding the language of "women's health." *Am J Obstet Gynecol.* 2018;219(6):585.e1-585.e5. doi:10.1016/j.ajog.2018.09.018

17. Delemarre-van de Waal HA, Cohen-Kettenis PT. Clinical management of gender identity disorder in adolescents: a protocol on psychological and paediatric endocrinology aspects. *Eur J Endocrinol.* 2006;155(suppl 1):S131-S137. doi:10.1530/eje.1.02231

18. Kanj RV, Conard LAE, Corathers SD, Trotman GE. Hormonal contraceptive choices in a clinic-based series of transgender adolescents and young adults. *Int J Transgend.* 2019;20(4):413-420. doi:10.1080/15532739.2019.1631929

19. American Psychological Association. Guidelines for psychological practice with transgender and gender nonconforming people. *Am Psychol.* 2015;70(9):832-864. doi:10.1037/a0039906

20. Shumer DE, Nokoff NJ, Spack NP. Advances in the care of transgender children and adolescents. *Adv Pediatr.* 2016;63(1):79-102. doi:10.1016/j.yapd.2016.04.018

21. Rosenthal SM. Transgender youth: current concepts. *Ann Pediatr Endocrinol Metab.* 2016;21(4):185-192. doi:10.6065/apem.2016.21.4.185

22. Copen CE, Chandra A, Febo-Vazquez I. Sexual behavior, sexual attraction, and sexual orientation among adults aged 18-44 in the United States: data from the 2011-2013 National Survey of Family Growth. *Natl Health Stat Report.* 2016;(88):1-14.

23. Bonnington A, Dianat S, Kerns J, et al. Society of Family Planning clinical recommendations: contraceptive counseling for transgender and gender diverse people who were female sex assigned at birth. *Contraception.* 2020; 102(2):70-82. doi:10.1016/j.contraception.2020.04.001

24. Krempasky C, Harris M, Abern L, Grimstad F. Contraception across the transmasculine spectrum. *Am J Obstet Gynecol.* Published online August 5, 2019. doi:10.1016/j. ajog.2019.07.043

25. Pradhan S, Gomez-Lobo V. Hormonal contraceptives, intrauterine devices, gonadotropin-releasing hormone analogues and testosterone: menstrual suppression in special adolescent populations. *J Pediatr Adolesc Gynecol.* 2019;32(suppl 5):S23-S29. doi:10.1016/j.jpag.2019.04.007

26. Cleland K, Harris M. *Emergency Contraception for Transgender and Nonbinary Patients* [Fact Sheet]. American Society for Emergency Contraception; Published January 2021. https://www.ec-ec.org/wp-content/ uploads/2021/01/ASEC-Factsheet_EC-for-transgender-patients.pdf

27. Grimstad F, Kremen J, Shim J, Charlton BM, Boskey ER. Breakthrough bleeding in transgender and gender diverse adolescents and young adults on long-term testosterone. *J Pediatr Adolesc Gynecol.* 2021;34(5):706-716.

28. Grimstad FW, Fowler KG, New EP, et al. Uterine pathology in transmasculine persons on testosterone: a retrospective multicenter case series. *Am J Obstet Gynecol.* 2019; 220(3):257.e1-257.e7.

29. Emans SJ, Laufer MR. *Emans, Laufer, Goldstein's Pediatric and Adolescent Gynecology.* 6th ed. Wolters Kluwer Health, Lippincott Williams & Wilkins; 2011.

30. American College of Obstetricians and Gynecologists. ACOG committee opinion no. 557: management of acute abnormal uterine bleeding in nonpregnant reproductive-aged women. *Obstet Gynecol.* 2013;121(4):891-896.

31. Charlton BM, Reynolds CA, Tabaac AR, et al. Unintended and teen pregnancy experiences of trans masculine people living in the United States. *Int J Transgend Health.* 2021;22(1-2):65-76. doi:10.1080/26895269.2020.1824692

32. Nahata L, Chen D, Moravek MB, et al. Understudied and under-reported: fertility issues in transgender youth—A narrative review. *J Pediatr.* 2019;205:265-271.

33. Lierman S, Tilleman K, Braeckmans K, et al. Fertility preservation for trans men: Frozen-thawed in vitro matured oocytes collected at the time of ovarian tissue processing

exhibit normal meiotic spindles. *J Assist Reprod Genet.* 2017;34(11):1449-1456. doi:10.1007/s10815-017-0976-5

34. Amir H, Yaish I, Samara N, Hasson J, Groutz A, Azem F. Ovarian stimulation outcomes among transgender men compared with fertile cisgender women. *J Assist Reprod Genet.* 2020;37(10):2463-2472.

35. Adeleye AJ, Cedars MI, Smith J, Mok-Lin E. Ovarian stimulation for fertility preservation or family building in a cohort of transgender men. *J Assist Reprod Genet.* Published online August 21, 2019.

36. Light AD, Obedin-Maliver J, Sevelius JM, Kerns JL. Transgender men who experienced pregnancy after female-to-male gender transitioning. *Obstet Gynecol.* 2014;124(6):1120-1127.

37. Joshi VB, Behl S, Pittock ST, et al. Establishment of a pediatric ovarian and testicular cryopreservation program for malignant and non-malignant conditions: The Mayo Clinic experience. *J Pediatr Adolesc Gynecol.* 2021;34(5): 673-680.

38. Boskey ER, Ganor O. Sexual orientation and attraction in a cohort of transmasculine adolescents and young adults. *Transgend Health.* 2022;7(3):270-275. doi:10.1089/trgh.2020.0190

39. Centers for Disease Control and Prevention. A Guide to Taking a Sexual History. https://www.cdc.gov/std/treatment/SexualHistory.pdf

40. Grimstad F, McLaren H, Gray M. The gynecologic examination of the transfeminine person after penile inversion vaginoplasty. *Am J Obstet Gynecol.* 2021;224(3):266-273. doi:10.1016/j.ajog.2020.10.002

41. Centers for Disease Control and Prevention, U.S. Public Health Service. *Preexposure Prophylaxis for the Prevention of HIV Infection in the United States—2021 Update: A Clinical Practice Guideline.* Centers for Disease Control and Prevention; 2021.

42. de Blok CJM, Wiepjes CM, Nota NM, et al. Breast cancer risk in transgender people receiving hormone treatment: Nationwide cohort study in the Netherlands. *BMJ.* 2019;365:l1652. doi:10.1136/bmj.l1652

43. Iwamoto SJ, Grimstad F, Irwig MS, Rothman MS. Routine screening for transgender and gender diverse adults taking gender-affirming hormone therapy: a narrative review. *J Gen Intern Med.* 2021;36(5): 1380-1389. doi:10.1007/s11606-021-06634-7

44. Peitzmeier SM, Reisner SL, Harigopal P, Potter J. Female-to-male patients have high prevalence of unsatisfactory Paps compared to non-transgender females: implications for cervical cancer screening. *J Gen Intern Med.* 2014;29(5):778-784. doi:10.1007/s11606-013-2753-1

45. Committee on Practice Bulletins—Gynecology. Practice bulletin no. 168: cervical cancer screening and prevention. *Obstet Gynecol.* 2016;128(4):e111-e130. doi:10.1097/AOG.0000000000001708

46. Ingham MD, Lee RJ, MacDermed D, Olumi AF. Prostate cancer in transgender women. *Urol Oncol.* 2018; 36(12):518-525. doi:10.1016/j.urolonc.2018.09.011

47. U.S. Preventive Services Task Force, Grossman DC, Curry SJ, et al. Screening for prostate cancer: US Preventive Services Task Force recommendation statement. *JAMA.* 2018;319(18):1901-1913. doi:10.1001/jama.2018.3710

Pediatric Gynecologic Examination

Tania Dumont

INTRODUCTION

The pediatric gynecologic examination (PGE) should only be performed when indicated. Unnecessary PGE in both the child and adolescent can lead to overmedicalization of their conditions, feelings of exploitation, and even trauma. If you are an unskilled trainee in the PGE, it is best to only do one examination where both you and the provider are present at the same time for the PGE. This will decrease the time the patient is in this vulnerable examination position and subject to touch by both you and the provider. Ideally, you should be taught how to perform the PGE on models during simulation sessions before doing them for the first time on a patient. Many simulation curriculums exist.[1-4] In what follows you will find the indications for a PGE based on age and pubertal status.[5]

Indications for Examination in the Child/Prepubertal Patient

- Confirmation of normal anatomy
- Vulvar complaints
- Abnormal vaginal discharge
- Suspected abuse
- Vulvovaginal trauma
- Prepubertal vaginal bleeding
- Precocious puberty/assessment of pubertal status

Indications for Examination in the Adolescent/Postpubertal Patient

- Confirmation of normal anatomy
- Vulvar complaints
- Abnormal vaginal discharge

- Suspected abuse
- Vulvovaginal trauma
- Abnormal uterine bleeding such as postcoital bleeding
- Intrauterine device/intrauterine system insertion (IUD/IUS)
- Suspected pelvic inflammatory disease (PID) or sexually transmitted infection (STI)
- Hyperandrogenic symptoms
- Delayed puberty/primary amenorrhea/assessment of pubertal status
- Dyspareunia
- Inability to insert tampons
- Pregnancy

APPROACH TO THE EXAMINATION

Having a systematic approach to the PGE is important. It should be performed in a consistent fashion such that one does not forget any parts of the PGE, which could then entail a repeat examination for the patient. The PGE should be tailored to the patient's age and maturity and their previous experiences.[6] Trauma-informed care should always be practiced. Restraining a patient to examine them should be avoided unless they are under 2 years of age and caregivers are agreeable.[7] Consent should always be obtained from patients and/or caregivers before performing a PGE. It is important to explain that the examination will not be painful nor change the look or function of the hymen.[8]

Explain to the patient how to self-position and offer alternative positions. Ensure the patient is draped appropriately and only exposes body parts that need to be. Before starting, ask the patient if they want to see the instruments/swabs you will be using and, if so, take the time to do this. They may also benefit from seeing images before the examination or using a mirror to watch you do the examination.

Labial separation and labial retraction (somewhat firm downward retraction while grasping the labia majora bilaterally) are very helpful in the prepubertal population for assessment of the hymen and lower vagina (Fig. 4.1). Similarly, it is important in the postpubertal

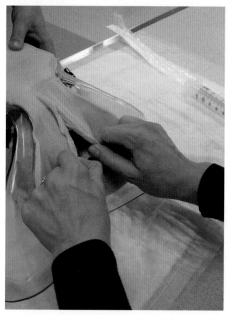

Fig. 4.1 Resident demonstrating the proper technique for labial retraction on a genital model.

patients when assessing for hymenal anomalies (e.g., imperforate hymen, septate hymen), vaginal agenesis (assessing for a dimple), and vaginal septa. Trainees providing gynecologic care should learn this part of the PGE on a pediatric and/or simulated model before attempting them on a patient (see Fig. 4.1). Finally, it is important to know what is normal on a PGE before being able to identify pathology (Table 4.1, Figs. 4.2 and 4.3).

Approach to the Pediatric/Prepubertal Examination

Consent for the examination should be obtained from the caregiver and assent from the child based on their age and maturity (Box 4.1). It is a good opportunity to review with the child what "private parts" are, who is allowed to see and touch them, and in what context.

We typically position in the child in the frog-leg or butterfly position (Fig. 4.4). If the child is uncomfortable with this position, ask them to do it sitting on their caregiver or consider the knee-chest position as seen in Fig. 4.4. Some children prefer to not be draped. Gowns are usually not necessary, as you are only exposing the bottom half of their bodies. As they are undressing, examine their diaper or underwear, looking for any bleeding or discharge.[9]

If the patient is presenting with vulvar pain, consider starting with a "Q-tip" test to assess the various vulvar dermatomes and innervation. In Table 4.2, you will find the typical areas you would examine in a prepubertal PGE.

A speculum examination in a prepubertal child in the office setting is NEVER appropriate. If you suspect

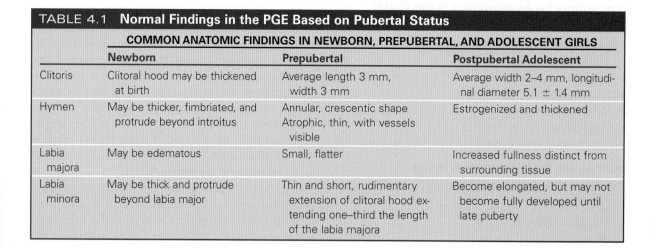

TABLE 4.1	Normal Findings in the PGE Based on Pubertal Status		
	COMMON ANATOMIC FINDINGS IN NEWBORN, PREPUBERTAL, AND ADOLESCENT GIRLS		
	Newborn	**Prepubertal**	**Postpubertal Adolescent**
Clitoris	Clitoral hood may be thickened at birth	Average length 3 mm, width 3 mm	Average width 2–4 mm, longitudinal diameter 5.1 ± 1.4 mm
Hymen	May be thicker, fimbriated, and protrude beyond introitus	Annular, crescentic shape Atrophic, thin, with vessels visible	Estrogenized and thickened
Labia majora	May be edematous	Small, flatter	Increased fullness distinct from surrounding tissue
Labia minora	May be thick and protrude beyond labia major	Thin and short, rudimentary extension of clitoral hood extending one–third the length of the labia majora	Become elongated, but may not become fully developed until late puberty

TABLE 4.1	Normal Findings in the PGE Based on Pubertal Status—cont'd		
	COMMON ANATOMIC FINDINGS IN NEWBORN, PREPUBERTAL, AND ADOLESCENT GIRLS		
	Newborn	Prepubertal	Postpubertal Adolescent
Vagina	Thickened vaginal mucosa, with white physiologic secretions Length 3–6 cm	Length 4–7 cm Atrophic walls, red and thin	Length 8+ cm Moist, dull pink, rugated
Cervix	Prominent, with fundus-cervix ratio 1/2	Flush with vagina with small central opening	Adult shape, usually dull pink, may have a prominent ectropion
Uterus	Average uterine length 3.5 cm, maximal thickness 1.4 cm, echogenic endometrium	Length including cervix 3.2 cm, thickness 1 cm, thin endometrium may not be visible	Length 4.72 cm at Tanner stage 2 breasts, 7.4 cm at Tanner stage 4 breasts
Ovaries	Intraabdominal location Volume 1.0 cm^3	Intraabdominal location Volume 0.54 ± 0.25 cm^3	Pelvic location Volume 1.9 cm^3 at Tanner stage 2 breasts, 4.19 cm^3 at Tanner stage 4 breasts

Reproduced from Simms-Cendan J. Examination of the pediatric adolescent patient. *Best Pract Res Clin Obstet Gynaecol.* 2018;48:3-13. doi:10.1016/j.bpobgyn.2017.08.005. Epub 2017 Sep 1. PMID: 29056510.

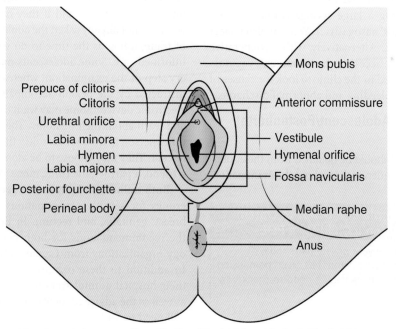

Fig. 4.2 Normal female genital anatomy. (From Zitelli and Davis' Atlas of Pediatric Physical Diagnosis, 8th Edition; Copyright © 2023 by Elsevier, Inc. All rights reserved.)

an infection, then vaginal swabs or lavage can be performed to obtain a culture. If you are worried about a foreign body or lesion, then vaginoscopy either at the bedside or in the operating room should be performed.[9]

To obtain vaginal cultures via swabs, it is best done with two providers. One should perform labial retraction while the other swabs the lower vagina without touching the hymen (see Fig. 4.5). Use the smallest swab that your institution has for cultures. If you

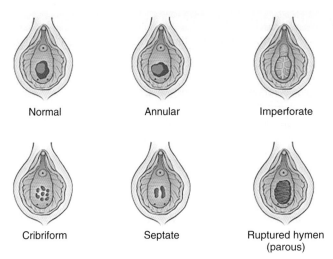

Normal   Annular   Imperforate

Cribriform   Septate   Ruptured hymen
                                     (parous)

Fig. 4.3 Various types of hymen. (From Dehn RW, Asprey DP. *Essential Clinical Procedures.* 4th ed. Elsevier Inc; 2021.)

suspect a foreign body and have a cooperative child, you can try and flush it out by injecting warm water or saline into the vagina using a large syringe connected to a catheter (e.g., urinary, nasogastric). You can also collect this fluid for cultures. Alternatively, with a cooperative child, and if you have access to the equipment, vaginoscopy can be performed in the clinic to look for causes of prepubertal vaginal bleeding and abnormal discharge.

Approach to the Adolescent/Postpubertal Examination

Consent for the PGE should be obtained from the adolescent and reviewed frequently throughout the examination.

BOX 4.1   Example of a Script to Obtain Assent and Position a Child for a PGE

- "Is it ok if I examine your private parts today?"
- "I am a doctor and your parent has given permission for this examination because we need to check why you are bleeding."
- "Do you agree?"
- "Lie down on the table on your back."
- "Now bend your knees."
- "Make sure your feet are close to your bottom. Pretend your legs are butterfly wings and open them wide."
- Use basic language that is appropriate to the child's developmental state.
- Use simple terms and short phrases to get them correctly positioned.

It is important to ask about any history of previous examinations and how they went, what the patient would like done differently, and if they have any questions. If you have not already asked the adolescent about a history of trauma, now is the time to do so and apply trauma-informed care. Some adolescents may want to know every step of the examination, whereas others prefer to be distracted by the person accompanying them or by an electronic device.[5] Some may want to watch with a mirror and learn about their anatomy. The decision to have another person in the room is solely the decision of the adolescent. They may choose to be alone or to have a parent, a friend, a partner, the clinic nurse, or a chaperone.

Both trainees and physicians need to consider chaperones for sensitive examinations, which include the breast, genitalia, and rectum. In Box 4.2 you will find the recommendations for both pediatric and gynecology organizations from Canada and the United States. In addition to these organizations, one should review their hospital administration's policies and procedures as well as the advice of their respective colleagues.[1,2] You will need to find out if having a chaperone is an opt-in, opt-out, or mandatory policy.[1] Chaperones may be a friend, a partner, a clinic nurse, or another staff member. You should always document in the medical record who the chaperone was or if a chaperone was declined.[1,2]

If only a vulvar examination is indicated, follow the steps in Table 4.2. If a complete genital examination is indicated, including assessment of the vagina, cervix, uterus,

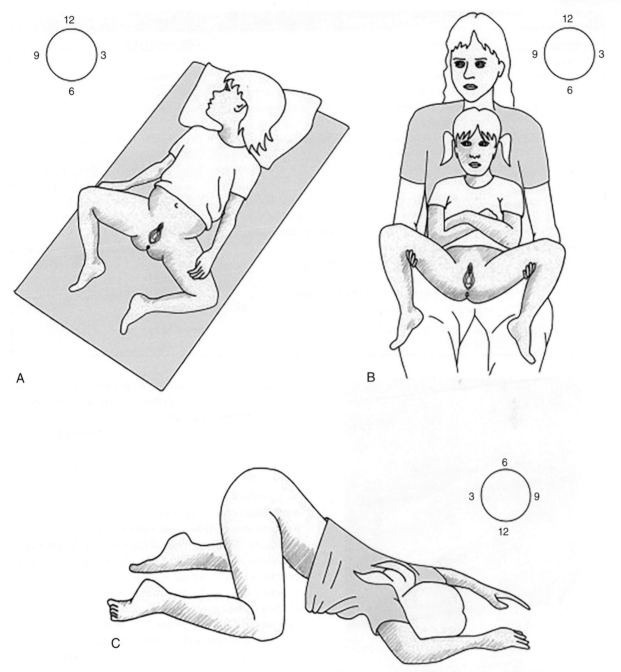

Fig. 4.4 Various positions for the prepubertal exam, including the frog-leg or butterfly position (alone or on a caregiver) and the knee-chest position. (From Jean Price; Injuries in prepubertal and pubertal girls; Best Practice & Research Clinical Obstetrics & Gynaecology Volume 27, Issue 1, February 2013, Pages 131-139.)

TABLE 4.2	Approach to the Prepubertal PGE	
Anatomy	**What You Are Looking For (and Why)**	**Tips and Tricks**
Mons pubis	Hair (Tanner staging)	See Chapter 5
Labia majora	Hair (Tanner staging) Lesions/excoriations/discoloration (vulvar dermatoses)	See Chapter 5 and 15
Labia minora	Lesions/excoriations/discoloration (vulvar dermatoses) Hypotrophic/absent (lichen sclerosis)	See Chapter 15
Clitoris, clitoral hood	Hypertrophy (hyperandrogenism, virilization) Phimosis (lichen sclerosis)	See Chapter 15 and Chapter 19
Introitus, hymen	Patency (imperforate/septate hymen) Erythema (infection) Abnormal discharge (infection, precocious puberty) Estrogenization status (prepubertal vs. postpubertal)	Use labial separation and retraction techniques (see Fig. 4.1)—asking the child to cough can help increase visualization; see Chapter 6
Urethra	Erythema, bleeding, prolapsus (urethral prolapse)	See Chapter 7 and 15
Lower vagina	Abnormal discharge (infection) Bleeding (infection, precocious puberty) Foreign body **Never use a speculum in the clinic setting**	Use labial retraction and knee-chest position (see Fig. 4.1, Fig. 4.4 and Chapter 7)
Perineum	Lesions/excoriations/discoloration (vulvar dermatoses)	See Chapter 15
Anus	Lesions/excoriations/discoloration (vulvar dermatoses) Pinworms	See Chapter 15

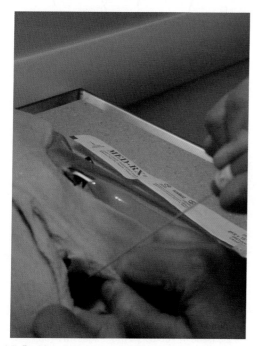

Fig. 4.5 Resident performing labial retraction and vaginal sampling on a pelvic model. (From Dumont T, Hakim J, Black A, Fleming N. Enhancing postgraduate training in pediatric and adolescent gynecology: evaluation of an advanced pelvic simulation session. *J Pediatr Adolesc Gynecol.* 2014;27[6]:360-370. doi:10.1016/j.jpag.2014.01.105. Epub 2014 Sep 23. PMID: 25256870.)

and adnexa, consider adding a speculum and bimanual examination. When you perform these, take into consideration whether your patient has ever inserted anything into their vagina before. This could be a tampon, fingers, toys, or through penetrative intercourse. If they have never inserted anything into their vagina before, reconsider your need for a speculum examination in the office.

Speculum examination: If you chose to proceed with a speculum examination (see indications earlier), chose a narrow one such as a medium Pederson or a Huffman speculum. "Medium" typically refers to the length of the speculum, and the name to its width (Fig. 4.6A–C). In comparison, a Pederson speculum is ⅞ inches wide, a Graves 1 inch, and a Huffman ½ inch[6] (see Fig. 4.6A). Despite certain speculums being described as pediatric, they should (1) never be used in the office setting in the prepubertal patient and (2) not be used in adolescents, as they are often not long enough to be able to see the cervix. The rest of the speculum examination is as you would perform in an adult patient, including inspection of the vaginal walls and cervix and obtaining vaginal/cervical swabs.

Bimanual examination: When performing a bimanual examination on the adolescent population, consider only inserting one finger into the vagina, especially if they have not previously had penetrative intercourse. The examination should be done in the same order

BOX 4.2 Organizational Recommendations for Chaperones

Organizations and Title of Statement	Recommendations
American Academy of Pediatrics (AAP; 2011) Policy Statement—Protecting Children From Sexual Abuse by Health Care Providers	Pediatricians must explain to parents and verbal children why they are performing each element of the examination and respect their need for modesty by providing appropriate draping and allowing privacy while changing. They should offer chaperones and provide them whenever requested or required as part of standard practice and local regulations or when the provider feels that a chaperone is needed. In general, examinations of younger children should be chaperoned by the child's parent or caregiver. As children become older, their caregivers and the children themselves should participate in the decision of whether to use a chaperone.
American College of Obstetricians and Gynecologists Committee Opinion Summary (ACOG; 2020) Sexual Misconduct)	It is recommended that a chaperone be present for all breast, genital, and rectal examinations. The need for a chaperone is irrespective of the sex or gender of the person performing the examination and applies to examinations performed in the outpatient and inpatient settings, including labor and delivery, as well as during diagnostic studies such as transvaginal ultrasonography and urodynamic testing.
Society of Obstetricians and Gynaecologists of Canada Guideline (SOGC; 2017)—The Presence of a Third Party During Breast and Pelvic Examinations	1. It is a reasonable and acceptable practice to perform a physical examination, including breast and pelvic examination, without the presence of a third person in the room unless the woman or health care provider indicates a desire for a third party to be present. 2. When a third party is present, it is recommended that the name of the person and his or her relationship to the patient and/or health care provider be documented in the patient's medical record. 3. If the health care provider chooses to have a third person present during all examinations, the health care provider should explain this policy to the woman. 4. If the woman wants a third party to be in the room, her wishes should be respected. She may choose the person she wants to be in the room. 5. Discussion about the presence of a third person in an examination room should stress that both the woman and the health care provider can choose to have a third person present during the examination. A woman should be offered that choice by one or more of the following means: • The health care provider may display a sign within the office that explains the choice. • The woman may be verbally offered the presence of a third person in the examination room. • The staff may document, within the office chart, the woman's choice with respect to third-party presence, so that the health care provider is made aware of the woman's choice before seeing her. 6. In the absence of a private area where the woman may disrobe (e.g., a curtained area or a separate office), the health care provider should leave the room before the woman undresses. Proper gowns or drapes should be available for the woman undergoing a pelvic and breast examination. 7. The health care provider should respect the wishes of the woman regarding privacy during history-taking and physical examination. Many women may not wish to have a third person in the examination room so that they can discuss personal or intimate matters with the health care provider alone. Health care providers should be sensitive to this wish and respect it as much as possible. However, the health care provider should use caution at all times to avert any potentially compromising situation. 8. If the situation is deemed to be too sensitive for breast and pelvic examinations to be conducted without the presence of a third party and a third party is not available or is refused by the patient, the health care provider should decline to conduct the examination. 9. If the health care provider or the woman wishes to have a third party present, the health care facility must comply with this request and provide an individual who is acceptable to both the patient and the health care provider.

From ACHA Guidelines Best Practices for Sensitive Exams. Published October 2019. https://www.acha.org/documents/resources/guidelines/ACHA_Best_Practices_for_Sensitive_Exams_October2019.pdf; CMPA. Is It Time to Rethink Your Use of Chaperones? Published March 2019. https://www.cmpa-acpm.ca/en/advice-publications/browse-articles/2019/is-it-time-to-rethink-your-use-of-chaperones; Laskey A, Haney S, Northrop S; Council on Child Abuse and Neglect. Protecting children from sexual abuse by health care professionals and in the health care setting. *Pediatrics*. 2022;150(3):e2022058879. doi:10.1542/peds.2022-058879; American College of Obstetricians and Gynecologists. Sexual misconduct: ACOG committee opinion, no. 796. *Obstet Gynecol*. 2020135(1):e43-e50. doi:10.1097/AOG.0000000000003608; No. 266-The presence of a third party during breast and pelvic examinations. *J Obstet Gynaecol Can*. 2017;39(11):e496-e497. doi:10.1016/j.jogc.2017.09.005

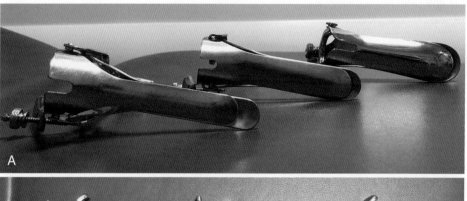

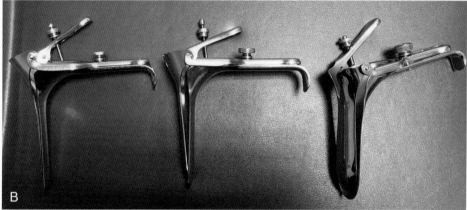

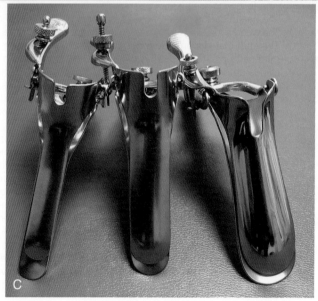

Fig. 4.6 Comparison between Huffman *(left)*, Pederson *(middle)*, and Graves speculum *(right)*. (A) View demonstrating speculum width (from narrow to wide). (B) View demonstrating speculum length (all are medium and the same length). (C) View demonstrating speculum width and length for comparison.

every time. Following is an example; however, what is important is that you develop your own routine that you will do in the same way every time so as to avoid omitting any steps that may help in providing your patient with the correct diagnosis.

After completing the steps in Table 4.2, move on to these steps.

1. Assess the sensitivity of the hymen as you enter.
2. Palpate the pelvic floor for contraction (hypotonicity or hypertonicity) and tenderness. This is especially useful in patients presenting with dyspareunia or the inability to insert tampons.
3. Palpate the anterior wall just under the urethra. This is important in patients with dyspareunia, dysuria, and other voiding dysfunction symptoms.
4. Mobilize the cervix gently to elicit any cervical motion tenderness that could help make the diagnosis of pelvic inflammatory disease.
5. Now add the abdominal hand to assess the shape, size, position, and tenderness of the uterus and adnexa.
6. As you remove your vaginal hand, palpate for any nodules or uterosacral tenderness that could be indicative of endometriosis.

EXAMINATION IN THE OPERATING ROOM

When an examination is indicated, its findings would change your management plan, and the patient cannot be examined in the clinic, the patient should be taken to the operating room for an examination under anesthesia (EUA) with possible vaginoscopy. The EUA should be performed as described previously. In a prepubertal patient who needs examination of their vagina (e.g., ruling out a foreign body or tumor), a vaginoscopy should be carried out. A cystoscope or small hysteroscope can be used with either normal saline or water. Care must be taken to not traumatize the hymen. As the instrument is advanced just past the hymen, the labia should be held together to provide vaginal distension and visualization of the vagina and cervix. Remember that the prepubertal vagina is short and one could perforate it with the instrument; thus it is of the utmost importance to observe the surgical screen/monitor when advancing your instrument. Once vaginal distention is achieved, you can assess the vagina and cervix. Biopsies can be taken as needed and foreign objects removed. The fluid can even be collected for culture and sensitivity. Once complete, reassess the hymen to ensure it was not traumatized.

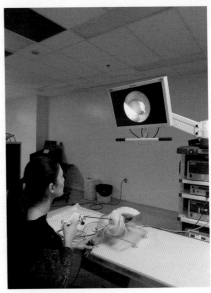

Fig. 4.7 Resident performing simulated vaginoscopy. On the screen you can see the most common foreign body in the vagina: toilet paper.

Vaginoscopy can be practiced in a simulated setting before being performed on a patient, as seen in Fig. 4.7.

SUMMARY

The physical examination is an important part of patient care. When indicated, it should be performed with consent and skillfully. Ensure you have an approach so that your examination is only done once and done in an efficient manner that will optimize patient comfort and provide you with the diagnostic information that you need. Improve your skills by performing these examinations in a simulation setting before performing them on a patient.

KEY POINTS

- The PGE is of the utmost importance in the diagnosis of most pediatric and adolescent gynecology conditions.
- The PGE should be performed when indicated and tailored to the patient's age, maturity level, pubertal status, and past experiences with a PGE.
- Consent and/or assent should always be obtained and trauma-informed care provided.
- Simulating the PGE before performing it on the patient will minimize patient and provider discomfort.
- When the PGE is indicated and cannot be performed in the clinic, the patient should be brought to the operating room.

REVIEW QUESTIONS

1. The pediatric gynecologic examination contains all of the following steps when examining a prepubertal child of 8 years old, except:
   a. Obtaining consent from the child and their caregiver
   b. Explaining the steps of the examination
   c. Holding the patient down on the table even if they are screaming so that you can obtain a good view of their vulva to make the correct diagnosis
   d. Performing labial separation and retraction in order to see the hymenal opening and lower vagina

2. When preparing to perform a pediatric gynecologic examination in the prepubertal child with malodorous discharge, which of the following does not need to be prepared?
   a. Vaginal swab
   b. Huffman speculum
   c. Gloves
   d. Nasogastric tube with warmed sterile water in a large syringe

3. Which of the following is not an indication to perform a pediatric gynecologic examination in a 15-year-old adolescent?
   a. Patient request for sexually transmitted infection screening given recent unprotected intercourse
   b. Insertion of intrauterine device for contraception
   c. Expanding vulvovaginal mass
   d. Pap test

REFERENCES

1. Loveless MB, Finkenzeller D, Ibrahim S, Satinet AJ. A simulation program for teaching obstetrics and gynecology residents the pediatric gynecology examination and procedures. *J Pediatr Adolesc Gynecol.* 2011;24(3):127-136.

2. Dumont T, Hakim J, Black A, Fleming N. Enhancing postgraduate training in pediatric and adolescent gynecology: evaluation of an advanced pelvic simulation session. *J Pediatr Adolesc Gynecol.* 2014;27(6):360-370. doi:10.1016/j.jpag.2014.01.105

3. Damle LF, Tefera E, McAfee J, et al. Pediatric and Adolescent Gynecology Education through Simulation (PAGES): development and evaluation of a simulation curriculum. *J Pediatr Adolesc Gynecol.* 2015;28(3):186-191. doi:10.1016/j.jpag.2014.07.008

4. Torres A, Horodeńska M, Witkowski G, Bielecki T, Torres K. High-fidelity hybrid simulation: a novel approach to teaching pediatric and adolescent gynecology. *J Pediatr Adolesc Gynecol.* 2019;32(2):110-116. doi:10.1016/j.jpag.2018.12.001

5. Simms-Cendan J. Examination of the pediatric adolescent patient. *Best Pract Res Clin Obstet Gynaecol.* 2018;48:3-13. doi:10.1016/j.bpobgyn.2017.08.005

6. Breech L. Tips for clinicians – The "well girl exam." *J Pediatr Adolesc Gynecol.* 2005;18:289-291.

7. Tipton AC. Child sexual abuse: physical examination techniques and interpretation of findings. *Adolesc Pediatr Gynecol.* 1989;2:1-25.

8. Emans SJ. Chapter 1 – Office evaluation of the child and adolescent. In: Herriot Emans SJ, Laufer MR, eds. *Emans, Laufer, Goldstein's Pediatric and Adolescent Gynecology.* 6th ed. Lippincott Williams & Wilkins; 2012:1-28.

9. Bacon JL. Pediatric vulvovaginitis. *Adolesc Pediatr Gynecol.* 1989;2:86-93.

10. National Cancer Institute. *ACS's Updated Cervical Cancer Screening Guidelines Explained.* September 18, 2020. https://www.cancer.gov/news-events/cancer-currents-blog/2020/cervical-cancer-screening-hpv-test-guideline

11. Choosing Wisely Canada. *Pap Tests.* https://choosingwiselycanada.org/pamphlet/pap-tests/

Normal Puberty

Hannah Canter and Megan Jacobs

INTRODUCTION

The period of human growth and development that occurs during adolescence is commonly referred to as *puberty*. This chapter focuses on normal pubertal changes, including sexual maturity and physical growth, as well as the underlying endocrinologic systems responsible for these processes. It is important for clinicians to understand these expected changes and the timing at which they occur.

HPG AXIS

The hypothalamic-pituitary-gonadal (HPG) axis is responsible for many of the physical changes that occur during puberty. A change from constant to pulsatile release of gonadotropin-releasing hormone (GnRH) from the hypothalamus signals the secretion of luteinizing hormone (LH) and follicle-stimulating hormone (FSH) from the anterior pituitary, which in turn stimulate the production of estradiol or testosterone from the ovaries or testes, respectively (Fig. 5.1). For the purposes of this chapter, individuals with ovaries will be referred to as assigned female at birth (AFAB).

AFAB PUBERTAL CHANGES

Estradiol, produced in the ovaries, plays an important role in pubertal changes for those AFAB. Breast development, changes in genitalia, and skeletal maturation are all influenced by estradiol and other circulating estrogens. Pubertal changes related to estrogen happen sequentially.

Thelarche, or breast budding, is typically the earliest recognizable sign of puberty in AFAB. These changes occur at a median age of 8.8 to 10 years and, as with many pubertal findings, may vary depending on race and ethnicity. Black and Hispanic youth have been noted to experience earlier initiation of puberty.[1] Adrenarche, or onset of pubic hair development, occurs at a similar time, between the ages 8.8 and 10.5 years. Thelarche and adrenarche are followed closely by the height spurt, with an average onset at 9.5 years and peak velocity around 11.5 years. Finally, menarche occurs at 12.5 years of age on average, with height growth potential continuing for 2 to 2.5 years after menarche with a maximum gain of ~2 inches.[1]

SMR: Breast Stages

The sexual maturity rating (SMR) scale describes different stages of pubertal development in three areas: breast, genitalia, and pubic hair. This staging is used as a common notation for clinicians and in some texts is also known as *Tanner staging*. Breast staging and pubic hair staging can be used in those AFAB. The SMR stages of breast development are described next (Fig. 5.2A):

- SMR 1 – Prepubertal. Only the papilla is elevated above the chest wall.
- SMR 2 – Breast bud. There is elevation of the breasts and papillae and increased diameter of the areolas.
- SMR 3 – The breasts and areolas continue to enlarge, but there is no separation of contour.
- SMR 4 – Mound on mound. The areolas and papillae elevate above the breasts.
- SMR 5 – Mature female breasts. The areolas have receded, and the papillae may extend slightly above the contour of the breasts.[2]

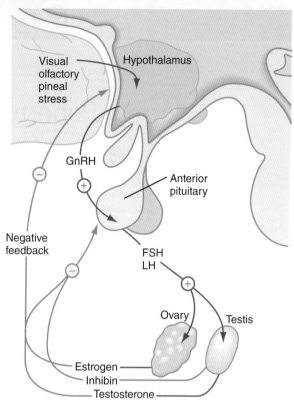

Fig. 5.1 Hypothalamic-pituitary-gonadal axis. *GnRH,* Gonadotropin-releasing hormone; *FSH,* follicle-stimulating hormone; *LH,* luteinizing hormone. From Basil j. Zitelli: Zitelli and Davis' Atlas of Pediatric Physical Diagnosis. Eighth Edition. Copyright © 2023 by Elsevier, Inc. All rights reserved.

Genital Changes

External genitalia changes also occur in AFAB during puberty in response to an increase in estrogen and other hormones; however, there are not specific SMR stages to describe this. In general, the external portion of the clitoris and the labia grow and widen, and the vulva may also change in color.[3] In adults, the color can range from light pink to red, dark brown, or black and can vary with different ethnicities. Overall, the vulval mucosa becomes less erythematous with estrogen exposure. Internally, the vagina and cervix also grow in size, and vaginal secretions are produced. This thin, white discharge is referred to as *physiologic leukorrhea,* and it typically precedes menarche by approximately 6 to 12 months.[4]

HPA AXIS

In addition to the gonadal axis, the hypothalamus and pituitary also signal to the adrenal glands (hypothalamic-pituitary-adrenal [HPA] axis) to produce adrenal androgens (dehydroepiandrosterone [DHEA], dehydroepiandrosterone sulfate [DHEAS], and androstenedione). This process occurs in AFAB between age 6 and 8 years and is referred to as *adrenarche.* The primary physical manifestation of adrenarche is the growth of axillary and pubic hair, or pubarche. Onset of hair growth typically occurs after age 8 in AFAB youth.[2]

In addition to sexual hair growth, youth experience other physical changes related to adrenal androgens. For example, DHEAS is converted in the apocrine and sebaceous glands, contributing to the development of body odor and acne, respectively.[1]

SMR: Pubic Hair Stages (see <u>Fig. 5.2</u>B)

- SMR 1 – Vellus hair develops over the mons pubis similar to the rest of the body. There is no sexual hair.
- Stage 2 – Sparse, long, pigmented, downy hair, which is straight or only slightly curled, appears on the labia majora or base of the phallus and scrotum.
- Stage 3 – A moderate amount of darker, coarser, and curlier sexual hair appears. The hair has spread laterally over the pubic hair.
- Stage 4 – The hair distribution is adult in type but decreased in total quantity. There is no spread to the medial surface of the thighs.
- Stage 5 – Hair is adult in quantity and type. There is spread to the medial surface of the thighs.

HPS AXIS

Another important aspect of puberty is linear growth and bone maturation. This is primarily driven by growth hormone (GH) via the hypothalamic-pituitary-somatotropic (HPS) axis. The hypothalamus signals to the pituitary via alternating GH-releasing hormone and somatostatin, leading to pulsatile release of GH (Fig. 5.3). Influences of many other factors are involved in stimulation and inhibition of GH release. The biologic effects of GH include increases in linear growth, bone thickness, and soft tissue growth.[5]

The pubertal growth spurt is a period of rapid growth that is mediated by GH via insulin growth factor hormones (IGF-1/somatomedin-C and IGF-2) as well as sex hormones: estradiol and testosterone.[1]

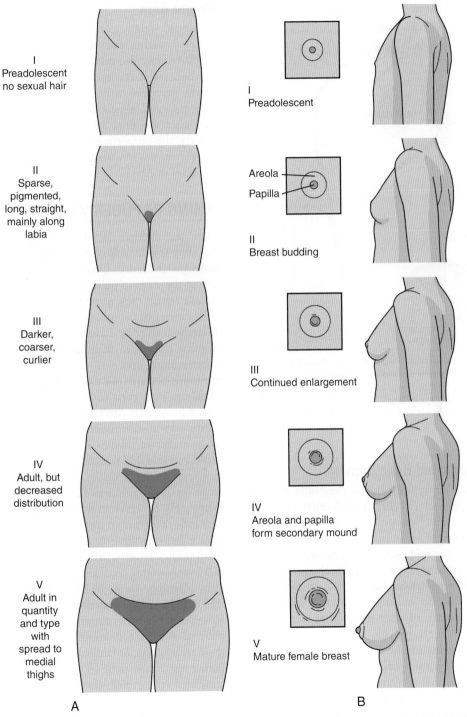

Fig. 5.2 Sexual maturity rating (SMR) staging for pubic hair (A) and breasts (B). (A. From Basil J. Zitelli: Zitelli and Davis' Atlas of Pediatric Physical Diagnosis. Eighth Edition. Copyright © 2023 by Elsevier, Inc. All rights reserved.)

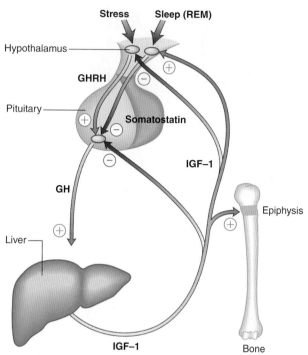

Fig. 5.3 Hypothalamic-pituitary-somatotropic axis. *GH,* Growth hormone; *GHRH,* growth hormone–releasing hormone; *IGF-1,* insulin growth factor hormone 1; *REM,* rapid eye movement. (From Adam Feather: Kumar and Clark's Clinical Medicine. Tenth Edition © 2021, Elsevier Limited. All rights reserved.[6])

Linear Growth and Bone Density

Linear growth during this time accelerates in puberty, with a peak height velocity (PHV) of 8.3 cm/yr, occurring between SMR 2 and 3, or age 11.5 years on average.[1]

Final adult height for an individual can be estimated using the following mid-parental height formulas[1]:

AFAB mid-parental height = [(paternal height − 13 cm or 5 in) + maternal height] / 2

It is important to remember that this calculation provides an estimate and that many other factors contribute to final adult height. For this reason, it is best to present this information to patients as a target height range, equal to the mid-parental height ± 2 standard deviations (SD) (1 SD = 5 cm or 2 in).

 Linear growth continues until there is closure of the growth plates, a process primarily driven by estrogen. This effect is also important for bone density, of which significant deposition is laid in childhood and adolescence. Bone density creation is completed at the latest by 30 years of age and will remain stable and eventually decrease with age.[7]

Weight Gain

Continued weight gain along the growth curve is also expected during puberty. Similar to height velocity, weight velocity also peaks during adolescence. This is in part because of the linear growth and increasing bone density described earlier. Additionally, increases in lean body mass and adipose tissue contribute to weight gain, even after the final adult height is reached. During puberty, the proportion of lean body mass vs. adipose tissue increases in assigned male at birth (AMAB) and decreases in AFAB.[1]

TIMING OF PUBERTAL ONSET

There are multiple factors affecting pubertal timing, including genetic and epigenetic factors as well as environmental influences. Genetics likely accounts for 50% to 80% of the onset of puberty; however, pinpointing what cascade signals these genes has yet to be fully identified.[8]

In developed nations, younger age trends for onset of thelarche (earlier by 1 year) and menarche (earlier by 4 months) have been demonstrated in the Copenhagen Puberty Study over a 15-year time span.[9] Although, as previously noted in this chapter, pubertal onset and menarchal age have been documented as occurring slightly earlier in African American/Black and Hispanic youth compared with Caucasian/White youth, the reality is often a matter of months difference. Between the mid-1800s and mid-1900s, average menarchal age decreased by 4 years. In the 1960s the average reported age of menarche for Black girls was 12.5 years and 12.8 years for White girls. However, in the 1970s in a Louisiana study, very little difference in menarchal age was found related to race. Between the 1970s and 1990s there were multiple small studies demonstrating a decrease in menarchal age of 0.7 years among Black girls and 0.1 years among White girls. Menarche seems to be the most notable stage in AFAB puberty and therefore has been studied more. However, it is a late occurrence in the sequence of AFAB pubertal changes, and skeletal maturation may have more to do with genetic or familial differences than menarche. Earlier age of menarche (<11 years of age) seems to be correlated with overall shorter status and higher weight (up to 5.5 kg heavier), with possible increased risk of breast cancer.[10] Race is a social construct, and it should be noted that in available studies race may have inappropriately been used to represent other variables, including weight, environmental exposures, and stressors including but not limited to racism.[11] Diagnosis of early or

TABLE 5.1	Endocrine-Disrupting Chemicals and Pubertal Effects		
Chemical	**Exposure**	**Hormonal Effect**	**Pubertal Effect**
Phthalates	Plasticizer intake orally, dermally, or via inhalation	Antiandrogenic activity (small estrogenic activity)	More research needed. Possible delayed or precocious pubertal effects.
Bisphenol A (BPA)	Plastics and epoxy resins on food and beverage packaging	Estrogen-like endocrine disruptor	More research needed. Possible precocious puberty or no effect on puberty.
Pesticides	Water, air, food, vertical transmission, and breast milk	Endocrine disruptor	Earlier thelarche or menarche to those exposed prenatally. Other studies without these findings.
Flame-retardant chemicals	Plastics, textiles, coatings Organohalogen: polybrominated diphenyl ethers (PBDEs)	Endocrine disruptor	May delay menarche, especially if higher body mass index (BMI).

precocious puberty should not be made on the basis of someone's racial or ethnic background, and treatments should not be withheld or offered differentially.

Physiology of Pubertal Onset

As outlined earlier, pulsatile GnRH secretion from the hypothalamus initiates the hormonal cascade, marking the onset of puberty. However, the events leading to the trigger of this pulse remain obscure overall.

Three neuropeptides act as activators of GnRH secretion: kisspeptin, neurokinin B, and dynorphin are produced by KNDy neurons in the arcuate nucleus of the hypothalamus and have direct projections to GnRH cell bodies. Kisspeptin pulses seem to be required for episodic LH secretion and occur simultaneously with GnRH pulses. In loss-of-function mutations of the *KISS1* gene coding kisspeptin, pubertal development does not occur (idiopathic hypogonadotropic hypogonadism). Neurokinin B dysfunction also leads to delayed pubertal development when encoding *TAC3* or *TACR3* genes have mutations.[12]

Inhibitors of GnRH secretion, or "silencers" of the polycomb group (PcG), repress the *KISS1* gene. The decreased expression from the hypothalamus of silencer genes along with increased methylation of silencers proceeds the onset of puberty. If these processes are blocked, pubertal failure can occur.[13] This also means that if there is dysfunction in the silencer genes at earlier ages, precocious puberty may occur. Mutations in puberty inhibition pathways and genes that have been identified include neurotransmitter gamma-aminobutyric acid (GABA) receptor, *MKRN3* gene loss of function (one-third of familial precocious puberty cases), and *DLK1* gene deletion.

Nongenetic Influences of Puberty

Delayed pubertal onset has been related to overall poor health in cases of children with chronic disease affecting nutrition and inflammation. Social and environmental stressors, including those within the family unit, have been suggested to have variable effects on pubertal timing.

Increased weight has been associated with earlier pubertal onset and progression. The leptin hormone, made in adipocytes, can affect the activity of the GnRH pulse generator, but is likely one of many influences. The theory is that leptin levels likely signal a sufficient store of metabolic fuel.[14]

Endocrine-disrupting chemicals in the environment have also been linked to affecting the age or advancement of puberty. They are further listed in Table 5.1.

PUBERTAL EXAMINATIONS

Pubertal examinations are recommended at preadolescent well visits, as pubertal changes may start as early as 8 years of age. These examinations assist in providing reassurance that changes are occurring in an appropriate timeline and order and can provide appropriate anticipatory guidance for youth and families of upcoming changes. This part of the encounter can be uncomfortable for patients, and it is important for clinicians to approach the subject with care. The components of the pubertal examination and the rationale behind them should be explained before visual or physical inspection. The patient's developmental status should be assessed appropriately for this examination; however, examinations should not be significantly delayed, as abnormalities may be missed. The provider should also ask the patient's permission before performing the examination and reassure them of their bodily autonomy. A chaperone is highly encouraged to be present during all breast, genital, and rectal examinations.[15] Appropriate chaperones include clinic staff members, such as medical assistants or nurses. Adolescents should be allowed the opportunity to determine if they would like their guardians in the examination room or not, but guardians or family members should not be used as chaperones. Youth should also be offered the opportunity to change into a gown or drape privately.

At early pubertal ages, physical examination of the breast is helpful to differentiate breast tissue from adipose chest tissue to determine SMR 2. Visual breast examinations are appropriate at older ages to assess SMR stages, as the changes are primarily visual.

AFAB pubic hair evaluation can be performed with the patient supine and looking quickly to assess thickness and distribution to assess SMR stage. Palpating inguinal folds for lymphadenopathy and assessing femoral pulses are also appropriate. A pelvic examination in a youth AFAB is not often indicated if menses are occurring normally and the patient has no concerns. In prepubertal patients, it can be helpful to assess estrogenization and any hymenal concerns or if there is a concern for female genital mutilation. However, there is no pelvic examination to determine "virginity," and this should be discouraged if requested.

PUBERTAL HEALTH CONCERNS

Apart from examination of appropriate growth and stages of puberty, office examinations should also consider how pubertal body changes can affect other health concerns, such as blood levels, a higher risk for sports injuries, and the psychological well-being of adolescents, including cosmetic and body image concerns. Anemia and iron deficiency are extremely common in adolescents. Hemoglobin with ferritin level concentrations tend to decrease in AFAB youth because of menstrual bleeding and, in some cases, insufficient iron intake.[16] During pubertal PHV, or "growth spurt," is the time of highest deposition of bone mineral density and highest risk for epiphysial growth plate damage. Adolescents experience higher incidence of sprains or strains of joints related to rapid bone changes, immediately followed by an increase in muscle mass leading to periods of range-of-motion limitation. Screening for scoliosis during this time of axial skeletal growth is extremely important.

Acne is also common and a regular occurrence in puberty; however, severe acne, especially early in puberty,

with other signs of hyperandrogenism, may signal a need for further evaluation for sources of androgen excess.

Further, youth AFAB who undergo earlier pubertal changes than their peers have been reported to have a greater decrease in self-esteem and body satisfaction, as well as increased rates of depression and antisocial behaviors. Additional considerations should include visual changes, with rates of myopia increasing during puberty.[17]

CONCLUSION

Puberty is a complex process involving multiple endocrinologic systems driving sexual maturity and physical growth. Fig. 5.4 provides a summary of these changes and the timing at which they occur. Puberty changes occur over the course of approximately 4 years, typically between the ages of 8 and 16;[1] however, there can be significant variation between individuals based on sex assigned at birth, race, ethnicity, and other genetic and

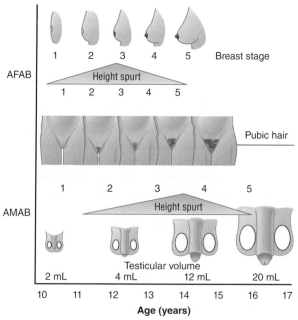

Fig. 5.4 The age of development of features of puberty, including sexual maturity rating and linear growth. Stages and testicular size show mean ages, and all vary considerably between individuals. The same is true of the height spurt, shown here in relation to other data. Numbers 2–5 indicate SMR stages of development. *AFAB,* Assigned female at birth; *AMAB,* assigned male at birth; *SMR,* sexual maturity rating. (From Adam Feather: Kumar and Clark's Clinical Medicine. Tenth Edition © 2021, Elsevier Limited. All rights reserved.[6])

environmental factors. Understanding how to assess pubertal changes on history and physical examination will help clinicians know when to provide reassurance about this normal variation vs. when pubertal changes may be abnormal and require further evaluation. These abnormalities, along with embryologic disorder of sexual development, are further discussed in Chapter 6.

PUBERTY INFORMATION FOR PATIENTS AND FAMILIES

- From the American Academy of Pediatrics (AAP):
  - https://www.healthychildren.org/English/ages-stages/gradeschool/puberty/Pages/default.aspx
  - You-ology: A Puberty Guide for Every Body: https://publications.aap.org/aapbooks/book/708/You-ology-A-Puberty-Guide-for-Every-Body?autologincheck5redirected
- From the American College of Obstetrics and Gynecology (ACOG): https://www.acog.org/womens-health/faqs/your-changing-body-puberty-in-girls
- From the American Academy of Family Physicians (AAFP): http://familydoctor.org/familydoctor/en/teens/puberty-sexuality.html
- From Planned Parenthood: https://www.planned-parenthood.org/learn/teens/puberty

---

KEY POINTS

- Pubertal evaluations are vital to providing appropriate anticipatory guidance.
- Knowledge of normal puberty stages aids in understanding when changes are abnormal, requiring intervention.
- There is still much to learn about the effects of genetic and environmental impacts on pubertal timing.

■ REVIEW QUESTIONS

1. A 11-year-old youth assigned female at birth has a breast sexual maturity rating stage of 3, reports breast budding about 1.5 years ago, and has just gained 1.5" in height in the past 1 year. The patient is complaining of white vaginal discharge for the past 2 months without odor or vaginal discomfort symptoms. The fluid is negative for pseudohyphae, clue cells, and white blood cells. The fluid has a normal pH. The patient denies any sexual activity. Maternal menarche occurred at 13 years. This patient and their parent would like to know when to expect menarche. What would be the most appropriate response based in the information provided?
   a. Menarche should have already occurred; a workup should be performed for delayed puberty.
   b. This patient should be advised to begin carrying menstrual supplies with them, as menarche is likely to start in the next 6 to 12 months.
   c. Provide guidance that the patient's menarche will occur at 13 years of age, just like their mother's menarche.
   d. Provide guidance that menarche should occur after the patient reaches their final adult height.

2. An 8-year-and-1-month-old girl (AFAB) is brought in by her parent with concern for pubertal hair growth. The parents are concerned for early puberty and are wondering if an intervention is needed. Height and weight are appropriate based on previous growth curves at the fiftieth percentile. Your examination reveals several fine, straight, soft, nonpigmented hairs on the mons pubis. No notable axillary hair is visible. No body odor is noted. Breast SMR stage is 1, and vulva by visual inspection demonstrates erythematous mucosa and normal structures without discharge. What is the next step in the workup for this patient?
   a. Order DHEAS, testosterone, androstenedione, and 17-hydroxyprogesterone (17-OHP) levels to evaluate for biochemical evidence of precocious adrenarche.
   b. Offer a GnRH agonist for pubertal suppression to delay progression of further pubertal changes at this age.
   c. Reassure parents that their child is normal by examination and is not demonstrating signs of premature puberty.
   d. Order a pelvic ultrasound to evaluate for ovarian mass.

3. On breast examination, your 13-year-old patient's breast contour is confluent with that of the areolas. She declines a genitourinary examination. She is 5'2" tall and weighs 90 pounds. What would be the most helpful piece of information to determine if she is SMR III or SMR V?
   a. If she has had menarche.
   b. If she has gained <2 cm (about 0.79 in) in height in the past 1 year.
   c. If she tells you she has pubic hair
   d. If she reports breast tenderness.

REFERENCES

1. Carswell JM, Stafford DEJ. Normal physical growth and development. In: Neinstein LS, Katzman DK, eds. *Neinstein's Adolescent and Young Adult Health Care, A Practical Guide*. 6th ed. Wolters Kluwer; 2016:28-37.

2. Escobar O, Gurtunca N, Viswanathan P, Feldman Witchel S. Pediatric endocrinology. In: Zitelli B, McIntire S, Nowalk A, Garrison J, eds. *Zitelli and Davis' Atlas of Pediatric Physical Diagnosis*. 8th ed. Elsevier; 2021:342-381.

3. Iezzi ML, Lasorella S, Varriale G, Zagaroli L, Ambrosi M, Verrotti A. Clitoromegaly in childhood and adolescence: behind one clinical sign, a clinical sea. *Sex Dev*. 2018;12:163-174. doi:10.1159/000489385

4. Farage M, Maibach H. Lifetime changes in the vulva and vagina. *Arch Gynecol Obstet*. 2006;273(4):195-202. doi:10.1007/s00404-005-0079-x

5. Felner EI, Patterson BC. Hormones of the hypothalamus and pituitary. In: Kliegman RM, St. Geme J, eds. *Nelson Textbook of Pediatrics*. 21st ed. Elsevier; 2019:2876-2880.

6. Gleeson H, Reddy N, Levy M. Endocrinology. In: Feather A, Randall D, Waterhouse D, eds. *Kumar and Clark's Clinical Medicine*. 10th ed. Elsevier; 2021:583-650.

7. Tanner JM, Goldstein H, Whitehouse RH. Standards for children's height at ages 2-9 years allowing for heights of parents. *Arch Dis Child*. 1970;45(244):755-762. doi:10.1136/adc.45.244.755

8. Papadimitriou A, Papadimitriou DT. Endocrine-disrupting chemicals and early puberty in girls. *Children (Basel)*. 2021;8(6):492. doi:10.3390/children8060492

9. Aksglaede L, Sørensen K, Petersen JH, Skakkebaek NE, Juul A. Recent decline in age at breast development: The Copenhagen Puberty Study. *Pediatrics*. 2009;123(5):e932-e939. doi:10.1542/peds.2008-2491

10. Freedman DS, Kahn LK, Serdula MK, Dietz WH, Srinivasan SR, Berenson GS. Relation of age at menarche to race, time period, and anthropometric dimensions: the Bogalusa Heart Study. *Pediatrics*. 2002;110(4):e43. doi:10.1542/peds.110.4e43

11. Osinubi AA, Lewis-de Los Angeles CP, Poitevien P, Topor LS. Are black girls exhibiting puberty earlier? Examining implications of race-based guidelines. *Pediatrics*. 2022;150(2):e2021055595.

12. Lehman MN, Coolen LM, Goodman RL. Minireview: Kisspeptin/neurokinin B/dynorphin (KNDy) cells of the arcuate nucleus: a central node in the control of gonadotropin-releasing hormone secretion. *Endocrinology*. 2010;151(8):3479-3489. doi:10.1210/en.2010-0022

13. Lomniczi A, Loche A, Castellano JM, et al. Epigenetic control of female puberty. *Nat Neurosci*. 2013;16(3):281-289. doi:10.1038/nn.3319

14. Roemmich JN, Rogol AD. Role of leptin during childhood growth and development. *Endocrino Metab Clin North Am*. 1999;28(4):749-764, viii. doi:10.1016/s0889-8529(05)70100-6

15. Curry ES; Committee on Practice and Ambulatory Medicine. Use of chaperones during the physical examination of the pediatric patient. *Pediatrics*. 2011;127(5):991-993. doi:10.1542/peds.2011-0322

16. Bergstrom E, Hernell O, Lonnerdal B, Persson LA. Sex differences in iron stores of adolescents: what is normal? *J Pediatr Gastroenterol Nutr*. 1995;20(2):215-224. doi:10.1097/00005176-199502000-00013

17. Tanner J. *Growth at Adolescence*. Blackwell Scientific Publications; 1962.

Abnormal Puberty

Ellen Lancon Connor and Lauren A. Kanner

INTRODUCTION

Puberty can be a source of much concern for adolescents. As children become more self-aware, they also become more aware of comparisons: *Why don't I have breasts yet? My friend does. When are my periods going to start?* The clinician's role is to educate the young person about their body and to guide them through puberty, being well-versed in potential signs that may herald underlying causes of atypical puberty. Genetic context is important: many forms of earlier or later puberty are heritable. When evaluating pubertal progression, the clinician must consider family history, the child's medical history, and a careful review of systems that could suggest underlying disease; examine the child thoroughly while explaining findings; and develop a plan for evaluation if pubertal aberrations are suspected.

TIMING VERSUS TEMPO OF PUBERTY

Both timing and tempo must be considered in diagnosing puberty occurring outside of two standard deviations of average[1] (Table 6.1). Pubertal concerns frequently arise about the timing of pubertal changes. Normal and abnormal pubertal variants change the timing of puberty's initiation or its sequence. In general, thelarche is considered normal after the age of 8 years and has been suggested as normal after 7 years old in African American girls. However, scrutiny of ascribing normalcy or abnormality for a physical condition based on race or ethnicity has led to the recognition that this is a source of implicit bias that can prevent or delay the evaluation of someone with a pathologic finding.[2] Thus it is prudent to evaluate children who present with

thelarche before the age of 8 years. Similarly, the child who has not had thelarche by the age of 13 years should be evaluated. Menarche, on average, occurs by the age of 12 to 12.5 years. The child who has not achieved menarche by 14 to 15 years should undergo thoughtful evaluation. These are examples of considering the *timing* of the pubertal event.

Pubertal tempo is also important to consider when evaluating pubertal development. Menarche typically follows true thelarche in 2.5 to 4 years. The child whose thelarche occurred 5 years ago without subsequent menarche might have an underlying health condition preventing this milestone. Similarly, the child who progresses from thelarche to menarche in 6 months, or who has menarche before thelarche, deserves evaluation.

CENTRAL VERSUS PERIPHERAL CAUSES OF ABNORMAL PUBERTY

When delayed or precocious puberty is identified, the clinician can delineate the cause of the abnormality with a careful history, review of systems and examination, and selective use of imaging and laboratory evaluation. Perhaps the most important consideration when sorting out causes is determining whether a pubertal anomaly is *central* or *peripheral*. Use of ultrasensitive luteinizing hormone (LH), follicle-stimulating hormone (FSH), estradiol and androgen assays are essential, as routine adult assays cannot detect the very low levels of estradiol in early puberty or the initial rise in LH that heralds puberty. Ultrasensitive estradiol and testosterone levels should be determined using liquid chromatography–tandem mass spectrometry.

TABLE 6.1   Timing Versus Tempo: Reasons to Evaluate for Abnormal Puberty

Precocious timing
  Thelarche before age 7-8 years
  Menarche before age 10 years
Precocious tempo
  Menarche occurring less than 2 years after
    thelarche or before thelarche
Delayed timing
  No thelarche by age 13 years
  No menarche by age 15 years
Delayed tempo
  Greater than 4 years after thelarche without
    menarche

Ultrasensitive measurements of LH and FSH should use two site electrochemiluminescent assays, which are more sensitive than standard immunoassays. Measuring gonadotropins is key in noting whether a pubertal timing or tempo aberration has arisen in the central nervous system (CNS) or stems from concerns elsewhere.

PRECOCIOUS PUBERTY

A child with a uterus and ovaries who has precocious puberty may present with (1) advanced bone age because of estrogen secretion, (2) breast development, and (3) even menarche. The uterus may be enlarged to a size commensurate with bone age, as both depend on estrogen secretion. Linear growth acceleration is seen with pubertal-level growth velocity. Adrenarchal signs of puberty arising from the adrenal gland often follow, with resultant acne, oiliness of the skin, apocrine body odor, and axillary and pubic hair.

Precocity can occur in isolation or in a complete fashion. Isolated forms include premature thelarche, premature adrenarche, or premature menarche. Complete forms are delineated into central precocious and peripheral sexual precocity based on the causative etiologies.

Premature thelarche (PT) refers to isolated breast tissue development, which can be seen at an early age in a patient who shows no additional signs of precocious puberty.[3] The typical presentation of PT is the appearance of glandular tissue in girls age 3 years or younger,

with little increase over the period of many months.[4] Some authors recommend that PT can be managed without hormonal testing or imaging in most girls without continued breast development and/or rapid growth velocity.[4] However, because a small percentage of these patients do actually have true precocious puberty, especially in females age >2, others feel that an initial hormone workup and imaging for abnormal puberty are warranted (as PT can be hard to distinguish from true precocious puberty). Accordingly, assessing for rapidity of thelarche and other pubertal changes; increased growth velocity; changes in ultrasensitive estradiol, LH, and FSH; and serial bone age radiographs should be undertaken to identify patients who have true precocious puberty.[5]

Premature adrenarche (PA) refers to maturation of the adrenal androgen axis with elevations of dehydroepiandrosterone sulfate (DHEAS) and androstenedione and is associated with the onset of pubic hair, comedones, and/or apocrine body odor. When adrenarche occurs before the age of 8 years in girls but is associated with a normal growth velocity, minimal or no bone age acceleration, and no evidence of clitoromegaly, the diagnosis of premature adrenarche can be made. This diagnosis is more common in girls with eventual polycystic ovary syndrome (PCOS) or those born small for gestational age, and some authors report African American girls.[4] However, a diagnosis of PA should not be overly influenced by ethnicity or race and should be determined carefully.

Typical laboratory findings include a modestly elevated DHEAS for age, commensurate with Tanner hair staging, but prepubertal FSH, LH, and estradiol concentration. Adrenal tumors, late-onset congenital adrenal hyperplasia (CAH; diagnosed with measurement of 17-OH progesterone), exogenous androgen exposure, and true precocious puberty must be eliminated as possible causes before the final diagnosis of PA can be made. Isolated PA has been associated with later hyperandrogenism, decreased ovulatory function, PCOS, hyperinsulinemia, and elevated triglyceride levels in adulthood. Therefore patients with PA should be monitored for these conditions through adolescence into adulthood.[6]

Premature menarche may occur in a child with a uterus who otherwise is experiencing normal puberty or has not even begun puberty. Early bleeding in this situation is likely the result of irregular patterns of

TABLE 6.2 McCune-Albright Syndrome: Clinical Characteristics

Characteristic	Associated Findings
Peripheral precocious puberty (gonadotropin-independent precocity)	Sudden-onset vaginal bleeding with or without breast development, but bleeding usually precedes significant breast growth Accelerated growth and skeletal maturation with adult height affected if prolonged exposure to sex steroid
Unilateral ovarian cysts	Detectable estradiol with prepubertal gonadotropins or enlarged ovary ± cyst visible on ultrasonography
Café-au-lait macules	Irregular borders, "coast of Maine"
Fibrous dysplasia	Ground-glass appearance and shepherd's crook deformity on x-ray
Other endocrinopathies associated with Guanine nucleotide binding protein, alpha stimulating (GNAS) activation	Thyrotoxicosis, gigantism or acromegaly, Cushing syndrome, hypophosphatemic rickets
Other nonendocrinopathies associated with GNAS activation	Cholestasis, hepatitis, intestinal polyps, cardiac arrhythmias, increased risk of malignancy

(Adapted from Javaid MK, Boyce A, Appelman-Dijkstra N, et al. Best practice management guidelines for fibrous dysplasia/McCune-Albright syndrome: a consensus statement from the FD/MAS international consortium. Orphanet J Rare Dis 2019; 14:139.)

hormone secretion seen before puberty is completed. However, other causes of early bleeding must be considered, including infection, foreign body, genitourinary trauma, sexual assault, ovarian mass or cyst, prolapse of the urethra, rectal bleeding mistaken for vaginal bleeding, or vaginal or cervical tumor. Munchausen by proxy (also known as *factitious disorder imposed on another*) is also a possible cause in a child who shows no other signs of puberty. McCune-Albright syndrome (MAS) may present with bleeding in a preschool child. Sedation or anesthesia may be needed to adequately examine the vagina and cervix in the younger child. If no etiology can be found, premature menarche is the presumed diagnosis, and the family can be reassured, with follow-up dependent on whether the bleeding recurs (Table 6.2). See Chapter 7 for more information on prepubertal vaginal bleeding.

Central Precocious Puberty

Central precocious puberty (CPP), also known as *gonadotropin-dependent precocious puberty,* is the development of complete isosexual pubertal changes caused by premature reactivation of the hypothalamic-pituitary-ovary axis, which has been quiet since the mini-puberty of infancy resolved (Table 6.3). A child may have central precocious puberty because of a genetic

TABLE 6.3 Causes of Central Precocious Puberty

Genetic etiology
  Loss of the *MKRN3* gene
  Mutations in the Kisspeptin gene (rare)
CNS abnormalities, congenital or acquired
  Congenital
  • Hydrocephalus, septic-optic dysplasia, tuberous sclerosis, CV infarction/bleed
  Acquired
  • Brain tumors, particularly with some genetic syndromes
  • Encephalitis
  • Brain injury
  • Some endocrine disruptors (DDT or DDE)
  • Some tumors (ovarian, pineal, hepatic)
Activation of HPO axis by peripheral precocity most commonly the result of:
  • Adrenocortical tumors
  • Ovarian tumors
  • CAH
  • Exogenous sex steroid exposure
Idiopathic

CAH, Congenital adrenal hyperplasia; *CNS,* central nervous system; *CV,* cardiovascular; *DDT,* dichlorodiphenyltrichloroethane; *DDE,* dichlorodiphenyldichloroethylene; *HPO,* hypothalamic-pituitary-ovarian.

mutation, exogenous exposure to sex steroids, a CNS lesion, or activation of the hypothalamic-pituitary-ovarian (HPO) axis, although often an etiology cannot be determined (idiopathic CPP). As imaging modalities and genetic testing improve, the incidence of the "idiopathic" form of precocity will likely decrease. It is also of note that multiple countries worldwide saw a significant increase in CPP during the COVID-19 pandemic.[7]

The most common genetic cause of central precocity is a loss-of-function mutation in the *MKRN3* gene.[8] This is the gene on chromosome 15 coding for the makorin RING finger protein 3. MKRN3 protein deficiency disinhibits the hypothalamus, leading to gonadotropin-releasing hormone pulses that activate pituitary secretion of LH and FSH. Rarely, mutations in the genes for kisspeptin (*KISS1*) or the kisspeptin receptor (*KISS1R*) may result in CPP. Routine genetic testing for CPP is not currently recommended, as it does not influence outcome.

CNS lesions, whether congenital or acquired, may result in CPP. Among prenatal or congenital causes are hydrocephalus, septo-optic dysplasia (also known as *optic nerve hypoplasia sequence*), tuberous sclerosis, and cerebrovascular infarction or bleed. Cerebral palsy, hydrocephalus, and spina bifida are known to sometimes be accompanied by precocious puberty of central origin. Postnatally, CPP can arise with brain tumors, particularly in patients with genetic syndromes such as neurofibromatosis type 1, DICER1 mutation, and Li-Fraumeni syndrome. Russell-Silver syndrome, or temple syndrome, can have central precocity as a finding, which can compromise final height. Acquired causes can include encephalitis, perinatal brain injury, or endocrine disruptor exposures, such as the pesticide dichlorodiphenyltrichloroethane (DDT) or its derivative, dichlorodiphenyldichloroethylene (DDE). Astrocytoma, optic nerve gliomas, and ependymomas are some of the tumors more commonly associated with central precocity. Teratomas, hepatoblastomas, choriocarcinomas, or pineal tumors may produce gonadotropins ectopically. Peripheral precocity related to adrenocortical carcinoma, ovarian virilizing tumors, CAH, or exogenous sex steroids may lead to central precocity by activating the HPO axis.

Evaluation starts with a thorough history and physical examination, including discussion of maternal age of menarche, evaluation for etiologies as noted earlier, and sexual maturity rating. Additional evaluation for CPP includes a bone age radiograph and laboratory testing with FSH, LH, and estradiol.[9] An ultrasensitive random LH level above 0.3 IU/L heralds puberty's initiation by the CNS. In the absence of this rise in LH, either observed spontaneously or with a luteinizing hormone–releasing hormone (LHRH) or gonadotropin-releasing hormone (GnRH) analogue stimulation test, evidence points to a peripheral source of precocity. Classically, with stimulation testing, the 20- or 60-minute LH sample should be at or above 5 to 8 IU/L if puberty is underway.[10] If CPP is diagnosed, magnetic resonance imaging (MRI) of the brain is warranted, especially in a child less than 6 years of age at presentation[11,12] (Fig. 6.1).

Treatment for CPP

The goals of therapy in CPP include allowing the patient to attain a normal adult height, ideally meeting the genetic potential range, and attaining pubertal completion when the child has the psychosocial and physical mechanisms for dealing with puberty. An additional goal for therapy is to delay menarche until an appropriate developmental age, as early menarche and sexual development can lead to psychosocial stress in the child and family.

CPP in a child with a uterus and ovaries can be temporarily delayed with a GnRH agonist (Table 6.4). GnRH agonists work by providing continuous stimulation of pituitary gonadotrophs, preventing the physiologic pulsatile stimulation by GnRH to the pituitary gland that would lead to FSH and LH secretion. GnRH can be offered for idiopathic CPP and for CPP related to an intracranial pathology.[13] Additionally, if the patient has an identifiable, intracranial lesion, treatment of the underlying lesion may be necessary. This may involve monitoring, as with a hypothalamic hamartoma, or chemotherapy, radiation, and/or surgery in the cases of tumors.

The decision of whether to give a GnRH agonist should be based on the age of presentation, pubertal tempo, height velocity, and estimated adult height from bone age as compared with the mid-parental height. For those presenting with precocious puberty after age 6 years, the recovery in height potential may be less, and so providers must ensure that the benefits of therapy outweigh the risks before initiating therapy.[14] The younger that a child presents with CPP, or the more rapid the pubertal progression, the more benefit the child could potentially have from initiation of a GnRH

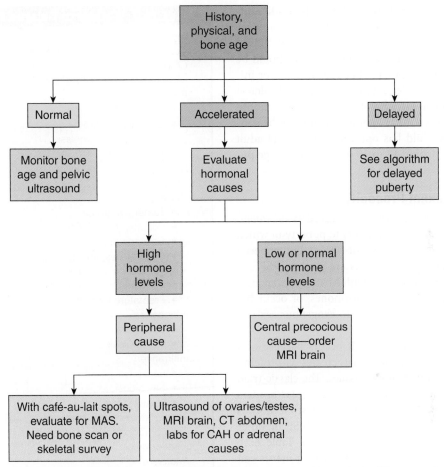

Fig. 6.1 Complete precocious puberty roadmap. *CAH,* Congenital adrenal hyperplasia; *CT,* computed tomography; *MAS,* McCune-Albright syndrome; *MRI,* magnetic resonance imaging.

TABLE 6.4	**Causes of Peripheral Precocity**
Genetic:	
McCune-Albright syndrome	
Late-onset congenital adrenal hyperplasia	
Other rare causes include Russell-Silver syndrome or temple syndrome	
Ovarian tumor	
Adrenal tumor	
Exogenous sex steroid exposure	
Lavender or tea tree oils	
Obesity	
Van Wyk Grumbach syndrome (rare)	

(From Cisternino M, Arrigo T, Pasquino AM, et al. Etiology and age incidence of precocious puberty in girls: a multicentric study. *J Pediatr Endocrinol Metab.* 2000;13(suppl 1):695-701.)

agonist. If the CPP presents after 6 years of age, the average height gained with therapy will decrease from 9 to 10 cm (seen in younger children) to only 4 to 7 cm of height increase.

GnRH agonist therapy is given as either as sustained-release depot formulations monthly, every 3 months, or every 6 months, or as a subcutaneous implant, which is changed according to standards for the individual implant, although the implants will have enough medication to last for 18 to 24 months without waning effects. Longer use of implants may carry a risk of implant retrieval difficulty.

While receiving GnRH agonists, patients must have evaluation of height velocity and puberty progression every 3 to 6 months, as well as repeat bone age measurements at 6- to 12-month intervals. Studies differ in recommendations of whether to monitor routine serum LH and sex steroid concentrations, but clinical evidence of continued pubertal progression should be investigated in this manner. After implantation or initial injection, GnRH adequacy should initially be determined with LH and estradiol measurement at 1 month and 3 to 4 months. GnRH agonist therapy can be continued until the child has optimized their final adult height and/or is within 12 to 18 months of average pubertal onset age.

Peripheral Sexual Precocity

Peripheral sexual precocity (PSP), also called *gonadotropin-independent sexual precocity,* refers to puberty in which gonadotropin signals are low or absent but pubertal levels (or higher) of sex steroids are present. PSP can have a genetic origin, such as with MAS or CAH, arise as a result of tumor-secreting hormones, or occur because of unintentional exposure to exogenous sex steroids (Table 6.5).

MAS can present with PSP. It occurs because of a postzygotic *GNAS* mutation that creates G-protein–coupled activation in multiple tissues. The classic triad of MAS is café-au-lait macules with irregular borders (typically unilateral on the body), polyostotic fibrous dysplasia predisposing to fractures, and PSP or other hyperfunctioning endocrine glands[15] (see Table 6.2). Puberty in children with MAS who have a uterus can present with ovarian cysts and/or premature menarche. Children may also have hyperthyroidism, Cushing syndrome, or growth hormone excess, depending on which tissues are affected by the mutation.

CAH, particularly late onset, can also present as peripheral precocity with accelerated growth velocity and bone age. For a child with a uterus, CAH may present as virilization with increased musculature, clitoromegaly, and premature pubic and axillary hair. Usually, late-onset CAH is the result of a partial enzyme defect involving 21-hydroxylase and can be diagnosed based on morning 17-OH progesterone level. DHEAS and androstenedione may be elevated, along with 11-ketotestosterone. In adolescents, late-onset CAH may have a phenotype consistent with PCOS.

Adrenal and ovarian tumors may secrete excess androgens or estrogen and initially present as precocity. Estrogen levels are usually more elevated in estrogen-secreting ovarian tumors, generally >100 pg/mL, than

TABLE 6.5 Causes of Delayed Puberty

Hypogonadotropic hypogonadism
  Constitutional delay of growth and puberty
  Chronic illness
  Malnutrition (weight loss, anorexia)
  Genetic syndromes
   • Kallmann syndrome
   • CHARGE syndrome
   • Optic nerve hypoplasia
   • Pituitary gene deficiencies
Hypergonadotropic hypogonadism (peripheral delayed puberty)
  Genetic
   • Turner syndrome
   • Peripheral X deletion
   • Galactosemia
   • Gonadal dysgenesis
  Surgical resection of ovaries
  Autoimmune
   • Premature ovarian failure
  Infectious
   • Coxsackie virus
   • Tuberculosis
  Infiltrative
   • Leukemia
   • Sarcoidosis
   • Histiocytosis
  Related to oncologic therapy (i.e., postchemotherapy or radiation)
Eugonadotropic
  Anatomic
   • Imperforate hymen
   • Vaginal septum
   • Müllerian anomalies (i.e., MRKH)

MRKH, Mayer-Rokitansky-Kuster-Hauser syndrome.
(From Sedlmeyer IL, Palmert MR. Delayed puberty: analysis of a large case series from an academic center. *J Clin Endocrinol Metab.* 2002;87(4):1613-1620; Saengkaew T, Howard SR. Genetics of pubertal delay. *Clin Endocrinol (Oxf).* 2022;97(4):473-482.)

in CPP. Hyperandrogenism may be seen in either ovarian or adrenal tumors, resulting in elevated total testosterone, DHEAS, and/or 11-ketotestosterone, typically above ranges expected for Tanner staging. Nonclassical CAH, caused by partial 21-hydroxylase deficiency, typically presents with morning 17-OH progesterone >200 ng/dL. Though sometimes initially difficult to discern, exposure to exogenous steroids through oral or transdermal routes can also lead to sexual precocity.

Families should be asked about possible home or daycare exposures to estrogen-, testosterone-, or DHEAS-containing creams, transdermal patches, or pills.

Precocity may also be seen with lavender or tea tree oils leading to thelarche, which has also been described with hair products containing placental or estrogen extracts.[16] Additionally, obesity is known to drive earlier puberty in girls, presenting with advanced bone age and increased height velocity in addition to signs of both estrogenization and adrenarche. A rare cause of precocity is the Van Wyk Grumbach syndrome, in which severe primary hypothyroidism is accompanied by delayed bone age and yet sexual precocity with low LH and FSH and extremely elevated thyrotropin (thyroid-stimulating hormone [TSH]). In this situation, alpha unit homology between TSH and FSH may permit binding of TSH to some FSH receptors.[17]

Evaluation for PSP is via the same route as for CPP noted earlier. If a peripheral component is suspected, additional testing would include evaluation for CAH with a 17-hydroxyprogesterone value, a DHEAS value to evaluate for adrenal pathology, and an ultrasound of the pelvis (see Fig. 6.1).

Treatment of Peripheral Sexual Precocity

Compared with CPP, PSP does not respond to a GnRH agonist, as the excess sex steroids are not the result of stimulation of the gonads by gonadotrophs.[13] Thus treatment is targeted to the underlying etiology and/or the gonads themselves. For those with MAS, treatment with an aromatase inhibitor or estrogen blocker such as selective estrogen receptor modulators can be used. For CAH, treatment is with corticosteroids that suppress excess adrenal androgen production by replacing cortisol to physiologic glucocorticoid levels, generally 10 to 15 mg/m^2/day of hydrocortisone or equivalent. The dose must suppress adrenocorticotropic hormone (ACTH) levels. In the future, corticotropin-releasing hormone (CRH) inhibitors may be used to suppress ACTH to decrease androgens.

If a tumor is the etiology of precocity, the tumor should be resected, and a multidisciplinary team with expertise in gynecologic surgery, endocrinology, and oncology should collaborate in care. For peripheral precocity secondary to exogenous sex steroids, identification and removal of the source of steroids should lead to regression of pubertal symptoms.

DELAYED PUBERTY

Approximately 2% of children have delayed puberty.[18] Sometimes the child with delayed puberty presents for evaluation because they are smaller than their peers. Otherwise, the child may present at a later age because they have not developed thelarche or had menses, whereas their unaffected friends or siblings have. Evaluation is warranted for the child who:

- Has not had thelarche by 13 years
- Still has an absence of menarche at 15 years

Two important questions should lead the evaluation of the child with delayed puberty:

1. Is the delay temporary or permanent?
2. Is the delay caused by a CNS issue with low gonadotropins, end-organ failure or absence of gonads with resulting high gonadotropins, or anatomic abnormalities?

Worldwide, the most common reason for pubertal delay is malnutrition, which can be because of lack of access to food or to caloric restriction. In the United States, constitutional delay of growth and puberty is the leading cause for delayed puberty and is a diagnosis of exclusion. As family history may aid in the diagnosis, a family history of pubertal timing and genetic diseases should be sought (Table 6.6).

Delayed puberty can be delineated into:

1. Hypogonadotropic hypogonadism
2. Hypergonadotropic hypogonadism
3. Eugonadotropic

Evaluation begins with examining growth records and obtaining a thorough history and review of systems. Signs and symptoms suggesting chronic disease, inadequate nutrition, genetic origins, or abnormal pubertal tempo (initiation of puberty without normal progression) should be sought. Physical examination for pubertal staging, inspection for associated craniofacial or skeletal abnormalities, and hymenal patency should be sought. Imaging may be needed to verify whether a uterus, vagina, and ovaries are present.

Laboratory evaluation starts with FSH, LH, and estradiol to assess the gonadotropic status and also should rule out thyroid, adrenal, and pituitary abnormalities at baseline, measuring prolactin TSH, 17-OH progesterone, and total serum testosterone.

Bone age radiograph is part of the initial evaluation. Pituitary or adrenal imaging may be needed, based on laboratory results. Genetic testing or chromosome testing may be done to diagnose causes (Fig. 6.2).

TABLE 6.6   Therapy for Central Precocious Puberty

Drug	Dose	Route
Leuprolide acetate	3.75, 7.5, 11.25, or 15 mg monthly **11.25 or 30 mg every 3 mo** **45 mg every 6 mo**	Intramuscular depot injection Subcutaneous injection
Triptorelin acetate	3.75 mg every 28 days 11.25 mg every 3 mo **22.5 mg every 6 mo**	Intramuscular depot injection
Histrelin acetate	**50-mg implant inserted every** **12 mo**—releases approximately 65 mcg daily for 12 mo	Subcutaneous implant

GnRH agonist dosing regimens.
Bolded is most common dosing in practice.
Dosing frequency may be adjusted based on success of pubertal suppression.
(From Bangalore Krishna K, Fuqua JS, Rogol AD, et al. Use of gonadotropin-releasing hormone analogs in children: update by an international consortium. *Horm Res Paediatr.* 2019;91(6):357-372.)

Hypogonadotropic Hypogonadism

Hypogonadotropic hypogonadism is hypogonadism that is the result of a central cause, with the lack of pubertal signaling from the pituitary gland or hypothalamus. This form of delayed puberty encompasses permanent deficiency of GnRH, LH, or FSH, as well as the temporary deficiencies caused by chronic illness, malnutrition, or constitutional delay of growth and puberty (see Table 6.3). In a female, a bone age of at least 10 years of age with low estradiol, LH, and FSH, measured by a laboratory with ultrasensitive assays, is consistent with hypogonadotropic hypogonadism. Conversely, if the spontaneous LH is at least 0.5 mIU/mL, central activation of puberty has begun.[19] With ultrasensitive assays for pubertal hormones, the traditional long LHRH stimulation test is not frequently needed. In the past, this test was carried out by administering GnRH or an LHRH analogue and obtaining estradiol, LH, and FSH at 0, 1, 2, 3, and 24 hours. It was often used to distinguish constitutional delay of growth and puberty from permanent hypogonadotropic hypogonadism.

Hypogonadotropic hypogonadism may be the result of congenital or acquired tumors, particularly craniopharyngioma, dysgerminoma, and prolactinoma. Genetic syndromes can occur leading to hypogonadotropic hypogonadism, including Kallmann syndrome, CHARGE syndrome, optic nerve hypoplasia, pituitary gene deficiencies, and many others. Kallmann syndrome has multiple genetic forms and is the most commonly recognized of the genetic etiologies of hypogonadotropic hypogonadism. It can be accompanied by anosmia or hyposmia, the hallmark of the disease. Also hearing impairment, cleft lip and palate, synkinesia, ectrodactyly, and hypodontia can be seen with Kallmann syndrome.

Hypergonadotropic Hypogonadism (Boxes 6.1 & 6.2)

Peripheral delayed puberty is also known as *hypergonadotropic hypogonadism,* and many causes of it exist (see Table 6.5). An elevated FSH is indicative of premature ovarian insufficiency (POI), and a workup is warrented. Causes may be genetic, including Turner syndrome, surgical, autoimmune ovarian insufficiency, infectious, infiltrative, or related to oncologic therapy. Once a diagnosis of POI is made, a karyotype of 30 to 50 cells is recommended.

Among the genetic causes of hypergonadotropic hypogonadism are Turner syndrome (affecting at least 1/2000 female infants), peripheral X_q deletion, galactosemia, and partial or complete gonadal dysgenesis. Surgical oophorectomy may occur with ovarian torsion, extensive malignant abdominal pathology, or in response to gonads containing a Y lineage or ovotestes. Infectious causes are uncommon but may occur with some viral infections such as mumps or coxsackie virus, tuberculosis, or severe pelvic inflammatory disease.[20] Infiltrative causes such as leukemia, sarcoidosis, or histiocytosis may occur. Chemotherapy and radiation both may lead to gonadal failure.

Eugonadotropic Delayed Puberty

Anatomic causes of delayed puberty will be accompanied by pubertal gonadotropin levels. Anatomic reasons for

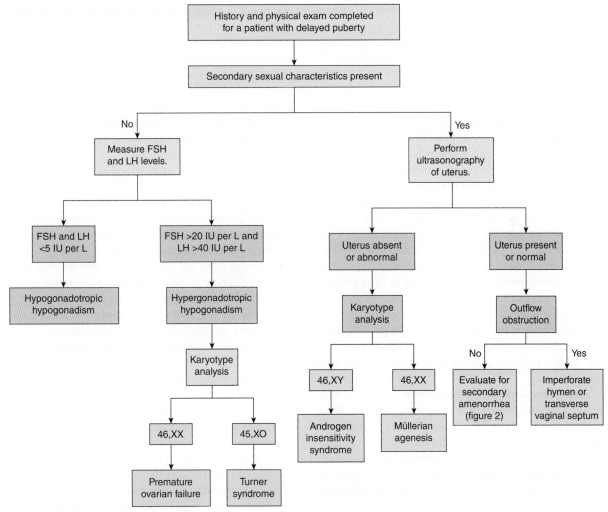

Fig. 6.2 Algorithm for the evaluation of precocious puberty. *FSH,* Follicle-stimulating hormone; *LH,* luteinizing hormone. (From https://www.aafp.org/pubs/afp/issues/2006/0415/p1374.html).

BOX 6.1 Hypogonadotropic Hypogonadism: Causes

Chronic illness
Malnutrition
Stress
Constitutional delay
Brain tumors (craniopharyngioma, dysgerminoma, prolactinoma)
Genetic syndromes (Kallmann, CHARGE)

BOX 6.2 Kallmann Syndrome: Clinical Features

Anosmia
Cleft lip/palate
Hearing impairment
Synkinesia, ectrodactyly, and hypodontiass

delayed menses may include imperforate hymen, vaginal septa, or other outflow obstructions such as müllerian agenesis (Mayer-Rokitansky-Kuster-Hauser syndrome [MRKH]) or androgen insensitivity syndrome (AIS).

Treatment of Delayed Puberty

Treatment for delayed puberty is determined by the etiology of the pubertal delay.[21,22]

Constitutional delay of growth and puberty: For children in which a full workup has been done and who have the diagnosis of constitutional delay of growth and puberty, as this is a transient condition, no specific treatment is required. However, considerations for catch-up in linear growth must be taken into account, as these patients frequently present initially for short stature and then have concerns about delayed puberty when they do not progress with secondary sexual characteristics at the same time as their peers.[23] Counseling regarding the expected course of constitutional growth and pubertal delay can alleviate parental and patient fears, including adult height goals and realistic expectations as well as appropriate timing for the child's pubertal development based on familial pubertal tempos.[23,24]

Hypogonadotropic hypogonadism: For those with delayed puberty caused by a chronic medical condition leading to a functional hypogonadotropic hypogonadism, the goal of treatment of the delayed puberty is to control their underlying health concerns, such as reducing inflammation from rheumatologic conditions or providing thyroid hormone replacement via levothyroxine for those with hypothyroidism.

For those with isolated GnRH deficiency at the level of the hypothalamus or with pituitary abnormality causing secondary hypogonadism, replacement of sex steroids will be first-line treatment. If the bone age has reached a pubertal age (10 years for girls), initiation of secondary sexual characteristics should begin with low-dose transdermal estrogen, with gradual increases in dose every 6 months. Progesterone should be added when the patient experiences spotting or at approximately 12 to 18 months after initiation of estrogen.

Transdermal estrogen is the preferred route of delivery for pubertal induction in females, as it bypasses the liver to reduce the first-pass effect, and transdermal estrogen has been shown in studies to provide greater support for bone mineralization.[25] Initial doses of transdermal estrogen will be lower than those used for re-

placement in adults to aid in linear growth and to attain optimal secondary sexual characteristics. Estradiol acts initially to stimulate growth via increased growth hormone secretion but ultimately closes epiphyses and ends growth at a bone age of 14 to 15 years. Using a 17-beta-estradiol transdermal patch, initial low doses can be increased over the course of 1 to 2 years up to adult levels of 0.5 or 1.0 mg/day for most women. Pelvic transabdominal ultrasound can be used to assess adequacy of the endometrial stripe.

Progestin therapy can be given as micronized progesterone 200 mg daily for 10 to 14 days (preferred) or medroxyprogesterone 5 to 10 mg daily for 10 to 14 days monthly. Longer courses of estradiol without monthly progesterone can also be contemplated, to have menses occur on a 2- to 3-month schedule.

Although there are many options and medical regimens to promote puberty, common options are noted next. Transdermal estrogen is preferable.

1. Initiate 0.3 mg conjugated estrogen or 0.5 mg micronized estradiol daily. After 6 months to a year, move to a monthly program with 0.625 mg conjugated estrogen or 1.0 mg estradiol and 5 to 10 mg medroxyprogesterone acetate for the first 10 to 14 days of each month.
2. Start transdermal estrogen patch at 6.5 to 12 mcg (matrix estrogen patches can be cut into one-half or one-quarter segments to start) and gradually increase the dose over 12 to 24 months. Once breast development has started and the transdermal estrogen has been increased to a 50-mcg patch, or menses spontaneously occurs, begin progesterone addback. A 10- to 14-day course of micronized progesterone or medroxyprogesterone given at the same time monthly is optimal for patients to achieve predictable cycles.

Hypergonadotropic hypogonadism: With primary gonadal failure or POI, estrogen replacement therapy can also begin at a bone age of 10 years, choosing estrogen therapy at gradually increasing doses to mimic spontaneous puberty's pattern, adding progesterone when spotting occurs or 12 to 18 months of estrogen therapy has been received. Some possible protocols are noted earlier.

Sometimes the etiology of hypogonadotropic hypogonadism (i.e., whether it is transient or permanent) is unclear. If planning a short trial of estrogen replacement, estradiol should be prescribed for 3 to 6 months, followed by repeat laboratory assessment of gonadotropins.

The goal of estradiol therapy, whether permanent or temporary, is to maintain serum concentrations of estradiol to support secondary sexual characteristics, bone health, and cardiovascular health. After a female patient has received estrogen replacement for 1.5 to 2 years or is having breakthrough bleeding, cyclic progesterone should be added for uterine protection to induce menstruation.

Of important note, for patients with a uterus but with hypogonadotropic or hypergonadotropic hypogonadism, fertility can be possible with reproductive endocrinology and high-risk obstetric involvement at the time of desired conception.

Eugonadotropic Causes

Children with an imperforate hymen or other surgical anomalies preventing menstruation may present with a history of other sexual characteristics without menarche, cyclic pelvic abdominal pain, abdominal mass, and a bulging of hymenal tissue without an apparent opening. Examination and referral to a pediatric adolescent gynecologist is warranted. Please see Chapter 37 obstructive mullerian anomalies.

KEY POINTS

- Precocious puberty can be central or the result of peripheral causes.
- Precocious puberty may be characterized by early timing and/or accelerated tempo.
- Delayed puberty may be the result of CNS causes, chronic disease, or end-organ abnormalities.
- Anatomic abnormalities may cause primary amenorrhea despite secondary sexual characteristics.
- Evaluation of puberty-related laboratory tests should be done using ultrasensitive assays to detect low hormonal levels of early puberty.

■ REVIEW QUESTIONS

1. A 14-year-old girl presents with a history of no thelarche but having had pubic hair since the age of 11 years. Her height is less than the third percentile. Weight is 50th percentile. She has a history of bicuspid aortic valve. Mother reports that she herself had menarche at age 12 years and is 68 inches tall. Examination reveals Tanner stage 1 breasts, a grade 2/6 systolic ejection click at the left upper sternal border, multiple pigmented nevi, and Tanner stage 3 pubic hair. Bone age is 12 years. What laboratory finding supports a diagnosis of gonadal failure in Turner syndrome?
   a. FSH 9 IU/L
   b. LH <0.1 IU/L
   c. FSH 95 IU/L
   d. Estradiol 96 pg/mL

2. A 14-year-old girl presents with a history of thelarche at age 10 years and pubic hair at age 11 years. She has had generalized pelvic pain every 21 to 35 days for the last 20 months. She has not had any spotting. She has Tanner stage 5 breasts and Tanner stage 5 pubic hair. What physical finding would explain all of this presentation?
   a. Webbed neck
   b. Delta-shaped ears
   c. Small mandible with triangular-shaped facies
   d. Imperforate hymen

3. A 4-year-old girl has presented to the office with early thelarche and menarche, as well as a history of laughing (gelastic) seizure episodes. Her primary care provider has obtained an MRI that demonstrated a hypothalamic hamartoma. Bone age is 9 years. What option is available to temporarily stop menarche and bone age advancement and allow more time for physical and emotional growth?
   a. Hormone replacement with transdermal estrogen and oral progesterone
   b. GHRH analogue given every 1, 3, or 6 months
   c. Aromatase inhibitor
   d. Intramuscular depot progesterone every 3 months

REFERENCES

1. Wei C, Davis N, Honour J, Crowne E. The investigation of children and adolescents with abnormalities of pubertal timing. *Ann Clin Biochem*. 2017;54(1):20-32. doi:10.1177/0004563216668378
2. Ioannidis JPA, Powe NR, Yancy C. Recalibrating the use of race in medical research. *JAMA*. 2021;325(7):623-624. doi:10.1001/jama.2021.0003
3. De Silva NK. Breast development and disorders in the adolescent female. *Best Pract Res Clin Obstet Gynaecol*. 2018;48:40-50. doi:10.1016/j.bpobgyn.2017.08.009
4. Kaplowitz P, Bloch C, Section on Endocrinology, American Academy of Pediatrics. Evaluation and referral of children with signs of early puberty. *Pediatrics*. 2016; 137(1). Epub 2015 Dec 14.

5. Emans SJ, Laufer MR. Precocious and delayed puberty. In: *Pediatric and Adolescent Gynecology*. 6th ed. Lippincott Williams and Wilkins; 2012:114-137.

6. Alvero, R, Schlaff WD. Normal and abnormal puberty. In: *Reproductive Endocrinology and Infertility: The Requisites and Obstetrics and Gynecology*. Mosby; 2007:33-48.

7. Oliveira Neto CP, Azulay RSS, Almeida AGFP, et al. Differences in puberty of girls before and during the COVID-19 pandemic. *Int J Environ Res Public Health*. 2022;19(8):4733. doi:10.3390/ijerph19084733

8. Latronico AC, Brito VN, Carel JC. Causes, diagnosis, and treatment of central precocious puberty. *Lancet Diabetes Endocrinol*. 2016;4(3):265-274.

9. Kaplowitz P, Bloch CA, the Section on Endocrinology, et al. Evaluation and referral of children with signs of early puberty. *Pediatrics*. 2016;137(1):e20153732.

10. Chen M, Eugster EA. Central precocious puberty: update on diagnosis and treatment. *Paediatr Drugs*. 2015;17:273.

11. Ng SM, Kumar Y, Cody D, Smith CS, Didi M. Cranial MRI scans are indicated in all girls with central precocious puberty. *Arch Dis Child*. 2003;88:414-418.

12. Kaplowitz PB. Do 6-8 year old girls with central precocious puberty need routine brain imaging? *Int J Pediatr Endocrinol*. 2016;2016:9. doi:10.1186/s13633-016-0027-5

13. Vargas Trujillo M, Dragnic S, Aldridge P, Klein KO. Importance of individualizing treatment decisions in girls with central precocious puberty when initiating treatment after age 7 years or continuing beyond a chronological age of 10 years or a bone age of 12 years. *J Pediatr Endocrinol Metab*. 2021;34:733.

14. Giabicani E, Lemaire P, Brauner R. Models for predicting the adult height and age at first menstruation of girls with idiopathic central precocious puberty. *PLoS One*. 2015;10(3):e0120588. doi:10.1371/journal.pone.0120588

15. Javaid MK, Boyce A, Appelman-Dijkstra N, et al. Best practice management guidelines for fibrous dysplasia/McCune-Albright syndrome: a consensus statement from the FD/MAS international consortium. *Orphanet J Rare Dis*. 2019;14(1):139. doi:10.1186/s13023-019-1102-9

16. Henley DV, Lipson N, Korach KS, Bloch CA. Prepubertal gynecomastia linked to lavender and tea tree oils. *N Engl J Med*. 2007;356(5):479-485. doi:10.1056/NEJMoa064725

17. Baranowski E, Hogler W. An unusual presentation of acquired hypothyroidism: The Van Wyk–Grumbach syndrome. *Eur J Endocrinol*. 2012;166(3):537-542.

18. Harrington J, Palmert MR. An approach to the patient with delayed puberty. *J Clin Endocrinol Metab*. 2022;107(6):1739-1750. doi:10.1210/clinem/dgac054

19. Bangalore Krishna K, Fuqua JS, Rogol AD, et al. Use of gonadotropin-releasing hormone analogs in children: update by an international consortium. *Horm Res Paediatr*. 2019;91:357.

20. Cui L, Sheng Y, Sun M, Hu J, Qin Y, Chen ZJ. Chronic pelvic inflammation diminished ovarian reserve as indicated by serum anti müllerian hormone. *PLoS One*. 2016;11(6):e0156130. doi:10.1371/journal.pone.0156130

21. Young J, Xu C, Papadakis GE, et al. Clinical management of congenital hypogonadotropic hypogonadism. *Endocr Rev*. 2019;40:669.

22. Carel JC, Léger J. Clinical practice. Precocious puberty. *N Engl J Med*. 2008;358(22):2366-2377. doi:10.1056/NEJMcp0800459

23. Raivio T, Falardeau J, Dwyer A, et al. Reversal of idiopathic hypogonadotropic hypogonadism. *N Engl J Med*. 2007;357(9):863-873. doi:10.1056/NEJMoa066494

24. Zhu J, Choa RE, Guo MH, et al. A shared genetic basis for self-limited delayed puberty and idiopathic hypogonadotropic hypogonadism. *J Clin Endocrinol Metab*. 2015;100:E646.

25. Gravholt CH, Andersen NH, Conway GS, et al. Clinical practice guidelines for the care of girls and women with Turner syndrome: proceedings from the 2016 Cincinnati International Turner Syndrome Meeting. *Eur J Endocrinol*. 2017;177(3):G1-G70. doi:10.1530/EJE-17-0430

26. Buyukgebiz A, Hindmarsh PC, Brook CGD. Treatment of constitutional delay of growth and puberty with oxandrolone compared with growth hormone. *Arch Dis Child*. 1990;65(4):448-449.

Prepubertal Vaginal Bleeding

Clara Tang, Laura Hollenbach, and Kathryn Stambough

INTRODUCTION

Prepubertal vaginal bleeding is the onset of vaginal bleeding that occurs before the normal age of puberty and may occur both with and without preceding pubertal milestones. Although many etiologies of prepubertal vaginal bleeding are benign and self-limiting, exclusion of malignancy and treatment for nonmalignant but persistent sources of bleeding may be indicated. Common causes of prepubertal vaginal bleeding include trauma, infection, anatomic/structural, hematologic, hormonal, and neoplastic etiologies,[1-4] which are further delineated in Table 7.1.

STRADDLE INJURY/GENITAL TRAUMA

Trauma accounts for up to 45% of cases of prepubertal vaginal bleeding,[4-7] which is typically accidental. Pediatric perineal injuries account for <1% of all pediatric injuries.[8] A straddle injury is compression of the soft tissues of the perineum between the bony pelvis and an object during trauma. This injury generally involves the mons pubis, clitoris, and labia, and in the absence of a penetrating mechanism of injury, rarely involves the hymen or vagina.

Typically patients will present with some history concerning for accidental trauma. In general, patients complain of pain and bright red vaginal bleeding. Associated symptoms may include pain with urination, an inability to void or defecate, pain with ambulation, and perineal edema and ecchymosis. Evaluation of genital trauma should include an examination of the external genitalia, and analgesia and/or procedural sedation can be considered for patient comfort and cooperation. Any concern for penetration may require a sedated examination with vaginoscopy. Providers should be aware of the possibility of abuse and try to rule this out of the differential diagnosis whenever genital trauma is noted (see Table 7.1). In the setting of a superficial straddle injury with well-visualized laceration borders, application of pressure and ice packs can reduce both bleeding and edema. Surgical repair may not be required, and conservative management with sitz baths, oral analgesia, and topical anesthetic may be adequate. Medical skin adhesive can be considered for small lacerations, particularly in settings in which avoidance of sedation is desired.

For injuries that do not achieve hemostasis with the aforementioned conservative management or for deep and/or extensive lacerations, surgical repair is required. Labial hematomas generally tamponade with application of pressure and ice, although incision and drainage may be required for expanding lesions. Consideration should be given to indwelling urethral catheterization in the setting of urinary retention and inability to void until edema and pain improve. Penetrating injuries may require vaginal packing (Fig. 7.1). Refer to Chapter 17 for further information on traumatic genital injury.

INFECTIOUS CAUSES OF PREPUBERTAL VAGINAL BLEEDING

Group A *beta-hemolytic streptococcus* is one of the more common pathogens isolated in the evaluation of vulvovaginitis and prepubertal vaginal bleeding.[9] Concurrent pharyngeal colonization occurs in up to 95% of individuals.[10] Other potential infectious etiologies for prepubertal vaginal bleeding include *Shigella, Enterobius vermicularis,* and vaginal leeches.[11-13] Clinicians should be suspicious of this etiology in the face of a recent

TABLE 7.1   Causes of Prepubertal Vaginal Bleeding

PREPUBERTAL VAGINAL BLEEDING			
Etiology	**Evaluation**	**Differential Diagnosis**	**Treatment**
Straddle injury/genital trauma	History, physical examination (may include sedated vaginoscopy)	Nonaccidental trauma, failure of midline fusion (perineal groove)	Application of pressure and ice, surgical repair, urethral catheterization, pain control
Urethral prolapse	History, physical examination (may include sedated vaginoscopy ± cystoscopy)	Sarcoma botryoides, Skene duct cyst, urethral polyp or caruncle, prolapsed ureterocele, uterine prolapse	Sitz baths, treatment of constipation, topical estrogen therapy, rarely surgical resection
Vaginal foreign body	History, physical examination (may include sedated vaginoscopy or in-office vaginal irrigation); rarely plain film, pelvic sonography, or MRI	Vulvovaginitis, müllerian papilloma, vaginal or cervical polyp, malignant vaginal tumor	Vaginoscopy with removal of vaginal foreign body
Sarcoma botryoides	History, physical examination, biopsy, imaging (MRI)	Germ cell tumor, carcinoma, müllerian papilloma, urethral polyp or caruncle, urethral prolapse, prolapsed ureterocele, Skene duct cyst, uterine prolapse, adenomyosis, extragonadal yolk sac tumor	Surgical resection, chemotherapy
Hemangioma	History, physical examination	Infantile hemangioma, capillary hemangioma, pyogenic granuloma, capillary malformation, macrocystic lymphatic malformation, venous malformation, rhabdomyosarcoma, cutaneous metastatic disease	Observation, topical and/or oral beta-blocker, corticosteroid therapy, laser therapy, surgical excision
Precocious puberty	History, physical examination, laboratory evaluation, imaging (x-ray bone age, pelvic sonography, MRI brain), GnRH stimulation test	Premature thelarche, premature adrenarche, isolated premature menarche, poorly controlled congenital adrenal hyperplasia, congenital hypothyroidism, ovarian or adrenal tumors	Central precocious puberty: GnRH analogue treatment
Vulvovaginitis	History, physical examination	Vaginal foreign body, vulvar dermatoses, müllerian papilloma, sarcoma botryoides	Improved vulvovaginal hygiene, use of emollients, antibiotics

GnRH, Gonadotropin-releasing hormone; *MRI,* magnetic resonance imaging.

infection. Evaluation is via vaginal culture with antibiotic treatment geared toward the offending organism.

URETHRAL PROLAPSE

Urethral prolapse has been reported in 1 in 3000 patients.[14,15] Although often seen in prepubertal females, it can also present in postmenopausal women or hypoestrogen states. Urethral prolapse is more common in patients of African descent.[14,15]

Urethral prolapse is prolapse of the redundant urethral mucosa through the meatus. Although the etiology for urethral prolapse is likely multifactorial, episodic increases in intraabdominal pressure in conditions like constipation and chronic cough are likely contributory. The distal female urethra has high concentrations of estrogen receptors and therefore may be more susceptible to prolapse in estrogen deficiency.[16]

Although urethral prolapse may be incidentally noted and otherwise asymptomatic, many patients typically

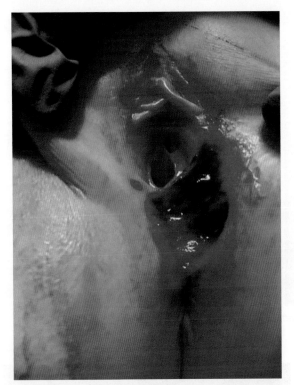

Fig. 7.1 Perineal straddle injury, unrepaired.

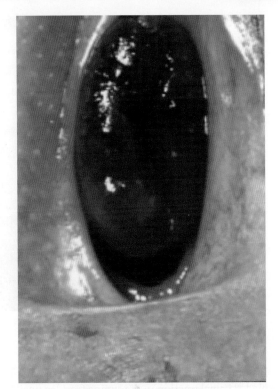

Fig. 7.2 Urethral prolapse.

present with painless, bright red vaginal bleeding. Other symptoms may include concurrent constipation. A history should include evaluating for the presence of comorbid conditions that may increase intraabdominal pressure and assess for any other sources of prepubertal vaginal, including the presence of any secondary sexual characteristics.

Examination of the external genitalia is necessary for a diagnosis of urethral prolapse. A protruding donut-shaped mass is typically noted, and care should be taken to evaluate for a distinctly separate hymen and distal vagina. If the origin of the mass is not clear, sedated examination can be considered with cystoscopy and/or vaginoscopy for further clarification. Observation during urination or placement of a small urethral catheter can also be employed to verify urethral origin.

The differential diagnosis of a protruding interlabial mass includes urethral prolapse and sarcoma botryoides. Less common causes include Skene duct cyst, urethral polyp, prolapsed ureterocele, and uterine prolapse.

Conservative management of urethral prolapse includes sitz baths and addressing any underlying cause of increased intraabdominal pressure such as constipation. Application of topical estrogen is usually effective at treatment of the prolapse and resolution in symptoms. Surgical resection of the urethral mucosal edges is rarely needed (Fig. 7.2).[17]

VAGINAL FOREIGN BODY

The presence of a vaginal foreign body should be considered in the setting of persistent vaginal discharge with or without vaginal bleeding. The incidence of a vaginal foreign body has been reported in up to 10% of patients referred to a tertiary care center for persistent blood discharge and up to 25% of patients who required a procedure for evaluation.[18,19]

Patients with a vaginal foreign body typically present with chronic vaginal discharge, which may be bloody. Perineal irritation caused by associated vulvovaginitis may be present. A history assessing for any prior placement of a foreign body in a body orifice should be pursued along with the duration of bloody vaginal discharge, exposure to topical irritants, and review of hygiene techniques.

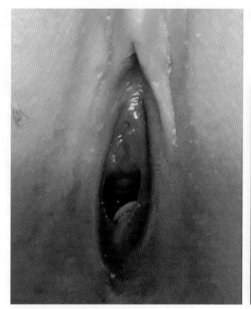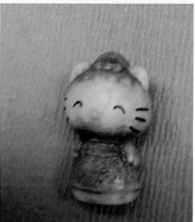

Fig. 7.3 Distal vagina with vaginal foreign body *(left)*. Vaginal foreign body after removal *(right)*.

Examination of the external genitalia should be performed.[20] Labial traction in the supine frog-leg position or knee-chest position may facilitate visualization of the foreign body in the distal vagina (Fig. 7.3) (refer to Chapter 4 for further information on examination of the prepubertal patient). A high index of suspicion in many cases will necessitate a sedated examination with vaginoscopy and removal of a possible foreign body.[18,21] Imaging studies may be limited in evaluating for the presence of a vaginal foreign body, but pelvic sonography,[22] pelvic x-ray,[23] or magnetic resonance imaging[24] may be considered. The differential diagnosis of bloody vaginal discharge includes vaginal foreign body, vulvovaginitis, müllerian papilloma, vaginal or cervical polyp, or malignant vaginal tumor. One of the most common vaginal foreign bodies is toilet paper, which typically involves the unintentional migration of toilet paper into the more proximal vagina with toileting. Other vaginal foreign bodies can similarly be unintentional (i.e., blade of grass), but some vaginal foreign bodies are intentionally placed in the vagina. Chronic inflammation of the vaginal mucosa caused by the presence of the foreign object results in symptoms. In severe cases, chronic pressure to the vaginal walls can result in fistula formation and stenosis. Vaginoscopy with removal of the vaginal foreign body remains the

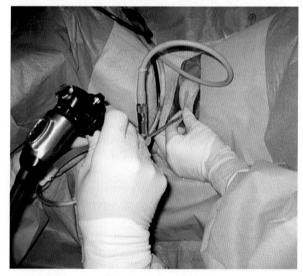

Fig. 7.4 Vaginoscopy.

mainstay of treatment (Fig. 7.4). This should be considered in all patients with bloody discharge and in patients with chronic discharge recalcitrant to improved perineal hygiene and medical management. Vaginal irrigation, which can be performed with vaginal placement of a pediatric Foley catheter and instillation of a reasonable amount (200 cc) of sterile saline within the vagina using moderate pressure,[18] can also be employed in appropriate patients.

SARCOMA BOTRYOIDES (OR BOTRYOID RHABDOMYOSARCOMA)

Malignancy remains a rare but important source of bleeding in the prepubertal female.[25,26] Rhabdomyosarcoma is the most common soft tissue tumor in children. It is also the most common malignancy of the pediatric female genital tract but accounts for less than 4% of all pediatric rhabdomyosarcomas. The majority of cases occur in children younger than 5 years of age.

The etiology of rhabdomyosarcoma is not well known, and most cases appear to be sporadic. *DICER1* mutations have been reported.[27] These highly malignant tumors are believed to arise from the developing skeletal muscle cells, or myoblasts. The botryoid subtype of rhabdomyosarcoma develops its typical "grapelike" presentation caused by proliferation of underlying tumor cells elevating the epithelium of hollow organs, creating polypoid masses.[26]

"Botryoides" is derived from thc Greek word "botrys," or "grapes," which describes the gross appearance of these tumors. Patients tend to present with painless vaginal bleeding and/or bloody discharge with a grapelike mass protruding from the vagina (Fig. 7.5). In infants and young children, these tumors are most commonly found in the vagina. In reproductive-aged women, the cervix is the most common site. Cross-striated rhabdomyoblasts ("strap cells") are the characteristic histopathologic finding.[25]

The differential diagnosis of a protruding vaginal mass has previously been addressed and includes genital tract malignancies such as sarcoma botryoides, germ cell (endodermal sinus) tumor, or carcinoma. Benign causes include müllerian papilloma, urethral polyp, urethral prolapse, prolapsed ureterocele, Skene duct cyst, or uterine prolapse.[28] Other etiologies for a pelvic mass that presents with prepubertal vaginal bleeding include extragonadal yolk sac tumors and benign uterine neoplasm (adenomyosis).[29,30]

Historically, the mainstay of treatment has been radical surgery, such as pelvic exenteration. However, this has been increasingly replaced with chemotherapy, more conservative and fertility-sparing surgical procedures, and radiation therapy. The basis of treatment has largely been based on the Intergroup Rhabdomyosarcoma

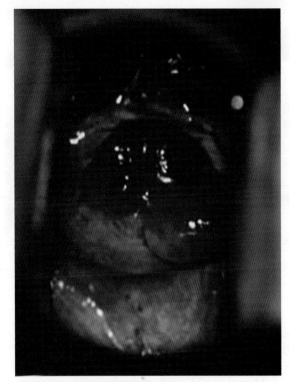

Fig. 7.5 Sarcoma botryoides.

Study Group (ISRG) trial results.[25] First-line treatment now consists of combination chemotherapy with reservation of surgical resection for persistent or local disease. Radiotherapy is avoided whenever possible because of its toxicity and long-term sequalae.[26] For patients with locoregional tumors, the estimated 5-year survival rate is 87%; in patients aged 1 to 9, the estimated 5-year survival is 98%.[31]

HEMANGIOMA

Infantile hemangioma (IH) is the most common benign vascular anomaly and occurs in 5% of the population.[32] They most commonly occur children.[33] Although usually sporadic, risk factors for IH include prematurity, advanced maternal age, placental abnormalities, female gender, and low birth weight.[34] Capillary hemangioma (CH) is less common than IH and typically presents at birth.

IH is caused by aberrant proliferation of endothelial cells and angiogenesis.[32] IH may be subtle or absent at birth and generally grows fastest during the first 6 months of life. IH typically spontaneously involutes in early childhood.[33]

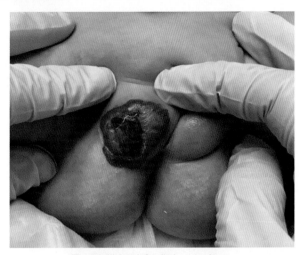

Fig. 7.6 Vulvar infantile hemangioma.

Patients with a hemangioma may present with vaginal bleeding in the setting of ulceration. An examination of the external genitalia typically demonstrates a well-defined vascular lesion (Fig. 7.6). A thorough history should explore the onset of the lesion(s), progression over time, ulceration, bleeding, and location. Hemangiomas can generally be diagnosed with examination alone, and routine imaging is often not indicated. The presence of five or more IHs should prompt abdominal imaging with ultrasound to assess for the concurrent presence of hepatic hemangioma.[35]

The differential diagnosis of a cutaneous vascular lesion includes both IH and CH. Other possible etiologies include pyogenic granuloma, capillary malformation, macrocystic lymphatic malformation, venous malformation, rhabdomyosarcoma, and cutaneous metastatic disease.

A majority of hemangiomas involute without the need for intervention. Almost 80% of hemangiomas achieve their final size by 3 months of age, and observation is usually the only indicated treatment for most lesions.

Treatment is indicated for life-threatening IH, which may cause cardiac or respiratory failure based on location and lesions that may result in anatomic distortion or functional risk such as loss of vision or ulceration.[36] Beta-blockade is the mainstay of treatment for IH, and over 90% of IH lesions demonstrate a decrease in size and color after initiation. Multimodal treatment may be indicated and typically includes corticosteroid therapy, laser therapy, and surgical excision.[33]

PRECOCIOUS PUBERTY

Concerns regarding precocious puberty are common, and most concerns are the result of nonpathologic causes.[37]

Precocious puberty generally presents with the onset of the development of secondary sexual characteristics before the normal age of puberty. A thorough history should evaluate for the timing of the onset of secondary sexual characteristic development and the tempo of maturation. An evaluation for exogenous hormone exposure and a thorough birth and medical history should be obtained. Examination should not only include an examination of the external genitalia to evaluate for a source of vaginal bleeding but also Tanner staging to evaluate for the presence and degree of secondary sexual characteristic development. Hormonal withdrawal caused by the mini-puberty of infancy should be considered in the setting of vaginal bleeding in the postnatal period. The presence of vaginal bleeding, growth acceleration, advancement of bone age, and clitoromegaly portend pathologic rather than benign causes of early pubertal development and necessitate further evaluation. Evaluation should include laboratory testing, assessment for skeletal maturation, and possibly a gonadotropin-releasing hormone (GnRH) stimulation test to confirm central precocious puberty (CPP). Imaging may also be required to evaluate for noncentral sources of estrogen production. See Chapter 6 for further information on abnormal puberty.

The differential diagnosis for CPP or peripheral precocious puberty (PPP) includes premature thelarche, premature adrenarche, and in the presence of prepubertal vaginal bleeding, premature menarche.[38,39] Isolated premature vaginal bleeding can occur in the absence of other pubertal milestones and may be cyclic, several days in duration, and without uterine and vaginal pathology.[40] Isolated premature menarche is generally self-limited.[39]

The management of CPP includes the use of long-acting GnRH analogue therapy for suppression of the hypothalamic-pituitary-gonadal (HPG) axis. Therapy is generally continued until the normal age of pubertal onset.

Treatment of PPP is dependent on the etiology. McCune-Albright syndrome accounts for up to 85% of PPP in females, and treatment may include the use of aromatase inhibitors, selective estrogen receptor modulators, or in cases of central escape to CPP, GnRH analogue therapy.[33] Autonomous ovarian cysts generally resolve without intervention, and surgical management with cystectomy is typically not required.[38] Poorly controlled congenital adrenal hyperplasia is improved with adherence to mineralocorticoid replacement and/or GnRH analogue therapy. Poorly controlled hypothyroidism can present with precocious puberty and generally improves with thyroid replacement. Ovarian or adrenal tumors causing PPP are treated with surgical resection.

Other causes of prepubertal vaginal bleeding are addressed elsewhere in this publication and include vulvovaginitis, vulvar ulcerations, and vulvar dermatoses. As previously mentioned, Group A *beta-hemolytic streptococcus* is one of the more common pathogens isolated in the evaluation of vulvovaginitis and prepubertal vaginal bleeding, and other potential infectious etiologies for prepubertal vaginal bleeding include *Shigella, E. vermicularis*, and vaginal leeches.[41-43] Also as mentioned, hormonal withdrawal caused by the mini-puberty of infancy should be considered in the setting of vaginal bleeding in the postnatal period.

KEY POINTS

- Prepubertal vaginal bleeding is often the result of a benign and self-limited process, but treatment for nonmalignant but persistent causes and exclusion of malignancy may be needed.
- A thorough history and physical examination should be considered first-line for evaluation. Supine frog-leg and prone knee-chest position with downward labial traction is generally well tolerated and sufficient for evaluation.
- Vaginoscopy can be considered if more complete evaluation is indicated. Consideration can be given for in-office vaginal irrigation, particularly in cases where a foreign body can be visualized in the distal vagina with labial traction.

REVIEW QUESTIONS

1. A common comorbidity associated with urethral prolapse is:
   a. Precocious puberty
   b. Allergic rhinitis
   c. Constipation
   d. Uterine prolapse

2. Risk factors for infantile hemangiomas include all of the following except:
   a. Prematurity
   b. Female gender
   c. Placental abnormalities
   d. Large for gestational age

3. Treatment of central precocious puberty includes:
   a. Gonadotropin-releasing hormone analogue
   b. Surgical cystectomy
   c. Aromatase inhibitor
   d. Selective estrogen receptor modulator

REFERENCES

1. Zhang J, Zhang B, Su Y, et al. Prepubertal vaginal bleeding: an inpatient series from a single center in Fujian China. *J Pediatr Adolesc Gynecol.* 2020;33(2):120-124. doi:10.1016/j.jpag.2019.11.009
2. Dwiggins M, Gomez-Lobo V. Current review of prepubertal vaginal bleeding. *Curr Opin Obstet Gynecol.* 2017;29(5):322-327. doi:10.1097/GCO.0000000000000398
3. Howell JO, Flowers D. Prepubertal vaginal bleeding: etiology, diagnostic approach, and management. *Obstet Gynecol Surv.* 2016;71(4):231-242. doi:10.1097/OGX.0000000000000290
4. Soderstrom HF, Carlsson A, Borjesson A, et al. Vaginal bleeding in prepubertal girls: etiology and clinical management. *J Pediatr Adolesc Gynecol.* 2016;29(3):280-285. doi:10.1016/j.jpag.2015.10.017
5. Hill NC, Oppenheimer LW, Motron KE. The etiology of vaginal bleeding in children. A 20-year review. *Br J Obstet Gynaecol.* 1989;96(4):467-470. doi:10.1111/j.1471-0528.1989.tb02424.x
6. Imai A, Horibe S, Tamaya T. Genital bleeding in premenarcheal children. *Int J Gynaecol Obstet.* 1995;49(1):41-45. doi:10.1016/0020-7292(94)02305-i
7. Heller ME, Savage MO, Dewhurst J. Vaginal bleeding in childhood: a review of 51 patients. *Br J Obstet Gynaecol.* 1978;85(10):721-725. doi:10.1111/j.1471-0528.1978.tb15590.x
8. Casey JT, Bjurlin MA, Cheng EY. Pediatric genital injury: an analysis of the National Electronic Injury Surveillance Survey. *Urology.* 2013;82(5):1125-1131. doi:10.1016/j.urology.2013.05.042
9. Stricker T, Navratil F, Sennhauser FH. Vulvovaginitis in prepubertal girls. *Arch Dis Child.* 2003;88(4):324-336. doi:10.1136/adc.88.4.324
10. Clegg HW, Giftos PM, Anderson WE, et al. Clinical perineal streptococcal infection in children: epidemiological

features, low symptomatic recurrence rate after treatment, and risk factors for recurrence. *J Pediatr.* 2015;167(3): 687-963.e1-e2. doi:10.1016/j.jpeds.2015.05.034

11. Gershman ML, Simms-Cendan J. Vaginal bleeding in prepubertal females: a case of Shigella vaginitis and review of literature. *BMJ Case Rep.* 2022;15(8):e251303. doi:10.1136/bcr-2022-251303

12. Smolyakov R, Talalay B, Yanai-Inbar I, et al. Enterobius vermicularis infection of female genital tract: a report of three cases and review of the literature. *Eur J Obstet Gynecol Reprod Biol.* 2003;107(2):220-222. doi:10.1016/s0301-2115(03)00003-4

13. Majidi S, Hiradfar M, Shojaian R, et al. Pediatric vaginal leech infestation with severe bleeding: a case report and review article. *J Pediatr Adolesc Gynecol.* 2019;32(4): 420-424. doi:10.1016/j.jpag.2019.03.007

14. Holbrook C, Misra D. Surgical management of urethral prolapse in girls: 13 years' experience. *BJU Int.* 2012;110(1): 132-134. doi:10.1111/j.1464-410X.2011.10752.x

15. Wei Y, Wu S, Lin T, et al. Diagnosis and treatment of urethral prolapse in children: 16 years' experience with 89 Chinese girls. *Arab J Urol.* 2017;15(3):248-253. doi:10.1016/j.aju.2017.03.004

16. McCaskill A, Inabinet CF, Tomlin K, et al. Prepubertal genital bleeding: examination and differential diagnosis in pediatric female patients. *J Emerg Med.* 2018;55(4):e97-e100. doi:10.1016/j.jemermed.2018.07.011

17. Valerie E, Gilchrist BF, Frischer J, et al. Diagnosis and treatment of urethral prolapse in children. *Pediatr Urol.* 1999;54(6):1082-1084. doi:10.1016/S0090-4295(99)00311-8

18. Smith YR, Berman DR, Quint EH. Premenarchal vaginal discharge: findings of procedures to rule out foreign bodies. *J Pediatr Adolesc Gynecol.* 2002;15(4):227-230. doi:10.1016/s1083-3188(02)00160-2

19. Capraro VJ. Vulvovaginitis and other local lesions of the vulva. *Clin Obstet Gynecol.* 1974;1(3):533-551.

20. Merritt DF. Evaluation of vaginal bleeding in the preadolescent child. *Semin Pediatr Sure.* 1998;7(1):35-42. doi:10.1016/s1055-8586(98)70004-6

21. Ekinci S, Karnak Y, Tanyel FC, et al. Prepubertal vaginal discharge: vaginoscopy to rule out foreign body. *Turk J Pediatr.* 2016;58(2):168-171. doi:10.24952/turkjped.2016.02.007

22. Yang X, Sun L, Ye J, et al. Ultrasonography in detection of vaginal foreign bodies in girls: a retrospective study. *J Pediatr Adolesc Gynecol.* 2017;30(6):620-625. doi:10.1016/j.jpag.2017.06.008

23. Wittich AC, Murray JE. Intravaginal foreign body of long duration: a case report. *Am J Obstet Gynecol.* 1993;169(1):211-212. doi:10.1016/0002-9378(93)90169-J

24. Kihara M, Sato N, Kimura H, et al. Magnetic resonance imaging in the evaluation of vaginal foreign bodies in a young girl. *Arch Gynecol Obstet.* 2001;265:221-222. doi:10.1007/s00404000016

25. Berek J, Hacker N. Chapter 14: vaginal cancer. In: Berek & Hacker's Gynecologic Oncology. Wolters Kluwer; 2015.

26. Fernandez-Pineda I, Spont SL, Parida L, et al. Vaginal tumor in childhood: the experience of St. Jude Children's Research Hospital. *J Pediatr Surg.* 2011;46(11):2071-2075.

27. Dural O, Kebudi R, Yavuz E, et al. DICER1-related embryonal rhabdomyosarcoma of the uterine corpus in a prepubertal girl. *J Pediatr Adolesc Gynecol.* 2020;33(2):173-176. doi:10.1016/j.jpag.2019.12.002

28. McQuillan SK, Grover SR, Pyman J, et al. Literature review of benign mullerian papilloma contrasted with vaginal rhabdomyosarcoma. *J Pediatr Adolesc Gynecol.* 2016;29(4):333-337. doi:10.1016/j.jpag.2015.02.114

29. Yin M, Wang T, Yang JX. Yolk sac tumor of the uterus in a 2-year-old girl: a case report and literature review. *J Pediatr Adolesc Gynecol.* 2022;35(2):177-181. doi:10.1016/j.jpag.2021.09.005

30. Khaja A, Shim JY, Laufer MR. Benign uterine neoplasm as a cause of prepubertal bleeding. *J Pediatr Adolesc Gynecol.* 2022;35(1):88-90. doi:10.1016/j.jpag.2021.06.010

31. Arndt CA, Donaldson SS, Anderson JR, et al. What constitutes optimal therapy for patients with rhabdomyosarcoma of the female genital tract? *Cancer.* 2001;91(12): 2454-2468.

32. Dickison P, Christou E, Wargon O. A prospective study of infantile hemangioma with a focus on incidence and risk factors. *Pediatr Dermatol.* 2011;28(6):663-669. doi:10.1111/j.1525-1470.2011.01568.x

33. DeHart A, Richter G. Hemangioma: recent advances. *F1000Res.* 2019;18(8):F1000 Faculty Rev-1926. doi:10.12688/f1000research.20152.1

34. Castren E, Salminen P, Vikkula M, et al. Inheritance patterns of infantile hemangioma. *Pediatrics.* 2016;138(5):e20161623. doi:10.1542.peds.2016-1623

35. Horri KA, Drolet BA, Frieden IJ, et al. Prospective study of the frequency of hepatic hemangiomas in infants with multiple cutaneous infantile hemangiomas. *Pediatr Dermatol.* 2011;28(3):245-253. doi:10.1111/j.1525-1470.2011.01420.x

36. Leaute-Labreze C, Harper JI, Hoeger PH. Infantile haemangioma. *Lancet.* 2017;390(10089):85-89. doi:10.1016/S0140-6736(16)00645-0

37. Eugster EA. Update on precocious puberty in girls. *J Pediatr Adolesc Gynecol.* 2019;32(5):455-459. doi:10.1016/j.jpag.2019.05.011

38. Nella A, Kaplowitz PB, Ramnitz MS, et al. Benign vaginal bleeding in 24 prepubertal patients: clinical, biochemical

and imaging features. *J Pediatr Endocrinol Metab.* 2014;27(9-10):821-825. doi:10.1515/jpem-2013-0415

39. Ejaz S, Lane A, Wilson T. Outcome of isolated premature menarche: a retrospective and follow-up study. *Horm Res Paediatr.* 2015;84(4):217-222. doi:10.1159/000435882

40. Merckx M, Weyers S, Santegoeds R, et al. Menstrual-like vaginal bleeding in prepubertal girls: an unexplained condition. *Facts Views Vis Obgyn.* 2011;3(4):267-270.

41. Herman-Giddens ME. Recent data on pubertal milestones in United States children: the secular trend toward earlier development. *Int J Androl.* 2006;29(1):241-246. doi:10.1111/j.1365-2605.00575.x

42. Cantas-Orsdemir S, Garb JL, Allen HF. Prevalence of cranial MRI findings in girls with central precocious puberty: a systemic review and meta-analysis. *J Pediatr Endocrinol Metab.* 2018;31(7):701-710. doi:10.1515/jpem-2018-0052

43. Chae HS, Rheu CH. Precocious pseudo puberty due to an autonomous ovarian follicular cyst: case report with a review of literatures. *BMC Res Notes.* 2013;6:319. doi:10.1186/1756-0500-6-319

8

The Normal Menstrual Cycle

Megan E. Harrison, Shelby H. Davies, and Andrew Lupo

INTRODUCTION

The menstrual period is a key marker of health. In fact, many professional medical organizations recommend that the menstrual cycle be considered a vital sign, as timely identification of abnormal menstrual patterns can assist in early identification of potential health issues. Treating menses as a vital sign also highlights its importance and significance to patients, caregivers, and other health care providers.[1-3]

Despite the fact that 1.8 billion people across the world menstruate each month,[4] stigma around periods still exists. Gender inequality, discriminatory social norms, cultural taboos, poverty, and lack of basic services like toilets and menstrual products can cause menstrual health and hygiene needs to go unmet.[4] Practitioners play an important role in reducing stigma and increasing sexual and reproductive health education by providing holistic care when it comes to assessing menstrual health. This chapter will review what is considered a "normal" menstrual cycle in adolescence and will share practical tips on how to take a complete, holistic menstrual history. Situations considered out of the range of normal will also be discussed.

PHYSIOLOGY

Fig. 8.1 describes the normal physiology of the menstrual cycle.

WHAT'S "NORMAL" FOR ADOLESCENTS?

Menarche

The age of menarche varies globally. Many variables have been identified as potential contributors to the timing of

menarche; for example, higher weight/body mass index (BMI), more robust nutritional status, and higher socioeconomic status have all been linked with earlier onset of menarche around the world.[7] Physical activity, sleep quality, and emotional stressors may also be important contributors to pubertal timing.[8] Onset of both puberty and menarche appears to occur later in lower-income countries (LICs), likely secondary to suboptimal nutritional status.[1,2,9] The median age of menarche across well-nourished individuals in high-income countries (HICs) has been relatively stable for several decades, at 12.4 years of age (Table 8.1).[9] Interestingly, new data show a possible trend to a lower median age of menarche of 11.9 years of age.[10] Studies have also shown that Black adolescents begin puberty and menstruation earlier than their White peers, whereas Latinx youth have menarche between the two.[9] The effect of structural racism on age of menarche has not been well researched and should be prioritized.[11,12]

Cycle Length

Menstrual periods are often irregular in adolescents in the years after menarche. The positive stimulatory feedback mechanism of estrogen on luteinizing hormone (LH) does not mature until 2 to 5 years after menarche, which can lead to irregular periods. In general, cycles become more regular after 2 to 3 years post menarche with 50% to 80% of the cycles being anovulatory and irregular during the first 2 years after menarche.[13] That said, 10% to 20% of cycles remain anovulatory up to 5 years after menarche. A menstrual cycle length between 21 and 45 days (mean 32 days) during adolescence is considered normal (see Table 8.1). The length of the interval between the onset of menses and the establishment of ovulatory cycles is associated with the age of menarche; those who are younger at

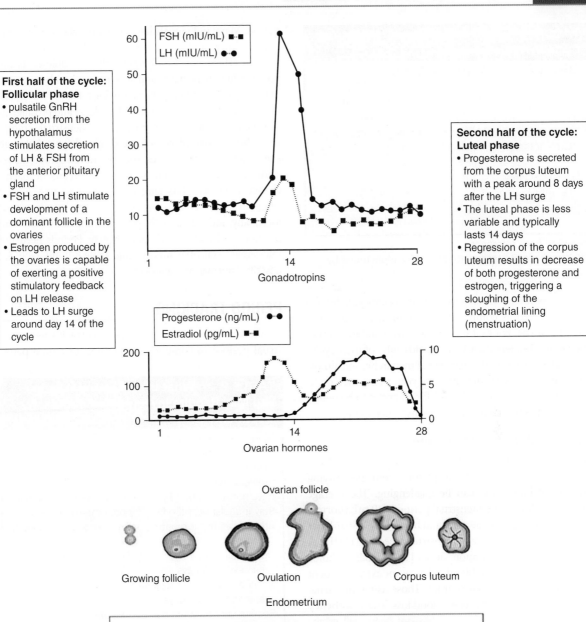

First half of the cycle: Follicular phase
- pulsatile GnRH secretion from the hypothalamus stimulates secretion of LH & FSH from the anterior pituitary gland
- FSH and LH stimulate development of a dominant follicle in the ovaries
- Estrogen produced by the ovaries is capable of exerting a positive stimulatory feedback on LH release
- Leads to LH surge around day 14 of the cycle

Second half of the cycle: Luteal phase
- Progesterone is secreted from the corpus luteum with a peak around 8 days after the LH surge
- The luteal phase is less variable and typically lasts 14 days
- Regression of the corpus luteum results in decrease of both progesterone and estrogen, triggering a sloughing of the endometrial lining (menstruation)

FSH (mIU/mL) ■··■
LH (mIU/mL) ●··●

Gonadotropins

Progesterone (ng/mL) ●··●
Estradiol (pg/mL) ■··■

Ovarian hormones

Ovarian follicle

Growing follicle   Ovulation   Corpus luteum

Endometrium

| 1 | 2 | 3 | 4 | 5 | 6 | 7 | 8 | 9 | 10 | 11 | 12 | 13 | 14 | 15 | 16 | 17 | 18 | 19 | 20 | 21 | 22 | 23 | 24 | 25 | 26 | 27 | 28 | 29 |

Days

Fig. 8.1 Physiology of the normal menstrual cycle.[5,6]

TABLE 8.1 What's a "Normal" Menstrual Cycle in Adolescents?[a]	
Menarche	Median age 12–12.5 y Occurs between 10 and 15 y[b] Occurs typically 2–3 y after thelarche/breast bud development
Menstrual Cycle Interval	Mean approximately 32 days in first gynecologic year Typically 21–45 days
Menstrual Flow Length/Volume	<7 days' duration 3–6 pads/tampons per day May have clots less than the size of a quarter

[a]Adapted from references 1, 2, 17.
[b]10% menstruate by age 10–11; >95% menstruate by age 15.[9,10]

the time of menarche achieve regular ovulatory cycles in a shorter period as compared with those who experience later menarche. For example, in those who undergo earlier menarche (i.e., less than 12 years old), 50% of their cycles are ovulatory within the first year of menarche, and almost all of their cycles are ovulatory by year 5 post menarche, whereas it can take over 5 years for all cycles to be ovulatory in individuals who had later-onset menarche.[13]

Menstrual Blood Flow/Volume

Individuals experience different amounts of vaginal bleeding during their menstrual periods, and quantifying volume of blood loss can be challenging. The average blood loss during the menstrual period is 40 mL (normal range between 25 and 69 mL), and blood loss >80 mL per period is considered heavy menstrual bleeding (HMB). A regular disposable tampon or pad fully soaked holds approximately 5 mL of blood, whereas an extraabsorbent tampon/pad holds about 10 mL.[14] Those using menstrual cups can more easily measure blood loss. The absorbency of reusable period underwear has not been well established. It is important to note that HMB at menarche can be the presenting sign for teens with inherited bleeding disorders; coagulopathies are found in 20% of patients presenting with HMB.[15–17] Heavy bleeding can also seriously affect an adolescent's quality of life from a physical, social, emotional, and material point of view.[6,15,17]

Other Symptoms

It is considered "normal" for individuals to have some associated symptoms sometimes before or during their period. Many individuals have dysmenorrhea—recurrent, crampy lower abdominal/pelvic pain that occurs during menses.[6] The majority of dysmenorrhea in adolescents and young adults is primary and is associated with a normal ovulatory cycle and no pelvic pathology. Primary dysmenorrhea is mitigated by prostaglandin release and prostaglandin-mediated uterine contractions.[13] Menstrual cramps may also be affected by volume of blood flow. Although everyone's experience varies, some common symptoms reported are lower back pain, bloating, sore breasts, headache, changes in bowel habits, fatigue, and mood swings.[6] Even if symptoms reported are considered "normal" or nonpathologic, any individual with period complaints needs to be supported and treated appropriately. Periods need not interfere in someone's functioning. Table 8.1 and Table 8.2 describe "normal" vs. "abnormal."

PERIOD TRACKING

Adolescents should be encouraged to track their menstrual periods in some form, whether it be on a paper

TABLE 8.2 What Is an Abnormal Period and May Require Investigation and/or Treatment?[a]
Menstrual periods that: Have not started within 3 y of thelarche Have not started by 13 y of age with lack of breast development Have not started by 15 y of age with breast development Stay irregular past the first 3 y post menarche Are regular, occur monthly, and then become markedly irregular Occur more often than every 21 days or less often than every 45 days Occur every 3 mo or less often Last longer than 7 days Require very frequent pad/tampon/product changes (bleeding through products in <2 h or have frequent leaking) Are so painful they lead to missed school or participation in activities Are associated with severe mental health concerns, like gender dysphoria, depression, and suicidal ideation Are associated with severe physical symptoms, like migraines/headaches, vomiting, syncope, shortness of breath, palpitations, and dizziness

[a]Adapted from references 1, 15.

calendar or journal or electronically. This allows the individual and their health care provider to note patterns in cycle interval length, total bleeding days, amount of bleeding, and any other symptoms they want to better understand in relation to their menstrual cycle.[16] Many patients use electronic apps to track their menses.[18] Some apps can track a multitude of things ranging from premenstrual syndrome (PMS) symptoms, cycle length, menstrual flow, sexual health, and fertility. Although these apps can help teens track important variables for their menstrual health, practitioners should be aware of the potential privacy concerns. There are also reports that some apps allow parents and peers to track a teen's data without their knowledge.[19] If they choose to use a period-tracking app, it is essential that adolescents research the security features to ensure that their personal health data are not being collected, shared, and/or sold without their explicit consent.[20]

PERIOD PRODUCTS

Many menstruators around the world do not have the luxury of choice when it comes to period products.[21] For those who do, many factors contribute to their decision making (Table 8.3), including product cost. Period poverty—the financial and material barriers to accessing menstrual products—affects nearly a quarter of all students in the United States.[22] It is essential that practitioners are sensitive to their patients' social and financial circumstances and understand how this may affect their menstrual hygiene practices.

The most used menstrual product worldwide is the disposable menstrual pad.[23] News investigations and online calculators show that disposable period products can cost between $8 to $10 per package.[24] Average prices rose 8.3% for a package of menstrual pads and 9.8% for tampons in 2022 alone, the biggest annual price jump since

TABLE 8.3 **Factors Contributing to Menstrual Hygiene Choice[21]**
Product availability
Cost
Reliability
Peer pressure/influence
Cultural considerations
Family
Environmental impact

TABLE 8.4 **Reusable Menstrual Products[a]**	
	Reusable pads can be made with synthetic or natural fibers and last about 5 y. Individuals who choose reusable pads also require access to clean water in order to be able to wash these products after use.
	Period underwear or pants can be made of synthetic or natural fibers and are quoted to last about 2 y; as with the reusable pads, period underwear must be washed after use.
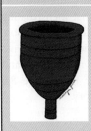	Menstrual cups are made of medical-grade silicone or rubber and can last up to 10 y; cups are placed internally by the user, and the cup collects menstrual blood. Individuals who use menstrual cups require access to water for washing the cup as well, although less water is required as compared with washing a reusable pad. The reusable menstrual cup has been estimated to have the lowest impact on the environment by far, especially in terms of waste.

Original artwork by Madelyn Frank.
[a]Table 8.4 used with permission.[21]

August 2012 according to the Bureau of Labor Statistics.[25] Some menstruators opt to use reusable menstrual products, such as reusable pads, period underwear/pants, and menstrual cups. Table 8.4 describes these reusable products in more detail. Reusable menstrual underwear can cost between $15 and more than $40 per pair,[21] commercial reusable menstrual pads between $9 and more than $40,[21,26] and menstrual cups approximately $25 per cup or more.[21,27] Although the up-front cost can be a major barrier for many individuals, reusable menstrual products may be a more cost-effective approach over time and more environmentally conscious.[28-30]

TAKING A COMPLETE, HOLISTIC MENSTRUAL HISTORY

Anticipatory guidance is an essential component of counseling young people about puberty and development. Individuals who have received education about what to expect regarding pubertal stages and what is considered "normal" (including menstruation) experience less anxiety and uncertainty about growth and development. Adolescents want menstrual health preparation that includes assurance that menstruation is normal and healthy and information on the pragmatics of menstrual hygiene management as well as the subjective experience of menstruation.[31,32]

In addition to screening for abnormalities and red flags on history, health care providers must also focus on the more personal, subjective, and immediate aspects of the menstruation experience, such as menstrual hygiene product choice and access. Once practitioners open the conversation on these practical aspects of menstruation, we start to destigmatize periods and reinforce that menstruating patients are worthy and deserving of this focused attention. Additionally, it is more likely for individuals to discuss their menses if these discussions are normalized and brought up by a health care provider first. Table 8.5 describes tips for taking a menstrual history.

A sexual history is another important part of a comprehensive menstrual history. The first sign of pregnancy for some can be a late menstrual period, and sexually transmitted infections (STIs) may present with breakthrough vaginal bleeding or abnormal periods. Sexual pleasure devices or foreign bodies can at times lead to injuries and vaginal bleeding that is mistaken for a menstrual period. Importantly, sexual trauma can also cause vaginal bleeding; it is essential therefore for practitioners to screen for sexual violence to ensure patient safety.

WRAP-UP

Menarche is a time of tremendous change for a young person and an opportunity for health care providers to help a young person feel comfortable and in control of their changing body. Menarche and menstrual periods should be framed as a sign of health (i.e., a vital sign) and not as a source of shame and burden. Health care

TABLE 8.5 **Taking a Menstrual History**	
Ask About	
Pubertal stages	Have you noticed your body changing at all lately; like breast bud development, emotional changes, pubic hair, axillary hair, body odor, and vaginal discharge?
Age of menarche	How old were you/what grade were you in when your period started for the first time?
Menses duration	Usually, how many days does the bleeding last?
Cycle length	How far apart do your periods come? **When was your LMP (first day of your last period)?**
Menstrual flow	On your heaviest bleeding days, how often do you change your menstrual product? Do you ever leak through to your clothes/PJs? Do you pass clots? Is there a family history of bleeding disorders?
Menstrual hygiene and product access	What products do you use (e.g., tampons, pads, reusable cup, reusable pads, period underwear)? Do you ever have any trouble accessing/buying your product of choice?
PMS symptoms	Do you have any symptoms in the week before or during your period, like pain (abdominal/pelvic/back), nausea, bloating, emotional changes/mood swings, headaches, or any other symptoms? If so, how do you manage them?
Pain	Do you have abdominal or pelvic pain before or during your periods? Do you take pain relievers?
Psychosocial	Does your period ever stop you from going to school or to work? Or doing things that you like to do (e.g., extracurricular activities, going out with friends)? If so, what is it about your period that holds you back (e.g., pain vs. no access to products vs. embarrassment vs. other symptoms)?
Emotional support	Who do you talk to if you have questions about your period? Where do you get your information?[a]
Sexual history	See text

[a]This is a good opportunity for practitioners to ensure individuals have a trusted person to speak with (can include the practitioner themselves), as well as making them aware of reputable resources (e.g., trusted website, patient handouts).

providers play a vital role in destigmatizing menses by taking a holistic approach to discussions around puberty and menstrual health.

KEY POINTS

- The menstrual period is a key marker of health and should be considered a vital sign.
- The mean age of menarche in HICs is 12 to 12.5 years, with a cycle interval range between 21 and 45 days in the first gynecologic year.
- Cycles often become more regular 2 to 3 years post menarche.
- Adolescents should be encouraged to track their menstrual periods in some fashion to gain more information about their cycles and any associated symptoms.
- A holistic menstrual history should also include the more personal and subjective aspects of the menstruation experience, such as menstrual hygiene product choice and access.

REVIEW QUESTIONS

1. One of the following indicators is a red flag on history that an individual may require further evaluation and/or treatment:
   a. Your 13-year-old patient, who started thelarche at age 12 years, has not had a first menstrual period
   b. Your 15-year-old patient reports that her menstrual period lasts for 12 days
   c. Your 16-year-old patient who experienced their first menstrual period at age 14 years has a menstrual cycle interval length of 34 days
   d. Your 14-year-old patient who experienced menarche 18 months ago reports menstrual periods every 2 months

2. The following is true about dysmenorrhea:
   a. Primary dysmenorrhea is mitigated by the release of LH and FSH
   b. Menstrual cramps that are NOT associated with heavy menstrual bleeding do not require treatment even if they are interfering in an individual's school attendance
   c. The majority of dysmenorrhea in adolescents and young adults is associated with a normal ovulatory cycle and no pelvic pathology
   d. Dysmenorrhea is not common in adolescents

3. The following is true about menarche:
   a. The age of menarche is the same in countries around the world
   b. Lower weight/BMI and lower socioeconomic status have been linked with earlier onset of menarche
   c. The median age of menarche in high-income countries (HICs) has been decreasing over the past 10 years
   d. Black adolescents appear to begin puberty and menstruation earlier than their White peers

REFERENCES

1. American Academy of Pediatrics, Committee on Adolescence, American College of Obstetricians and Gynecologists, Committee on Adolescent Health Care. Menstruation in girls and adolescents: using the menstrual cycle as a vital sign. *Pediatrics.* 2006;118(5):2245-2250. doi:10.1542/peds.2006-2481

2. ACOG. Committee opinion no. 651 summary: menstruation in girls and adolescents: using the menstrual cycle as a vital sign. *Obstet Gynecol.* 2015;126(6):1328. https://doi.org/10.1097/AOG.0000000000001210

3. Hillard PJA. Using the menstrual cycle as a vital sign: what we still want to know about adolescent menstrual cycles. *J Pediatr Adolesc Gynecol.* 2022;35(4):413-414. doi:10.1016/j.jpag.2022.06.004

4. UNICEF. Menstrual Hygiene. Accessed October 19, 2022. www.unicef.org/wash/menstrual-hygiene

5. Emans SJH, Laufer MR, Goldstein DP. *Pediatric and Adolescent Gynecology.* 6th ed. Wolters Kluwer Health/Lippincott Williams & Wilkins Health; 2011.

6. The Society of Obstetricians and Gynaecologists of Canada. Your Period: Menstrual Cycle Basics. Accessed October 29, 2022. https://www.yourperiod.ca/normal-periods/menstrual-cycle-basics/#cycleComprehensive

7. Karim A, Qaisar R, Hussain MA. Growth and socio-economic status, influence on the age at menarche in school going girls. *J Adolesc.* 2021;86(1):40-53. doi:10.1016/j.adolescence.2020.12.001

8. Yermachenko A, Dvornyk V. Nongenetic determinants of age at menarche: a systematic review. *BioMed Res Int.* 2014;2014:1-14. doi:10.1155/2014/371583

9. Chumlea WC, Schubert CM, Roche AF, et al. Age at menarche and racial comparisons in US girls. *Pediatrics.* 2003;111(1):110-113. doi:10.1542/peds.111.1.110

10. Martinez GM. *Trends and Patterns in Menarche in the United States: 1995 through 2013–2017.* U.S. Department of Health and Human Services, Centers for Disease

Control and Prevention, National Center for Health Statistics; 2020.

11. Osinubi AA, Lewis-de los Angeles CP, Poitevien P, Topor LS. Are black girls exhibiting puberty earlier? Examining implications of race-based guidelines. *Pediatrics.* 2022;150(2):e2021055595. doi:10.1542/peds.2021-055595

12. Creo AL, Pittock ST, Ameenuddin N. Reframing "normal" puberty: pivoting from a white standard. *J Adolesc Health.* 2022;71(1):8-9. doi:10.1016/j.jadohealth.2022.03.017

13. Harel Z. Dysmenorrhea in adolescents. *Ann N Y Acad Sci.* 2008;1135(1):185-195. doi:10.1196/annals.1429.007

14. Holland K, Nwadike VR. How much blood do you lose on your period? *Healthline.* Accessed October 30, 2022. https://www.healthline.com/health/how-much-blood-do-you-lose-on-your-period

15. ACOG. Committee opinion no. 785: screening and management of bleeding disorders in adolescents with heavy menstrual bleeding. *Obstet Gynecol.* 2019;134(3):e71-e83.

16. Hillard PJA. Menstruation in adolescents: what do we know? And what do we do with the information? *J Pediatr Adolesc Gynecol.* 2014;27(6):309-319. doi:10.1016/j.jpag.2013.12.001

17. Haamid F, Sass AE, Dietrich JE. Heavy menstrual bleeding in adolescents. *J Pediatr Adolesc Gynecol.* 2017;30(3):335-340. doi:10.1016/j.jpag.2017.01.002

18. Bradley S, Bacharach E, Martens A, Spanfeller J. The 11 best period tracker apps to get to know your cycle, according to ob-gyns. *Women's Health.* Published July 25, 2022. Accessed September 29, 2022. https://www.womenshealthmag.com/health/g26787041/best-period-tracking-apps/

19. Fowler LR, Gillard C, Morain S. Teenage use of smartphone applications for menstrual cycle tracking. *Pediatrics.* 2020;145(5):e20192954. doi:10.1542/peds.2019-2954

20. Garamvolgyi F. Why US women are deleting their period tracking apps. *The Guardian.* Published July 28, 2022. Accessed October 31, 2022. https://www.theguardian.com/world/2022/jun/28/why-us-woman-are-deleting-their-period-tracking-apps

21. Harrison ME, Tyson N. Menstruation: environmental impact and need for global health equity. *Int J Gynecol Obstet.* 2023;160(2):378-382. doi:10.1002/ijgo.14311

22. Period poverty: the launch pad. Published May 2021. Accessed October 1, 2022. https://period-action.org/periodpoverty

23. Cooper K. The people fighting pollution with plastic-free periods. *BBC News.* Published 2018. Accessed March 3, 2022. https://www.bbc.com/news/world-43879789

24. Smialek D, Zulawinska J. Period products cost calculator. Omni Calculator. Published April 6, 2022. Accessed October 19, 2022. https://www.omnicalculator.com/everyday-life/period-products-cost

25. Sirtori-Cortina D, Rockeman O. It's getting more expensive to have your period, thanks to inflation. Bloomberg. Published June 9, 2022. https://www.bloomberg.com/news/articles/2022-06-09/inflation-is-pushing-tampon-prices-up-10?leadSource=uverify%20wall

26. van Eijk AM, Jayasinghe N, Zulaika G, et al. Exploring menstrual products: a systematic review and meta-analysis of reusable menstrual pads for public health internationally. *PLoS One.* 2021;16(9):e0257610. doi:10.1371/journal.pone.0257610

27. Eveleth R. The best menstrual cup. New York Times Wirecutter. Published December 11, 2020. Accessed June 1, 2022. https://www.nytimes.com/wirecutter/reviews/best-menstrual-cup/

28. Luo OD, Huang J, Shen S. Counselling on reusable menstrual products: an opportunity to mitigate climate change and address period poverty in the doctor's office. *BMJ Opin.* Published July 30, 2021. Accessed May 20, 2022. https://blogs.bmj.com/bmj/2021/07/30/counselling-on-reusable-menstrual-products-an-opportunity-to-mitigate-climate-change-and-address-period-poverty-in-the-doctors-office/

29. Babagoli MA, Benshaul-Tolonen A, Zulaika G, et al. The cost-benefit and cost-effectiveness of providing menstrual cups and sanitary pads to schoolgirls in rural Kenya. Published Online June 2020. https://anjatolonen.files.wordpress.com/2020/06/ce_cb_analysis_mhm_si.pdf

30. van Eijk AM, Zulaika G, Lenchner M, et al. Menstrual cup use, leakage, acceptability, safety, and availability: a systematic review and meta-analysis. *Lancet Public Health.* 2019;4(8):e376-e393. doi:10.1016/S2468-2667(19)30111-2

31. Koff E, Rierdan J. Preparing girls for menstruation: recommendations from adolescent girls. *Adolescence.* 1995;30(120):795-811.

32. Schmitt ML, Hagstrom C, Nowara A, et al. The intersection of menstruation, school and family: experiences of girls growing up in urban cities in the U.S.A. *Int J Adolesc Youth.* 2021;26(1):94-109. doi:10.1080/02673843.2020.1867207

Common Menstrual Concerns in the Adolescent

Nancy Sokkary and Oluyemisi Adeyemi-Fowode

INTRODUCTION

Abnormal uterine bleeding (AUB) is the most common complaint among adolescents reporting to a gynecologist.[1] They may present with bleeding that lasts for several weeks at a time or concern that they go months between periods. Young girls and their caretakers can have difficulty assessing what constitutes normal menstrual cycles or patterns of bleeding. Although some irregularity is expected around menarche, it can be hard to assess what is concerning for a more severe problem. The American College of Obstetricians and Gynecologists (ACOG) has provided guidance on what constitutes normal menses in young girls and adolescents (Table 9.1). Please refer to Chapter 8 for further discussion of normal menses.

ABNORMAL UTERINE BLEEDING

AUB refers to bleeding from the uterine corpus that is abnormal in volume, regularity, frequency, or duration and occurs in the absence of pregnancy.[2]

Menstrual irregularities refer to a deviation in what is considered normal menstrual bleeding in adolescents or adult women. The most common menstrual irregularities are described in Table 9.2.[2-4]

Prevalence

Menstrual cycles are often irregular during adolescence. Immaturity of the hypothalamic-pituitary-ovarian (HPO) axis during the early years after menarche often results in anovulation, and cycles may be somewhat irregular. However, 90% of cycles will be within the range of 21 to 45 days, although short cycles of less than 20 days and long cycles of more than 45 days may occur. By the third year after menarche, 60% to 80% of menstrual cycles are 21 to 34 days long, as is typical of adults.[3]

There is a paucity of data in regard to the prevalence of specific menstrual irregularities (see Table 9.2) in the adolescent population. A cross-sectional study with 848 girls aged 12 to 18 years looked to characterize the menstrual cycle (regularity and menstrual flow length) in this population.[5] A total of 41.3% of the girls reported irregular cycles and 17.2% reported menstrual flow length of >6 days. Irregular cycles were noted to be more prevalent among young teens ages 12 to 14 (44.6%) than among teenagers ages 15 to 18 (39.2%). Also, a higher percentage of younger teens ages 12 to 14 reported longer menstrual flow (22.9%) compared with the teenagers ages 15 to 18 (13.7%).[5]

Etiology/Pathophysiology of AUB

Causes of AUB are numerous and often multifactorial.[2,6] In an effort to create a universally accepted system of nomenclature to describe AUB in nonpregnant women, a new classification system was introduced in 2011. This system classifies AUB into heavy menstrual bleeding (HMB) or intermenstrual bleeding (IMB). From there, causes are broken down into two main categories. The PALM acronym refers to structural causes of AUB, and the COEIN acronym is reserved for nonstructural causes of AUB (see PowerPoint recording).

Structural causes of AUB (PALM) could be the result of uterine polyps, adenomyosis, leiomyoma (also known as *fibroids*), and malignancy. Nonstructural causes of AUB are the case for the majority of adolescent patients—COEIN—and include coagulopathy,

TABLE 9.1	**Normal Menses**
Menarche (median age)	12.43
Mean cycle interval	32.2 days in first gynecologic year
Menstrual cycle interval	Typically 21–45 days
Menstrual flow length	7 days or less
Menstrual product use	Three to six pads or tampons per day

From American Academy of Pediatrics Committee on Adolescence; American College of Obstetricians and Gynecologists Committee on Adolescent Health Care, Diaz A, Laufer MR, Breech LL. Menstruation in girls and adolescents: using the menstrual cycle as a vital sign. *Pediatrics.* 2006;118(5):2245-2250.

TABLE 9.2	**Menstrual Irregularities**
Amenorrhea (pronounced *ey-men-uh-REE-uh*)	Absent menstrual periods Primary amenorrhea: No menses by age 15 or 2–3 y post thelarche Secondary amenorrhea: No menses for at least 6 mo in a nonpregnant patient who has already achieved menarche (started having periods)
Heavy menstrual bleeding (HMB)	See section on HMB
Irregular menstrual periods	Cycle-to-cycle variation of more than 20 days
Shortened menstrual bleeding	Less than 2 days in duration
Intermenstrual bleeding	Episodes of bleeding that occur between normally timed periods, also known as spotting

From American Academy of Pediatrics Committee on Adolescence; American College of Obstetricians and Gynecologists Committee on Adolescent Health Care, Diaz A, Laufer MR, Breech LL. Menstruation in girls and adolescents: using the menstrual cycle as a vital sign. *Pediatrics.* 2006;118(5): 2245-2250; Committee on Practice Bulletins—Gynecology. Practice bulletin no. 128: diagnosis of abnormal uterine bleeding in reproductive-aged women. *Obstet Gynecol.* 2012;120(1):197-206. (Reaffirmed 2021); Munro MG, Critchley HO, Fraser IS. The FIGO systems for nomenclature and classification of causes of abnormal uterine bleeding in the reproductive years: who needs them? *Am J Obstet Gynecol.* 2012;207(4):259-265.

ovulatory dysfunction, endometrial causes such as sexually transmitted infections, and iatrogenic reasons such as breakthrough bleeding from a contraception or side effect of hormone therapy. The N is the "not yet classified" subcategory where causes that do not fit well into any of the previously mentioned subcategories are located; an example of this would be arteriovenous malformations.

One of the most common reasons for AUB in the adolescent is ovulatory dysfunction. The differential diagnosis for anovulation in adolescents is broad and can be divided into physiologic versus pathologic causes. Physiologic causes of anovulation include the process of puberty or an immature HPO axis does not have the necessary hormonal feedback needed to regulate menses. Pregnancy or breastfeeding, which increases prolactin levels, can also result in anovulation.

Pathologic causes can be the result of elevated androgens such as in polycystic ovary syndrome (PCOS), congenital adrenal hyperplasia (CAH), or androgen-producing tumors. Hypothalamic dysfunction, which can occur because of eating disorders such as anorexia nervosa, and elevated prolactin from pathologic causes such as pituitary tumor, thyroid disease, and premature ovarian insufficiency (POI) are also possible causes. Iatrogenic causes stem from treatment of other ailments such as radiation to the brain or pelvis or chemotherapy with toxic effects to the ovaries. And finally, certain drugs or medications can cause increases in the prolactin level and/or menstrual disturbances such as risperidone.

Refer to the see PowerPoint recordings for further delineation of AUB.

Clinical Presentation and Classical Signs

The presentation for AUB will vary depending on the etiology. Determining the etiology of AUB is essential in choosing the most appropriate and effective management for the individual, and it is accomplished by obtaining a thorough history and physical examination and ordering relevant laboratory and imaging tests (Table 9.3).

Evaluation/Testing

A thorough history is perhaps the most important component and should be taken in a systematic manner, while taking the clinical setting into consideration.

TABLE 9.3 Evaluation of Abnormal Uterine Bleeding in Adolescents

History

- Menarche/gynecologic age
- Menstrual history (regular or irregular pattern, typical interval, duration, use of sanitary products per day, associated cramping);[a] if applicable, when did change in pattern occur and details of current episode
- Impact on quality of life
- Any history of past brain or pelvic radiation, chemotherapy
- Medications (specific attention to those that might cause AUB; e.g., anticoagulants, NSAID use, hormonal contraceptives)
- Sexual activity status, trauma, assault[b]
- See HMB section for specific HMB questions
- Review of systems:
  - Symptoms of anemia: headache, dizziness, syncope, fatigue, pica
  - Symptoms of pathologic causes of anovulation: unwanted hair growth, severe acne, eating habits, headaches, nipple discharge, constipation, diarrhea, cold or heat intolerance, hot flashes
  - Associated symptoms: fever, chills, pelvic pain, vaginal discharge

Physical Examination

- Temperature, blood pressure, heart rate, BMI, assessment of hemodynamic stability (if indicated)
- Dermatologic
- Signs of anemia and bleeding disorders (pallor, bruises, petechiae, ecchymosis)
- Signs of hyperandrogenism (acne, hirsutism)
- Signs of insulin resistance (acanthosis nigricans)
- Thyroid examination
- Abdominal examination (evaluate for presence of mass, hepatosplenomegaly)
- Sexual maturity rating (breast and pubic hair)
- External genitalia examination
- Speculum examination/bimanual (if clinically indicated and patient is able to tolerate)

Laboratory Tests

- Pregnancy test
- Assessment of anemia from blood loss: CBC, ferritin level
- TSH
- Testing for other causes as indicated:
  - Bleeding disorder evaluation (see later)
  - STI screening with gonorrhea and chlamydia if sexually active
  - Free/total testosterone, DHEAS, 17 hyrdoxyprogesterone prolactin if PCOS suspected
  - Liver function tests

Imaging
- Pelvic ultrasound depending on clinical judgement

AUB, Abnormal menstrual bleeding; *BMI,* body mass index; *CBC,* complete blood count; *DHEAS,* dehydroepiandrosterone sulfate; *HMB,* heavy menstrual bleeding; *NSAID,* nonsteroidal antiinflammatory drug; *PCOS,* polycystic ovarian syndrome; *STI,* sexually transmitted infection; *TSH,* thyroid-stimulating hormone.
[a]Can use a menstrual calendar app for patients being expectantly managed.
[b]It is best to ask sensitive questions privately.

Direct information regarding the timing, length, and heaviness of the cycle should be elicited:

1. When did you start your period?
2. How often do you bleed?
3. How many days do you bleed for?
4. How many pads or tampons do you use per day or per hour?

All the components of a physical examination are important depending on your clinical setting. However, attention should be paid to vital signs, checking the skin for any signs of unwanted hair growth, acne, thyroid abnormalities, Tanner staging, and an external genitalia examination. Speculum examination is often not necessary and may not be well tolerated in this population. The external genital examination can be accomplished via labial retraction in a down and out manner to evaluate the introitus, and in some cases, this technique exposes the distal third of the vagina. Refer to Chapter 4 for further information on pediatric gynecologic examination.

Laboratory tests for AUB with associated ovulatory dysfunction (AUB-O) include a pregnancy test, a complete blood count (CBC) to evaluate for anemia and platelet quantity, screening for thyroid hormone (as thyroid abnormalities are associated with menstrual abnormalities), and sexually transmitted infections (when appropriate). Bleeding disorder screening should also be performed if indicated (discussed later). Structural abnormalities account for only a small minority of cases of AUB in this population; thus clinical evaluation should guide the inclusion of a pelvic ultrasound. Although the transvaginal is considered the most accurate route to assess the female reproductive structures, the majority of adolescent patients will not tolerate it, and thus transabdominal pelvic imaging is the imaging modality of choice in nonsexually active females.

See Fig. 9.1 for important aspects to look for during the physical examination and Table 9.3 for detailed history, laboratory, and imaging testing for abnormal uterine bleeding.

TREATMENT

Determining the etiology of AUB is essential in choosing the most appropriate and effective management for the individual (Table 9.4).

TABLE 9.4 AUB Treatment

Etiology	Management
Coagulopathy[a]	Hormone therapy
Ovulatory Dysfunction	
Ovarian Failure, Premature[a]	Hormone therapy
Primary Pituitary Disease[a]	Treat underlying disease
Thyroid Disease	Treat underlying disease
Iatrogenic: chemotherapy/ radiation	Hormone therapy
Medications	Discuss alternatives, hormone therapy
Hyper**A**ndrogenic anovulation (PCOS, CAH)[a]	Hormone therapy
Hyperpro**L**actinemia	Treat underlying disease
Hypothalamic dysfunction (anorexia nervosa)	Treat underlying disease
Endometrial (e.g., STIs)	Treat underlying disease
Iatrogenic (e.g., BTB with contraception)	Optimize hormone therapy, offer alternatives
Not yet classified	Treat underlying disease

OPTIMAL-H is an acronym that can be used to remember causes of ovulatory dysfunction.
[a]Consider collaboration with hematology and endocrinology as indicated for optimal management of disease.
BTB, Breakthrough bleeding; *CAH,* congenital adrenal hyperplasia; *PCOS,* polycystic ovarian syndrome; *STI,* sexually transmitted infection.

TABLE 9.5 Hormone Therapy

Combined Hormonal Therapy (E + P)	Progestin Therapy (P Only)
Combined Oral Contraceptives (OCPs)	Oral Progestins
Transdermal Patches	Depot Medroxyprogesterone Acetate (DMPA)
Vaginal Ring	Levonorgestrel Intrauterine Device

Hormone Therapy

Hormone therapy comprises two main categories (Tables 9.5 and 9.6):

1. Combined hormonal therapy with estrogen and progestin
2. Progestin therapy only

TABLE 9.6 Strategies to Manage Unexpected Bleeding With Hormonal Medication

Method	Strategies[a]
Estrogen-containing methods (combined OCPs, patch, ring)	Make sure that the patient is compliant with medication If using in an extended or continuous fashion, can take a 4-day break or use traditionally for monthly menses Breakthrough bleeding is expected in the initial months and over time may continue with <30 mcg ethinyl estradiol pills
Oral progestins[b]	Make sure that the patient is compliant with medication; needs to take at same exact time daily Can perform a taper; increase dose for 7 days, then return to traditional dosing
Depot medroxyprogesterone acetate[b]	Rates of amenorrhea increase with more prolonged use NSAIDs (5–7 days of treatment) Addition of combined OCPs (if medically eligible) for 10–20 days (skip placebo pills of OCPs)
Implant[b]	NSAIDs (5–7 days of treatment) Addition of combined OCPs (if medically eligible) for 10–20 days (skip placebo pills of OCPs)
Progestin-containing intrauterine device[b]	Lower-dose IUDs associated with more bleeding Expert opinion supports a trial of NSAIDs, doxycycline, POPs, and continuous OCP use

[a]Evaluate for pregnancy if applicable.
[b]Counsel patient on alternative methods, given progestin-only methods are notorious for irregular bleeding; provide reassurance.
IUD, Intrauterine device; NSAID, nonsteroidal antiinflammatory drug; OCP, oral contraceptives; POP, progestin-only pill.
From American College of Obstetricians and Gynecologists. General approaches to medical management of menstrual suppression. Clinical consensus no. 3. Obstet Gynecol. 2022;140:528-541; U.S. Selected Practice Recommendations for Contraceptive Use, 2016. Recommendations and Reports. July 29, 2016;65(4):1–66. https://www.cdc.gov/mmwr/volumes/65/rr/rr6504a1.htm; Adeyemi-Fowode OA, Bercaw-Pratt JL. Intrauterine devices: effective contraception with noncontraceptive benefits for adolescents. J Pediatr Adolesc Gynecol. 2019;32(5S):S2-S6.

When counseling regarding hormonal therapy, an individualized approach with shared decision making is important, and one needs to take several factors into consideration such as the priorities, preferences (e.g., Can the patient commit to taking a pill daily or do they need a long-acting contraceptive method?), concerns of the patient, and the medical history.

Although generally safe in a healthy patient, there are some medical conditions where estrogen should be avoided such as in migraines with aura, uncontrolled hypertension, and hypercoagulable disorders, to mention a few. The US Medical Eligibility Criteria for Contraceptive Use (US MEC) was designed by the Centers for Disease Control and Prevention (CDC) to provide guidance on the safety of contraceptive options, especially in women with particular medical conditions. There is a free app that can be downloaded for quick access (https://www.cdc.gov/reproductivehealth/contraception/contraception-app.html). Refer to Chapter 21 for more detailed information on contraceptive choices in adolescents.

When starting hormonal therapy, it is important to discuss common side effects and set expectations regarding breakthrough bleeding, the patient should be reassured that if bothersome, there are treatment options available (see Table 9.6).

HEAVY MENSTRUAL BLEEDING

HMB is defined as excessive menstrual bleeding that negatively effects emotional, social, and material quality of life.[7] Objectively, it is described as greater than 80 mL of blood loss per cycle, which is difficult for a patient to assess, so greater than or equal to eight fully saturated pads a day and greater than or equal to 8 days of bleeding would also qualify as HMB. There are more and more menstrual products on the market including menstrual cups, sponges, and underwear, and the milliliters of blood that each product can hold is often found online.

Prevalence

The exact prevalence of HMB among adolescents is unknown, but surveys have reported that 15% to 40% of adolescents perceive their bleeding as abnormally heavy.[8,9] The frequency of HMB among adolescents with bleeding disorders is far higher. Females with von Willebrand disease (vWD), the most common bleeding disorder among women with HMB, report that HMB is the single most common bleeding symptom they experience. Approximately 95% of women with vWD report heavy menstrual bleeding, and over 50% of women with rare factor deficiencies report it.[10,11]

Etiology/Pathophysiology

There are multiple etiologies for HMB among reproductive-age women. These are well defined via the previously discussed ACOG mnemonics PALM and COEIN. Single episodes of heavy menstrual or vaginal bleeding may be attributed to trauma from abuse, foreign body or straddle injury, infections such as cervicitis, or pregnancy related. Persistent or recurrent HMB may be caused by anovulatory cycles, PCOS, or thyroid disease. Although uterine pathology such as polyps and fibroids are possible causes, they are much less common in this patient population.[2] Medications specifically used by adolescents that may result in heavy menses include various forms of contraception (AUB section). More individuals need to use direct-acting oral anticoagulants and other blood thinners that can certainly increase bleeding of any kind, including menstrual bleeding.[12] Patients receiving various forms of chemotherapy can experience thrombocytopenia, which may lead to HMB. Chemotherapeutic agents commonly associated with thrombocytopenia include carboplatin, cisplatin, gemcitabine, paclitaxel, and temozolomide.[13] Finally the risk of bleeding disorders is much higher in patients with heavy menses since menarche. Although vWD is the most common bleeding disorder, factor deficiency and platelet abnormalities should also be considered.[11] Clotting factor deficiencies are rare, including factor II, V, VII, X, and XI and hemophilia. As mentioned, thrombocytopenia can result in HMB, as can platelet dysfunction. Platelet dysfunction may be inherited such as Bernard-Soulier and Glanzmann syndromes or acquired from medication, liver disease, and myeloproliferative disorders.[14]

Clinical Presentation/Classic Signs

Adolescents with HMB will typically present with the complaint of bleeding too much or for too long during menstruation. Adolescents may complain of needing to be picked up from school because of soiling of their clothes or using towels at night so they do not bleed through onto their sheets. Classic signs or associated symptoms may help to identify the underlying etiology; for example, a history of prolonged gum bleeds may suggest an underlying bleeding disorder; fatigue and pallor reflect anemia; or skin changes and weight gain could be the presenting symptoms of thyroid disease (see Fig. 9.1).

Evaluation/Testing

A thorough history is important to establish the amount of bleeding and frequency (see earlier) and to evaluate for underlying causes. It can be helpful to use an app that tracks cycles for more accurate and objective data. The Sisterhood app, created by the Hemophilia Federation of America (https://www.sisterhoodapp.com/) can be a useful tool. The Pictorial Bleeding Assessment Tool (PBAC) has also been shown to help evaluate bleeding prospectively among patients (https://www.rch.org.au/uploaded-Files/Main/Content/rch_gynaecology/PBAC.pdf).

Additionally, several other menstrual products are now available, including period panties and menstrual cups. These alternatives often have estimated milliliters of blood loss that can be calculated based on use.[15]

A bleeding-specific history should be performed (Table 9.7). A family history of known bleeding disorders and heavy bleeding and need for transfusion should be elicited.

It is recommended to use a bleeding assessment tool (BAT) to evaluate patients who warrant further laboratory evaluation. These should specifically be used when presenting to a primary care setting such as a pediatrician or family medicine clinic; they are not recommended for subspecialist referral centers such as a pediatric hematologist. Based on the sensitivity and specificity of various BATs, the ACOG recommends a bleeding disorder workup for any *adolescent* who meets any of the following criteria[16,17]:

1. Duration of menses was greater than or equal to 7 days and reports either "flooding" or bleeding through a tampon or napkin in 2 hours or less with *most periods*
2. A history of treatment for anemia
3. A family history of a diagnosed bleeding disorder
4. A history of excessive bleeding with tooth extraction, delivery or miscarriage, or surgery

Physical Examination

The physical examination is also used to help elicit the cause of HMB. Evaluation of the skin may suggest a

TABLE 9.7 Bleeding History

Menses Specific	General Bleeding Symptoms	Medical History	Medication
Frequent soiling for clothes or bedding	Epistaxis >10 min	Known bleeding disorder	Anticoagulants
Large clots (>2 cm)	Frequent/prolonged gum bleeding	History of anemia	Chemotherapy
Changing saturated pad more than every 2 hours	Easy bruising Excessive bleeding associated with trauma or surgery	History of transfusion Chronic medical illness: systemic lupus erythematosus, liver disease, renal disease Postpartum hemorrhage	Hormonal Medication

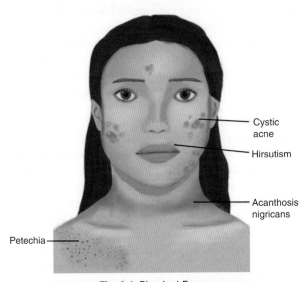

Fig. 9.1 Physical Exam

Labels: Cystic acne, Hirsutism, Acanthosis nigricans, Petechia

TABLE 9.8 Bleeding Disorder Workup

PT, PTT, INR
Fibrinogen
von Willebrand panel:
von Willebrand factor antigen
Factor VIII
von Willebrand factor activity[a]

[a]Historically von Willebrand factor activity was evaluated by a ristocetin cofactor activity, but because of high test result variability in addition to a nonclinically significant polymorphism, GPIbM will replace this ristocetin cofactor in the future.[19]

INR, International normalized ratio; *PT,* prothrombin time; *PTT,* partial thromboplastin time.

bleeding disorder with petechiae, poorly healed wounds, hematomas, or bruising (Fig. 9.1). Pallor can be seen in patients with chronic or significant anemia. The physical examination can also help rule out other causes such PCOS and thyroid disease (see AUB section). An examination of the genitalia is indicated for patients who are sexually active, if there is a concern for trauma, or if the source of bleeding is not confirmed to be vaginal.

Laboratory

The initial evaluation of a patient presenting with an acute episode of heavy menses should include having a CBC collected. A type and screen are warranted if transfusion is being considered. Iron studies, including ferritin, thyroid-stimulating hormone, and pregnancy test, should be checked upon presentation.[18]

Adolescents presenting with HMB who screen positive (affirmative response to any of the four BAT questions posed earlier) should undergo a bleeding disorder workup, which includes the labs in Table 9.8.

If a patient requires a transfusion, these laboratory studies should be drawn before the administration of blood products. However, several aspects of the bleeding disorder workup are acute-phase reactants, which means they can be falsely elevated during an acute bleed or in cases of severe anemia. For that reason, the bleeding disorder panel should always be drawn or repeated once the patient has stabilized and hemoglobin has returned to normal.

For cases of an abnormal bleeding disorder workup or persistent heavy bleeding that fails therapy, a hematology referral is recommended. Hematology may initiate further evaluation of more rare bleeding disorders such as factor deficiency and disorders of platelet function.[20]

Imaging

Ultrasound may be indicated for adolescents with HMB. In general, it is not part of the initial evaluation because structural causes such as cancer, polyps, and fibroids are so rare. However, it should be considered in individuals who fail initial medical management or in individuals who have a palpable abdominal mass or concern for müllerian or vaginal anomaly.[18] Transabdominal ultrasound is usually sufficient to assess ovarian and uterine structures. Magnetic resonance imaging (MRI) can be considered in cases of anomalous or complex anatomy.

Treatment/Management

Treatment can be divided into acute versus maintenance therapy. Several institutions have published protocols for acute heavy menses that are publicly available and can be accessed online, such as the ED Guidelines for Heavy Menstrual Bleeding https://www.choa.org/-/media/Files/Childrens/medical-professionals/clinical-practice-guidelines/heavy-menstrual-bleeding-ed.pdf.

Acute

Patients who are hemodynamically compromised or severely anemic (<8 g/dL) with active bleeding should be admitted, transfused as appropriate, and started on hormone therapy. Hormone therapy may include intravenous (IV) estrogen or a combined oral contraceptive pill or high-dose progesterone (Table 9.9). Several tapers exist, but there is little evidence to support one as being more effective than the other (Table 9.10).[21-23]

Patients who are anemic but hemodynamically stable with a hemoglobin of greater than 8 g/dL can typically be managed on an outpatient basis.[24] If they are actively bleeding, a taper should be initiated. Those who are not actively bleeding or have a normal hemoglobin can be started on maintenance therapy as discussed later.

There are specific hematologic agents to address heavy bleeding caused by specific deficiencies or disorders, including factor replacement, recombinant von Willebrand factor, and desmopressin. Hematology should guide the usage of these products.[25] A massive transfusion protocol is rarely indicated for HMB in the adolescent but may be implemented in collaboration with hematology or an intensivist.

Surgical intervention is usually not warranted in the adolescent with HMB. Most adolescents will respond to hormone and/or hematologic therapy. Additionally, dilation and curettage can worsen bleeding for women with an underlying bleeding disorder. Successful uterine tamponade with a 30-mL Foley balloon has been reported in cases of patients who were acutely hemorrhaging.[7] Uterine ablation, embolization and hysterectomy should only be considered in a life-threatening emergency.[20]

Antifibrinolytics. Antifibrinolytics such as tranexamic acid or aminocaproic acid help to stabilize blood clot formation, thereby decreasing blood loss. They may be used in isolation for HMB but are most often used as an adjunct to hormonal methods. They are effective for treating HMB even in patients with bleeding disorders.[26] Antifibrinolytics may be used in the acute bleed if there is insufficient response to hormone therapy or in patients who want to avoid hormones. Antifibrinolytics and hormonal therapy can safely be used together. The risk of thrombosis with combined hormonal contraception and tranexamic acid is theoretical and evidence of venous thromboembolic events when combined hormonal contraception and and tranexamic acid are used simultaneously has not been seen clinically.[27]

Maintenance

A wide variety of maintenance therapies can be initiated in patients who are transitioning off a taper or who present to an outpatient clinical setting in stable condition without anemia, or with mild anemia but no active bleeding (Table 9.11).

Combined oral contraceptive pills have been shown to decrease blood loss per cycle and can also be used safely and effectively to decrease the number of cycles per year.[28] There are no randomized controlled trials

TABLE 9.9	Acute HMB Protocol	
Actively Bleeding AND Hgb <8 OR Unstable	**Actively Bleeding AND Hgb 8-12 AND Stable**	**No Active Bleeding OR Not Anemic AND Stable**
• Admit/ observation • Transfuse as appropriate • Initiate taper	• Discharge home • Initiate taper • Outpatient follow-up	• Discharge home • Initiate maintenance therapy

TABLE 9.10 **Sample Taper**		
COC 30–50 mcg Ethinyl Estradiol[a,b]	**Medroxyprogesterone Acetate**[b]	**Norethindrone Acetate**[b]
TID × 7 days	20 mg BID × 5 days	10 mg TID until bleeding stops
BID × 7 days	20 mg QD × 5 days	10 mg BID × 7 days
Daily	10 mg daily	5–10 mg daily

BID, Twice a day; *COC,* combined oral contraceptive; *QD,* daily; *TID,* three times a day.
[a]Skip placebo week.
[b]The days and taper vary to illustrate options; note this is not the only acceptable taper for each medication.

TABLE 9.11 **Maintenance Therapy: Sample Medication Usage**
Combined oral contraceptive (COC) pills • COC 30-35 mcg ethinyl estradiol • 1 tab daily • May skip placebo week
Oral progesterone only • Norethindrone acetate 0.35-10 mg qday • 1-3 tabs daily
Depot medroxyprogesterone acetate • 150 mg IM every 3 months • 104 mg SQ every 3 months
Intrauterine device • 52 mg levonorgestrel for up to 8 y
Antifibrinolytic • Tranexamic acid • 1300 mg PO TID for up to 5 days for episodes of heavy bleeding

IM, intramuscular; *PO,* oral; *qday,* daily; *SQ,* subcutaneous; *TID,* three times a day

comparing efficacy of combined oral contraceptive pills for HMB, but generally lower ethinyl estradiol dosing (<20 mcg) may not control heavy bleeding as well.[18]

Oral progesterone therapy is very effective as a taper for acute bleeding episodes but can also be used cyclically or continuously for maintenance therapy in cases of HMB.[18] Although high-dose norethindrone acetate (≥5 mg) has high rate of amenorrhea, some may choose the progesterone-only pill, norethindrone (0.35 mcg), which can decrease bleeding but has a much higher rate—approximately 40%—of breakthrough bleeding.[23]

Depot medroxyprogesterone acetate generally has a high rate of amenorrhea, typically quoted as 70% or greater. In patients with severe bleeding disorders or other risk for hematoma with intramuscular injection, 104 mg subcutaneous can be used as an alternative, with similar bleeding and side effect profile.[29]

As stated earlier *levonorgestrel intrauterine devices (IUDs),* specifically those containing 52 mg of progesterone, result in high rates of amenorrhea. They are particularly effective for maintenance therapy for HMB, including in individuals with bleeding disorders.[30-32] Additionally, they can be used for up to 8 years with similar or improved bleeding profile.

Antifibrinolytics. Antifibrinolytics can be used in a cyclic fashion for patients who want to avoid hormones. Patients can be instructed to take a short course of antifibrinolytics for bleeding that lasts longer than 5 days, but if this is required every month, a hormonal option should likely be added to their regimen. Antifibrinolytics can also be used for excessive breakthrough bleeding if it occurs with other maintenance therapies.

SPECIAL CONSIDERATIONS

AUB, including HMB, is the most common gynecologic problem among adolescent females. It can have a significant impact on their quality of life, academic performance, and participation in extracurricular activities. There is a broad differential for adolescents with AUB, but a thorough history and appropriate workup can help guide therapy. Additionally, irregular or heavy bleeding may be the presenting symptoms of a more serious underlying illness such as thyroid disease or a bleeding disorder. Although there are several therapeutic options to regulate the menstrual cycle and decrease bleeding, the most effective option for a given clinical scenario is yet to be determined. Proper evaluation, referral, and treatment can have a significant impact on a young menstruating female.

KEY POINTS

- AUB is common in adolescents.
- An immature HPO axis is the most common cause of AUB in adolescents.
- A thorough history and physical examination will drive additional workup.
- Treatment of AUB should address the underlying cause.
- HMB in the adolescent may be the presenting symptom of a bleeding disorder.
- Most adolescents with HMB should undergo laboratory screening for a bleeding disorder, which includes CBC, ferritin, PT/PTT, and von Willebrand panel.
- Hormones are the most commonly used and effective form of treatment for both acute episodes and chronic HMB.

REVIEW QUESTIONS

1. Which of the following is the most likely cause of abnormal uterine bleeding in an adolescent?
   a. Polyp
   b. Ovulatory dysfunction
   c. Adenomyosis
   d. Malignancy
2. Which of the following clinical scenarios would warrant a bleeding disorder workup?
   a. A 9-year-old with irregular menses that last for 6 days and uses 3 pads per day
   b. A 15-year-old with menses every 21 days that last for 8 days and has to change her pad between every class period and has frequent nosebleeds
   c. A 14-year-old who bled for 2 weeks on one occasion but otherwise normally has 5 days of menstrual bleeding and no associated bleeding symptoms
   d. A 7-year-old who has not started her period yet but her parents are concerned because the mother has endometriosis
3. Which of the following would be most effective at stopping an acute episode of vaginal bleeding?
   a. Ibuprofen 600 mg every 6 hours
   b. Immediate placement of a 52-mg intrauterine device
   c. Depot medroxyprogesterone acetate 150 IM
   d. Norethindrone acetate 10 mg PO TID

REFERENCES

1. Elmaoğulları S, Aycan Z. Abnormal uterine bleeding in adolescents. *J Clin Res Pediatr Endocrinol.* 2018;10(3): 191-197. doi:10.4274/jcrpe.0014
2. Committee on Practice Bulletins—Gynecology. Practice bulletin no. 128: diagnosis of abnormal uterine bleeding in reproductive-aged women. *Obstet Gynecol.* 2012;120(1):197-206.
3. American Academy of Pediatrics Committee on Adolescence; American College of Obstetricians and Gynecologists Committee on Adolescent Health Care; Diaz A, Laufer MR, Breech LL. Menstruation in girls and adolescents: using the menstrual cycle as a vital sign. *Pediatrics.* 2006;118(5):2245-2250.
4. Munro MG, Critchley HO, Fraser IS. The FIGO systems for nomenclature and classification of causes of abnormal uterine bleeding in the reproductive years: who needs them? *Am J Obstet Gynecol.* 2012;207(4):259-265.
5. Marques P, Madeira T, Gama A. Menstrual cycle among adolescents: girls' awareness and influence of age at menarche and overweight. *Rev Paul Pediatr.* 2022;40:e2020494.
6. Adeyemi-Fowode OA, Brander E. Understanding abnormal uterine bleeding in adolescents. *Contemporary OB/GYN J.* 2022;67(3):20-24.
7. Haamid F, Sass AE, Dietrich JE. Heavy menstrual bleeding in adolescents. *J Pediatr Adolesc Gynecol.* 2017;30(3): 335-340. doi:10.1016/j.jpag.2017.01.002. Erratum in: *J Pediatr Adolesc Gynecol.* 2017 Dec;30(6):665.
8. Agarwal A, Venkat A. Questionnaire study on menstrual disorders in adolescent girls in Singapore. *J Pediatr Adolesc Gynecol.* 2009;22:365-371.
9. Friberg B, Ornö AK, Lindgren A, Lethagen S. Bleeding disorders among young women: a population-based prevalence study. *Acta Obstet Gyn Scan.* 2006;85:200-206.
10. Data and Statistics on von Willebrand Disease. Centers for Disease Control and Prevention. January 16, 2022.
11. James AH. Women and bleeding disorders. *Haemophilia.* 2010;16(suppl 5):160-167.
12. Jaffray J, Young G. Direct oral anticoagulants for use in paediatrics. *Lancet Child Adolesc Health.* 2022;6(3):207-214. doi:10.1016/S2352-4642(21)00343-6
13. Kuter DJ. Treatment of chemotherapy-induced thrombocytopenia in patients with non-hematologic malignancies. *Haematologica.* 2022;107(6):1243-1263. doi:10.3324/haematol.2021.279512
14. Philip C. Platelet disorders in adolescents. *J Pediatr Adol Gyn.* 2010;23:S11.
15. van Eijk AM, Zulaika G, Lenchner M, et al. Menstrual cup use, leakage, acceptability, safety, and availability: a

systematic review and meta-analysis. *Lancet Public Health.* 2019;4(8):e376-e393. doi:10.1016/S2468-2667(19)30111-2

16. Philipp CS, Faiz A, Dowling NF, et al. Development of a screening tool for identifying women with menorrhagia for hemostatic evaluation. *Am J Obstet Gynecol.* 2008;198(2):163.e1-e8. doi:10.1016/j.ajog.2007.08.070

17. ACOG. Clinical, screening and management of bleeding disorders in adolescents with heavy menstrual bleeding. Committee Opinion No 785, September 2019.

18. Borzutzky C, Jaffray J. Diagnosis and management of heavy menstrual bleeding and bleeding disorders in adolescents. *JAMA Pediatr.* 2020;174(2):186-194. doi:10.1001/jamapediatrics.2019.5040

19. Flood VH, Gill JC, Morateck PA, et al. Common VWF exon 28 polymorphisms in African Americans affecting the VWF activity assay by ristocetin cofactor. *Blood.* 2010;116(2):280-286. doi:10.1182/blood-2009-10-249102

20. Moon LM, Perez-Milicua G, Dietrich JE. Evaluation and management of heavy menstrual bleeding in adolescents. *Curr Opin Obstet Gynecol.* 2017;29(5):328-336. doi:10.1097/GCO.0000000000000394

21. Asku F, Madazli R, Budak E, Cepni I, Benian A. High-dose medroxyprogesterone acetate for the treatment of dysfunctional uterine bleeding in 24 adolescents. *Aust NZ J Obstet Gynaecol.* 1997;37:228-231.

22. Munro M, Mainor N, Basu R, Brisinger M, Barreda L. Oral medroxyprogesterone acetate and combination oral contraceptives for acute uterine bleeding, a randomized controlled trial. *Obstet Gynecol.* 2006;108:924-929.

23. Santos M, Hendry D, Sangi-Haghpeykar H, Dietrich JE. Retrospective review of norethindrone use in adolescents. *J Pediatr Adolesc Gynecol.* 2014;27(1):41-44. doi:10.1016/j.jpag.2013.09.002

24. World Health Organization. Haemoglobin concentrations for the diagnosis of anemia and assessment of severity. In: *Vitamin and Mineral Nutrition System.* World Health Organization; 2011.

25. Peyvandi F, Kouides P, Turecek PL, Dow E, Berntorp E. Evolution of replacement therapy for von Willebrand disease: from plasma fraction to recombinant von Willebrand factor. *Blood Rev.* 2019;38:100572. doi:10.1016/j.blre.2019.04.001

26. Kouides PA, Byams VR, Philipp CS, et al. Multisite management study of menorrhagia with abnormal laboratory haemostasis: a prospective crossover study of intranasal desmopressin and oral tranexamic acid. *Br J Haematol.* 2009;145(2):212-220. doi:10.1111/j.1365-2141.2009.07610.x

27. Thorne JG, James PD, Reid RL. Heavy menstrual bleeding: is tranexamic acid a safe adjunct to combined hormonal contraception?. Contraception. 2018;98(1):1-3. doi:10.1016/j.contraception.2018.02.008

28. Teichmann A, Apter D, Emerich J, et al. Continuous, daily levonorgestrel/ethinyl estradiol vs. 21-day, cyclic levonorgestrel/ethinyl estradiol: efficacy, safety and bleeding in a randomized, open-label trial. *Contraception.* 2009;80(6):504-511. doi:10.1016/j.contraception.2009.05.128

29. Kaunitz A, Darney P, Ross D, et al. Subcutaneous DMPA vs. intramuscular DMPA: a 2-year randomized study of contraceptive efficacy and bone mineral density. *Contraception.* 2009;80:7.

30. Lu M, Yang X. Levonorgestrel-releasing intrauterine system for treatment of heavy menstrual bleeding in adolescents with Glanzmann's thrombasthenia: illustrated case series. *BMC Women Health.* 2018;18(1):45. doi:10.1186/s12905-018-0533-0

31. Adeyemi-Fowode OA, Santos XM, Dietrich JE, Srivaths L. Levonorgestrel-releasing intrauterine device use in female adolescents with heavy menstrual bleeding and bleeding disorders: single institution review. *J Pediatr Adolesc Gynecol.* 2017;30(4):479-483. doi:10.1016/j.jpag.2016.04.001

32. Jensen JT, Lukkari-Lax E, Schulze A, Wahdan Y, Serrani M, Kroll R. Contraceptive efficacy and safety of the 52-mg levonorgestrel intrauterine system for up to 8 years: findings from the Mirena Extension Trial. *Am J Obstet Gynecol.* 2022;227(6):873.e1-873.e12. doi:10.1016/j.ajog.2022.09.007

Dysmenorrhea and Endometriosis in the Adolescent Female

Christina Davis-Kankanamge and Alla Vash-Margita

INTRODUCTION

Dysmenorrhea, which is pain associated with menstrual cycles, has a significant impact on the day-to-day functioning of adolescents. This chapter aims to review dysmenorrhea and endometriosis (the most common cause of secondary dysmenorrhea in adolescent females).

DEFINITIONS

- **Dysmenorrhea** is pain associated with menstrual bleeding, often described as abdominal cramps.
- **Primary dysmenorrhea** is the presence of pain before or during cycles without an underlying pathology.
- **Secondary dysmenorrhea** is the presence of pain before or during cycles with an underlying pathology, commonly found to be endometriosis.
- **Endometrial cells** (found normally within the uterus) are located outside of the uterus. Common locations are the ovaries, fallopian tubes, and peritoneum.

PREVALENCE AND EPIDEMIOLOGY

The prevalence rates of dysmenorrhea vary across the globe but range from 16% to 93% of patients who menstruate.[1-4] The prevalence of endometriosis is 10% to 15% in reproductive-age women and 35% to 50% in women with pelvic pain. The true prevalence of endometriosis in adolescents is unknown. A majority of adolescent females with chronic pelvic pain or dysmenorrhea unresponsive to hormonal therapies and nonsteroidal antiinflammatory drugs (NSAIDs) will be diagnosed with endometriosis at the time of diagnostic laparoscopy.[5]

ETIOLOGY AND PATHOPHYSIOLOGY

Dysmenorrhea is subdivided into primary and secondary. We briefly describe primary dysmenorrhea, including pathophysiology, diagnosis, and treatment. Secondary dysmenorrhea, with a primary focus on endometriosis as the most common etiology, is covered in depth in this chapter.

The etiology of dysmenorrhea is poorly understood. Primary dysmenorrhea is primarily linked to two prostaglandins, prostaglandin F2α and prostaglandin E2. The changes in estrogen, progesterone, and prostaglandins levels are thought to trigger an inflammatory cascade that leads to myometrial hypercontractility.[6,7] The resultant hypoxia and ischemia of the uterine muscle thus lead to pain. The increased contractility of the musculature is also thought to be the cause of associated symptoms of nausea and diarrhea.[8]

In order to diagnose primary dysmenorrhea, careful attention to history regarding time of onset, characteristics, locations, and menstrual regularity is necessary. A common history for primary dysmenorrhea is a patient who started menses 1 to 2 years prior with minimal pain, and as the menstrual cycle becomes more predictable, the pain worsens. The pain of primary dysmenorrhea is closely associated with pain 1 to 2 days before menses onset and for the first 2 days, with improvement by the end of menses. Primary dysmenorrhea responds well to NSAIDs or hormonal suppression, or both, and does not have an underlying pathology.[5] To differentiate primary dysmenorrhea from secondary dysmenorrhea, it is key to note how the pain responds to antiinflammatory medications. If there is minimal response or a response followed by worsening pain or debilitating

TABLE 10.1	Variety of Possible Etiologies of Endometriosis			
Sampson's Theory	**Meyer's Theory**	**Halban's Theory**		
Retrograde menstruation	Embryologic totipotent cells	Vascular/lymphatic spread	Deficient cell-mediated immunity	Genetic predisposition
Transport of viable fragments of endometrium through fallopian tubes during menstruation	Cells undergo metaplastic transformation into functional endometrium	Endometrial cells spread via the vascular or lymphatic system, explains remote locations	Deficiency in cellular immunity allows proliferation	Polygenic/multifactorial predisposition, 7× higher greater risk of endometriosis if first-degree relative with endometriosis

pain, it is recommended to then proceed with additional testing and evaluation for secondary dysmenorrhea. The underlying pathology of secondary dysmenorrhea is discussed later. Various potential etiologies of endometriosis are listed in Table 10.1.

CLINICAL PRESENTATION AND EVALUATION FOR ENDOMETRIOSIS

A thorough history, including gynecologic, medical, surgical, and family history, is of paramount importance. Special attention is paid to the menstrual history—onset of menses (menarche), cyclicity, length of menses, and rate of flow (light, moderate, heavy). The onset of pelvic pain should be elicited, with astute attention paid to the fact whether pain has been the same in severity or has been getting worse. The latter may lead to workup for an obstructive müllerian anomaly, characterized by a slow building of the pain progressively with each cycle. The most common clinical presentation of endometriosis in adolescents is pain associated with the menstrual cycle and outside menses, cyclical and noncyclical pain, respectively. The levels and concentrations of active macrophages, interleukin (IL)-1β, IL-6, and IL-8; nerve growth factor (NGF); and other inflammatory factors are increased in peritoneal fluid (PF) and endometriotic lesions in patients with endometriosis.[9-11] These molecular changes contribute to dysmenorrhea, dyspareunia and pelvic pain.[12] Innervation is also altered, namely, there is increased number of total intact nerve fibers, increased sensory and decreased sympathetic nerve fiber density.[13]

In addition to dysmenorrhea, endometriosis is associated with dyspareunia in sexually active adolescents (pain during sexual intercourse), dyschezia (pain on bowel movement), and dysuria (pain on urination). Notably,

adolescent females with endometriosis commonly have both acyclic and cyclic pain in 62.5%, acyclic only in 28.1%, and cyclic only in 9.4%.[14] In the same cohort, the authors described multiple associated symptoms such as gastrointestinal (34.3%), urinary (12.5%), and irregular menses (9.4%). Fibromyalgia and chronic fatigue syndrome were found in 7% and 4%, respectively, in adolescent patients in one study.[15] Other associated symptoms may include migraines, nausea, frequent urination, and changes in bowel movement pattern[16-18] (Table 10.2).

Providers taking care of the adolescent patient presenting with vague complaints of pelvic or abdominal pain must entertain a diagnosis of endometriosis, as there is a notorious delay—up to 12.1 years—in the diagnosis, particularly in adolescent patients.[18-22] Pain characteristics vary, so careful history documentation via a pain dairy is helpful. Either a paper format or web-based application can be useful. Various characteristics of pain are described in Table 10.3. Of note, Wüest and colleagues report that young patients (ages ≤24 years) with clinically diagnosed endometriosis have significantly higher pain scores for dysmenorrhea, dyspareunia, and noncyclic pelvic pain compared with older patients.[23]

As mentioned earlier, various associated symptoms are common. Dun and colleagues describe a case series of 25 females (mean age 17.2 years) with laparoscopically diagnosed endometriosis of which 53% reported at least one genitourinary symptom and 56% reported at least one gastrointestinal symptom. A cross-sectional study reported that adolescents with endometriosis were more likely to experience migraines (69.3%) than those without endometriosis (30.7%).[18] Bowel health plays an important role in the pathophysiology of abdominal pain, especially functional abdominal pain. Functional constipation is highly prevalent in adolescents. A 2021 systematic

TABLE 10.2   Conditions and Symptoms Associated With Endometriosis

	Organ System	Condition/Symptom
Gynecologic		Dysmenorrhea – cyclic pelvic pain associated with menses
		Dyspareunia
		Pelvic pain – acyclic pain not associated with menses
		Vulvodynia
Nongynecologic	Gastrointestinal	Dyschezia (pain with bowel movement)
		Increased or decreased frequency of bowel movement
		Irritable bowel syndrome
		Nausea and/or vomiting
	Urologic	Dysuria (pain with urination)
		Painful bladder syndrome
	Neurologic	Migraines
	Psychological/psychiatric	Anxiety
		Depression
	Rheumatologic	Chronic fatigue syndrome
	Social	Short-term disability (missed work or school)

TABLE 10.3   Description of Pain Associated With Endometriosis

Pelvic and Abdominal Pain in Adolescent Females		Pelvic and Abdominal Pain in Adolescent Females	
Location	Abdomen – mid, upper	Associated symptoms	Constipation
	Lower back		Diarrhea
	Pelvis		Dysuria
	Thighs/lower extremities		Nausea
Severity	Mild, moderate, severe		Vomiting
	Scale of 1–10		Headache
Length/frequency	Minutes		Migraine
	Hours	Provoking factors	Bowel movements
	Days		Menses
	Months		Physical activity
Relation to menses	During or around menses		Sexual activity
	Not associated with menses		Urination
Type	Aching	Alleviating factors	Food intake
	Cramping		Heating pad
	Dull		Medications (variety, doses,
	Electric shock		and frequency)
	Intense		Rest
	Nagging		Sleep
	Pins and needles		Shower/bath
	Sharp		
	Shooting		
	Spasms		
	Splitting		
	Stabbing		
	Tender		
	Throbbing		
	Tingling		
	Tiring or exhausting		

review of functional gastrointestinal disorders (FGIDs) using the Rome IV criteria has demonstrated that functional constipation is the most common functional abdominal pain disorder (FAPD) in children older than age 4 years, with a prevalence of 3% to 28.7%.[24] Because of this high prevalence of FGIDs, routine screening for these conditions is part of the workup in any adolescent patient with pelvic pain.

Physical Examination

The physical examination is comprehensive and includes vital signs, body mass index (BMI) with assessment of growth chart, and overall health. A general examination, including abdominal examination, is performed, with attention paid to abdominal tenderness at rest, with palpation, presence of mass(es), and points of tenderness along the abdominal muscles (trigger points).[25]

In most adolescents, the pelvic examination will be limited to inspection of the external genitalia to assess Tanner stage, anatomy, and level of estrogenation of the vulva and the configuration and patency of the hymen. Speculum and/or digital vaginal examination is deferred in sexually naïve adolescents. If there is suspicion for reproductive tract obstruction (i.e., müllerian anomaly), a rectal abdominal examination may be better tolerated after informed consent is obtained. Additionally, a lubricated cotton swab can be inserted into the vagina to assess the vaginal length and patency. A bimanual pelvic examination assessing for palpable nodularity, thickened uterosacral ligaments, point tenderness in the rectovaginal space, pouch of Douglas, adnexa, and rectosigmoid space is reserved for sexually active females in the late stage of adolescence (ages 18–21 years). Abnormal bimanual examination findings are rare in early-stage endometriosis,[26] which most adolescents will be diagnosed with (stage I and II).[27]

Musculoskeletal etiologies of pelvic pain, including myofascial pain, can be evaluated by palpating for abdominal wall tenderness (e.g., Carnett sign) while asking patient to raise a straight leg. Left lower quadrant tenderness elicited during palpation should raise concern for constipation. In many cases abdominal examination and external inspection of the genitalia will not reveal any abnormalities.

Laboratory Assessment

Currently there are no approved specific blood tests or noninvasive biomarkers in the United States to identify endometriosis. Active ongoing research is directed toward the identification of noninvasive biomarkers such as CA-125, microRNAs, menstrual effluent, and proteomics.[28-32]

In specific cases if there is a suspicion for an inflammatory process, a complete blood count (CBC) or erythrocyte sedimentation rate (ESR) may be obtained. In adolescents with bowel symptoms such as diarrhea, bloating, constipation, abdominal pain, or weight loss, laboratory evaluation may include workup for celiac disease with tissue transglutaminase and endomysial and deamidated gliadin peptide antibodies.[33] If there are any symptoms associated with bladder function, urinalysis or urine culture should be obtained. In sexually active teens, a urine pregnancy test and/or sexually transmitted infection testing is indicated, specifically, nucleic acid amplification test (NAAT) for *Chlamydia trachomatis* and *Neisseria gonorrhoeae*. It should be noted that at this time there are no approved specific blood tests or markers to identify endometriosis in clinical practice in the United States.

Imaging Techniques and Findings

Transabdominal ultrasound (US) is the preferred modality for the evaluation of pelvic organs in adolescent females. The yield of detecting endometriosis is not high. According to a retrospective observational study, two-dimensional (2D), three-dimensional (3D), and power Doppler US pelvic examination (transvaginal or transrectal in pre–sexually active adolescents) identified at least one ultrasound feature of endometriosis in 36 (13.3%) of 270 cases.[34] Ovarian endometriomas were found in 22 (11%) patients, adenomyosis in 16 (5.2%), and deep infiltrating endometriosis (DIE) in 10 (3.7%).[34]

Comparison of the diagnostic accuracy of 2D and 3D transvaginal US in comparison with magnetic resonance imaging (MRI) for identification of DIE in one prospective observational study (albeit in women older than 18 years of age) showed that there was a statistically significant difference between 2D US and MRI for the intestinal location of DIE, whereas no differences were found among the techniques for the other locations (retrocervical septum, rectovaginal septum, uterosacral ligaments, and vaginal fornix).[35] There are no studies analyzing MRI utility in the diagnosis of endometriosis in adolescent females. Thus endometriosis remains predominantly a clinical diagnosis, with imaging studies reserved for cases in which structural anomalies are suspected and the standard treatment course is unsuccessful.

CLASSIC SIGNS

The 3 Ds: Dysmenorrhea/Dyschezia/Dyspareunia

Differential Diagnosis of Pelvic Pain in Adolescents

The differential diagnosis of endometriosis is extensive and is usually grouped into gynecologic and nongynecologic causes, with the latter including gastrointestinal, genitourinary, musculoskeletal, and psychological origins (Table 10.4). There may be a cross-section of a few diagnoses, and a multidisciplinary approach to diagnosis should be pursued.

MANAGEMENT/TREATMENT OPTIONS

Lifestyle Modifications and Medical Management

The management of dysmenorrhea should start with education and assessment of measures taken before presentation to relieve pain. Evidence shows that providing educational material on the physiology of the menstrual cycle, the best time to start and continue an analgesic, the necessity for taking the medication on a regular basis (not as-needed), and the selection of the most appropriate analgesic

drug improves the control of dysmenorrhea.[36-38] If poor posture and/or hypertonicity in the abdominal wall is suspected or diagnosed, physical therapy should be directed at the myofascial pain component such as trigger point injections with local anesthetics and/or corticosteroids.

First-line treatment for primary or secondary dysmenorrhea is NSAIDs.[5,39] Second-line treatment of the various formulations of hormonal preparations in the form of pills, patch, or a vaginal ring exists and has been used as treatment for dysmenorrhea associated with endometriosis (Table 10.5). The treatment approach should be tailored to individual needs. For example, in a patient who has not used tampons, a vaginal ring is probably not a viable option. Symptoms may recur if hormonal suppression is discontinued.

Third-line therapy may include gonadotropin-releasing hormone (GnRH) agonists (leuprolide acetate) or antagonist (elagolix), although both formulations are approved only for adolescents 18 years or older. There are scarce data on the effects of leuprolide acetate treatment in adolescents younger than 18 years. One study described positive effects of a treatment regimen of a GnRH agonist combined with add-back therapy in teens with mean age 17.9 years, including teens as young as

TABLE 10.4	**Differential Diagnosis of Pelvic Pain in Adolescents**			
Gastrointestinal	**Genitourinary**	**Musculoskeletal**	**Psychological**	**Gynecologic**
Appendicitis	Calculi	Bone and joint inflammation	Abuse (physical, emotional, sexual)	Adenomyosis[a]
Abdominal migraine/ functional abdominal pain	Cystitis	Congenital anomalies	Anxiety	Adnexal torsion
	Painful bladder syndrome	Fibromyalgia	Depression	Bartholin cyst abscess
Cholecystitis/ cholangitis	Pyelonephritis	Nerve entrapment	Somatization	Cysts – ovarian and paraovarian
Constipation	Ureteral obstruction	Pelvic orthopedic trauma	Substance abuse	Ectopic pregnancy
Diverticular disease	Ureteral diverticulum/polyp	Pelvic floor dysfunction		Endometriosis
Gastric ulcer		Tumors[a]		Endometrial polyp[a]
Gastritis				Hydrosalpinx/pyosalpinx
Inflammatory bowel disease				Lichen sclerosus
Irritable bowel syndrome				Leiomyomas[a]
Meckel diverticulum				Mittelschmerz
Mesenteric adenitis				Müllerian anomalies: obstructive and nonobstructive
				Pelvic inflammatory disease/tubo-ovarian abscess
				Vaginismus
				Vaginitis
				Vulvodynia

[a]Rare in adolescent age group.

TABLE 10.5 Treatment Modalities		
Estrogen-Progesterone–Containing Preparations[a]	Progesterone-Containing Preparations	Nonhormonal Preparations

• Pill: 20–35 mcg ethynyl estradiol (EE) + various progestins
• Patch: 0.30–0.35 mcg EE + various progestins
• Vaginal ring: 0.013–0.015 mg EE + various progestins
	• Norethindrone 0.35 mg[c]
	• Norethindrone acetate 5 mg, 10 mg (up to 20 mg PO/day)
	• Medroxyprogesterone acetate 150 mg IM q3mo[a,c]
	• Intrauterine system (IUS): levonorgestrel, various dosing regimens
		• GnRH agonists[b]:
		  Leuprolide acetate: 11.25 mg intramuscular injection every 3 mo or 3.75 mg intramuscular injection every month with add-back therapy: norethindrone acetate 5 mg daily
		  Nafarelin: nasal spray 400 μg per day
		• GnRH antagonist[b]:
		  Elagolix: 150 mg by mouth every day or 200 mg by mouth twice per day

[a]Risk of venous thrombotic event.
[b]Approved by the US Food and Drug Administration (FDA) for patients 18 years of age and older.
[c]Approved for birth control by FDA.
^^ [d]Only add-back therapy approved by the FDA.
GnRH, Gonadotropin-releasing hormone.

15.4 years. Importantly, add-back therapy in a form of norethindrone acetate or norethindrone acetate 5 mg daily plus conjugated equine estrogens 0.625 mg daily is usually offered because of concern of short-term side effects such as mood swings, hot flushes, and weight gain and long-term side effects, namely effects on bone mineral density if used over 6 months or longer.[40,41]

Just as during the diagnostic process, a multidisciplinary approach may be necessary during the treatment of endometriosis. Neuropathic medications (amitriptyline, serotonin-noradrenaline reuptake inhibitors, anticonvulsants, citalopram, imipramine, venlafaxine) have been used to treat chronic pelvic pain. A recent systematic review reported that most of the studies analyzed have shown pain improvement with the help of neuromodulators for chronic pain. However, no improvement was found in the study with the highest statistical power.[42] It is important to note that the majority of these studies addressed adult women with endometriosis.

Cognitive behavioral treatment and mindfulness training have been used in patients with chronic pelvic pain and endometriosis with positive results.[43,44] Transcutaneous electrical nerve stimulation (TENS) has been used for primary dysmenorrhea in adolescent patients ages 14 to 19 years with significant reduction of pain between the intervention group and control.[45] Acupuncture has been used as a means to alleviate dysmenorrhea. Currently, there are no large studies that address acupuncture as a treatment modality for pelvic pain in adolescents other than a few case reports. Only a few randomized, blinded clinical trials have addressed the efficacy of acupuncture in treating endometriosis-related pain. A meta-analysis by Xu and colleagues compared the variation in pain between the acupuncture and control groups and showed that acupuncture had a positive effect on the primary pain level as compared with the control groups.[46] As a result, this therapy could be applied as a complementary treatment for endometriosis-related pain.

Surgical Approach

Diagnostic laparoscopy is still considered the gold standard of diagnosis, as it yields a peritoneal biopsy with histologic diagnosis. However, this paradigm has been challenged, especially within the adolescent patient.[47]

When should the provider offer diagnostic laparoscopy? Or in other words, when is the patient likely to proceed with surgery? In one study that included adolescents older than 18 years, the authors concluded that older age (20–29 years), severe dysmenorrhea, a failed trial of hormonal treatment, a previous diagnosis of endometriosis, and previous abdominal or pelvic surgery were associated with scheduled surgery.[48]

Laparoscopy[49] may be offered to a patient with chronic pelvic pain as the next diagnostic modality if a conservative approach fails or the patient and guardian desire a definitive diagnosis.[49] Laparoscopy may establish the presence of the disease or refute it. It is important to emphasize that laparoscopy does not carry an absolute diagnostic utility: if histopathology was used as the gold standard, sensitivity for laparoscopic visualization was 90.1%, whereas specificity was 40.0% in a study conducted in adult women, with positive and negative predictive values of 81.0% and 58.8%, respectively, and the accuracy was 77%.[50] During surgery, a comprehensive survey of the pelvis and abdomen is recommended with visualization of the appendix as well as destruction of the visible implants via electrocautery, endocoagulation, laser ablation, or excision. Biopsy of the suspicious peritoneal lesions should be undertaken. The operator should be proficient in identifying endometriotic lesions, as these may appear as atypical small, 1- to 3-mm, clear, vesicular lesions scattered throughout the peritoneal lining (Figs. 10.1–10.3).[51] During surgery, the size and location of the endometriotic lesions are documented, thereby assigning the stage of the endometriosis as I to IV according to the revised classification of endometriosis by the American Society for Reproductive Medicine (Fig. 10.4).[26]

There is also an app for staging endometriosis from AAGL that can serve as a useful tool to document intraoperative findings: https://play.google.com/store/apps/details?id=br.com.medicinia.aagl&hl=en_US&gl=US&pli=1. According to a recent Cochrane review, there is very low-quality evidence that laparoscopic excision and ablation are similarly effective in relieving pain (only one study).[52] The same review offered no conclusion as to which laparoscopic surgical intervention is most effective and whether holistic or medical treatment modalities are more effective than laparoscopic surgery with regard to the treatment of severe endometriosis. Although laparoscopy has been considered the gold standard for the diagnosis of endometriosis to date, this recommendation has been challenged because of recent

evidence that the vast majority (92.2%) of adolescent patients with pelvic pain had improvement in symptoms after conservative treatment.[47]

Current evidence does not support the use of radical excisional surgery ("peritoneal stripping"—a technique described in adult women) for superficial endometriosis, as it may increase extensive adhesive formation. As such, peritoneal stripping should not be used in the adolescent population. Furthermore, at present there is no study that shows superiority of the laparoscopic technique for the treatment of superficial peritoneal disease. A trial of

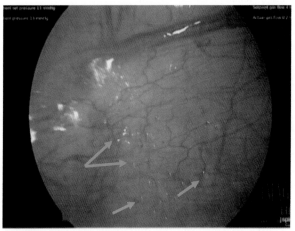

Fig. 10.2 Endometriotic lesions in a 15-year-old patient with pelvic pain: clear 1- to 2-mm vesicular lesions scattered over the peritoneum *(blue arrows)*. (Courtesy Alla Vash-Margita, MD.)

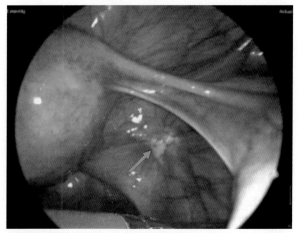

Fig. 10.1 Endometriotic lesions in a 19-year-old patient with pelvic pain: "powder-burn" lesion over the right uterosacral ligament *(blue arrow)*. (Courtesy Alla Vash-Margita, MD.)

Fig. 10.3 Calcified endometriotic lesion in an 18-year-old patient with pelvic pain: right posterior cul-de-sac *(blue arrow)*. (Courtesy Alla Vash-Margita, MD.)

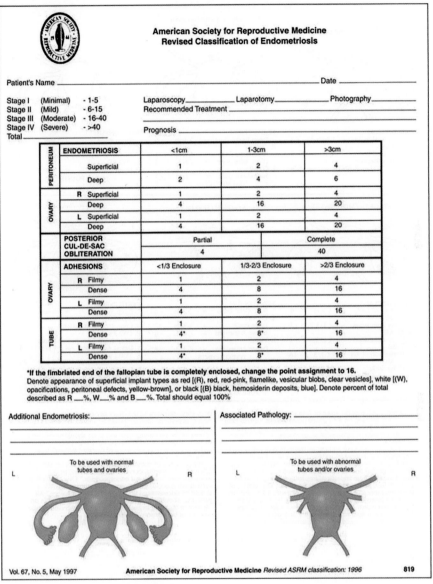

American Society for Reproductive Medicine
Revised Classification of Endometriosis

Patient's Name _____ Date _____

Stage I (Minimal) - 1-5
Stage II (Mild) - 6-15
Stage III (Moderate) - 16-40
Stage IV (Severe) - >40
Total _____

Laparoscopy _____ Laparotomy _____ Photography _____
Recommended Treatment _____
_____
Prognosis _____

PERITONEUM	ENDOMETRIOSIS	<1cm	1-3cm	>3cm
	Superficial	1	2	4
	Deep	2	4	6
OVARY	R Superficial	1	2	4
	Deep	4	16	20
	L Superficial	1	2	4
	Deep	4	16	20
	POSTERIOR CUL-DE-SAC OBLITERATION	Partial		Complete
		4		40
	ADHESIONS	<1/3 Enclosure	1/3-2/3 Enclosure	>2/3 Enclosure
OVARY	R Filmy	1	2	4
	Dense	4	8	16
	L Filmy	1	2	4
	Dense	4	8	16
TUBE	R Filmy	1	2	4
	Dense	4*	8*	16
	L Filmy	1	2	4
	Dense	4*	8*	16

*If the fimbriated end of the fallopian tube is completely enclosed, change the point assignment to 16.
Denote appearance of superficial implant types as red [(R), red, red-pink, flamelike, vesicular blobs, clear vesicles], white [(W), opacifications, peritoneal defects, yellow-brown], or black [(B) black, hemosiderin deposits, blue]. Denote percent of total described as R ___%, W ___% and B ___%. Total should equal 100%

Additional Endometriosis: _____

Associated Pathology: _____

L   To be used with normal
tubes and ovaries   R

L   To be used with abnormal
tubes and/or ovaries   R

Vol. 67, No. 5, May 1997   American Society for Reproductive Medicine *Revised ASRM classification: 1996*   819

Fig. 10.4 Revised classification of endometriosis. (From American Society for Reproductive Medicine: Revised American Society for Reproductive Medicine classification of endometriosis: 1996. Fertility and Sterility Volume 67, Issue 5, May 1997, Pages 817-821.)[26]

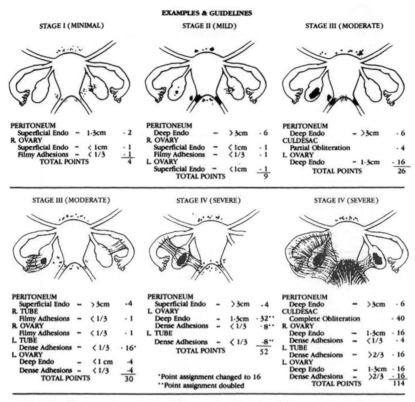

EXAMPLES & GUIDELINES

STAGE I (MINIMAL)	STAGE II (MILD)	STAGE III (MODERATE)

PERITONEUM
Superficial Endo – 1-3cm – 2
R. OVARY
Superficial Endo – < 1cm – 1
Filmy Adhesions – < 1/3 – 1
TOTAL POINTS   4

PERITONEUM
Deep Endo – > 3cm – 6
R. OVARY
Superficial Endo – < 1cm – 1
Filmy Adhesions – < 1/3 – 1
L. OVARY
Superficial Endo – < 1cm – 1
TOTAL POINTS   9

PERITONEUM
Deep Endo – > 3cm – 6
CULDESAC
Partial Obliteration   – 4
L. OVARY
Deep Endo – 1-3cm – 16
TOTAL POINTS   26

STAGE III (MODERATE)	STAGE IV (SEVERE)	STAGE IV (SEVERE)

PERITONEUM
Superficial Endo – > 3cm –4
R. TUBE
Filmy Adhesions – < 1/3 – 1
R. OVARY
Filmy Adhesions – < 1/3 – 1
L. TUBE
Dense Adhesions – < 1/3 – 16*
L. OVARY
Deep Endo – < 1 cm –4
Dense Adhesions – < 1/3 –4
TOTAL POINTS   30

PERITONEUM
Superficial Endo – > 3cm –4
L. OVARY
Deep Endo – 1-3cm – 32**
Dense Adhesions – < 1/3 –8**
L. TUBE
Dense Adhesions – < 1/3 –8**
TOTAL POINTS   52

PERITONEUM
Deep Endo – > 3cm – 6
CULDESAC
Complete Obliteration   – 40
R. OVARY
Deep Endo – 1-3cm – 16
Dense Adhesions – < 1/3 – 4
L. TUBE
Dense Adhesions – > 2/3 – 16
L. OVARY
Deep Endo – 1-3cm – 16
Dense Adhesions – > 2/3 – 16
TOTAL POINTS   114

*Point assignment changed to 16
**Point assignment doubled

Determination of the stage or degree of endometrial involvement is based on a weighted point system. Distribution of points has been arbitrarily determined and may require further revision or refinement as knowledge of the disease increases.

To ensure complete evaluation, inspection of the pelvis in a clockwise or counterclockwise fashion is encouraged. Number, size and location of endometrial implants, plaques, endometriomas and/or adhesions are noted. For example, five separate 0.5cm superficial implants on the peritoneum (2.5 cm total) would be assigned 2 points. (The surface of the uterus should be considered peritoneum.) The severity of the endometriosis or adhesions should be assigned the highest score only for peritoneum, ovary, tube or culdesac. For example, a 4cm superficial and a 2cm deep implant of the peritoneum should be given a score of 6 (not 8). A 4cm

deep endometrioma of the ovary associated with more than 3cm of superficial disease should be scored 20 (not 24).

In those patients with only one adnexa, points applied to disease of the remaining tube and ovary should be multiplied by two. **Points assigned may be circled and totaled. Aggregation of points indicates stage of disease (minimal, mild, moderate, or severe).

The presence of endometriosis of the bowel, urinary tract, fallopian tube, vagina, cervix, skin etc., should be documented under "additional endometriosis." Other pathology such as tubal occlusion, leiomyomata, uterine anomaly, etc., should be documented under "associated pathology." All pathology should be depicted as specifically as possible on the sketch of pelvic organs, and means of observation (laparoscopy or laparotomy) should be noted.

Fig. 10.4   cont'd.

hormonal management using combined hormonal or progestin-only therapy is advised for adolescents dealing with primary dysmenorrhea symptoms. It is worth considering the duration of the hormonal management trial and the persistence of symptoms. If a patient does not respond to medical management after 3 to 6 months of therapy, the primary approach is to proceed to laparoscopy for diagnosing and treating endometriosis. The timing of laparoscopy may depend on symptom severity and its impact on school and daily activities. Without a definitive diagnosis, adolescents and their families may

be distressed, and the potential improvement in pain symptoms postoperatively might be desirable. For patients who wish to avoid surgery, a presumptive clinical diagnosis of endometriosis can be considered through a combination of history, examination, and imaging. A clinical diagnosis may be warranted if a conversion from cyclic hormonal therapy to continuous hormonal therapy (e.g., decreasing withdrawal bleeds) is needed for optimal symptom management. Since adolescence is a time of peak bone accrual, it's not recommended to empirically use GnRH agonists in adolescents without a definitive diagnosis of endometriosis and failure of first-line hormonal management.[53]

SPECIAL CONSIDERATIONS FOR POPULATIONS WITH PELVIC PAIN AND/OR ENDOMETRIOSIS

Mental Health

Mental health conditions among adolescents with chronic pelvic pain are common. Smorgick and colleagues reported on comorbid pain syndromes in 56% of adolescents and young women who were less than age 24 years, as well as mood conditions (defined as anxiety and/or depression) in 48% of women.[15] In another study that compared women with endometriosis with those without, the adjusted hazard ratios and 95% confidence intervals were 1.38 (1.34, 1.42) for anxiety, 1.48 (1.44, 1.53) for depression, and 2.03 (1.60, 2.58) for self-directed violence; in addition, association with depression was stronger among women with endometriosis younger than 35 years.[54] Furthermore, in a large population-based study, Gao and colleagues investigated psychiatric comorbidities among women with endometriosis, including adolescents.[55] The authors demonstrated that after adjustment for birth characteristics and education, women with endometriosis had an increased risk of being diagnosed with depression, anxiety and stress-related disorders, alcohol/drug dependence, and attention-deficit/hyperactivity disorder compared with the general population and with their sisters without endometriosis.[55]

Abuse

In addition to a higher prevalence of psychiatric disorders among adolescents and adult women with endometriosis, studies show that early-life sexual and physical abuse is associated with an increased risk of endometriosis. Severity, chronicity, and accumulation of types of abuse are associated with greater risk.[56] In terms of the mechanisms underlying the association between abuse and endometriosis, the current literature suggests that early traumatic experiences induce persistent sensitization of the central stress response systems, including dysregulation of the hypothalamic-pituitary-adrenal (HPA) axis with resultant persistent lack of cortisol availability in traumatized or chronically stressed individuals. This may lead to an increased vulnerability for the development of stress-related bodily disorders.[57,58]

Trans male Individuals

Emerging evidence describes endometriosis in trans-male individuals. Endometriosis should be suspected in transmale people with pelvic pain even when the use of cross-hormone treatment is present.[59]

Research Gaps

At the present time there are no reliable diagnostic tools for endometriosis in adolescent females. Adolescents represent an underserved population with high morbidity and significant social impact.[51] Current and future research should place emphasis on the development of noninvasive biomarkers in adolescents and adult women and evaluation of the most effective treatment modalities.[60] Clarification of the etiology would be beneficial. Evaluation of the outcomes and/or success rates for surgical or medical treatments that aim to cure endometriosis, rather than manage it, should also be the focus of research.

ACKNOWLEDGMENTS

The authors would like to acknowledge the support of Alyssa Grimshaw, MSLIS, Harvey Cushing/John Hay Whitney Medical Library, Yale University.

KEY POINTS

- Careful history and physical examination are the main modalities of the diagnosis of dysmenorrhea and/or endometriosis in the adolescent female.
- Pelvic examination is reserved for the external inspection of the external genitalia with avoidance of the bimanual examination in sexually naïve patients.
- At this time, there is no laboratory test that is approved for the diagnosis of endometriosis in clinical practice in the United States.
- Referral to pain clinic and/or psychologist, lifestyle modification, physical therapy, and acupuncture may serve as adjunct treatment for chronic pelvic pain and/or endometriosis.
- NSAIDs and various hormonal preparations are the main treatment modalities for chronic pelvic pain and/or endometriosis.
- In adolescents, consider performing a laparoscopy to diagnose and treat endometriosis, with the timing influenced by the severity of the symptoms and responsiveness to medical treatment.

REVIEW QUESTIONS

1. Dysmenorrhea can lead to:
   a. Functional impairment
   b. Increased productivity at work
   c. Fertility issues
   d. Endometrial cancer
2. Endometriosis is found in which body parts?
   a. Abdominal cavity
   b. Bladder
   c. Surface of ovary
   d. Lung
   e. All of the above
3. What is the first-line treatment for suspected endometriosis in an adolescent patient?
   a. Diagnostic laparoscopy
   b. GnRH antagonist
   c. NSAIDs
   d. Oral contraceptive pill

REFERENCES

1. Hadjou OK, Jouannin A, Lavoue V, Leveque J, Esvan M, Bidet M. Prevalence of dysmenorrhea in adolescents in France: results of a large cross-sectional study. *J Gynecol Obstet Hum Reprod.* 2022;51(3):102302. doi:10.1016/j.jogoh.2021.102302
2. Banikarim C, Chacko MR, Kelder SH. Prevalence and impact of dysmenorrhea on Hispanic female adolescents. *Arch Pediatr Adolesc Med.* 2000;154(12):1226-1229. doi:10.1001/archpedi.154.12.1226
3. Hillen TI, Grbavac SL, Johnston PJ, Straton JA, Keogh JM. Primary dysmenorrhea in young Western Australian women: prevalence, impact, and knowledge of treatment. *J Adolesc Health.* 1999;25(1):40-45. doi:10.1016/s1054-139x(98)00147-5
4. De Sanctis V, Soliman A, Bernasconi S, et al. Primary dysmenorrhea in adolescents: prevalence, impact and recent knowledge. *Pediatr Endocrinol Rev.* 2015;13(2):512-520.
5. ACOG. ACOG committee opinion no. 760: dysmenorrhea and endometriosis in the adolescent. *Obstet Gynecol.* 2018;132(6):e249-e258. doi:10.1097/aog.0000000000002978
6. Monsivais D, Dyson MT, Yin P, et al. ERβ- and prostaglandin E2-regulated pathways integrate cell proliferation via Ras-like and estrogen-regulated growth inhibitor in endometriosis. *Mol Endocrinol.* 2014;28(8):1304-1315. doi:10.1210/me.2013-1421
7. Bulun SE, Yilmaz BD, Sison C, et al. Endometriosis. *Endocr Rev.* 2019;40(4):1048-1079. doi:10.1210/er.2018-00242
8. Kho KA, Shields JK. Diagnosis and management of primary dysmenorrhea. *JAMA.* 2020;323(3):268-269. doi:10.1001/jama.2019.16921
9. Zhang T, De Carolis C, Man GCW, Wang CC. The link between immunity, autoimmunity and endometriosis: a literature update. *Autoimmun Rev.* 2018;17(10):945-955. doi:10.1016/j.autrev.2018.03.017
10. Yu J, Francisco AMC, Patel BG, et al. IL-1β stimulates brain-derived neurotrophic factor production in eutopic endometriosis stromal cell cultures: a model for cytokine regulation of neuroangiogenesis. *Am J Pathol.* 2018;188(10):2281-2292. doi:10.1016/j.ajpath.2018.06.011
11. Arnold J, Barcena de Arellano ML, Rüster C, et al. Imbalance between sympathetic and sensory innervation in peritoneal endometriosis. *Brain Behav Immun.* 2012;26(1):132-141. doi:10.1016/j.bbi.2011.08.004
12. Tai FW, Chang CY, Chiang JH, Lin WC, Wan L. Association of pelvic inflammatory disease with risk of endometriosis: a nationwide cohort study involving 141,460 individuals. *J Clin Med.* 2018;7(11):379. doi:10.3390/jcm7110379
13. Wang G, Tokushige N, Markham R, Fraser IS. Rich innervation of deep infiltrating endometriosis. *Hum Reprod.* 2009;24(4):827-834. doi:10.1093/humrep/den464
14. Laufer MR, Goitein L, Bush M, Cramer DW, Emans SJ. Prevalence of endometriosis in adolescent girls with chronic pelvic pain not responding to conventional therapy. *J Pediatr Adolesc Gynecol.* 1997;10(4):199-202. doi:10.1016/s1083-3188(97)70085-8
15. Smorgick N, Marsh CA, As-Sanie S, Smith YR, Quint EH. Prevalence of pain syndromes, mood conditions, and asthma in adolescents and young women with endometriosis. *J Pediatr Adolesc Gynecol.* 2013;26(3):171-175. doi:10.1016/j.jpag.2012.12.006
16. DiVasta AD, Vitonis AF, Laufer MR, Missmer SA. Spectrum of symptoms in women diagnosed with endometriosis during adolescence vs adulthood. *Am J Obstet Gynecol.* 2018;218(3):324.e1-324.e11. doi:10.1016/j.ajog.2017.12.007
17. Miller JA, Missmer SA, Vitonis AF, Sarda V, Laufer MR, DiVasta AD. Prevalence of migraines in adolescents with endometriosis. *Fertil Steril.* 2018;109(4):685-690. doi:10.1016/j.fertnstert.2017.12.016
18. Dun EC, Kho KA, Morozov VV, Kearney S, Zurawin JL, Nezhat CH. Endometriosis in adolescents. *JSLS.* 2015;19(2):e2015.00019. doi:10.4293/jsls.2015.00019
19. Ballweg ML. Big picture of endometriosis helps provide guidance on approach to teens: comparative historical data show endo starting younger, is more severe. *J Pediatr Adolesc Gynecol.* 2003;16(suppl 3):S21-S26. doi:10.1016/s1083-3188(03)00063-9

20. Ballard K, Lowton K, Wright J. What's the delay? A qualitative study of women's experiences of reaching a diagnosis of endometriosis. *Fertil Steril.* 2006;86(5):1296-1301. doi:10.1016/j.fertnstert.2006.04.054

21. Hudelist G, Fritzer N, Thomas A, et al. Diagnostic delay for endometriosis in Austria and Germany: causes and possible consequences. *Hum Reprod.* 2012;27(12): 3412-3416. doi:10.1093/humrep/des316

22. Arruda MS, Petta CA, Abrão MS, Benetti-Pinto CL. Time elapsed from onset of symptoms to diagnosis of endometriosis in a cohort study of Brazilian women. *Hum Reprod.* 2003;18(4):756-759. doi:10.1093/humrep/deg136

23. Wüest A, Limacher JM, Dingeldein I, et al. Pain levels of women diagnosed with endometriosis: is there a difference in younger women? *J Pediatr Adolesc Gynecol.* 2023;36(2):140-147. doi:10.1016/j.jpag.2022.10.011

24. Vernon-Roberts A, Alexander I, Day AS. Systematic review of pediatric functional gastrointestinal disorders (Rome IV Criteria). *J Clin Med.* 2021;10(21):5087. doi:10.3390/jcm10215087

25. Ross V, Detterman C, Hallisey A. Myofascial pelvic pain: an overlooked and treatable cause of chronic pelvic pain. *J Midwifery Womens Health.* 2021;66(2):148-160. doi:10.1111/jmwh.13224

26. Revised American Society for Reproductive Medicine classification of endometriosis: 1996. *Fertil Steril.* 1997;67(5):817-821. doi:10.1016/s0015-0282(97)81391-x

27. Hirsch M, Dhillon-Smith R, Cutner AS, Yap M, Creighton SM. The prevalence of endometriosis in adolescents with pelvic pain: a systematic review. *J Pediatr Adolesc Gynecol.* 2020;33(6):623-630. doi:10.1016/j.jpag.2020.07.011

28. Nisenblat V, Prentice L, Bossuyt PM, Farquhar C, Hull ML, Johnson N. Combination of the non-invasive tests for the diagnosis of endometriosis. *Cochrane Database Syst Rev.* 2016;7(7):CD012281. doi:10.1002/14651858.Cd012281

29. Dabi Y, Suisse S, Puchar A, et al. Endometriosis-associated infertility diagnosis based on saliva microRNA signatures. *Reprod Biomed Online.* 2023;46(1):138-149. doi:10.1016/j.rbmo.2022.09.019

30. Bendifallah S, Suisse S, Puchar A, et al. Salivary microRNA signature for diagnosis of endometriosis. *J Clin Med.* 2022;11(3):612. doi:10.3390/jcm11030612

31. Anastasiu CV, Moga MA, Elena Neculau A, et al. Biomarkers for the noninvasive diagnosis of endometriosis: state of the art and future perspectives. *Int J Mol Sci.* 2020;21(5):1750. doi:10.3390/ijms21051750

32. Warren LA, Shih A, Renteira SM, et al. Analysis of menstrual effluent: diagnostic potential for endometriosis. *Mol Med.* 2018;24(1):1. doi:10.1186/s10020-018-0009-6

33. Caio G, Volta U, Sapone A, et al. Celiac disease: a comprehensive current review. *BMC Med.* 2019;17(1):142. doi:10.1186/s12916-019-1380-z

34. Martire FG, Lazzeri L, Conway F, et al. Adolescence and endometriosis: symptoms, ultrasound signs and early diagnosis. *Fertil Steril.* 2020;114(5):1049-1057. doi:10.1016/j.fertnstert.2020.06.012

35. Guerriero S, Alcázar JL, Pascual MA, et al. Deep infiltrating endometriosis: comparison between 2-dimensional ultrasonography (US), 3-dimensional US, and magnetic resonance imaging. *J Ultrasound Med.* 2018;37(6):1511-1521. doi:10.1002/jum.14496

36. Jung HS, Lee J. The effectiveness of an educational intervention on proper analgesic use for dysmenorrhea. *Eur J Obstet Gynecol Reprod Biol.* 2013;170(2):480-486. doi:10.1016/j.ejogrb.2013.07.004

37. Dawood MY, Khan-Dawood FS. Clinical efficacy and differential inhibition of menstrual fluid prostaglandin F2alpha in a randomized, double-blind, crossover treatment with placebo, acetaminophen, and ibuprofen in primary dysmenorrhea. *Am J Obstet Gynecol.* 2007;196(1):35.e1-e5. doi:10.1016/j.ajog.2006.06.091

38. Harel Z. Dysmenorrhea in adolescents and young adults: etiology and management. *J Pediatr Adolesc Gynecol.* 2006;19(6):363-371. doi:10.1016/j.jpag.2006.09.001

39. Marjoribanks J, Ayeleke RO, Farquhar C, Proctor M. Nonsteroidal anti-inflammatory drugs for dysmenorrhoea. *Cochrane Database Syst Rev.* 2015;2015(7):CD001751. doi:10.1002/14651858.CD001751.pub3

40. Sadler Gallagher J, Feldman HA, Stokes NA, et al. The effects of gonadotropin-releasing hormone agonist combined with add-back therapy on quality of life for adolescents with endometriosis: a randomized controlled trial. *J Pediatr Adolesc Gynecol.* 2017;30(2):215-222. doi:10.1016/j.jpag.2016.02.008

41. DiVasta AD, Feldman HA, Sadler Gallagher J, et al. Hormonal add-back therapy for females treated with gonadotropin-releasing hormone agonist for endometriosis: a randomized controlled trial. *Obstet Gynecol.* 2015;126(3):617-627. doi:10.1097/aog.0000000000000964

42. Andrade MA, Soares LC, Oliveira MAP. Efeito de neuromoduladores na intensidade da dor pélvica crônica em mulheres: revisão sistemática. [The effect of neuromodulatory drugs on the intensity of chronic pelvic pain in women: a systematic review.] *Rev Bras Ginecol Obstet.* 2022;44(9):891-898. doi:10.1055/s-0042-1755459

43. Boersen Z, de Kok L, van der Zanden M, Braat D, Oosterman J, Nap A. Patients' perspective on cognitive behavioural therapy after surgical treatment of endometriosis: a qualitative study. *Reprod Biomed Online.* 2021;42(4):819-825. doi:10.1016/j.rbmo.2021.01.010

44. Mikocka-Walus A, Druitt M, O'Shea M, et al. Yoga, cognitive-behavioural therapy versus education to improve quality of life and reduce healthcare costs in people with endometriosis: a randomised controlled

trial. *BMJ Open*. 2021;11(8):e046603. doi:10.1136/bmjopen-2020-046603

45. Manisha U, Anuradha L. Effect of high frequency transcutaneous electrical nerve stimulation at root level menstrual pain in primary dysmenorrhea. *J Bodyw Mov Ther*. 2021;26:108-112. doi:10.1016/j.jbmt.2020.12.025

46. Xu Y, Zhao W, Li T, Zhao Y, Bu H, Song S. Effects of acupuncture for the treatment of endometriosis-related pain: a systematic review and meta-analysis. *PLoS One*. 2017;12(10):e0186616. doi:10.1371/journal.pone.0186616

47. Sachedina A, Abu Bakar M, Dunford AM, Morris A, Nur Azurah AG, Grover SR. Dysmenorrhea in young people: experiences from a tertiary center with a focus on conservative management. *J Obstet Gynaecol Res*. 2021;47(1):352-358. doi:10.1111/jog.14532

48. Mirowska-Allen KL, Sewell M, Mooney S, Maher P, Ianno DJ, Grover SR. The characteristics of women recommended a laparoscopy for chronic pelvic pain at a tertiary institution. *Aust N Z J Obstet Gynaecol*. 2019;59(1):123-133. doi:10.1111/ajo.12836

49. Becker CM, Bokor A, Heikinheimo O, et al. ESHRE guideline: endometriosis. *Hum Reprod Open*. 2022;2022(2):hoac009. doi:10.1093/hropen/hoac009

50. Gratton SM, Choudhry AJ, Vilos GA, et al. Diagnosis of endometriosis at laparoscopy: a validation study comparing surgeon visualization with histologic findings. *J Obstet Gynaecol Can*. 2022;44(2):135-141. doi:10.1016/j.jogc.2021.08.013

51. Shah DK, Missmer SA. Scientific investigation of endometriosis among adolescents. *J Pediatr Adolesc Gynecol*. 2011;24(suppl 5):S18-S19. doi:10.1016/j.jpag.2011.07.008

52. Bafort C, Beebeejaun Y, Tomassetti C, Bosteels J, Duffy JM. Laparoscopic surgery for endometriosis. *Cochrane Database Syst Rev*. 2020;10(10):CD011031. doi:10.1002/14651858.CD011031.pub3

53. Shim JY, Laufer MR, King CR, Lee TTM, Einarsson JI, Tyson N. Evaluation and Management of Endometriosis in the Adolescent. *Obstet Gynecol*. 2024;143(1):44–51. doi:10.1097/AOG.0000000000005448.

54. Estes SJ, Huisingh CE, Chiuve SE, Petruski-Ivleva N, Missmer SA. Depression, anxiety, and self-directed violence in women with endometriosis: a retrospective matched-cohort study. *Am J Epidemiol*. 2021;190(5):843-852. doi:10.1093/aje/kwaa249

55. Gao M, Koupil I, Sjöqvist H, et al. Psychiatric comorbidity among women with endometriosis: nationwide cohort study in Sweden. *Am J Obstet Gynecol*. 2020;223(3):415.e1-415.e16. doi:10.1016/j.ajog.2020.02.033

56. Harris HR, Wieser F, Vitonis AF, et al. Early life abuse and risk of endometriosis. *Hum Reprod*. 2018;33(9):1657-1668. doi:10.1093/humrep/dey248

57. Heim C, Ehlert U, Hanker JP, Hellhammer DH. Abuse-related posttraumatic stress disorder and alterations of the hypothalamic-pituitary-adrenal axis in women with chronic pelvic pain. *Psychosom Med*. 1998;60(3):309-318. doi:10.1097/00006842-199805000-00017

58. Heim C, Ehlert U, Hellhammer DH. The potential role of hypocortisolism in the pathophysiology of stress-related bodily disorders. *Psychoneuroendocrinology*. 2000;25(1):1-35. doi:10.1016/s0306-4530(99)00035-9

59. Shim JY, Laufer MR, Grimstad FW. Dysmenorrhea and endometriosis in transgender adolescents. *J Pediatr Adolesc Gynecol*. 2020;33(5):524-528. doi:10.1016/j.jpag.2020.06.001

60. Rogers PA, Adamson GD, Al-Jefout M, et al. Research priorities for endometriosis. *Reprod Sci*. 2017;24(2):202-226. doi:10.1177/1933719116654991

Amenorrhea

Lauren A. Kanner and Emily Chi

INTRODUCTION

Puberty is defined as the acquisition of adult height, bone strength, sexual characteristics, and reproductive capacity. Female puberty is divided between multiple stages, the first of which is thelarche (breast budding). Thelarche typically occurs after 8 years of age and is followed by pubarche (pubic hair development), a growth spurt, and finally, menarche. Menarche occurs 2 to 3 years after thelarche, with the average age of onset at 12.4 years.[1] The determinants of menarcheal age are undergoing continuous study; however, research has shown that socioeconomic status, genetics, general health, nutrition, and exercise appear to play a role.[1-3] (See Chapter 5 on puberty for more information.)

Amenorrhea, or the absence of menses, may be either a transient or permanent phenomenon caused by disruption at any point in the hypothalamic-pituitary-gonadal (HPG) axis or female reproductive system. Amenorrhea is classified as either primary or secondary. Primary amenorrhea is defined as the absence of menarche in ≥15-year-old females with or without developed secondary sexual characteristics and normal growth or if there is a lack of menses 3 years after thelarche. Secondary amenorrhea is defined as the absence of menses for 6 months or the equivalent of three previous cycle intervals, whichever is longer, in adolescents who previously had menses.[4] The epidemiology, evaluation, and management of common causes of primary and secondary amenorrhea will be discussed in this chapter. Remember that some etiologies can present as either primary or secondary amenorrhea.

PRIMARY AMENNORHEA

The initial workup for a patient with primary amenorrhea is going to rely on the history and physical examination, specifically the absence or presence of secondary sexual characteristics (Fig. 11.1). This assessment will lead to laboratory work to assess for gonadotropin rise or evaluation of androgen levels, which may then lead to further laboratory work and/or pelvic ultrasounds (Table 11.1). Treatment will then be dependent on the diagnosis reached, but may involve estrogen replacement, caloric balancing, or surgical consultation.

Turner Syndrome

Turner syndrome is the most common cause of primary amenorrhea and occurs in approximately 1/2000 females.[5] In the most common form of Turner syndrome, the X chromosome is missing completely, and individuals have a 45,XO karyotype (40%–50% of cases). Turner mosaicism also exists in which there is a cell line with X monosomy and another with 46,XX (45,XO/46,XX; 15%–25% prevalence), a 46,XY cell line (45,XO/46,XY; 10%–12%), or a cell line with three X chromosomes (3%).[6] Of note, the genotype does not correlate with the severity of the phenotype.

Common associated phenotypic features, pictured in Fig. 11.2 and 11.3, include short stature, a webbed neck, low hairline, broad "shield" chest, congenital heart disease (bicuspid aortic valve, aortic coarctation), horseshoe kidney, and primary ovarian insufficiency (POI). In Turner syndrome, ovarian oocytes and follicles undergo accelerated apoptosis, often in utero, and are eventually replaced by fibrous tissue. This results in lack

Differentiating primary amenorrhea

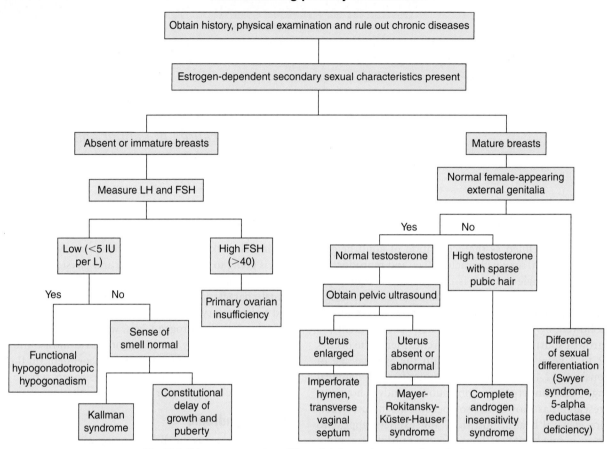

Fig. 11.1 Primary amenorrhea differential diagnosis workup flow chart.

of sufficient oocytes for menses by puberty, streak ovaries on ultrasound (Fig. 11.4), and early menopause.[7]

In Turner syndrome, the external female genitalia, uterus, and fallopian tubes develop normally until puberty, when estrogen-induced maturation fails to occur because of the absence of ovarian follicles.[8] Such individuals may lack secondary sexual characteristics, such as breast development, but should still progress normally through adrenarche (i.e., development of pubic hair, skin oiliness/acne, and body odor). There are some individuals who achieve menarche or spontaneous puberty with ovarian insufficiency by menarche.

Patients with suspected Turner syndrome based on history and examination should undergo a karyotype analysis. Other laboratory studies will show significantly elevated follicle-stimulating hormone (FSH) and luteinizing hormone (LH) levels because of the absence of ovarian oocytes and follicles. Anti-müllerian hormone may also be used as a marker for ovarian insufficiency and would be extremely low or undetectable.[9,10] Once the diagnosis is confirmed, all patients should also undergo a complete cardiac evaluation to evaluate for structural abnormalities.

Treatment of Turner syndrome focuses on hormonal therapy. Patients may receive growth hormone and estrogen to improve growth outcome, uterine length and volume, bone mineralization, and peak bone mass.[11] Given the risk for short stature, patients with Turner syndrome will be offered growth hormone, even if identified at a pubertal age, to attempt to optimize growth

TABLE 11.1 Diagnostic Features of Common Causes of Primary Amenorrhea

Anatomic Site	Etiology	Signs and Symptoms	Laboratory Findings	Imaging Findings	Karyotype
Hypothalamus	Kallmann syndrome	Anosmia, hearing loss, cleft lip/palate, synkinesis, unilateral renal agenesis, absent secondary sexual characteristics	Prepubertal low levels of LH and FSH, negative progesterone challenge, positive estrogen/progesterone challenge	No abnormalities	46,XX
Ovary	Turner syndrome	Short stature, webbed neck, widely spaced nipples, horseshoe kidney, streak ovaries	Elevated FSH and LH levels; low AMH and estradiol	Streak gonads on pelvic ultrasound	45,XO, can be mosaic 45,XO/46,XX, 45,XO/46,XY, or more rare X chromosome mosaics
	Swyer syndrome	Tall stature, functional female genitalia and structures, streak ovaries	Elevated FSH and LH levels, low estradiol levels		46,XY
Uterus	Müllerian agenesis (Mayer-Rokitansky-Küster-Hauser syndrome)	Typical female secondary sexual characteristics, short and blind-ended vagina	Normal LH, FSH, and testosterone levels	Small or absent uterus with ovaries present on pelvic ultrasound	46,XX
	Androgen insensitivity syndrome	Absence of the upper vagina, uterus, and fallopian tubes; testes may be palpable in the labia or inguinal area; sparse pubic and axillary hair	Normal or elevated LH, elevated testosterone	Abdominal or inguinal gonads on ultrasound or MRI	46,XY
Vagina	Transverse septum	Cyclic pelvic pain, possible vaginal or pelvic mass, typical secondary sexual characteristics	Normal laboratory tests	May be noted as hypointense on pelvic MRI	46,XX
Hymen	Imperforate hymen	Cyclic pelvic pain, hematocolpos, typical secondary sexual characteristics	Normal laboratory tests	Rarely indicated	46,XX
Miscellaneous	Constitutional delay of growth and puberty	Delayed adrenarche and gonadarche, family history of "late bloomers"	Lower levels of LH and FSH, delayed bone age	Normal except delayed bone age	46,XX
	5-Alpha reductase deficiency	Ambiguous genitalia at birth, virilization during puberty	Elevated serum testosterone-to-DHT ratio	Abdominal or inguinal gonads on ultrasound or MRI	46,XY

AMH, Anti-müllerian hormone; *DHT,* dihydrotestosterone; *FSH,* follicle-stimulating hormone; *LH,* luteinizing hormone; *MRI,* magnetic resonance imaging.

Phenotype of Turner syndrome

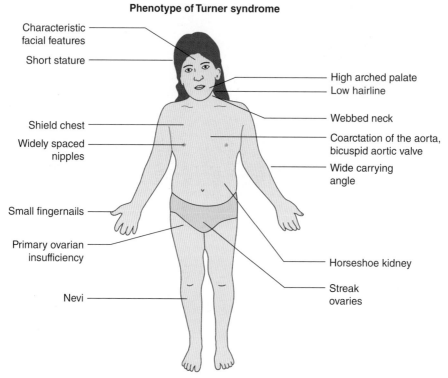

Characteristic facial features
Short stature
High arched palate
Low hairline
Webbed neck
Shield chest
Coarctation of the aorta, bicuspid aortic valve
Widely spaced nipples
Wide carrying angle
Small fingernails
Primary ovarian insufficiency
Horseshoe kidney
Streak ovaries
Nevi

Fig. 11.2 Phenotypic presentation of Turner syndrome.

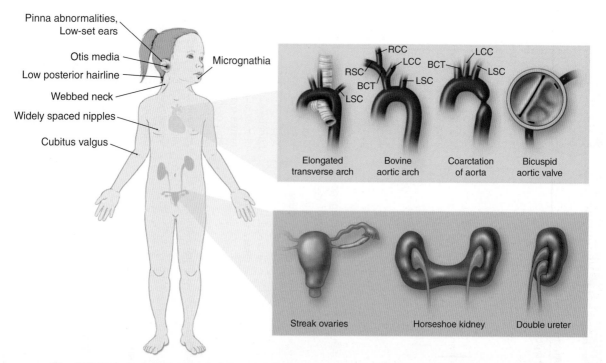

Pinna abnormalities, Low-set ears
Otis media
Micrognathia
Low posterior hairline
Webbed neck
Widely spaced nipples
Cubitus valgus

RCC
LCC
LCC
BCT
RSC
LSC
BCT
LSC
LSC

Elongated transverse arch
Bovine aortic arch
Coarctation of aorta
Bicuspid aortic valve

Streak ovaries
Horseshoe kidney
Double ureter

Fig. 11.3 Typical physical characteristics and findings associated with Turner syndrome. (Image from Granger et al.[12])

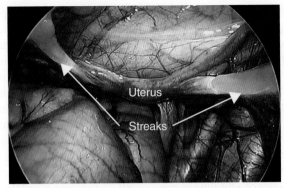

Fig. 11.4 Bilateral streak ovaries found in patients with complete lack of gonadal development. (From Claire M. de la Calle, Sunghoon Kim, Laurence S. Baskin: Diagnosis and treatment of the intra-abdominal gonad in the pediatric population: Testes, ovaries, dysgenetic gonads, streaks, and ovotestes. Journal of Pediatric Surgery, Volume 55, Issue 11, November 2020, Pages 2480-2491.)

before initiation of pubertal estrogen to maximize linear growth before growth plate closure but estrogen replacement for those identified younger may start early at a low dose to also help optimize height attainment.[13,14] (See Chapter 18 on POI/Turner syndrome for more information.)

Swyer Syndrome

Swyer syndrome, or 46,XY gonadal dysgenesis, is significantly less common than Turner syndrome and occurs in approximately 1/100,000 births.[15] In complete 46,XY gonadal dysgenesis, the fibrous streak gonads resemble ovarian tissue but cannot secrete anti-müllerian hormone, resulting in persistent müllerian structures and a female phenotype. Individuals are born with functional female genitalia and structures, including a vagina, uterus, and fallopian tubes. Patients often present during adolescence or early adulthood with lack of pubertal development or primary amenorrhea, although adrenarche and stature are normal.

The presentation of Swyer syndrome and Turner syndrome can be similar, but there are phenotypic differences as well as the genetic differences (Table 11.2).

If Swyer syndrome is suspected based on examination and history, the patient should undergo a karyotype analysis and laboratory tests for FSH, LH, prolactin, thyroid-stimulating hormone (TSH), free thyroxine (T_4), androstenedione, estradiol, and testosterone. FSH and LH levels will be elevated with low estradiol levels, suggestive of hypergonadotropic hypogonadism. Swyer syndrome patients will also have low androgen levels.

Treatment for Swyer syndrome involves hormonal replacement therapy with estrogen and progesterone from puberty onward. In addition to helping with the development of secondary sexual characteristics, hormone replacement therapy can also assist in the prevention of bone loss and osteoporosis.[16] Completely undeveloped streak gonads (see Fig. 11.4) are associated with an increased risk of abdominal tumors (most commonly dysgerminoma), so a gonadectomy is recommended at the time of diagnosis.

Mayer-Rokitansky-Küster-Hauser Syndrome

Mayer-Rokitansky-Küster-Hauser syndrome, or müllerian agenesis, occurs in approximately 1/5000 adolescents.[17] Due to the failure of müllerian duct development, females

TABLE 11.2 Differences and Similarities Between Turner Syndrome and Swyer Syndrome	
Turner Syndrome	**Swyer Syndrome**
• Short stature	• Tall stature with long arms and legs
• Lack of secondary sexual characteristics	• Lack of secondary sexual characteristics
• Streak ovaries developing over time	• Streak gonads from birth
• Variable uterine size depending on time of ovarian insufficiency onset	• Hypoplastic uterus
• Typical external female genitalia	• Typical external female genitalia

with a 46,XX karyotype undergo agenesis of the uterus and upper two-thirds of the vagina. Because these individuals have functional ovaries, secondary sexual characteristics develop normally and external genitalia are typical female but the vagina is short and blind-ended.

Patients typically present with primary amenorrhea despite normal secondary sexual characteristics. Laboratory findings include normal LH, FSH, and testosterone levels. A chromosome analysis can be performed to rule out Turner syndrome and androgen insensitivity syndrome. Abdominal or translabial imaging can be performed to assess for the presence of a midline uterus. Magnetic resonance imaging (MRI) will demonstrate rudimentary müllerian structures in a majority of patients with müllerian agenesis.[18]

Treatment includes vaginal and surgical care. Vaginal agenesis is treated by noninvasive vaginal dilatation (first-line therapy) or vaginoplasty.[19,20] Genetic motherhood is possible by using gestational surrogacy. (See Chapter 26 on nonobstructive müllerian anomalies for more information).

Complete Androgen Insensitivity Syndrome

This is an X-linked recessive disorder that affects 2 to 5 per 100,000 individuals who are genetically male.[21] 46,XY patients with this disease will appear to have a normal external female phenotype. Due to a defect in the androgen receptor, patients fail to develop all of the male sexual characteristics that are dependent on testosterone. Their external genitalia are typically female in appearance, but testes may be palpable in the labia or inguinal area. This is because their testes make müllerian-inhibiting substance, causing regression of all müllerian structures (fallopian tubes, uterus, and upper third of the vagina). At puberty, breast development occurs, but pubic and axillary hair are sparse.

Diagnosis is based on the absence of the upper vagina, uterus, and fallopian tubes on physical examination and pelvic ultrasonography, high serum testosterone concentrations (in the range for normal men), and a male (46,XY) karyotype.

Treatment involves surgical excision of the testes after puberty if located intraabdominally because of the increased risk (2%–5%) of developing testicular cancer after 25 years of age.[22]

Constitutional Delay of Growth and Puberty

 Constitutional delay is the most common cause of delayed puberty and menarche in girls, comprising up to

~30% of females with primary amenorrhea.[2] Characterized by both delayed adrenarche and gonadarche, it is often difficult to distinguish clinically from congenital gonadotropin-releasing hormone (GnRH) deficiency.

Constitutional delay of growth and puberty is a diagnosis of exclusion, and one must first rule out hormonal deficiencies, systemic illness, or syndromes associated with growth impairment. Laboratory workup should include other causes of short stature and amenorrhea, including TSH, T_4, insulin-like growth factor-1 (IGF-1), insulin-like growth factor binding protein-3 (IGF-BP-3), karyotype, and the growth hormone (GH) stimulation test, which would all be expected to be in the normal range. Low levels of LH and FSH are expected in adolescents with younger skeletal age caused by physiologic hypogonadotropic hypogonadism. Bone age is usually delayed compared with chronologic age, but the developmental milestones are achieved at usual bone ages.[23] Parents or siblings may give a history of being "late bloomers," with a late growth spurt or late puberty compared with their peers.

There is no treatment for constitutional growth delay other than reassurance and monitoring. These individuals will eventually progress through spontaneous puberty and menarche and do not require treatment.

Kallmann Syndrome

Kallmann syndrome, or isolated GnRH deficiency with anosmia, occurs in approximately 1/125,000 females. This condition develops because of the lack of migration of gonadotropes in the hypothalamus through the olfactory node. Approximately 50% of patients have a demonstrable genetic mutation that is identifiable but occurs in multiple genes.[24] Because of the absence of hypothalamic GnRH, laboratory findings are notable for pulsatile and prepubertal low serum gonadotropin concentrations (LH, FSH).

Secondary sexual characteristics are often completely absent, and adolescents will have an inability to smell. Associated congenital anomalies include midline defects (cleft lip/palate), neurosensory hearing loss, synkinesis (alternating mirror movements), unilateral renal agenesis, and skeletal defects including syndactyly and ectrodactyly (lobster claw deformity).

Diagnosis is made via hormone evaluation, olfactory function testing, and imaging such as MRI of the brain to evaluate the olfactory bulbs. Patients will also have a negative progesterone challenge test if an attempt to invoke menses is undertaken. This test involves administration of medroxyprogesterone, which leads to secretory transformation of the endometrium and withdrawal bleeding within a week of finishing the medroxyprogesterone course. Adolescents with a profound decrease in estrogen who lack an estrogen-primed endometrium, including patients with Kallmann syndrome or idiopathic hypogonadotropic hypogonadism, are unlikely to respond. This is in contrast to administration of estrogen followed by medroxyprogesterone, which is typically followed by withdrawal bleeding in most adolescents with amenorrhea secondary to hypogonadism, including Kallmann syndrome or idiopathic hypogonadotropic hypogonadism. A lack of withdrawal bleeding with administration of estrogen and medroxyprogesterone suggests the presence of abnormal endometrium (including uterine synechiae) or outflow obstruction.

Treatment for Kallmann syndrome involves hormone replacement therapy with exogenous GnRH administered in a pulsatile regimen designed to mimic endogenous GnRH secretion.[25]

5-Alpha Reductase Deficiency

This is a rare autosomal recessive disorder occurring in genetic 46,XY males and is also known as *huevos a las doce* based on a Dominican community with high incidence. In this community, these individuals are recognized as having their own gender. These patients have bilateral testes and normal testosterone production, but they have impaired virilization during embryogenesis caused by an inability to convert testosterone via 5-alpha reductase to its more potent metabolite, dihydrotestosterone (DHT). As a result, at birth, these neonates may appear phenotypically female or have ambiguous genitalia. Later during puberty, the disorder is more recognizable because of the onset of virilization (male-pattern hair growth, increased muscle mass, and voice deepening) caused by the normal peripubertal increase in testosterone secretion in males. These individuals do not undergo DHT-dependent masculinization (enlargement of the male external genitalia and prostate).[26]

Diagnosis is typically made in the newborn period when neonates present with ambiguous genitalia. These individuals may also present during puberty with clear signs of virilization. Laboratory evaluation includes a karyotype, 17-hydroxyprogesterone, FSH, LH, testosterone, DHT, anti-müllerian hormone, electrolytes, and urinalysis. Elevated serum testosterone-to-DHT ratio is the hallmark of 5-alpha reductase deficiency. An abdominopelvic ultrasound should also be obtained to assess for the presence of internal male/female structures.

Treatment includes a multidisciplinary discussion regarding the long-term effects of gender assignment, including gender identity, gender role, and sexuality. In patients with 5-alpha reductase deficiency who are raised as male, testosterone or DHT therapy may increase penile length.[27] If testosterone is used in a prepubertal patient for a prolonged course, parents should be counseled over the possibility of decreasing final adult height secondary to androgen-associated skeletal advancement. In such patients who are raised female, estrogen replacement therapy may be started at a bone age of 12 years or once an increase in gonadotropins is observed. Cycling of estrogen therapy or progesterone is not required because of the lack of a uterus.

ANATOMIC CAUSES OF PRIMARY AMENORRHEA

Imperforate Hymen

The incidence of an imperforate hymen is estimated to be 1 in 1000 female births. Patients may present with cyclic pelvic pain and a bulging, blue-colored mass caused by the retained blood in the vagina, referred to as a *hematocolpos*.[28] This is diagnosed with a physical examination and easily corrected with surgery.

Transverse Vaginal Septum

The incidence of transverse vaginal septum is estimated to be 1 in every 70,000 females. This condition occurs because of the failed fusion of the vaginal plate and the urogenital sinus.[29]

After menarche, symptoms are similar to those associated with an imperforate hymen, with cyclic pelvic pain and possible vaginal or pelvic mass, but this may depend on the location of the septum (transverse vs. longitudinal). Laboratory findings are normal, and patients will develop typical secondary sexual characteristics and undergo typical puberty and adrenarche, but present with amenorrhea or dysmenorrhea. Diagnosis is by physical examination, and management is surgical.[30] (See Chapter 27 on obstructive müllerian anomalies for more information.)

SECONDARY AMENORRHEA

The initial workup for a patient with secondary amenorrhea will also rely on the history and physical examination in addition to a need for confirmatory laboratory work with gonadotropin levels, thyroid function monitoring, and pituitary function screening, which may then lead to further workup with imaging (Fig. 11.5, Table 11.3). Treatment will then be dependent on the diagnosis reached.

Functional Hypothalamic Amenorrhea

Functional hypothalamic amenorrhea (FHA) occurs in approximately 20% of females with delayed puberty or incomplete pubertal development.[33] Due to a decrease in hypothalamic GnRH secretion, serum concentrations of FSH and LH remain in the prepubertal range. This results in absent midcycle surges in LH secretion, lack of normal follicular development, anovulation, and decreased serum estradiol concentrations. Risk factors for FHA include eating disorders (such as anorexia nervosa), excessive exercise, and stress.

The diagnosis of FHA is based on the findings of amenorrhea, low serum gonadotropins and estradiol (E2), and, usually, evidence of a precipitating factor (exercise, low weight, stress).[34] Adolescents suspected to have FHA should undergo biochemical testing for other causes of amenorrhea, including human chorionic gonadotropin (hCG) to rule out pregnancy, as well as serum prolactin, TSH and free T$_4$, and FSH to rule

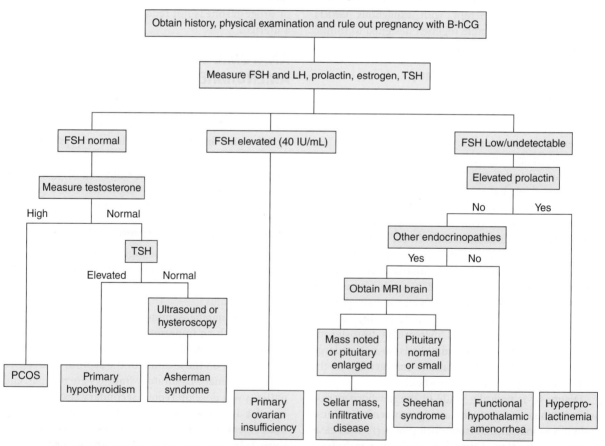

Fig. 11.5 Secondary amenorrhea differential diagnosis workup flow chart. *B-hCG*, Beta human chorionic gonadotropin; *FSH*, follicle-stimulating hormone; *LH*, luteinizing hormone; *MRI*, magnetic resonance imaging; *PCOS*, polycystic ovary syndrome; *TSH*, thyroid-stimulating hormone.

TABLE 11.3 **Diagnostic Features of Common Causes of Secondary Amenorrhea**

Anatomic Site	Etiology	Signs or Symptoms	Laboratory Findings	Imaging
Hypothalamus	Functional hypothalamic amenorrhea	Anorexia nervosa, other eating disorder, excessive exercise, weight loss, stress, psychiatric illness	Prepubertal low levels of FSH and LH, low estradiol	Usually normal brain MRI. Pelvic ultrasound may show thin uterine stripe.
Pituitary gland	Prolactinoma (lactotroph adenomas)	Galactorrhea, headache, visual disturbances	Elevated prolactin; decreased FSH, LH, and estradiol	Notable on brain MRI or CT depending on size, but macroprolactinoma sometimes not seen initially if caught early.
	Other sellar masses (other kinds of pituitary adenoma, craniopharyngioma, germinoma, cyst)[31]	Headache, visual disturbances	Elevated pituitary hormones depending on the type of pituitary adenoma; decreased FSH, LH, and estradiol	Notable on brain MRI or CT.
Thyroid	Hypothyroidism	Fatigue, cold intolerance, weight gain, constipation, dry skin, coarse hair	Elevated TSH, low free T_4	Not often needed, but may note abnormality on thyroid ultrasound, such as enlargement or heterogenous texture.
Ovary	Polycystic ovary syndrome	Hirsutism, acne, may be overweight, polycystic ovaries	Elevated LH and FSH, increased androgens, hyperinsulinemia	Ultrasound not indicated in <8 years postmenarchal and cannot be used for diagnosis.[32]
	Acquired primary ovarian insufficiency (autoimmune oophoritis, irradiation or surgery, chemotherapy, infection)	Symptoms of estrogen deficiency (hot flashes, vaginal dryness, osteoporosis)	Elevated LH and FSH, estrogen deficiency	On ultrasound or MRI may show streak gonad, lack of ovarian follicles, thin endometrial stripe.

CT, Computed tomography; *FSH,* follicle-stimulating hormone; *LH,* luteinizing hormone; *MRI,* magnetic resonance imaging; T_4, thyroxine.

out hyperprolactinemia, thyroid dysfunction, and primary ovarian insufficiency (POI), respectively. If there is evidence of hyperandrogenism, obtain serum androgens. Although many individuals with polycystic ovary syndrome (PCOS) are overweight, athletic adolescents with PCOS may present with a leaner phenotype and/or less obvious signs of hyperandrogenism.[35,36] For example, an athlete with PCOS who also has very low weight may have hormonal suppression of androgens and estrogen until weight is restored. At a higher weight, the same athlete may then demonstrate increased androgens on laboratory testing. A progestin challenge test may be useful in differentiating between FHA, a condition associated with E2 deficiency and scant or no withdrawal bleeding, and conditions such as PCOS in which E2 levels are not low and bleeding occurs after administration of exogenous progestin.

Treatment of adolescents with FHA involves treating the underlying cause of hypogonadotropic hypogonadism and potential long-term consequences, such as infertility, sexual dysfunction caused by genitourinary symptoms such as vaginal dryness and dyspareunia, and/or low bone mineral density (BMD). It is also important to screen for and treat common comorbid conditions such as anxiety and other mood disorders. Recovery is related to low energy availability (EA), as this is the driver of FHA. It is important to note that low EA can occur in a patient with normal body mass index (BMI). Recovery involves the reversal of the inciting factor (eating disorder, low EA, or stress).[37] There is currently no evidence that supplemental calcium and vitamin D prevent bone loss—food is the best source to obtain the recommended daily allowances.

The 2017 Endocrine Society guidelines recommend the administration of physiologic doses and formulations of estrogen to prevent further bone loss and improve bone density in adult patients. There are no specific recommendations for adolescents. Current studies demonstrate that transdermal estrogen may aid in bone recovery, especially in the case of an eating disorder with amenorrhea >12 months and signs of low BMD. There may be a role for estrogen in these adolescents.[38-40]

Polycystic Ovary Syndrome

PCOS is one of the most common endocrinopathies in adolescents, affecting between 5% and 10%. This condition accounts for an estimated 20% of the cases of amenorrhea.[41] There are currently three sets of diagnostic criteria for PCOS in adults (summarized in Table 11.4), which can be extrapolated for use in adolescents. Whereas in adults, the Rotterdam criteria is recommended, in adolescents, the International PCOS guidelines recommend using the National Institutes of Health (NIH) criteria. The Rotterdam guidelines accept any two out of three criteria: oligomenorrhea and primary/secondary amenorrhea, hyperandrogenism, and polycystic ovaries on ultrasound, whereas the NIH criteria exclude ultrasound evaluation. Ultrasound is not recommended in the diagnosis of adolescents, as it is

believed that the current adult sonographic diagnostic criteria may not properly differentiate PCOS from normal adolescent ovarian morphology. Therefore until normative ovarian features and specific PCOS distinguishing features have been examined in adolescents, the application of adult ultrasound criteria for diagnosing PCOS is not recommended until 8 years post menarche.[32] If an adolescent meets one of the two NIH diagnostic criteria, they may be considered "at risk" for PCOS and should be followed and offered symptom-based management.[42,43]

Hyperandrogenism is usually manifested clinically as acne or hirsutism and sometimes as a high serum concentration of at least one androgen (testosterone, androstenedione, dehydroepiandrosterone [DHEA], DHEA-sulfate, or DHT). It is important to note that diagnosis of this condition is difficult in adolescence because of the overlap between normal pubertal physiologic changes and adult PCOS diagnostic criteria, including irregular menstrual cycles and acne.[32] Forty to 60% percent of adolescents with PCOS are overweight or obese, but even those with normal weight may have insulin resistance. Insulin resistance is hypothesized to alter normal hypothalamic hormonal feedback, causing an elevation in LH and FSH, increased androgens (e.g., testosterone) from theca interna cells, and a decreased rate of follicular maturation, resulting in unruptured follicles (cysts) and anovulation.

The mainstay of PCOS treatment includes weight loss and targeted symptomatic care. Weight loss can occur through lifestyle changes, pharmacotherapy, and when necessary, bariatric surgery.[45] This reduces hyperinsulinemia and subsequently hyperandrogenism, thus restoring ovulatory cycles, and improves metabolic risk. Chronic anovulation in PCOS is associated with an

TABLE 11.4   Comparison of the Current Diagnostic Criteria for PCOS in Adults[44]

Clinical Finding	National Institutes of Health Criteria, 1990 (Must Have Both of the Findings Marked)	Rotterdam Criteria, 2003 (Must Have Any Two of the Findings Marked)	Androgen Excess and PCOS Society, 2009 (Must Have A Plus Either B or C)
Hyperandrogenism*	X	X	A
Oligomenorrhea	X	X	B
Polycystic ovaries		X	C

*Clinical or biochemical evidence of excess androgen.
PCOS, Polycystic ovary syndrome.
(Wiliams T, Mortada R, Porter M. Diagnosis and Treatment of Polycystic Ovary Syndrome. American Family Physician. 2016; 94 (2): 106–113.)

increased risk of endometrial hyperplasia and endometrial cancer, so regular shedding of the endometrium with cyclic progestins or combined estrogen-progestin hormonal contraceptives is recommended. (For more information on PCOS diagnosis and treatment, see Chapter 19.)

Prolactinoma

Among pituitary causes of secondary amenorrhea, prolactinomas (lactotroph adenomas) are the most common and are responsible for approximately 13% of cases of secondary amenorrhea.[42] An elevated level of prolactin suppresses hypothalamic GnRH secretion, resulting in low gonadotropin and estradiol concentrations and amenorrhea. Physical examination findings include chiasmal syndrome symptoms (e.g., bitemporal field loss, headaches, nausea and vomiting).[46,47]

When measuring serum prolactin concentration, it is important to note that other factors, including stress, sleep, and intercourse, can also raise serum prolactin.[48] Therefore it is recommended to measure serum prolactin at least twice before sellar imaging is obtained, especially in adolescents with borderline high values (20–50 ng/mL). Further workup with consideration for treatment should occur if a serum prolactin is >100 mcg/L SI units or if presenting with symptoms for other endocrinopathies, such as short stature or galactorrhea.[49] In general, hyperprolactinemia causes primary amenorrhea 14% to 41% of the time and secondary amenorrhea 29% to 45% of the time, although this is more common with idiopathic hyperprolactinemia than with a prolactinoma.[49,50]

Hyperprolactinemia may also be caused by a multitude of other factors, including chest wall injuries, conditions that cause decreased dopaminergic inhibition of prolactin secretion, or disease in or near the hypothalamus or pituitary that interferes with the secretion of dopamine or its delivery to the pituitary gland. Chest wall injuries, such as severe burns, increase prolactin secretion because of a neural mechanism similar to that of suckling.[51] Drug-induced hyperprolactinemia may also be caused by antipsychotics (especially risperidone), selective serotonin reuptake inhibitors (SSRIs), D_2 receptor agonists (metoclopramide and domperidone), and dopamine synthesis inhibitors (methyldopa).[52] Severe clinical hypothyroidism also predisposes to hyperprolactinemia, although the mechanism is unknown.

Treatment for hyperprolactinemia should be aimed at removal of the offending agent, treatment of underlying disease, or pharmacotherapy with dopamine agonists (cabergoline and bromocriptine) to shrink the size of the prolactinoma. Surgery and radiation may be required if dopamine agonists are ineffective at reducing the prolactinoma.

Also note that any sellar mass (e.g., other kinds of pituitary adenomas, craniopharyngiomas, meningiomas, cysts) can also cause deficient gonadotropin secretion. Only a pituitary adenoma can cause hypersecretion of other pituitary hormones, but any mass lesion in the area of the sella can cause hyposecretion of one or more pituitary hormones. To evaluate for hypersecretion, obtain serum insulin-like growth factor (IGF)-1 (somatotroph adenomas) and adrenocorticotropic hormone (ACTH; corticotroph adenomas). Additional endocrine testing is needed when a gonadotroph or thyrotroph adenoma is suspected (LH, FSH, T_4, and TSH).

Primary Ovarian Insufficiency

POI, also known as *premature ovarian failure*, may be the result of complete or partial loss of an X chromosome (Turner syndrome), a fragile X premutation, autoimmune ovarian destruction, or, most commonly, idiopathic causes.[53] It may also be iatrogenic and secondary to chemotherapy or radiation. POI is defined as the depletion of oocytes before 40 years of age. This may present with variable-timing menses, and even if the patient is not menstruating, she may still have some fertility. In complete POI, lack of ovarian function results in estrogen deficiency, endometrial atrophy, and cessation of menstruation.

Loss of the negative feedback effects of estradiol and inhibin on the hypothalamus and pituitary results in high serum FSH concentrations, which distinguishes ovarian insufficiency from hypothalamic amenorrhea (low or normal FSH). Diagnosis is based on FSH >40 on two laboratory tests at least 1 month apart and amenorrhea for at least 3 months.[54]

Treatment for POI centers around issues that arise from estrogen deficiency. Estrogen therapy is given to prevent osteoporosis and relieve hot flashes along with other symptoms of estrogen deficiency. Calcium and vitamin D supplements are also recommended for prevention of osteoporosis.[55] For more information on POI, refer to Chapter 18 primary ovarian insufficiency and turner syndrome.

KEY POINTS

- Primary amenorrhea is defined as the absence of menarche in ≥15-year-old females with or without developed secondary sexual characteristics and normal growth or if there is a lack of menses 3 years after thelarche. Etiologies include but are not limited to Turner syndrome, Swyer syndrome, müllerian agenesis, androgen insensitivity syndrome, Kallmann syndrome, 5-alpha reductase deficiency, transverse septum, imperforate hymen, and constitutional delay of growth and puberty.
- Primary amenorrhea is evaluated initially by determining the presence or absence of secondary sexual characteristics (a marker of estrogen activity and therefore ovarian function), the presence or absence of a uterus, and the serum FSH level.
- Secondary amenorrhea is defined as the absence of menses for 6 months or the equivalent of three previous cycle intervals, whichever is longer, in adolescents who previously had menses. Etiologies include but are not limited to FHA, sellar masses including prolactinoma, PCOS, acquired POI, thyroid disease, and systemic illnesses such as rheumatologic conditions, celiac disease, or type 1 diabetes mellitus.
- After a thorough history, physical examination, and ruling out pregnancy, initial laboratory testing for adolescents with secondary amenorrhea includes FSH, prolactin, androgens, and TSH.
- Treatment of amenorrhea is directed at correcting the underlying pathology (if possible), helping the woman to achieve fertility (if desired), and preventing complications of the disease process.

REVIEW QUESTIONS

1. A 17-year-old patient presents to the clinic concerned that she has not had her period in 8 months despite a previous history of monthly menses. A pregnancy test is negative. The patient is 5′9″ and weighs 100 pounds. She mentions that she is a model and battles anorexia nervosa. The patient's history suggests which of the following causes for her amenorrhea?
   a. Systemic illness
   b. Swyer syndrome
   c. Hypothalamic-pituitary dysfunction
   d. Primary ovarian insufficiency

2. An 18-year-old woman who has never been pregnant presents for the evaluation of 3 months of amenorrhea. Her menstrual periods started at age 13 and had been regular up until this time. She complains of fatigue, nausea, and breast tenderness. Which of the following tests would be the most appropriate first step in the laboratory evaluation of this patient?
   a. Serum prolactin
   b. Pregnancy test
   c. Serum FSH
   d. Serum TSH

3. A 17-year-old female presents with Tanner stage IV breast development but no menses. Ultrasound confirms a blind vaginal vault and no uterus or cervix. What laboratory test would be most helpful in determining the etiology of her problem?
   a. Serum FSH
   b. Serum TSH
   c. Serum prolactin level
   d. Karyotype

4. A 15-year-old female presents with no period for the past 6 months and irregular periods since menarche at the age of 13. She is obese with normal vital signs, and you notice significant lower abdominal and facial hair in addition to acne over her shoulders and back. Which of the following pathogenetic mechanisms are involved in her case?
   a. Hyperandrogenism causing follicular arrest and anovulation
   b. Defects in insulin signaling for glucose transport and lipolysis
   c. Insulin and LH working synergistically in a stimulatory fashion on thecal cells
   d. All of the above

REFERENCES

1. Lacroix AE, Gondal H, Shumway KR, et al. Physiology, Menarche. [Updated 2022 Mar 17]. In: *StatPearls* [Internet]. Treasure Island, FL: StatPearls Publishing; 2022.
2. Sedlmeyer IL, Palmert MR. Delayed puberty: analysis of a large case series from an academic center. *J Clin Endocrinol Metab*. 2002;87(4):1613-1620. doi:10.1210/jcem.87.4.8395.
3. Ramraj B, Subramanian VM, Vijayakrishnan G. Study on age of menarche between generations and the factors associated with it. *Clin Epidemiol Global Health*. 2021;11:1–5.

4. Mushlin SB, Greene HL. *Decision Making in Medicine: An Algorithmic Approach*. 3rd ed. Elsevier; 2009.

5. Gravholt CH. Clinical practice in Turner syndrome. *Nat Clin Pract Endocrinol Metab*. 2005;1(1):41-52. doi:10.1038/ncpendmet0024.

6. Gravholt CH, Andersen NH, Conway GS, et al. Clinical practice guidelines for the care of girls and women with Turner syndrome: Proceedings from the 2016 Cincinnati International Turner Syndrome Meeting. *Eur J Endocrinol*. 2017;177:G1-G70.

7. Haber HP, Ranke MB. Pelvic ultrasonography in Turner syndrome: standards for uterine and ovarian volume. *J Ultrasound Med*. 1999;18(4):271-276. https://doi.org/10.7863/jum.1999.18.4.271

8. Sokol ER, Sokol AI. *General Gynecology: The Requisites in Obstetrics and Gynecology*. Mosby; 2007.

9. Lunding SA, Aksglaede L, Anderson RA, et al. AMH as predictor of premature ovarian insufficiency: a longitudinal study of 120 Turner syndrome patients. *J Clin Endocrinol Metab*. 2015;100:E1030-E1038. doi:10.1210/jc.2015-1621.

10. Hamza RT, Mira MF, Hamed AI, Ezzat T, Sallam MT. Anti-Müllerian hormone levels in patients with turner syndrome: relation to karyotype, spontaneous puberty, and replacement therapy. *Am J Med Genet A*. 2018;176(9):1929-1934. doi:10.1002/ajmg.a.40473.

11. Ross JL, Quigley CA, Cao D, et al. Growth hormone plus childhood low-dose estrogen in Turner's syndrome. *N Engl J Med*. 2011;364(13):1230-1242. doi:10.1056/NEJMoa1005669.

12. Granger A, Zurada A, Zurada-Zielińska A, Gielecki J, Loukas M. Anatomy of Turner syndrome. *Clin Anat*. 2016;29(5):638-642. https://doi.org/10.1002/ca.22727

13. Davenport ML. Evidence for early initiation of growth hormone and transdermal estradiol therapies in girls with Turner syndrome. *Growth Horm IGF Res*. 2006;16(suppl A):S91-S97. doi:10.1016/j.ghir.2006.04.002.

14. Kriström B, Ankarberg-Lindgren C, Barrenäs ML, Nilsson KO, Albertsson-Wikland K. Normalization of puberty and adult height in girls with Turner syndrome: results of the Swedish Growth Hormone trials initiating transition into adulthood. *Front Endocrinol (Lausanne)*. 2023;14:1197897. doi:10.3389/fendo.2023.1197897.

15. Behtash N, Karimi Zarchi M. Dysgerminoma in three patients with Swyer syndrome. *World J Surg Oncol*. 2007;5:71. doi:10.1186/1477-7819-5-71.

16. *Swyer Syndrome*. National Organization of Rare Disorders; 2019. https://rarediseases.org/rare-diseases/swyer-syndrome/

17. Fontana L, Gentilin B, Fedele L, Gervasini C, Miozzo M. Genetics of Mayer-Rokitansky-Kuster-Hauser (MRKH) syndrome. *Clin Genet*. 2017;91:233-246.

18. Preibsch H, Rall K, Wietek BM, et al. Clinical value of magnetic resonance imaging in patients with Mayer-Rokitansky-Kuster-Hauser (MRKH) syndrome: diagnosis of associated malformations, uterine rudiments and intra-uterine endometrium. *Eur Radiol*. 2014;24:1621-1627.

19. Roberts CP, Haber MJ, Rock JA. Vaginal creation for müllerian agenesis. *Am J Obstet Gynecol*. 2001;185:1349-1352; discussion 1352-1353.

20. Herlin MK, Petersen MB, Brännström M. Mayer-Rokitansky-Küster-Hauser (MRKH) syndrome: a comprehensive update. *Orphanet J Rare Dis*. 2020;15(1):214. doi:10.1186/s13023-020-01491-9.

21. Fulare S, Deshmukh S, Gupta J. Androgen insensitivity syndrome: a rare genetic disorder. *Int J Surg Case Rep*. 2020;71:371-373. doi:10.1016/j.ijscr.2020.01.032.

22. Ko JK, King TF, Williams L, Creighton SM, Conway GS. Hormone replacement treatment choices in complete androgen insensitivity syndrome: an audit of an adult clinic. *Endocr Connect*. 2017;6(6):375-379.

23. Aguilar D, Castano G. Constitutional growth delay. [Updated 2022 Jun 27]. In: StatPearls [Internet]. Treasure Island, FL: StatPearls Publishing; 2022. https://www.ncbi.nlm.nih.gov/books/NBK539780/

24. Laitinen EM, Vaaralahti K, Tommiska J, et al. Incidence, phenotypic features and molecular genetics of Kallmann syndrome in Finland. *Orphanet J Rare Dis*. 2011;6:41. doi:10.1186/1750-1172-6-41.

25. Silveira LFG, Latronico AC. Approach to the patient with hypogonadotropic hypogonadism. *J Clin Endocrinol Metab*. 2013;98(5):1781-1788. https://doi.org/10.1210/jc.2012-3550

26. Okeigwe I, Kuohung W. 5-Alpha reductase deficiency: a 40-year retrospective review. *Curr Opin Endocrinol Diabetes Obes*. 2014;21(6):483-487. doi:10.1097/MED.0000000000000116.

27. Praveen EP, Desai AK, Khurana ML, et al. Gender identity of children and young adults with 5alpha-reductase deficiency. *J Pediatr Endocrinol Metab*. 2008;21(2):173-179.

28. Laghzaoui O. Congenital imperforate hymen. *BMJ Case Rep*. 2016;2016:bcr2016215124. doi:10.1136/bcr-2016-215124.

29. Doğan E, Yavuz O, Altay C, Özmen S. Asymptomatic microperforated transverse vaginal septum presenting with primary infertility: a rare form of mullerian anomaly. *Turk J Obstet Gynecol*. 2019;16(2):140-142. doi:10.4274/tjod.galenos.2019.32956.

30. Williams CE, Nakhal RS, Hall-Craggs MA, et al. Transverse vaginal septae: management and long-term outcomes. *BJOG*. 2014;121(13):1653-1658. doi:10.1111/1471-0528.12899.

31. Karaca Z, Hacioglu A, Kelestimur F. Neuroendocrine changes after aneurysmal subarachnoid haemorrhage. *Pituitary*. 2019;22(3):305-321.

32. Peña AS, Witchel SF, Hoeger KM, et al. Adolescent poly-cystic ovary syndrome according to the international evidence-based guideline. *BMC Med.* 2020;18(1):72. doi:10.1186/s12916-020-01516-x.

33. Seppä S, Kuiri-Hänninen T, Holopainen E, Voutilainen R. Management of endocrine disease: diagnosis and management of primary amenorrhea and female delayed puberty. *Eur J Endocrinol.* 2021;184(6):R225-R242.

34. Gordon CM, Ackerman KE, Berga SL, et al. Functional hypothalamic amenorrhea: an Endocrine Society clinical practice guideline. *J Clin Endocrinol Metab.* 2017;102(5):1413-1439. doi:10.1210/jc.2017-00131.

35. Carmina E, Fruzzetti F, Lobo RA. Features of polycystic ovary syndrome (PCOS) in women with functional hypothalamic amenorrhea (FHA) may be reversible with recovery of menstrual function. *Gynecol Endocrinol.* 2018;34(4):301-304. doi:10.1080/09513590.2017. 1395842.

36. Teede HJ, Misso ML, Costello MF, et al. Recommendations from the International evidence-based guideline for the assessment and management of polycystic ovary syndrome. *Clin Endocrinol (Oxf).* 2018;89(3):251-268.

37. Falsetti L, Gambera A, Barbetti L, Specchia C. Long-term follow-up of functional hypothalamic amenorrhea and prognostic factors. *J Clin Endocrinol Metab.* 2002;87(2):500-505. doi:10.1210/jcem.87.2.8195.

38. Ackerman KE, Singhal V, Baskaran C, et al. Oestrogen replacement improves bone mineral density in oligo-menorrhoeic athletes: a randomized clinical trial. *Br J Sports Med.* 2019;53:229-236.

39. Nose-Ogura S, Yoshino O, Kanatani M, et al. Effect of transdermal estradiol therapy on bone mineral density of amenorrheic female athletes. *Scand J Med Sci Sports.* 2020;30(8):1379-1386.

40. Ackerman KE, Singhal V, Slattery M, et al. Effects of estrogen replacement on bone geometry and microarchitecture in adolescent and young adult oligoamenorrheic athletes: a randomized trial. *J Bone Miner Res.* 2020;35(2): 248-260.

41. Sheehan MT. Polycystic ovarian syndrome: diagnosis and management. *Clin Med Res.* 2004;2(1):13-27. doi: 10.3121/cmr.2.1.13.

42. Reindollar RH, Novak M, Tho SP, McDonough PG. Adult-onset amenorrhea: a study of 262 patients. *Int J Gynaecol Obstet.* 1987;25(4):347. https://doi. org/10.1016/0020-7292(87)90323-7

43. Teede HJ, Tay CT, Laven JJE, et al. Recommendations From the 2023 International Evidence-based Guideline for the Assessment and Management of Polycystic Ovary Syndrome. *J Clin Endocrinol Metab.* 2023;108(10):2447-2469. doi:10.1210/clinem/dgad463.

44. Wiliams T, Mortada R, Porter M. Diagnosis and treatment of polycystic ovary syndrome. *Am Fam Physician.* 2016;94(2):106-113.

45. Moghetti P, Castello R, Negri C, et al. Metformin effects on clinical features, endocrine and metabolic profiles, and insulin sensitivity in polycystic ovary syndrome: a randomized, double-blind, placebo-controlled 6-month trial, followed by open, long-term clinical evaluation. *J Clin Endocrinol Metab.* 2000;85(1):139-146. doi:10.1210/ jcem.85.1.6293.

46. Colao A, Loche S, Cappa M, et al. Prolactinomas in children and adolescents. Clinical presentation and long-term follow-up. *J Clin Endocrinol Metab.* 1998;83:2777-2780.

47. Fideleff HL, Boquete HR, Suárez MG, Azaretzky M. Prolactinoma in children and adolescents. *Horm Res.* 2009;72:197-205.

48. Petakov MS, Damjanović SS, Nikolić-Durović MM, et al. Pituitary adenomas secreting large amounts of prolactin may give false low values in immunoradiometric assays. The hook effect. *J Endocrinol Invest.* 1998;21(3):184-188. doi:10.1007/BF03347299.

49. Matalliotakis M, Koliarakis I, Matalliotaki C, Trivli A, Hatzidaki E. Clinical manifestations, evaluation and management of hyperprolactinemia in adolescent and young girls: a brief review. *Acta Biomed.* 2019;90(1): 149-157. doi:10.23750/abm.v90i1.8142.

50. Lee DY, Oh YK, Yoon BK, Choi DS. Prevalence of hyperprolactinemia in adolescents and young women with menstruation-related problems. *Am J Obstet Gynecol.* 2012;206(3):213.e1-213.e2135. doi:10.1016/j. ajog.2011.12.010.

51. Morley JE, Dawson M, Hodgkinson H, Kalk WJ. Galactorrhea and hyperprolactinemia associated with chest wall injury. *J Clin Endocrinol Metab.* 1977;45(5): 931-935. doi:10.1210/jcem-45-5-931.

52. Kleinberg DL, Noel GL, Frantz AG. Galactorrhea: a study of 235 cases, including 48 with pituitary tumors. *N Engl J Med.* 1977;296(11):589-600. doi:10.1056/ NEJM197703172961103.

53. Bakalov VK, Anasti JN, Calis KA, et al. Autoimmune oophoritis as a mechanism of follicular dysfunction in women with 46,XX spontaneous premature ovarian failure. *Fertil Steril.* 2005;84(4):958-965. doi:10.1016/j.fertnstert.2005.04.060.

54. Cox L, Liu JH. Primary ovarian insufficiency: an update. *Int J Womens Health.* 2014;6:235-243. doi:10.2147/IJWH. S37636.

55. Sullivan SD, Sarrel PM, Nelson LM. Hormone replacement therapy in young women with primary ovarian insufficiency and early menopause. *Fertil Steril.* 2016;106(7):1588-1599. doi:10.1016/j.fertnstert.2016.09.046.

Menstrual and Reproductive Concerns in Adolescents With Disabilities

Elisabeth H. Quint and Monica Woll Rosen

The Centers for Disease Control and Prevention (CDC) reports that over 12 million children and adolescents have a diagnosed developmental disability.[1] This number is on the rise, especially with the increase in autism spectrum disorder (ASD) in recent years. One in 44 children have a diagnosis of ASD according to the CDC.[1] This increased prevalence in children and adolescents with disabilities means that generalist providers will see significantly more patients with a variety of disabilities in the coming years. Unfortunately, traditional medical education often lacks specific training on how to best care for this cohort of patients, and many barriers often arise. According to the American College of Obstetricians and Gynecologists (ACOG), "excellent gynecologic healthcare for women and adolescents with disabilities is comprehensive; maintains confidentiality; is an act of dignity and respect toward the patient; maximizes the patient's autonomy; avoids harm; and assesses and addresses the patient's knowledge of puberty, menstruation, sexuality, safety, and consent."[2]

DISEASE/DEFINITION

There are many different types of disabilities. According to the CDC, a disability is any condition of the body or mind (impairment) that makes it more difficult for the person with the condition to do certain activities (activity limitation) and interact with the world around them (participation restrictions).[3] Disabilities can be physical—affecting, for example, mobility, dexterity, vision, or hearing—or intellectual—affecting thinking, remembering, learning, or communicating. Many people have challenges in both. Although patients with disabilities are often grouped together in discussing health care needs, it is imperative to remember that this group is quite diverse with a range of needs.

Whereas some disabilities are present at birth, others may occur because of an injury or are developmental, becoming apparent during childhood or adolescence. Disabilities can be static, or they may improve or progress over time.

With respect to reproductive health care, adolescence is the time when a disability may become more challenging because of growth, patient awareness, cyclical changes like seizure activity or moods, and, of course, menstruation and fertility. Although sexual activity, orientation, education, and safety are complicated issues for all teenagers, they are often ignored in adolescents with any disability.

PREVALENCE AND EPIDEMIOLOGY

Sixty-one million adults in the United States have a disability.[1] According to the CDC, 1 in 6 children have a developmental disability, with 1 in 345 having cerebral palsy.[1]

Most patients with disabilities go through puberty in a similar manner to their nondisabled peers, but the rate of maturation may vary. When patients go through puberty early (e.g., with spina bifida and cerebral palsy), they may have needs that are not yet anticipated.[4]

The overall prevalence of sexual activity is similar for reproductive-aged women with and without disabilities.[5] Women with disabilities have been victims of disproportionate incidences of sexual violence and inadequate sexual education counseling that have led to higher rates of sexually transmitted infections and unplanned pregnancies.[6] Recent research suggests that young persons with disabilities are three times as likely to experience sexual violence as those without disabilities, with the highest rates of violence occurring in those aged 12 to 15.[7,8] In a survey of about 8000 eleventh graders, 34% identified as having a disability. In this group, 20% self-reported that they had ever been forced to have sex, compared with 7% in the nondisabled group.[9]

There are only minimal data on gender issues in these adolescents, but parents and gender clinics have reported more gender variance in teens with ASD and attention-deficit/hyperactivity disorder, and in the study of eleventh graders, only 72% of the students with disabilities self-identified as heterosexual, compared with 91% in the nondisabled group.[9-12]

Reproductive health education is too often overlooked in this population, where despite experiencing these increased risks, adolescents with disabilities receive far less education on this topic from parents, schools, and providers compared with their peers.[13]

BARRIERS TO CARE AND COMMUNICATION CHALLENGES

Patients with disabilities often face multiple barriers to receiving adequate reproductive health care. Physical barriers include facilities that are inaccessible because of lack of elevators or ramps, lifts or lift teams are not available, or examination tables do not move up or down. Other barriers include need for longer appointment times and financial concerns.

Communication is another challenge. When talking to a patient with—or about a patient with—a disability, it is imperative to remember that a person is not a disability, condition, or diagnosis, but rather a person who *has* a disability, condition, or diagnosis. One should use neutral language that defines a patient's intellectual and cognitive abilities, rather than their disabilities. Certain phrases can be offensive to persons with disabilities including words such as *retardation, challenged,* and *wheelchair-bound*. It is important that a provider not assume, but rather assess, a patient's competence and ability to communicate without only letting caregivers speak on a patient's behalf. As with any patient, providers should give as much autonomy as possible to the patient, based on age and level of competence.

A survey showed that persons with a disability are significantly more likely than those without a disability to perceive that the physician does not listen to them,

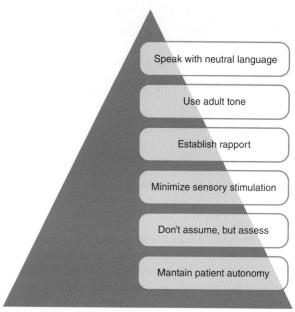

Fig. 12.1 Tips for conducting an interview and physical exam in adolescents with disabilities.

does not explain treatment so that they understand, does not treat them with respect, does not spend enough time with them, and does not involve them in treatment decisions.[14] Unfortunately, training in medical school and residency is lacking in disability care.[15] Both practicing pediatricians and obstetrics and gynecology providers have acknowledged discomfort and inadequate training.[16,17]

Providers may also have personal biases and therefore offer reproductive services less often to patients with disabilities.[18] Therefore education for providers should be improved so they can consider creative ways to communicate, respect autonomy, and ensure equitable access to reproductive health care (Fig. 12.1, Table 12.1).

CLINICAL PRESENTATION/EVALUATION

For patients with disabilities, adolescence can be a challenging time. The most common reasons why patients with disabilities present for reproductive health care include anticipatory pubertal guidance, behavioral changes with menses, issues around menstruation like suppression and hygiene, and safety and sexuality.[19,20] See Fig. 12.2. A recent study shows that adolescents with disabilities who present to their health care provider for anticipatory guidance typically present 13.5 months

TABLE 12.1 Common Phrases Misinterpreted by Patients With Disabilities and a Better Way to State Them	
Do Not Say	**Do Say**
Disabled person	Person with a disability
What happened to you?	How should I describe your disability?
Confined to a wheelchair, wheelchair bound	Wheelchair user, person who uses a wheelchair or mobility device
Nonverbal, mute	Person who uses an alternative method of communication, communicates nonverbally
Suffering from (disability)	Living with/has (disability)
Hearing impaired	Person who is hard of hearing
Slow learner	Has a learning disability
Brain damaged	Has a brain injury
Seeing eye dog	Service animal or dog
Able-bodied	Nondisabled
Handicapped parking, disabled restroom	Accessible parking or restroom
Mentally handicapped, retarded	Intellectually disabled
Afflicted by, victim of, suffers from (name of condition)	Has (name of condition)

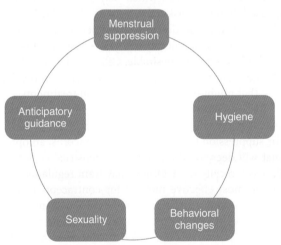

Fig. 12.2 Common reasons for patients with disabilities to present for reproductive health care.

who need help with toileting, menstrual management is handled by a parent or caretaker. Menstrual products can be hard to use or too personal to get help with (e.g., tampons and menstrual cups). Additionally, if a patient uses a wheelchair, pads may be uncomfortable and may require an adjustment period.[22] Period-absorbing underwear is a wonderful option to share with patients who struggle with hygiene. Another product called Tina, is a tampon inserter which is bioengineered to help those who are disabled or not able to insert a tampon on their own. See here for more information: tinahealthcare.com.

With the start of puberty—and especially with menstruation—families struggle with sexuality, safety, and fertility. Parents often think of their children with disabilities as asexual, when in fact, that is not the case. Parents are often uncomfortable addressing these issues and are looking to care providers for help.

SEXUAL HEALTH EDUCATION

At a reproductive health visit, sexuality and sex education needs should be assessed. Discussions should first evaluate the patient's understanding and knowledge of sexuality and sex. Next, providers should assess the patient's safety and ability to consent to any intimate contact, as well as any previous unwanted experiences. After an initial assessment, education can then include anatomic

before menarche, so starting anticipatory guidance at the time of breast development is recommended.[19]

Patients feel a sense of separation from their peers, but mood changes may be especially challenging for families who might already be struggling with emotional regulation.[21] Cyclical behavioral changes can also be associated with dysmenorrhea, which may be hard to assess in nonverbal patients. Menstruation can lead to hygiene concerns, as for many patients with disabilities

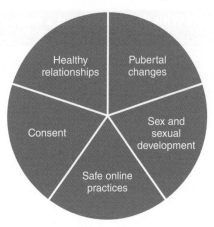

Fig. 12.3 Topics in sexual health education in adolescents with disabilities.

and physiologic changes of puberty, sex and sexual development, gender identity, healthy relationships, safe online practices, consent, and sexual abuse.[23] Some excellent resources are available for providers.[24-28] A resource for patients and their guardians, entitled Healthy Bodies: A Parent's Guide on Puberty for Girls with Disabilities, can be found at https://vkc.vumc.org/healthybodies/files/HealthyBodies-Girls-web.pdf. Girlology: You-Ology. A puberty guide for every body by Melissa Holmes.

It is helpful, if possible, to involve a social worker, sexual health educator, or nurse in these discussions to ensure developmentally appropriate teaching and to provide resources for the families to continue the discussions at home. Repeated messages with basic language and safety concepts like NO-GO-TELL are important to be taught and then repeated by the family.[29] NO-GO-TELL is a simple phrase that children can easily remember when in uncomfortable situations. They are taught to say "no," then "go" (i.e., remove themselves from the situation), and finally "tell" an adult.[29] If appropriate, a confidential interview to discuss sexual health should be considered, as it is for all teenagers. Lastly, with the increase of patients with disabilities using the Internet, providers should make an effort to address what types of online communication are safe (Fig. 12.3).

PHYSICAL EXAMINATION

Breast examinations can be started at age 21 or when deemed indicated. Pelvic examinations are not often needed in adolescents, except for the usual gynecologic indications like discharge, vulvar concerns, and so on. Cervical screening recommendations should be discussed with the patient and family and shared decision-making used to decide if and when this is appropriate. Consider these screenings in conjunction with other procedures, like dental procedures. Human papilloma virus (HPV) vaccinations are also recommended, as in the general population.

MENSTRUAL MANAGEMENT/TREATMENT OPTIONS

When discussing menstrual suppression and management, there are special considerations for patients with disabilities. First, it is important to be aware of the impact of menses on the patient's daily life.[30] Does menses prohibit an individual from participating in normal activities? Does it cause pain? Does it lower their seizure threshold? See Table 12.2 for more questions to consider discussing. Second, it is important to consider if a patient has significant mobility challenges and uses a wheelchair exclusively, which may put them at an increased baseline risk of a venous thrombotic event (VTE). If they additionally have other medical comorbidities, such as significant obesity, an estrogen-containing method may be less desirable. Often, patients with disabilities also take medications, like certain antiepileptics, that might interact with hormonal treatments.

Just as with any patient, treatment for menstrual management should be individualized. If there is a need for suppression because of hygiene concerns, an option that will decrease the number of menstrual cycles and flow is typically used. Others may want regulation only or the most effective method for contraception. Each option for menstrual regulation has unique benefits and drawbacks that need to be addressed. Menstrual suppression is not recommended before menarche.[2] See Table 12.3[31] for a complete list of hormonal options with some specific advantages and disadvantages.

Combined Hormonal Contraceptives

Options for menstrual suppression with both ethinyl estradiol and a progestin include a combined oral contraceptive pill (COCP), transdermal patch, or vaginal ring.

The pill can be an easy option for those looking for a noninvasive method of hormonal regulation. This is especially effective for patients already taking other pills at the same time every day. For those who are unable to swallow pills, there are chewable options, and

TABLE 12.2   Some Questions to Consider When Discussing Menstrual Management With Patients With Disabilities

Question	Significance
Does menses prohibit the patient from participating in normal activities?	If yes, shows that this is affecting daily life; if no, shows that may not be a huge issue
Does menses cause pain or behavior changes?	May want to consider continuous use
Does menses affect seizure activity?	Seizures may worsen with menses and therefore may want to consider continuous use
Do they use a wheelchair?	Can increase risk of blood clots if immobile
Are they on medications that can interact with hormonal management?	May reduce contraceptive efficacy or efficacy of antiepileptic drugs in particular
Are they sexually active?	Need to ensure compliance and tolerability
Do they want complete suppression, or do they desire a monthly cycle?	Different hormonal options can offer cyclic versus continuous use

TABLE 12.3   Options for Menstrual Suppression in Patients With Disabilities

Method	Disadvantages in Patients With Disabilities	Amenorrhea Rate[31]
COCP	Increases VTE risk; can interfere with certain antiepileptic drugs	70% at 1 y
Patch	Increases VTE risk; patient can remove	70% at 1 y
Vaginal ring	Increases VTE risk; requires placement by others	Not well-studied
Oral progestin	Breakthrough bleeding	75%–80% at 2 y
DMPA	Increases VTE risk, bone mineral density loss, weight gain	50%–60% at 1 y; 70% at 2 y
Implant	Breakthrough bleeding; patient might pick at device	11%–22% at 1 y
LNG-IUD	Insertion may require anesthesia	50% at 1 y; 60% at 5 y
Endometrial ablation	Not recommended in adolescents	No data in adolescents
Hysterectomy	Major surgery with ethical implications	100% immediately

COCP, Combined oral contraceptives; *DMPA,* depot medroxyprogesterone acetate; *LNG-IUD,* levonorgestrel intrauterine device; *VTE,* venous thromboembolism.

those pills can be crushed through a gastrostomy tube if necessary.

The patch is a good option, as it only needs to be applied weekly. However, patients with sensory issues may not be comfortable with a patch on their body and might pick at it or pull it off. One way to avoid this is to place it high on the patient's back or somewhere on their body that is out of reach.

Although the vaginal ring has the benefit of lasting for 3 to 4 weeks, it can be difficult to place and remove for many adolescents with dexterity and mobility issues, and placement by caregivers is controversial because of the intimate nature.

It is important to note that certain antiepileptic drugs can affect how well estrogen-containing medications work

as contraceptives. Estrogen does not alter the antiepileptic effect of these drugs, except for lamotrigine, in which it can decrease the levels. In addition to the common side effects of breakthrough bleeding, nausea, and headaches, a specific concern in patients with disabilities is VTE risk. Combined hormonal contraceptives (CHCs) increase the risk of VTEs in adolescents who take them—about two to three times the baseline risk for adolescents of 1 to 2/10,000.[32,33] Although there are no data on VTE in adolescents who use wheelchairs, minimal data on VTE in adults with mobility issues suggest a small increase in VTE risk.[34,35] When counseling adolescents with mobility concerns, consider all VTE risk factors together, such as obesity and family history.[36] Most young women who sustained a VTE on oral contraceptives (OCPs) have multiple risk factors.[37]

Progestin-Only Methods

VTEs should be discussed with families before initiating a progestin-only method. Even though the risk is lower than in estrogen-containing methods, a recent meta-analysis of women ages 15 to 49 concluded that although there was no increased risk of VTE for most progestin contraceptives, including the levonorgestrel intrauterine device (LNG-IUD), oral norethindrone, etonogestrel implant, and oral progesterone, there was a two to three times increased VTE risk with the use of depot medroxyprogesterone acetate (DMPA) and high doses of oral medroxyprogesterone and oral norethindrone acetate.[38,39]

Options for menstrual management with a progestin-only method, especially when estrogen may be contraindicated, include a pill, an injection, and an implant in the arm or uterus.

There are currently five oral progestin formulations in the US: norethindrone, norethindrone acetate, drospirenone, medroxyprogesterone acetate and megestrol. The benefit of pills is that dose adjustments can be made for adequate menstrual suppression. Additionally, the pill can be crushed for those who are unable to swallow pills. Unexpected bleeding, particularly at lower doses of progestins and with norethindrone, are common. These side effects can be difficult for patients with disabilities who seek timely menstrual suppression. Anticipatory counseling can often mitigate cessation of use.

DMPA is a well-tolerated intramuscular injection given every 10 to 12 weeks that leads to a 60% to 70% amenorrhea rate.[40] Side effects of DMPA include loss of bone mineral density, which is often already a concern in adolescents with disabilities, especially because of mobility concerns and other medications. Weight gain can be significant, especially in obese adolescents, and may lead to difficulty with transfers. The effects of DMPA on the menstrual cycle can last for as long as 9 months, so if significant mood concerns already exist, trying oral medroxyprogesterone first may be an option, as it can be stopped when desired.

The etonogestrel implant is Food and Drug Administration (FDA)-approved for 3 years; however, studies have shown that the contraceptive effect lasts for up to 5 years.[41] Patients with disabilities may struggle with the insertion of the device in the office, so it may need to be done with sedation. Additionally, those with sensory issues might pick at the device and not tolerate its placement. There is currently a clinical trial underway to see if an alternate scapular site in one's back may offer the same degree of efficacy. If shown to be effective, this may have significant benefit for patients with disabilities who may not tolerate having the device in the arm. Similar to other progestin-only forms of contraception, this can cause significant unplanned breakthrough bleeding (amenorrhea rates of only 11%–22%).

The LNG-IUD is an excellent long-acting hormonal method and one of the most effective options for contraception, with a high amenorrhea rate. There are several LNG-IUDs, with different amounts of LNG and variable bleeding patterns.[42] One drawback of this method in patients with disabilities is that they may not be able to describe discomfort or pain if the IUD is mispositioned. It also can expel 3% to 5% of the time. Another challenge with the LNG-IUD is that insertion is generally not tolerated in an office setting for adolescents with disabilities, so most require intravenous (IV) sedation or general anesthesia for placement. A recent study looking at 159 females under age 22 found that in 185 IUD placements over a 10-year period, 96% were done in the operating room.[43] This same study showed that most adolescents were satisfied with the IUD and kept them long term—95% at 1 year and 73% at 5 years. It can be useful to alert patients and families that if they are ever undergoing anesthesia for another reason, an IUD placement can typically be performed at the same time.

Surgical Options for Menstrual Suppression

The two surgical options for patients with disabilities are endometrial ablation and hysterectomy. According to ACOG, endometrial ablation is never recommended in adolescents and is specifically designed for older women who have completed childbearing.[2] Despite some families of children with significant disabilities requesting a hysterectomy for menstrual management, this is usually reserved only for medically indicated reasons such as cancer or as a last result when all other options are exhausted and the patient's health is compromised. Not only is a hysterectomy a major surgery with significant risks and recovery time, but it is also a complex issue with significant legal and ethical concerns.[44]

Choosing the Best Method

In a 2021 study of 262 adolescents with disabilities and menstrual concerns, final methods of treatment included

CHCs (30.9%), oral progestins (19.8%), DMPA (8.0%), etonogestrel implant (1.9%), and LNG-IUD (16.8%). Eighty-five percent of patients were satisfied with their final bleeding pattern, but no specific hormone was superior to another.[45] Individualized patient-centered care, taking into consideration the patient's and family's goals for menstrual management, will determine the optimal method and bleeding pattern outcomes.

KEY POINTS

- One in six children in the United States has a disability.
- The risk of sexual violence and coercion is up to threefold higher in this population.
- Though they are often at the highest need, sexual health education is addressed less often in this population; providers should help but need more education.
- Puberty is often in line with nondisabled peers but can be more isolating.
- The main reproductive health issues are safety, menstrual effect on daily life, and moods.
- There are several options for menstrual suppression and contraception, each with unique benefits and risks.

▌REVIEW QUESTIONS

1. A mom brings her 10-year-old daughter with DiGeorge syndrome to you for anticipatory guidance on menarche. The mom says that her daughter started having breast development 1 year ago. She has not had a period. The mother is wondering if we can start her daughter on birth control pills to suppress her from having periods before they start, as she knows that her daughter will not respond well to the sight of blood. You tell her:
   a. Definitely. We can start today to suppress her first period from ever coming.
   b. Her first period is late, as it should occur at the same time as breast development.
   c. It is best to place an intrauterine device instead of starting pills at her age.
   d. Menarche typically occurs 2 to 2.5 years after breast development begins. We do not consider starting medication for suppression until after this occurs.

2. A 15-year-old girl with spina bifida presents to discuss birth control. She has a history of a deep venous thrombosis. She would like to use a method that is noninvasive, and she is scared of needles. You recommend:
   a. Combined hormonal contraceptive pills
   b. Progestin-only pills
   c. No method, as she will never be able to have intercourse
   d. Vaginal ring

3. A 17-year-old girl with autism had menarche 6 months ago and presents to you with dysmenorrhea. In addition to addressing her pain, it is important to discuss:
   a. Sexuality and sex education
   b. Safety and healthy relationships
   c. Gender identity
   d. All of the above

REFERENCES

1. Centers for Disease Control and Prevention. Increase in Developmental Disabilities Among Children in the United States. 2021. Accessed November 8, 2022. https://www.cdc.gov/ncbddd/developmentaldisabilities/features/increase-in-developmental-disabilities.html
2. American College of Obstetricians Gynecologists' Committee on Adolescent Health Care. Committee opinion no. 668: menstrual manipulation for adolescents with physical and developmental disabilities. *Obstet Gynecol.* 2016;128(2):e20-e25.
3. Centers for Disease Control and Prevention. Disability and Health Overview. 2020. Accessed November 15, 2022. https://www.cdc.gov/ncbddd/disabilityandhealth/disability.html
4. Corbett BA, Schwartzman JM, Libsack EJ, et al. Camouflaging in autism: examining sex-based and compensatory models in social cognition and communication. *Autism Res.* 2021;14(1):127-142.
5. Haynes RM, Boulet SL, Fox MH, Carroll DD, Courtney-Long E, Warner L. Contraceptive use at last intercourse among reproductive-aged women with disabilities: an analysis of population-based data from seven states. *Contraception.* 2018;97(6):538-545.
6. Legano LA, Desch LW, Messner SA, et al. Maltreatment of children with disabilities. *Pediatrics.* 2021;147(5):e2021050920.
7. Iezzoni LI, Mitra M. Transcending the counternormative: sexual and reproductive health and persons with disability. *Disabil Health J.* 2017;10(3):369-370.
8. Ballan MS, Freyer MB. The sexuality of young women with intellectual and developmental disabilities: a neglected focus in the American foster care system. *Disabil Health J.* 2017;10(3):371-375.

9. Horner-Johnson W, Senders A, Higgins Tejera C, McGee MG. Sexual health experiences among high school students with disabilities. *J Adolesc Health.* 2021;69(2):255-262.

10. Wilson NJ, Macdonald J, Hayman B, Bright AM, Frawley P, Gallego G. A narrative review of the literature about people with intellectual disability who identify as lesbian, gay, bisexual, transgender, intersex or questioning. *J Intellect Disabil.* 2018;22(2):171-196.

11. Strang JF, Kenworthy L, Dominska A, et al. Increased gender variance in autism spectrum disorders and attention deficit hyperactivity disorder. *Arch Sex Behav.* 2014;43(8):1525-1533.

12. de Vries AL, Noens IL, Cohen-Kettenis PT, van Berckelaer-Onnes IA, Doreleijers TA. Autism spectrum disorders in gender dysphoric children and adolescents. *J Autism Dev Disord.* 2010;40(8):930-936.

13. Michielsen K, Brockschmidt L. Barriers to sexuality education for children and young people with disabilities in the WHO European region: a scoping review. *Sex Educ.* 2021;21(6):674-692.

14. Smith DL. Disparities in patient-physician communication for persons with a disability from the 2006 Medical Expenditure Panel Survey (MEPS). *Disabil Health J.* 2009;2(4):206-215.

15. Long-Bellil LM, Robey KL, Graham CL, et al. Teaching medical students about disability: the use of standardized patients. *Acad Med.* 2011;86(9):1163-1170.

16. Taouk LH, Fialkow MF, Schulkin JA. Provision of reproductive healthcare to women with disabilities: a survey of obstetrician-gynecologists' training, practices, and perceived barriers. *Health Equity.* 2018;2(1):207-215.

17. Holmes LG, Himle MB, Sewell KK, Carbone PS, Strassberg DS, Murphy NA. Addressing sexuality in youth with autism spectrum disorders: current pediatric practices and barriers. *J Dev Behav Pediatr.* 2014;35(3):172-178.

18. Streur CS, Schafer CL, Garcia VP, Quint EH, Sandberg DE, Wittmann DA. "If everyone else is having this talk with their doctor, why am I not having this talk with mine?": The experiences of sexuality and sexual health education of young women with spina bifida. *J Sex Med.* 2019;16(6):853-859.

19. Fei YF, Ernst SD, Dendrinos ML, Quint EH. Preparing for puberty in girls with special needs: a cohort study of caregiver concerns and patient outcomes. *J Pediatr Adolesc Gynecol.* 2021;34(4):471-476.

20. Kirkham YA, Allen L, Kives S, Caccia N, Spitzer RF, Ornstein MP. Trends in menstrual concerns and suppression in adolescents with developmental disabilities. *J Adolesc Health.* 2013;53(3):407-412.

21. Patel DR, Greydanus DE, Calles Jr JL, Pratt HD. Developmental disabilities across the lifespan. *Dis Mon.* 2010;56(6):304-397.

22. Wilbur J, Torondel B, Hameed S, Mahon T, Kuper H. Systematic review of menstrual hygiene management requirements, its barriers and strategies for disabled people. *PLoS One.* 2019;14(2):e0210974.

23. Breuner CC, Mattson G, Committee on Adolescence, Committee on Psychosocial Aspects of Child and Family Health. Sexuality education for children and adolescents. *Pediatrics.* 2016;138(2):e20161348.

24. Rosen M. Pediatric and Adolescent Gynecology, Part 1 – Patients with Disabilities [Internet]. University of Michigan; 2022. Podcast. https://www.obgyndelivered.com/podcast/episode/1a44732e/pediatric-and-adolescent-gynecology-part-1-patients-with-disabilities

25. Leanage A, Burgess R, Ogrodnik M, Malik P. Sexual Health and Sexual Education for Women with Disabilities: Challenges & Opportunities. 2018. https://docs.wixstatic.com/ugd/b2d084_4b5e683f5921486f9a76a7a5bc4dad8b.pdf

26. World Health Organization, United Nations Population Fund. Promoting Sexual and Reproductive Health for Persons with Disabilities. 2009. Accessed November 17, 2022. https://www.unfpa.org/publications/promoting-sexual-and-reproductive-health-persons-disabilities

27. Vanderbilt Kennedy Center, Vanderbilt Leadership in Neurodevelopmental Disabilities (LEND). Healthy Bodies: A Parent's Guide on Puberty for Girls with Disabilities. 2021. https://vkc.vumc.org/healthybodies/files/HealthyBodies-Girls-web.pdf

28. Autism Speaks Autism Treatment Network, Autism Intervention Research Network on Physical Health. Parent's Guide to Puberty and Adolescence for Children with Autism. 2014. Accessed November 17, 2022. https://www.autismspeaks.org/sites/default/files/2018-08/Puberty%20and%20Adolescence%20Resource.pdf

29. Pollio E, Deblinger E. Trauma-focused cognitive behavioural therapy for young children: clinical considerations. *Eur J Psychotraumatol.* 2017;8(suppl 7):1433929.

30. Albanese A, Hopper NW. Suppression of menstruation in adolescents with severe learning disabilities. *Arch Dis Child.* 2007;92(7):629-632.

31. Hillard PA. Menstrual suppression: current perspectives. *Int J Womens Health.* 2014;6:631-637.

32. Hennessey CA, Patel VK, Tefera EA, Gomez-Lobo V. Venous thromboembolism in female adolescents: patient characteristics. *J Pediatr Adolesc Gynecol.* 2018;31(5):503-508.

33. Stein PD, Kayali F, Olson RE. Incidence of venous thromboembolism in infants and children: data from the National Hospital Discharge Survey. *J Pediatr.* 2004;145(4):563-565.

34. Oedingen C, Scholz S, Razum O. Systematic review and meta-analysis of the association of combined oral contraceptives on the risk of venous thromboembolism: the

role of the progestogen type and estrogen dose. *Thromb Res.* 2018;165:68-78.

35. Spentzouris G, Scriven RJ, Lee TK, Labropoulos N. Pediatric venous thromboembolism in relation to adults. *J Vasc Surg.* 2012;55(6):1785-1793.

36. Srivaths L, Dietrich JE. Prothrombotic risk factors and preventive strategies in adolescent venous thromboembolism. *Clin Appl Thromb Hemost.* 2016;22(6):512-519.

37. Maher KN, Quint EH, Weyand AC. Management of contraception in adolescent females with hormone-related venous thromboembolism. *J Adolesc Health.* 2022;71(1):127-131.

38. Tepper NK, Whiteman MK, Marchbanks PA, James AH, Curtis KM. Progestin-only contraception and thromboembolism: a systematic review. *Contraception.* 2016;94(6):678-700.

39. Cockrum RH, Soo J, Ham SA, Cohen KS, Snow SG. Association of progestogens and venous thromboembolism among women of reproductive age. *Obstet Gynecol.* 2022;140(3):477-487.

40. Raidoo S, Pearlman Shapiro M, Kaneshiro B. Contraception in adolescents. *Semin Reprod Med.* 2022;40(1-02):89-97.

41. McNicholas C, Maddipati R, Zhao Q, Swor E, Peipert JF. Use of the etonogestrel implant and levonorgestrel intrauterine device beyond the U.S. Food and Drug Administration-approved duration. *Obstet Gynecol.* 2015;125(3):599-604.

42. American College of Obstetricians and Gynecologists. Practice bulletin no. 110: noncontraceptive uses of hormonal contraceptives. *Obstet Gynecol.* 2010;115(1):206-218.

43. Schwartz BI, Alexander M, Breech LL. Intrauterine device use in adolescents with disabilities. *Pediatrics.* 2020;146(2):e20200016.

44. Quint EH, O'Brien RF, Committee on Adolescence, North American Society for Pediatric and Adolescent Gynecology. Menstrual management for adolescents with disabilities. *Pediatrics.* 2016;138(1):e20160295.

45. Frances Fei Y, Ernst SD, Dendrinos ML, Quint EH. Satisfaction with hormonal treatment for menstrual suppression in adolescents and young women with disabilities. *J Adolesc Health.* 2021;69(3):482-488.

Relative Energy Deficiency in Sports

Mary E. Romano and Debra K. Braun-Courville

INTRODUCTION

Relative energy deficiency in sports (RED-S) is a more comprehensive term for the condition previously known as the *female athlete triad (FAT)* (Fig. 13.1). In 2014 the International Olympic Committee (IOC) issued a consensus statement outlining and expanding FAT to a broader definition known as RED-S, which describes the sequelae of the energy imbalance that can occur in athletes (both recreational and professional) who do not meet their daily nutritional needs.[1] This expanded definition reflects emerging evidence that[1] the condition can occur in both males and females and[2] the physiologic impairments extend beyond the components of the triad—energy availability, menstrual function, and bone health. The IOC also suggested that low energy availability can have direct effects on physical health but also overall athletic performance. RED-S recognizes that symptoms occur along a spectrum and that identification of subclinical symptoms should prompt early intervention and treatment to minimize the risks of long-term disease.[1,2]

This chapter will provide an overview of RED-S, including existing definitions, epidemiology and risk factors, proposed pathophysiology, clinical signs and symptoms, screening evaluation, and management. We also provide information about research gaps and special considerations when treating this population. Of note throughout the chapter, male and female refers to sex assigned at birth to reflect the existing literature. This chapter will focus on females given that this is a book covering important topics in pediatric and adolescent gynecology.

MANAGEMENT/TREATMENT

RED-S is defined as any impairment in physiologic functioning caused by relative energy deficiency. This can include menstrual function, bone health, gastrointestinal conditions, hematologic findings, immune function, cardiovascular health, physical injury, impaired athletic performance, and psychological stress. The energy deficiency may be an unintentional mismatch between energy intake and energy spent through exercise or may be intentional because of the presence of disordered eating. Low energy availability (EA) is the hallmark of RED-S; energy availability can be defined as follows[3]:

$$\text{Energy Availability} = \frac{\substack{\text{Energy Intake (in kcal)} \\ -\text{Exercise Energy} \\ \text{Expenditure (in kcal)}}}{\text{Fat-Free Mass (in kg)}}$$

PREVALENCE AND EPIDEMIOLOGY

It is hard to assess the overall prevalence of RED-S due to the spectrum of the disease as athletes may have any number of the components and not necessarily all at the same time. Although any athlete can have issues with energy deficiency, athletes in individual sports and those that focus on weight class, leanness, size/appearance, and endurance are thought to be most at risk. There are also concerns that focusing on a single sport at an earlier age can also increase the athlete's risk of inadequate/low EA.[4] Several large-scale studies have looked at the population thought to be at most risk—elite

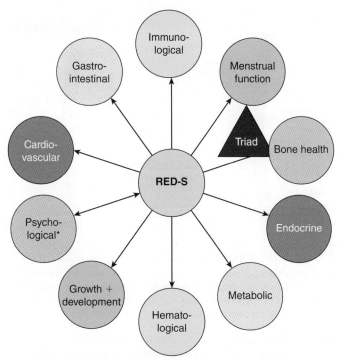

Fig. 13.1 Relative energy deficiency in sports (RED-S), a more comprehensive term for the condition previously known as female athlete triad (TRIAD), reflecting all systems affected by low energy availability (EA). (Mountjoy M, Sundgot-Borgen J, Burke L, et al. The IOC consensus statement: beyond the female athlete triadrelative energy deficiency in sport [RED-S]. *Br J Sports Med.* 2014;48[7]:491-497.)

female collegiate athletes. Earlier studies looking at triad components in this population found that 27% of athletes reported menstrual disturbance, 6% had low bone mineral density (BMD), and 16% had sustained at least one stress fracture.[5] Later studies looking at the broader RED-S criteria in elite female athletes found that 50% to 80% of athletes reported some component of RED-S, with menstrual dysfunction, bone health, and anxiety being the most common symptoms.[6] It is also important to note that one does not have to be an elite athlete to be at risk for low EA, as one study demonstrated a risk of low EA in up to 45% of recreational athletes.[7]

ETIOLOGY AND PATHOPHYSIOLOGY

Low EA is the primary driver and etiology of RED-S. A mismatch between energy taken in through diet and calories expended through exercise results in the downstream sequelae observed in athletes. It can be difficult to

accurately assess EA in a person because of the reliability of self-reported intake data and the specialized tools needed for accurate EA measurement. Therefore measuring EA is not routinely recommended. Data suggest that in an active female, adequate energy availability is ≥45 kcal/kg of fat-free mass (FFM) per day, and negative physiologic changes are observed when EA is ≤30 kcal/kg/FFM per day.[1] Low EA may be voluntary, with intentional inadequate oral intake. But for some athletes, inadequate intake is unintentional and not the result of disordered eating, compulsive exercise, or weight control behaviors. Athletes who involuntarily underfuel and fail to increase caloric and nutritional intake when they increase exercise through additional training or competition requirements may also be predisposed to RED-S (Fig. 13.2).

Although every bodily system is affected by low EA, the triad components have been most studied and described in the literature. Low EA appears to alter the function of the hypothalamic-pituitary-ovarian (HPO)

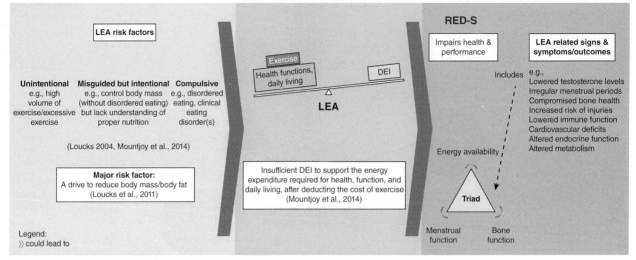

Fig. 13.2 Unintentional, misguided but intentional, and compulsive behaviors are risk factors for low energy availability (LEA). These risk factors can result in a decrease in dietary energy intake (DEI) and/or increase in exercise energy expenditure (EEE). Over time, these lead to relative energy deficiency in sport (RED-S), with concomitant health and performance consequences. These can present as signs, symptoms, and outcomes in both male (e.g., lowered testosterone levels) and female (e.g., irregular menstrual cycle) athletes. RED-S encompasses the earlier identified condition female athlete triad (Triad). (Sim A, Burns F. Review: questionnaires as measures for low energy availability [LEA] and relative energy deficiency in sport [RED-S] in athletes. *J Eat Disord.* 2021;9:41).

axis by disrupting the pulsatile secretion of gonadotropin-releasing hormone (GnRH), which then affects the downstream secretion of luteinizing hormone (LH) and follicle-stimulating hormone (FSH). Loss of pulsatile LH and FSH secretion results in ovulatory dysfunction and decreased estradiol production (Fig. 13.3). Physiologically, menstrual suppression is an adaptive conservation mechanism to the low EA state, whereby available energy is directed to more essential bodily functions.[1,2] This disruption is referred to as *functional hypothalamic amenorrhea (FHA),* and restoration of EA will restore HPO axis function and ovulation. The exact mechanism is unclear, as there is variability among athletes in terms of the degree or duration of low EA that triggers HPO dysfunction. Other RED-S endocrine effects described include alterations in thyroid function, decreases in insulin secretion, and elevations in cortisol secretion. The anorexigenic and orexigenic hormones of leptin, peptide YY, and ghrelin can also be affected (see Fig. 13.3).[1]

Optimal hormonal status (estrogen, testosterone, growth hormone, insulin, and insulin-like growth factor [IGF]-1) is needed to establish and maintain healthy bones.[8] Estrogen plays a critical role in bone development, particularly internal endocortical bone. Estrogen also affects both bone osteoblastic and osteoclastic activity, forming healthy bone and achieving peak bone mass. FHA leads to overall reduced ovarian estradiol production, which can disrupt bone development. Impaired bone health in female athletes with low EA is well established.[9-11] Although exercise and mechanical loading are known to improve bone health,[8,12,13] physical activity in the face of inadequate EA will ultimately decrease bone strength.[14] Athletes with menstrual dysfunction are more than twice as likely to develop a stress fracture compared with their eumenorrheic counterparts.[15] Studies have found that low EA as a consequence of calorie restriction may be more harmful for bones compared with excessive exercise.[16] Athletes with low EA demonstrate documented decreases in BMD and disruptions to bone turnover markers and bone microarchitecture; these changes are associated with an increased risk of bone stress injury.[10] Female athletes with low EA and impaired menstrual function have been shown to have lower BMD at the hip, femoral

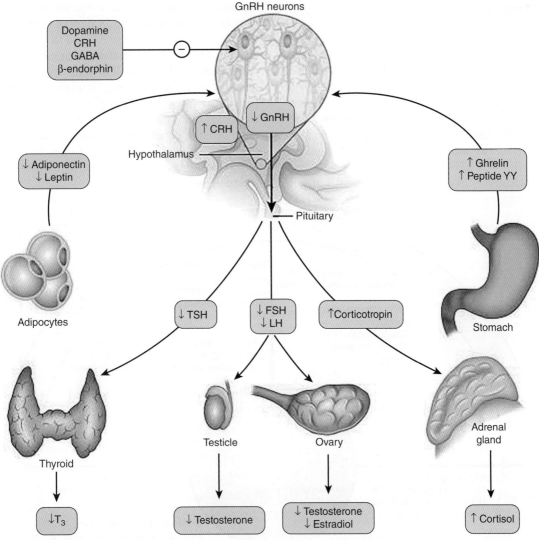

Fig. 13.3 Low energy availability (EA) causes disruptions in hormones that decrease the secretion of gonadotropin-releasing hormone (GnRH). There is overactivity of the hypothalamic-pituitary-adrenal axis, causing an increase in corticotropin-releasing hormone (CRH) and corticotropins/cortisol. There is decreased activity of the hypothalamic-pituitary-gonadal axis, causing a decrease in follicle-stimulating hormone (FSH), luteinizing hormone (LH), estrogen, and testosterone. There are also changes to thyroid hormones including thyroid-stimulating hormone (TSH) and triiodothyronine (T_3). (From Donaldson, A. Gordon C. Skeletal complications of eating disorders. *Metabolism*. 2015;64[9]:943-951.)

neck, spine, and whole body.[2,11] This impairment is associated with menstrual dysfunction, which can range from oligomenorrhea to amenorrhea; these bone changes are not seen in eumenorrheic athletes.[1] The resulting changes in BMD may lead to increased fracture risk.[11,17] Although low EA may occur independent of low weight and body mass index (BMI), there is an increased incidence of low BMD observed in females with BMI <17.5 kg/m^2 or weight <85th percentile for age/sex. The risk for injury is higher in athletes with low EA who also have the triad of disordered eating, menstrual dysfunction, and low BMD.[10]

SCREENING

Screening requires that coaches, trainers, and health care providers working with athletes have an awareness and a high index of clinical suspicion about the manifestations of low EA, which may or may not be associated with disordered eating behaviors (Fig. 13.4). Prior research has shown a general lack of awareness of the disorder.[18-20] Annual preparticipation examinations should include an assessment of symptoms associated with low EA and RED-S, including regular screenings for any change or disruption in menstrual function,

recurrent or nonhealing stress injuries, and disordered or restrictive eating patterns. A normal weight does not exclude the possibility of low EA, and all athletes should be comprehensively asked about their eating and exercise behaviors. The American Academy of Pediatrics preparticipation history form (https://www.aap.org/en/patient-care/preparticipation-physical-evaluation/) incorporates questions looking at specific risk factors, and the IOC has developed a Clinical Assessment Tool (RED-S CAT) that assesses risk factors for RED-S as well as outlining criteria for sports participation and/or return to play[21,22] (Fig. 13.5).

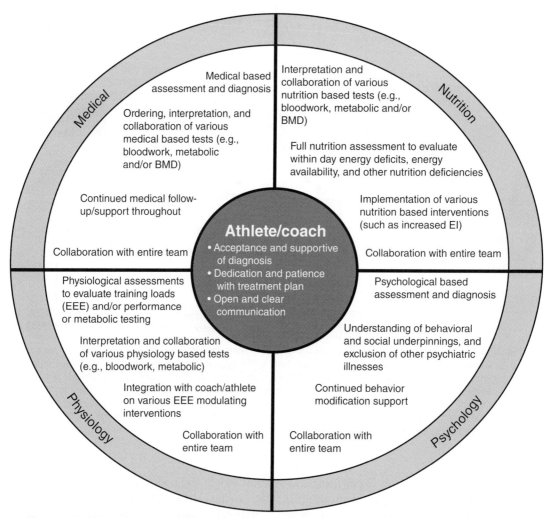

Fig. 13.4 Multidisciplinary approach to relative energy deficiency in sports (RED-S). Approach to be used in screening, treatment, and prevention of RED-S. (From Stellingwerff T, Heikura IA, Meeusen R, et al. Overtraining syndrome (OTS) and relative energy deficiency in sport (RED-S): shared pathways, symptoms and complexities. *Sports Med.* 2021;51:2251-2280.)

This form should be placed into the athlete's medical file and should *not* be shared with schools or sports organizations. The Medical Eligibility Form is the only form that should be submitted to a school or sports organization.

Disclaimer: Athletes who have a current Preparticipation Physical Evaluation (per state and local guidance) on file should not need to complete another History Form.

■ **PREPARTICIPATION PHYSICAL EVALUATION (Interim Guidance)**

HISTORY FORM

Note: Complete and sign this form (with your parents if younger than 18) before your appointment.

Name: _____ Date of birth: _____

Date of examination: _____ Sport(s): _____

Sex assigned at birth (F, M, or intersex): _____ How do you identify your sex? (F, M, non-binary, or another sex): _____

Have you had COVID-19? (check one): ☐ Y ☐ N

Have you been immunized for COVID-19? (check one): ☐ Y ☐ N   If yes, have you had: ☐ One shot ☐ Two shots ☐ Three shots ☐ Booster date(s) _____

List past and current medical conditions. _____

Have you ever had surgery? If yes, list all past surgical procedures. _____

Medicines and supplements: List all current prescriptions, over-the-counter medicines, and supplements (herbal and nutritional). _____

Do you have any allergies? If yes, please list all your allergies (i.e., medicines, pollens, food, stinging insects). _____

Patient Health Questionnaire Version 4 (PHQ-4)

Over the last 2 weeks, how often have you been bothered by any of the following problems? (Circle response.)

	Not at all	Several days	Over half the days	Nearly every day
Feeling nervous, anxious, or on edge	0	1	2	3
Not being able to stop or control worrying	0	1	2	3
Little interest or pleasure in doing things	0	1	2	3
Feeling down, depressed, or hopeless	0	1	2	3

(A sum of ≥3 is considered positive on either subscale [questions 1 and 2, or questions 3 and 4] for screening purposes.)

GENERAL QUESTIONS (Explain "Yes" answers at the end of this form. Circle questions if you don't know the answer.)	Yes	No
1. Do you have any concerns that you would like to discuss with your provider?		
2. Has a provider ever denied or restricted your participation in sports for any reason?		
3. Do you have any ongoing medical issues or recent illness?		
HEART HEALTH QUESTIONS ABOUT YOU	Yes	No
4. Have you ever passed out or nearly passed out during or after exercise?		
5. Have you ever had discomfort, pain, tightness, or pressure in your chest during exercise?		
6. Does your heart ever race, flutter in your chest, or skip beats (irregular beats) during exercise?		
7. Has a doctor ever told you that you have any heart problems?		
8. Has a doctor ever requested a test for your heart? For example, electrocardiography (ECG) or echocardiography.		

HEART HEALTH QUESTIONS ABOUT YOU (*CONTINUED*)		Yes	No
9. Do you get light-headed or feel shorter of breath than your friends during exercise?			
10. Have you ever had a seizure?			
HEART HEALTH QUESTIONS ABOUT YOUR FAMILY	Unsure	Yes	No
11. Has any family member or relative died of heart problems or had an unexpected or unexplained sudden death before age 35 years (including drowning or unexplained car crash)?			
12. Does anyone in your family have a genetic heart problem such as hypertrophic cardio-myopathy (HCM), Marfan syndrome, arrhyth-mogenic right ventricular cardiomyopathy (ARVC), long QT syndrome (LQTS), short QT syndrome (SQTS), Brugada syndrome, or catecholaminergic polymorphic ventricular tachycardia (CPVT)?			
13. Has anyone in your family had a pacemaker or an implanted defibrillator before age 35?			

Fig. 13.5 American Academy of Pediatrics preparticipation history form (https://www.aap.org/en/patient-care/preparticipation-physical-evaluation/). Questions 2, 14, 25 through 32 are most pertinent to this population.

BONE AND JOINT QUESTIONS	Yes	No
14. Have you ever had a stress fracture or an injury to a bone, muscle, ligament, joint, or tendon that caused you to miss a practice or game?		
15. Do you have a bone, muscle, ligament, or joint injury that bothers you?		
MEDICAL QUESTIONS	Yes	No
16. Do you cough, wheeze, or have difficulty breathing during or after exercise?		
17. Are you missing a kidney, an eye, a testicle, your spleen, or any other organ?		
18. Do you have groin or testicle pain or a painful bulge or hernia in the groin area?		
19. Do you have any recurring skin rashes or rashes that come and go, including herpes or methicillin-resistant *Staphylococcus aureus* (MRSA)?		
20. Have you had a concussion or head injury that caused confusion, a prolonged headache, or memory problems?		
21. Have you ever had numbness, had tingling, had weakness in your arms or legs, or been unable to move your arms or legs after being hit or falling?		
22. Have you ever become ill while exercising in the heat?		
23. Do you or does someone in your family have sickle cell trait or disease? **Unsure**		
24. Have you ever had or do you have any problems with your eyes or vision?		

MEDICAL QUESTIONS (*CONTINUED*)		Yes	No
25. Do you worry about your weight?			
26. Are you trying to or has anyone recommended that you gain or lose weight?			
27. Are you on a special diet or do you avoid certain types of foods or food groups?			
28. Have you ever had an eating disorder?			
MENSTRUAL QUESTIONS	N/A	Yes	No
29. Have you ever had a menstrual period?			
30. How old were you when you had your first menstrual period?			
31. When was your most recent menstrual period?			
32. How many periods have you had in the past 12 months?			

Explain "Yes" answers here.

I hereby state that, to the best of my knowledge, my answers to the questions on this form are complete and correct.

Signature of athlete: _____

Signature of parent or guardian: _____

Date: _____

© 2023 American Academy of Family Physicians, American Academy of Pediatrics, American College of Sports Medicine, American Medical Society for Sports Medicine, American Orthopaedic Society for Sports Medicine, and American Osteopathic Academy of Sports Medicine. Permission is granted to reprint for noncommercial, educational purposes with acknowledgment.

Fig. 13.5, cont'd

When there are concerns for disordered eating behaviors or other psychiatric diagnoses, it is appropriate to have those athletes further assessed by a provider with expertise in the treatment of eating disorders. Several questionnaires have been developed to assess eating behaviors and attitudes in athletes, although they have not been universally validated for all ages, sexes, and levels of athletes. These include the SCOFF, the Eating Attitudes Test (EAT), the Eating Disorder Screen for Primary Care (ESP), the Eating Disorder Examination Questions (EDE-Q), the Brief ED in Athletes Questionnaire (BEDA), and the Low Energy Availability in Females Questionnaire (LEAF-Q)[23-25] (Table 13.1).

A menstrual history should be taken in all female athletes with attention to questions about contraceptive use that may alter bleeding patterns. Age at menarche, menstrual frequency, episodes of missed menses, and duration of periods should be evaluated. Many athletes assume that amenorrhea is normal. However, it is not appropriate for athletes to have a change in their

TABLE 13.1 Questionnaires Used or Developed to Measure Low Energy Availability

Questionnaire	Validated	Behavior Based[1]	Symptom Based[2]	Diagnostic vs. Screening Tool
Low Energy Availability in Females Questionnaire (LEAF-Q)	Yes, with endurance-trained female athletes	N/A	Provider assessment of symptoms related to low energy availability—GI symptoms, menstrual dysfunction, injury history	Screening
Eating Disorder Inventory (EDI) – Drive for Thinness (DT)	No	Self-report of disordered eating attitudes	N/A	Screening
Eating Disorder Examination – Questionnaire (EDE-Q)	Yes, for nonactive males and females	Self-report of eating disorder behaviors	N/A	Screening
Brief Eating Disorder in Athletes Questionnaire – BEDA-Q	Yes, in adolescent female elite athletes	Self-reported assessment of weight loss intention and history of dieting	Self-reported assessment of body image concerns, desire for weight loss	Screening
RED-S Risk Assessment	No	Provider assessment of eating disorder behaviors	Provider assessment of symptoms related to low energy availability—GI symptoms, menstrual dysfunction, injury history	Screening and return-to-play guidelines
Eating Disorder Screen for Primary Care (ESP)	Yes: primary care patients, university students, and athletes	Provider assessment of eating disorder behaviors	N/A	Screening

Question Examples:

[1]Behavior based:

- Do you restrict your intake to change your weight?
- Do you ever eat in secret or hide/hoard food?
- Do you ever binge, overeat, or feel like you lose control when eating?
- Do you ever do anything to "get rid of" food/calories that you've taken in—purging, excessive exercise, diet pills, or laxatives?
- Are you actively trying to lose weight?

[2]Symptom based:

- Does your weight affect the way you feel about yourself?
- Do you feel guilty after eating?
- Are you preoccupied with the desire to be thinner?
- Do you have any dizziness with standing?
- Do you have fatigue or headaches?
- Do you have frequent abdominal pain, fullness, or bloating?
- Do you have any issues with constipation?
- Do you have any missed periods or prolonged periods of amenorrhea?
- Have there been any significant changes in your weight in the last 6 months?
- Have you had absences from your athletic training or been restricted from participation in sports because of injury?

menstrual pattern or amenorrhea when their activity levels increase, and those who experience this should be further assessed for the presence of low EA and/or disordered eating. FHA in RED-S is a diagnosis of exclusion, and other causes of menstrual dysfunction, including pregnancy or contraceptive use, should be assessed before making a RED-S diagnosis.

MANIFESTATIONS AND CLINICAL PRESENTATION

Athletes with RED-S can present with a variety of symptoms given all the bodily systems that are affected by low EA. Athletes may present with alterations in their vital signs, including bradycardia, hypotension, orthostasis, or hypothermia. They may also present with decreased energy, fatigue, near syncope, or syncope. Bradycardia may be difficult to assess based on the low resting heart rate present in many elite athletes. Resting metabolic rate is often reduced in athletes with EA as an energy conservation mechanism.[26-28] As outlined earlier, athletes may also present with changes to their menstrual pattern, which can range from shorter/lighter periods to complete amenorrhea. Athletes may also present with a stress fracture and/or stress injury. Weight loss may be a presenting feature for some individuals, and even in athletes in whom weight loss is appropriate, it is important to ask how patients are losing weight and monitor for precipitous changes in weight, especially if they are associated with other signs of low EA as described earlier. In athletes who have not yet completed their growth and development, particularly those athletes less than 18 years of age, lack of weight gain or arrest of growth should always be a concern. Patients may present with gastrointestinal symptoms such as nausea, early satiety, abdominal pain, constipation, or bloating (Table 13.2).

Patients with RED-S may also present with psychological symptoms such as depressed or anxious mood, body image dissatisfaction, obsessive thoughts, compulsive behaviors, or disordered eating. Disordered eating behaviors include restrictive eating, self-induced vomiting, binging, and compulsive and excessive exercise behaviors. For many athletes with RED-S there are psychological and/or psychiatric comorbidities that may present before or at the onset of symptoms. However, there is some evidence that low EA itself can contribute to psychological symptoms. Adolescents who have a

diagnosis of FHA have been reported to have higher rates of depressive symptoms and other psychosomatic disorders, as well as decreased ability to handle stress. These symptoms occurred in those without a diagnosis of anorexia nervosa, although they were higher in the group with a diagnosed restrictive eating disorder.[2]

In addition to physical and psychological health manifestations, overall sports performance may be negatively affected by RED-S. The IOC outlined several possible athletic performance changes that may be associated with RED-S (Fig. 13.6).

TABLE 13.2 **Manifestations/Clinical Presentations of RED-S**
Vital Signs
Bradycardia
Hypothermia
Orthostasis
Systemic Symptoms
Fatigue
Syncope
Dizziness
Menstrual Changes
Oligomenorrhea
Amenorrhea
Musculoskeletal
Stress fracture
Stress/overuse injury
Decreased endurance/poor performance
Growth/Development
Weight loss
Arrest of growth
Pubertal arrest/delay
Gastrointestinal
Nausea
Vomiting
Early satiety
Constipation
Bloating
Psychological
Depressed or anxious mood
Obsessive thoughts and/or compulsive behaviors
Body image dissatisfaction

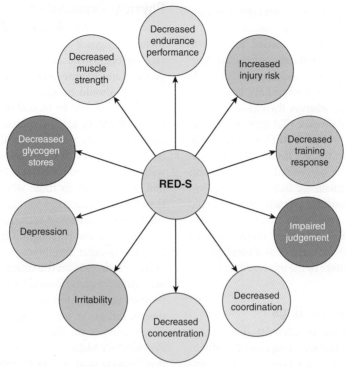

Fig. 13.6 Potential effects of relative energy deficiency in sports (RED-S) and low energy availability (EA). (Adapted from Constantini NW. Medical concerns of the dancer. Book of Abstracts, XXVII FIMS World Congress of Sports Medicine, Budapest, Hungary, 2002:151.)

EVALUATION

A thorough history should prompt and guide the evaluation and physical examination. When possible, obtaining and reviewing growth charts, particularly during annual preparticipation examinations, can alert providers to any significant and concerning changes in weight. Attention to abnormal vital signs, including last menstrual period, can also raise concerns for low EA. In athletes where there are concerns about intake, providers should specifically ask about daily eating habits including special diets, description of meals and snacks, food group exclusions, or other restrictive eating behaviors. A 24-hour diet recall can be helpful to provide a more specific record of whether an athlete is meeting their daily nutritional needs. Providers should also explicitly ask about daily exercise levels, including duration and intensity (considering organized sports participation, recreational activities, and at-home exercise training). During the history, providers are simultaneously assessing for signs of low EA as well as symptoms of other illnesses that may be

contributing, such as inflammatory bowel disease, celiac disease, diabetes, or thyroid disease. If there are concerns for disordered eating behaviors, providers should ask specifically about binge and purge behaviors and any concerns the athlete has about body size, shape, or weight. An assessment of mood is also important, and specific questionnaires exist to assess for the presence of depression or anxiety (Patient Health Questionnaire-9: https://www.apa.org/depression-guideline/patient-health-questionnaire.pdf and Generalized Anxiety Disorder-7: https://adaa.org/sites/default/files/GAD-7_Anxiety-updated_0.pdf).[29,30] Special consideration should be given to adolescents and young adults, particularly family members who can corroborate or provide additional history as needed. If parents are present, it is always important to query about their concerns regarding the adolescent's intake, exercise, or other behaviors. It is also important to make sure that the adolescent has a safe space to share any confidential information they may not feel comfortable disclosing in front of parents or family.

Each state has laws that govern adolescent confidentiality and what is considered protected information.

No specific laboratory tests are needed to evaluate RED-S; as a corollary, no single test can confirm the diagnosis. As a diagnosis of exclusion, blood tests are frequently ordered. Individuals with low EA often have suppressed triiodothyronine (T_3) levels, whereas thyroid-stimulating hormone (TSH) and free thyroxine (T_4) may be normal. LH and FSH are often suppressed in RED-S patients with menstrual dysfunction. If measured, insulin, IGF-1, cortisol, and leptin levels can be suppressed in patients with RED-S. Peptide YY and ghrelin are increased in the low EA state. Endothelial dysfunction and alterations in lipid profiles have been noted in amenorrheic as compared with eumenorrheic athletes.[28] Iron deficiency anemia may be detected in patients with low EA, either as a consequence of reduced micronutrient intake or the increased metabolic demand caused by athletics.

Imaging Technique and Findings

If concerns for impaired bone health exist, dual energy x-ray absorptiometry (DEXA) scanning can be useful to measure BMD. Although there are no standard recommendations on when to obtain a DEXA scan, indications may include athletes who have been amenorrheic for >12 months, patients with eating disorders or those at risk for low EA, or individuals with concerning or multiple fractures.[31] The International Society for Clinical Densitometry recommends spine and whole body as the preferred skeletal measurement sites in adolescents and young adults.[29] Whereas adult DEXA results are provided as T-scores, adolescent bone mineral content and areal density results are reported as Z-scores, which is the number of standard deviations above or below the median according to age and sex norms.[32] DEXA provides an areal measurement of bone, not necessarily volume. Bone microarchitecture, volume, and strength can be measured with high-resolution peripheral quantitative computed tomography (HR-pQCT), but this may not be as readily available as a DEXA scan.

Classic Signs

Given the variability and understanding of RED-S as a spectrum, clinical manifestations can be subtle, and there are few classic signs of the disorder. A high index of suspicion among athletes by coaching, training staff, dieticians, providers, and parents should prompt appropriate evaluation and management.

Physical Examination

Providers should carefully review anthropometric and metabolic signs if concerns for RED-S exist. A low heart rate and orthostatic vital signs may point to medical compromise and require urgent intervention. Weight, height, and BMI should be measured. Individuals less than 20 years of age should be plotted on growth charts, with particular attention to BMI percentile. While RED-S may exist in patients with a normal BMI, providers should have a high index of suspicion in patients with low body weight, unexpected weight loss, lack of appropriate growth and development, or those who have a median BMI less than the 85th percentile for age/sex. As discussed earlier, RED-S is a diagnosis of exclusion, so appropriate medical evaluation should be sought if there are concerns for the presence of other conditions or pathology. Physical signs of hyperandrogenism (hirsutism, acne, male pattern baldness, clitoromegaly) should be assessed, as they may point to other etiologies for menstrual dysfunction. As thyroid disease can cause weight loss or menstrual irregularities, examination of the thyroid gland should be undertaken. Providers should also look for clinical signs of malnutrition (muscle wasting, bradycardia, lanugo, bruising, hair loss) that may be a consequence of low EA. Sexual maturity rating and pubertal evaluation should be measured for younger patients to monitor for arrest of development or indications of differences in sex development for patients with amenorrhea or menstrual concerns.

DIFFERENTIAL DIAGNOSIS

FHA is a diagnosis of exclusion. Therefore an appropriate medical workup for amenorrhea should be instituted. Pregnancy testing should be encouraged for all sexually active individuals who present with oligomenorrhea. Other causes of menstrual irregularities include uterine pathology or outflow tract obstruction, primary ovarian insufficiency, chronic anovulation, polycystic ovarian syndrome, and other endocrinologic disorders (Fig. 13.7). Underlying endocrinologic conditions that may affect bone health should also be considered. As mentioned earlier, inadequate oral intake to meet daily needs may be intentional or unintentional, and screening for eating disorders should be carefully considered. Adolescents and young adults who fulfill the *Diagnostic and Statistical Manual of Mental Disorders, Fifth Edition* (DSM-5) criteria for an eating disorder may require more intensive medical evaluation.

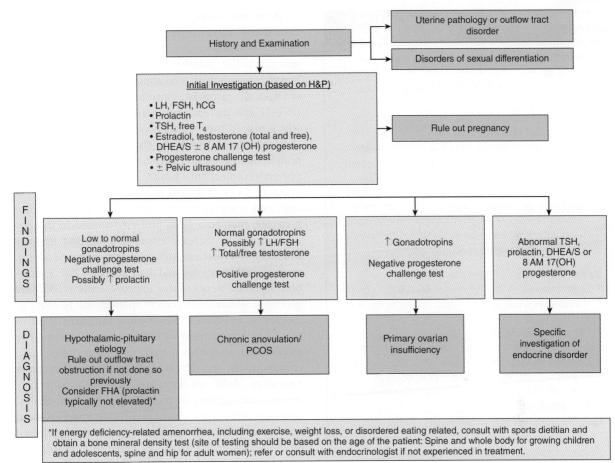

Fig. 13.7 Evaluation of the patient with amenorrhea or oligomenorrhea. *LH,* Luteinizing hormone; *FSH,* follicle stimulating hormone; *TSH,* thyroid stimulating hormone; *DHEAS,* dehydroepiandrosterone sulfate; *PCOS,* polycystic ovarian syndrome; *HCG,* human chorionic gonadotropin. (From Jameson JL, De Groot LJ, Illingworth P. Amenorrhea, anovulation, and dysfunctional uterine bleeding. In Jameson JL, De Groot LJ, editors: Endocrinology adult and pediatric, ed 6, St. Louis, MO, 2010, Saunders, pp 2341-2355.)

MANAGEMENT/TREATMENT OPTIONS

Once a diagnosis of RED-S has been established, treatment should be geared toward correcting the energy imbalance (Table 13.3). If food restriction or inadequate oral intake is the primary cause, then referral to a registered dietitian for nutrition education and meal planning may be adequate. Increasing energy intake is of critical importance for patients with identified energy deficits. Prior literature has shown that increases of 250 to 360 kcal/day may be sufficient to restore menstrual function in women with FHA.[33] Providers and dietitians should advocate for increasing caloric intake with food first (either augmenting meals or the addition of snacks), but nutritional supplements may

be needed for certain athletes. Daily caloric goals need to be created, but the athlete should also be aware of macronutrient choices and metabolic needs. Carbohydrate and essential fat intake may need to be adjusted to provide a more balanced approach. Micronutrient intake such as vitamin D, iron, and calcium should also be evaluated. Recommended dietary vitamin D intake in adolescents and young adults is 600 to 800 IU/day; calcium is 1000 to 1300 mg/day.[13,14] There are no specific guidelines to recommend increased micronutrient intake for athletes; however, vitamin D deficiency should be corrected, if needed. Serum vitamin D levels less than 30 ng/mL have been associated with risk for bone injury.[34] In patients with identified eating disorders, a multidisciplinary approach may be

TABLE 13.3 **Management and Treatment RED-S**
Restoration of Energy Availability (Mainstay of Treatment)
• Referral to registered dietitian for education and meal planning.
• Attention to adequate intake AND macronutrient choices (quantity and quality).
• Consider decrease/cessation in activity if unable to meet caloric needs and/or increase intake to meet caloric needs.
• Consider the need for psychological support in patients who are unable to increase intake or who demonstrate signs/symptoms suggestive of disordered eating; may also be necessary in those athletes with co-occurring mood symptoms.
Bone Health
• Supplementation with vitamin D 600–800 IU (more if laboratory evidence of vitamin D deficiency) and calcium 1000–1300 mg/day.
• Consider dual energy x-ray absorptiometry (DEXA) scan in athletes with amenorrhea ≥12 mo.
• Consider transdermal estrogen/cyclic progesterone in athletes with documented loss of bone density.
• Bisphosphonates are not routinely recommended for adolescents.
Note: Resumption of menses through restoration of adequate energy availability is the preferred approach for optimal bone health/bone density.
Menstrual Dysfunction
• Nonpharmacologic resumption of menses through restoration of adequate daily energy availability.
• Offer contraception when indicated or if desired. May use oral contraceptive pills if athlete preference, but these do not offer any bone-protective benefits. Oral contraceptive pills may negatively affect bone health given their effects on insulin-like growth factor (IGF)-1.

required, with input from medical providers, dietitians, and mental health professionals specializing in the treatment of patients with eating disorders. If EA is not improved with increases in intake, then reductions in energy expenditure should be considered. This may be achieved with alterations in physical activity, competition, and/or training schedules. Certain athletes may require a complete cessation of exercise until EA is restored.

Hormonal therapies for menstrual function and bone health are controversial. Although initiating combined hormonal contraception can induce menses, it only masks the underlying problem. Owing to first-pass hepatic metabolism, combined oral contraceptives (COCs) downregulate insulin-like growth factor 1 (IGF-1) and increase sex hormone–binding globulin, which may further impair bone growth in oligomenorrheic athletes.[35] COCs do contain estrogen, but the nonphysiologic ethinyl estradiol in COCs has not been proven to protect bone health.[17,20] However, if there are concerns for bone density loss and hormonal therapy is indicated, transdermal estrogen paired with cyclic progesterone may be a more preferred approach; this has been shown to increase estradiol levels and improve BMD and microarchitecture in oligomenorrheic adolescents and athletes[17,36-38] and does not affect IGF-1 secretion. It should be noted that improvements in BMD are greater in athletes who achieve spontaneous recovery of menses, as opposed to those using transdermal estrogen.[37] Therefore improving energy availability should be emphasized, even if hormonal therapies are used. These considerations should be made while simultaneously evaluating adolescent sexual practices. If the patient requires contraception for pregnancy prevention, adolescents should be counseled appropriately, and COCs can and should be considered if that is the method preferred by the adolescent. It should be noted that transdermal estrogen and cyclic progesterone are not sufficient for pregnancy prevention. Bisphosphonates have been used in adult women with osteoporosis. However, the evidence for adolescents and young adults is limited.[39] Similarly, the use of recombinant parathyroid hormone, insulin, and testosterone supplementation is not recommended.[2] It should be re-emphasized that the greatest improvements in body weight and BMD are achieved with correction of the energy imbalance, not hormonal treatments. Resumption of menses has been proven to reduce risk to bones and normalize bone health.[10,31,40] Improved EA will also allow for recovery of the hypothalamic-pituitary-gonadal axis and other hormonal profiles to further decrease fracture risk[2,33,38] (Fig. 13.8). Although these treatments may be indicated for certain patients, first-line management for RED-S is still restoration of EA and elimination of the energy-deficient state.

Even in the absence of a confirmed eating disorder diagnosis, cognitive behavioral therapy has been used in the treatment of FHA with resumption of menses.[41,42]

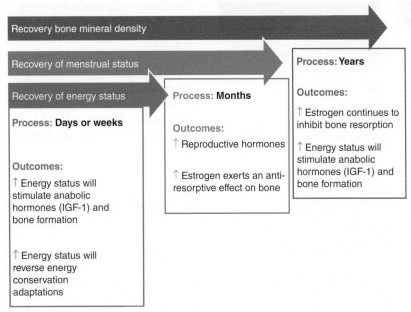

Fig. 13.8 Timeline to recovery of energy availability (EA), menstrual function and bone mineral density (BMD). *IGF-1,* Insulin-like growth factor 1. (From De Souza MJ, Nattiv A, Joy E, et al. 2014 Female Athlete Triad Coalition Consensus Statement on Treatment and Return to Play of the Female Athlete Triad: 1st International Conference held in San Francisco, California, May 2012 and 2nd International Conference held in Indianapolis, Indiana, May 2013. *Br J Sports Med.* 2014;48(4):289.)

SPECIAL CONSIDERATIONS FOR THIS POPULATION

Ninety percent of BMD accrual occurs in adolescence; peak bone mass is usually attained by 18 years of age.[43] Therefore special consideration should be given to adolescent athletes at risk for low EA and consequential bone loss. As they may have already achieved full bone development, young adults with RED-S may be less vulnerable to the consequences of bone issues, but they are certainly not protected. Even with recovery of menstrual function, bone loss may be irreversible in former amenorrheic athletes.[44] Although weight-bearing activity is known to increase BMD through bone modeling and remodeling, this beneficial effect may be lost in those with RED-S and impaired menstrual function.[45] Normal body weight is not necessarily protective either. Prior studies have found that normal-weight athletes with menstrual abnormalities have more drive for thinness and disordered eating behaviors compared with nonathletes or athletes with normal menstrual patterns.[46]

The psychological effects of RED-S should be taken seriously. In addition to impaired sports performance,

the hypoestrogenic state affects verbal memory and executive functioning. This may be particularly concerning for high school and collegiate student athletes.[2]

If an individual has been treated for RED-S, return to sports participation needs careful consideration. A stepwise red light/green light approach has been suggested, modeled after sport concussion return-to-play guidelines. This is known as the *RED-S Clinical Assessment Tool (RED-S CAT).*[22] The RED-S CAT provides a framework for clinical decision making, overall risk assessment, and return-to-play guidelines. Athletes are evaluated for a variety of clinical parameters (injury status, menstrual standing, BMD, and laboratory data) and then categorized as low, moderate, or high risk of developing/experiencing morbidity (Fig. 13.9). The return-to-play model can be helpful for medical providers in determining whether EA has been restored and if the athlete is ready to return to sports participation.

RESEARCH GAPS

Increased research looking at the direct relationship between low EA and health effects beyond the triad is

High risk: No start red light	Moderate risk: Caution yellow light	Low risk: Green light
- Anorexia nervosa and other serious eating disorders - Other serious medical (psychological and physiological) conditions related to low energy availability - Use of extreme weight loss techniques leading to dehydration induced hemodynamic instability and other life threatening conditions.	- Prolonged abnormally low % body fat measured by DXA* or anthropometry - Substantial weight loss (5–10% body mass in one month) - Attenuation of expected growth and development in adolescent athlete	- Appropriate physique that is managed without undue stress or unhealthy diet/exercise strategies
	- Low **EA of prolonged and/or severe nature	- Healthy eating habits with appropriate EA
	- Abnormal menstrual cycle: Functional hypothalamic amenorrhea >3 months - No menarche by age 15y in females	- Healthy functioning endocrine system
	- Reduced bone mineral density (either in comparison to prior DXA or Z-score <-1 SD) - History of 1 or more stress fractures associated with hormonal/menstrual dysfunction and/or low EA	- Healthy bone mineral density as expected for sport, age, and ethnicity - Healthy musculoskeletal system
- Severe ECG abnormalities (i.e., bradycardia)	- Athletes with physical/psychological complications related to low EA+/- disordered eating - Diagnostic testing abnormalities related to low EA +/- disordered eating	
	- Prolonged relative energy deficiency - Disordered eating behavior negatively affecting other team members - Lack of progress in treatment and/or noncompliance	

*dual energy X-ray absorptiometry
**EA: Energy availability=Energy intake – Energy cost of exercise (additional energy expended in undertaking exercise).

Fig. 13.9 RED-S clinical assessment tool used to assess risk of return to activity and sports. Data from history and physical examination, will place athletes into high, moderate, or low risk categories. **High risk:** Sports participation likely to cause significant risks to health and treatment participation. **Moderate risk:** Clearance for sports with supervision from treatment team; regular follow-up intervals to monitor progress and any clinically significant changes to health and/or nutrition status. **Low risk:** Clear for full sports participation. *ECG*, Electrocardiogram; *SD*, standard deviation. (From Relative Energy Deficiency in Sport (RED-S). British Journal of Sports Medicine (https://doi.org/10.1136/bjsports-2014-094559.)

needed. This would also increase the understanding of other RED-S endpoints to be aware of outside of the triad components of osteoporosis, amenorrhea, and disordered eating. Long-term effects on fertility and bone health are generally lacking in adults who have a previous or current diagnosis of RED-S; however, some of these data exist based on studies of patients with anorexia nervosa. There has also been little done to

correlate bone health or the status of bone health as reported in DEXA scans and the effect on both short- and long-term fracture risk. Further, research on medical treatment options has primarily focused on the role of hormonal supplementation and its effect on bone health. There have been few data on the benefits of hormonal treatment in addressing other physiologic dysfunction and systems affected by low EA. We also have a limited understanding of the psychological consequences of RED-S.

KEY POINTS

- RED-S is defined as any impairment in physiologic functioning caused by relative energy deficiency. This can include menstrual function, bone health, gastrointestinal conditions, hematologic findings, immune function, psychological stress, and cardiovascular health.
- Optimal EA is important for top athletic performance, but also injury and illness prevention.
- Low energy availability (EA is the hallmark of RED-S).

$$\text{Energy Availability} = \frac{\text{Energy Intake (in kcal)} - \text{Exercise Energy Expenditure (in kcal)}}{\text{Fat Free Mass (in kg)}}$$

- There is no practical, standardized tool to measure EA. Measurement is variable and often dependent on patient-reported measures. Twenty-four-hour diet recalls and 3- or 7-day dietary logs facilitated by a sports dietitian may help with accuracy.
- Low EA with or without disordered eating behaviors can cause alterations in endocrinologic function, leading to poor bone health and menstrual abnormalities.
- RED-S prevention can be facilitated through awareness and education for medical providers, athletes, coaches, and dieticians (see Fig. 13.4).
- Treatment of RED-S is primarily nonpharmacologic; restoration of energy imbalance is key.

REVIEW QUESTIONS

1. Energy availability is defined as:
   a. Daily dietary caloric intake
   b. Amount of calories expended each day through activity and exercise
   c. Energy remaining for bodily functions and physiologic processes after energy for exercise has been used
   d. Energy released through carbohydrate metabolism

2. Which of the following is true regarding RED-S?
   a. Menstrual pattern changes are a normal consequence of sports participation for females.
   b. Athletes with RED-S have a low body weight.
   c. Intentional food restriction is the cause of the low energy availability state.
   d. An imbalance between energy intake and expenditure results in hormonal disruption.
3. What would be the most appropriate treatment for a patient in RED-S to ensure optimal bone health and protect bone health?
   a. Initiation of combined oral contraceptive pills
   b. Vitamin D supplementation
   c. Restoration of adequate daily energy availability
   d. Cessation of all physical activity

SUPPLEMENTAL MATERIALS FOR CHAPTER

Supplemental Screening Questionnaires for Providers: Eating Disorder Screening Tools:

SCOFF (https://www.psychtools.info/scoff/)

LEAF-Q (https://www.sportsmedicinebroadcast.com/wp-content/uploads/2019/12/Martinsen-2014-BEDA-q-dvelopement.pdf)

BEDA (https://www.mdpi.com/2077-0383/10/17/3976)

*It is recommended that LEAF-Q and BEDA be used together for RED-S screening.

Mood Screening Tools:

PHQ-9 (https://www.apa.org/depression-guideline/patient-health-questionnaire.pdf)

GAD-7 (https://adaa.org/sites/default/files/GAD-7_Anxiety-updated_0.pdf)

REFERENCES

1. Mountjoy M, Sundgot-Borgen J, Burke L, et al. The IOC consensus statement: beyond the Female Athlete Triad—Relative Energy Deficiency in Sport (RED-S). *Br J Sports Med*. 2014;48(7):491-497.
2. Mountjoy M, Sundgot-Borgen JK, Burke LM, et al. IOC consensus statement on relative energy deficiency in sport (RED-S): 2018 update. *Br J Sports Med*. 2018;52:687-697.
3. Loucks AB. Energy balance and body composition in sports and exercise. *J Sports Sci*. 2004;22:1-14.
4. Weiss Kelly AK, Hecht S, Council on Sports Medicine and Fitness. The female athlete triad. *Pediatrics*. 2016;138(2): e20160922.
5. Tenforde AS, Carlson JL, Chang A, et al. Association of the female athlete triad risk assessment stratification to the development of bone stress injuries in collegiate athletes. *Am J Sports Med*. 2017;45(2):302-310.
6. Carson TL, West BT, Sonneville K, et al. Identifying latent classes of Relative Energy Deficiency in Sport (RED-S) consequences in a sample of collegiate female cross country runners. *Br J Sports Med*. 2023;57(3):153-159.
7. Slater J, McLay-Cooke R, Brown R, Black K. Female recreational exercisers at risk for low energy availability. *Int J Sport Nutr Exerc Metab*. 2016;26:421-427.
8. Weaver CM, Gordon CM, Janz KF, et al. The National Osteoporosis Foundation's position statement on peak bone mass development and lifestyle factors: a systematic review and implementation recommendations. *Osteoporos Int*. 2016;27(4):1281-1386. Epub 2016 Feb 8. Erratum in: *Osteoporos Int*. 2016;27(4):1387.
9. Nose-Ogura S, Yoshino O, Dohi M, et al. Low bone mineral density in elite female athletes with a history of secondary amenorrhea in their teens. *Clin J Sport Med*. 2020;30(3):245-250. doi:10.1097/JSM.0000000000000571
10. Ackerman KE, Sokoloff NC, DeNardo Maffazioli G, Clarke HM, Lee H, Misra M. Fractures in relation to menstrual status and bone parameters in young athletes. *Med Sci Sports Exerc*. 2015;47(8):1577-1586.
11. De Souza MJ, Nattiv A, Joy E, et al. 2014 Female Athlete Triad Coalition consensus statement on treatment and return to play of the female athlete triad: 1st International Conference held in San Francisco, California, May 2012 and 2nd International Conference held in Indianapolis, Indiana, May 2013. *Br J Sports Med*. 2014;48(4):289.
12. Carey DE, Golden NH. Bone health in adolescence. *Adolesc Med State Art Rev*. 2015;26(2):291-325.
13. Golden N. Optimizing bone health in children and adolescents. *Pediatrics*. 2014;134(4):e1229.
14. Christo K, Prabhakaran R, Lamparello B, et al. Bone metabolism in adolescent athletes with amenorrhea, athletes with eumenorrhea, and control subjects. *Pediatrics*. 2008; 121(6):1127-1136.
15. Bennell K, Matheson G, Meeuwisse W, Brukner P. Risk factors for stress fractures. *Sports Med*. 1999;28(2):91-122.
16. Papageorgiou M, Dolan E, Elliott-Sale KJ, Sale C. Reduced energy availability: implications for bone health in physically active populations. *Eur J Nutr*. 2018;57(3):847-859. doi:10.1007/s00394-017-1498-8
17. Ackerman KE, Singhal V, Baskaran C, et al. Oestrogen replacement improves bone mineral density in oligo-amenorrhoeic athletes: a randomized clinical trial. *Br J Sports Med*. 2019;53:229-236.
18. Pantano KJ. Knowledge, attitude, and skill of high school coaches with regard to the female athlete triad. *J Pediatr Adolesc Gynecol*. 2017;30(5):540-545.

19. Kroshus E, DeFreese JD, Kerr ZY. Collegiate athletic trainers' knowledge of the female athlete triad and relative energy deficiency in sport. *J Athl Train.* 2018;53(1):51-59. doi:10.4085/1062-6050-52.11.29

20. Ackerman KE, Stellingwerff T, Elliott-Sale KJ, et al. #REDS (Relative Energy Deficiency in Sport): time for a revolution in sports culture and systems to improve athlete health and performance. *Br J Sports Med.* 2020; 54(7):369-370. doi:10.1136/bjsports-2019-101926

21. MacDonald J, Schaefer M, Stumph J. The preparticipation physical evaluation. *Am Fam Physician.* 2021;103(9): 539-546.

22. Mountjoy M, Sundgot-Borgen J, Burke L, et al. The IOC relative energy deficiency in sport clinical assessment tool (RED-S CAT). *Br J Sports Med.* 2015;49(21):1354.

23. Morgan JF, Reid F, Lacey JH. The SCOFF questionnaire: a new screening tool for eating disorders. *West J Med.* 2000;172(3):164-165.

24. Martinsen M, Holme I, Pensgaard A, Torstveit MK, Sundgot-Borgen J. The development of the Brief Eating Disorder in Athletes Questionnaire. *Med Sci Sports Exerc.* 2014;46(8):1666-1675.

25. Sim A, Burns SF. Review: questionnaires as measures for low energy availability (LEA) and relative energy deficiency in sport (RED-S) in athletes. *J Eat Disord.* 2021;9(1):41.

26. Melin A, Tornberg ÅB, Skouby S, et al. Energy availability and the female athlete triad in elite endurance athletes. *Scand J Med Sci Sports.* 2015;25(5):610-622. doi:10.1111/sms.12261

27. Logue DM, Madigan SM, Melin A, et al. Low energy availability in athletes 2020: an updated narrative review of prevalence, risk, within-day energy balance, knowledge, and impact on sports performance. *Nutrients.* 2020;12(3):835.

28. Rickenlund A, Eriksson MJ, Schenck-Gustafsson K, Hirschberg AL. Amenorrhea in female athletes is associated with endothelial dysfunction and unfavorable lipid profile. *J Clin Endocrinol Metab.* 2005;90(3):1354-1359.

29. Kroenke K, Spitzer RL, Williams JB. The PHQ-9: validity of a brief depression severity measure. *J Gen Intern Med.* 2001;16(9):606-613.

30. Kroenke K, Williams JB, Löwe B. A brief measure for assessing generalized anxiety disorder: the GAD-7. *Arch Intern Med.* 2006;166(10):1092-1097.

31. Krugh M, Langaker MD. Dual energy x-ray absorptiometry. 2022 Jun 11. In: *StatPearls* [Internet]. Treasure Island, FL: StatPearls Publishing; 2022.

32. International Society for Clinical Densitometry. 2019 Official Positions. https://iscd.org/wp-content/uploads/2021/09/2019-Official-Positions-Pediatric-1.pdf

33. Ciadella-Kam L. Dietary intervention. *Nutrients.* 2014;3:3018-3039.

34. Moreira CA. Stress fractures: concepts and therapeutics. *J Clin Endocrinol Metab.* 2017;102:525-534.

35. Singhal V, Ackerman KE, Bose A, Flores LPT, Lee H, Misra M. Impact of route of estrogen administration on bone turnover markers in oligomenorrheic athletes and its mediators. *J Clin Endocrinol Metab.* 2019;104:1449-1458.

36. Misra M, Katzman D, Miller KK, et al. Physiologic estrogen replacement increases bone mineral density in adolescent girls with anorexia nervosa. *J Bone Miner Res.* 2011;26:2430-2438.

37. Nose-Ogura S, Yoshino O, Kanatani M, et al. Effect of transdermal estradiol therapy on bone mineral density of amenorrheic female athletes. *Scand J Med Sci Sports.* 2020;30(8):1379-1386.

38. Ackerman KE, Singhal V, Slattery M, et al. Effects of estrogen replacement on bone geometry and microarchitecture in adolescent and young adult oligoamenorrheic athletes: a randomized trial. *J Bone Miner Res.* 2020;35(2):248-260.

39. Eghbali-Fatourechi G. Bisphosphonate therapy in pediatric patients. *J Diabetes Metab Disord.* 2014;13(1):109.

40. De Souza MJ, Stock NC, Ricker EA, et al. The path towards progress: a critical review to advance the science of the female and male athlete triad and relative energy deficiency in sport. *Sports Med.* 2022;52:13-23.

41. Misra M, Prabhakaran R, Miller KK, et al. Weight gain and restoration of menses as predictors of bone mineral density change in adolescent girls with anorexia nervosa-1. *J Clin Endocrinol Metab.* 2008;93(4):1231-1237. doi:10.1210/jc.2007-1434

42. Michopoulos V, Mancini F, Loucks TL, Berga SL. Neuroendocrine recovery initiated by cognitive behavioral therapy in women with functional hypothalamic amenorrhea: a randomized, controlled trial. *Fertil Steril.* 2013;99(7):2084-2091.e1.

43. Berga SL, Loucks TL. Use of cognitive behavior therapy for functional hypothalamic amenorrhea. *Ann N Y Acad Sci.* 2006;1092:114-12x9.

44. Whiting SJ, Vatanparast H, Baxter-Jones A, Faulkner RA, Mirwald R, Bailey DA. Factors that affect bone mineral accrual in the adolescent growth spurt. *J Nutr.* 2004;134(3):696S-700S.

45. Keen AD, Drinkwater BL. Irreversible bone loss in former amenorrheic athletes. *Osteoporos Int.* 1997;7(4):311-315.

46. Cano Sokoloff N, Eguiguren ML, Wargo K, et al. Bone parameters in relation to attitudes and feelings associated with disordered eating in oligo-menorrheic athletes, eumenorrheic athletes and nonathletes. *Int J Eat Disord.* 2015;48:522-526.

Breast Concerns

Kim Hoover and Amy Boone

INTRODUCTION

Breast development is an essential component of the pubertal transformation. It is imperative for a pediatric provider to recognize normal and abnormal breast development. Although the majority of pediatric breast concerns are benign, familiarity with specific conditions is important for diagnosis and patient counseling.

Typically breast development begins at 4 to 6 weeks' of gestational age along the anterior body wall in what is typically referred to as the "milk line" (Fig. 14.1). Nipple development occurs at 8 months' of gestation, and breast buds may be palpable at 34 weeks' of gestation. These buds are resultant from exposure to maternal estrogen and typically regress within the first few months of life. During puberty, thelarche occurs as the ductal tissue grows because of endogenous estrogen exposure and lobular/areolar tissue expand because of progesterone exposure.[1,2] Timing of thelarche can vary by body mass index (BMI) and ethnicity; however, consensus groups have determined thelarche at age less than 8 years or no breast development by age 13 warrant investigation for normal BMI and a general population.[1,3,4]

In what follows we will discuss common conditions and variants seen with adolescent breast development.

BREAST ABSCESS

A breast abscess is a purulent, fluctuant mass. Inflammatory lesions comprise around 4% of all breast lesions in nonlactating adolescents.[5,6] It may result from local infection, epidermoid cysts, foreign bodies, trauma, nipple piercing, and folliculitis often stemming from the

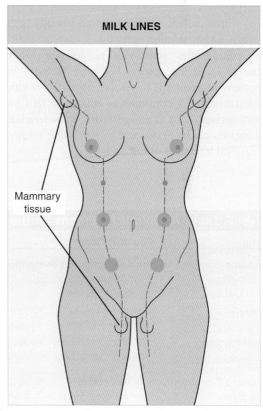

MILK LINES

Mammary tissue

Fig. 14.1 Natural milk lines. (From Lorenzo Cerroni, Jean L. Bolognia, Julie V. Schaffer, Dermatology, Fifth Edition; fig 64.22.)

shaving of periareolar hair.[7] Infants less than 2 months may develop mastitis or even an abscess from bacterial spread through the nipple (https://www.youtube.com/watch?v=DUsHZv4rNKc). The most common organisms identified in breast abscesses are *Staphylococcus aureus,* beta-hemolytic streptococcus, *Escherichia coli,* and *Pseudomonas aeruginosa.*[5] A patient with a breast abscess typically presents with localized tenderness and induration followed by erythema and then a fluctuant mass. Associated symptoms may include fever, axillary adenopathy, and/or nipple discharge. A breast ultrasound helps to distinguish between cellulitis and a blocked duct or abscess. On physical examination, a tender, indurated, or fluctuant erythematous breast mass is typically seen. The most common location is the areolar/periareolar area.[7] The differential diagnosis includes cellulitis and cystic breast disease. Management includes local care with warm compresses and pain relief with nonsteroidal antiinflammatory drugs (NSAIDs), acetaminophen, or acetaminophen with codeine. Antimicrobial coverage should initially include coverage for methicillin-resistant *S. aureus* (MRSA) until culture and sensitivity results are available (Table 14.1). If the abscess becomes fluctuant or if symptoms progress/fail to resolve, aspirate for culture and sensitivity. If it continues to enlarge or fails to respond, incision and drainage (with consideration of packing) should be performed by a provider trained in the surgical treatment of the breast.[7]

BREAST VARIATIONS

There are many variants of breast/nipple shape and size, the majority of which are benign and do not require intervention.

Tuberous Breasts

Tuberous breasts are described as having a constricted breast base, decrease in breast volume, abnormal elevation of the inframammary fold, and areolar herniation. The etiology and pathophysiology are controversial; however, most agree they are embryonal in origin with anomaly of the areolar fascia.[8] The condition manifests as a tuberous root-shaped or mushroom-shaped breast developing in early breast growth (Figs. 14.2 and 14.3). This variant is seen to arise in puberty, and prevalence can be as high as 27%.[8] There is no other testing required relevant to the condition unless a unilateral tuberous shape is noted. In this situation, ruling out an underlying breast mass is prudent. Additional caution should be taken with estrogen when given during delayed pubertal induction, as tuberous changes can occur when initiating induction at adult levels of estrogen at greater than 20 mcg/day.[9] Management and treatment

TABLE 14.1	**Antibiotic Regimens for the Treatment of a Breast Abscess**	
Drug	**Pediatric Dose**[a]	**Considerations**
Immune Competent, Well Appearing, no Systemic Symptoms		
Amoxicillin-clavulanate	25 mg/kg/day PO of the amoxicillin component in 2 divided doses	
Cephalexin	25–50 mg/kg/day PO divided in 3–4 doses (Max = 2 g/day)	
Clindamycin	30–40 mg/kg/day PO divided in 3–4 doses (Max = 1.8 g/day)	Suggested in areas of increased MRSA
Immune Compromised, Ill Appearing		
Nafcillin or oxacillin	100–150 mg/kg/day IV in 4 divided doses	IV drug of choice when MRSA less likely
Vancomycin	40 mg/kg/day IV in 4 divided doses	Use if high concern for MRSA or life-threatening PCN allergy
Clindamycin	25–40 mg/kg/day IV in 3 divided doses	IV drug of choice if high concern for MRSA or life-threatening PCN allergy

[a]Dose not appropriate for neonates.
IV, Intravenous; *MRSA,* methicillin-resistant *Staphylococcus aureus*; *PCN,* penicillin; *PO,* orally.
(Adapted from Stevens DL, Bisno AL, Chambers HF, et al. Practice guidelines for the diagnosis and management of skin and soft tissue infections: 2014 update by the Infectious Diseases Society of America. *Clin Infect Dis.* 2014;59:147-159.)

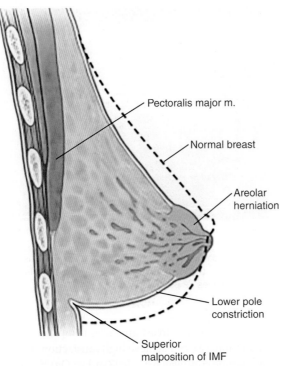

Fig. 14.2 Tubular breast with constricted base. (From Atlas of Reconstructive Breast Surgery. Kolker, Adam R.; Shay, Paul L.. Published January 1, 2020. Pages 293-309. © 2020; fig 24.2B.)

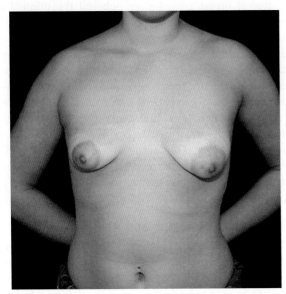

Fig. 14.3 Tubular breast with constricted base. (From Lee L.Q, Pu, Nolan S Karp: Atlas of Reconstructive Breast Surgery. First edition, © 2020, Elsevier Inc. All rights reserved.)

options are surgical. High levels of satisfaction are seen with surgical correction by a plastic surgeon with expertise with this particular breast variant (https://www.youtube.com/watch?v=TeUOLEuiNjE).[10]

Accessory Breast Tissue and Nipple

The most common area for accessory nipple to be located is inferior to the breast, and the most common location for accessory breast glandular tissue is in the axilla (Figs. 14.4–14.6). The prevalence of accessory nipple is 1% at birth; however, accessory nipples are not often recognized until puberty.[11] Accessory nipples can occur anywhere along the milk line and are the result of failed

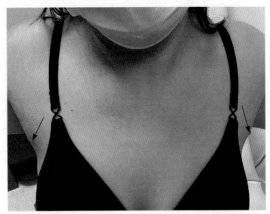

Fig. 14.4 Axillary accessory nipple. (From Case report: multiple supernumerary nipples in a young woman. *Am Fam Physician*. 2022;106[1]:11A-11B.)

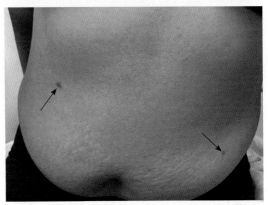

Fig. 14.5 Nipple on abdominal wall. (From Case report: multiple supernumerary nipples in a young woman. *Am Fam Physician*. 2022;106[1]:11A-11B.)

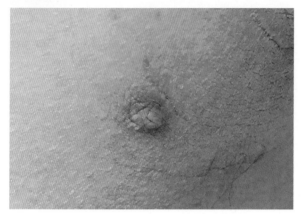

Fig. 14.6 Axillary accessory nipple. (From Case report: multiple supernumerary nipples in a young woman. *Am Fam Physician.* 2022;106[1]:11A-11B.)

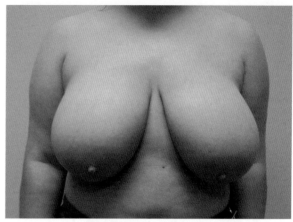

Fig. 14.7 Macromastia. (From Christina N. Canzoneri MD, Kurtis E. Moyer MD Challenges in Breast Evaluation: Breast Asymmetry, Macromastia, and the Surgically Altered Breast; Obstetrics and Gynecology Clinics of North America Volume 49, Issue 1, March 2022, Pages 73-85.)

regression during embryonic development.[11,12] They present as darkened areolar tissue anywhere along milk lines that can often mimic dermatologic nevi. Small studies suggest that accessory nipples could coincide with renal anatomic pathology, and imaging of the complete genitourinary tract may be considered, as renal and müllerian anomalies can occur concurrently.[12] Accessory nipples are generally asymptomatic; however, they can become painful and swollen with breastfeeding and pregnancy. Surgical removal can be performed when symptomatic (https://www.youtube.com/watch?v=gzXRXe-g7YE).

Macromastia (Juvenile Breast Hypertrophy)

Macromastia (Fig. 14.7), also known as *juvenile breast hypertrophy,* is a very rare condition with unknown prevalence.[13] The etiology and pathophysiology are unknown; however, it is theorized that it may be the result of an inappropriate response to endogenous hormones or autoimmune mediated.[13] The process usually occurs proximal to menarche, with bilateral rapid breast growth. Breasts may weigh up to 50 pounds each. Stretch marks often occur during rapid growth. Patients frequently report breast and upper back pain. Though no further testing is needed, ruling out the use of exogenous hormones is prudent. Additionally, many argue that the use of imaging is helpful to eliminate the notion of an underlying mass effect.[13] Management with supportive undergarments is beneficial. Consider the use of NSAIDs for pain and progesterone or antiestrogens to

slow growth.[1,2] Once breast growth is complete, referral for mammoplasty can achieve high satisfaction (https://www.youtube.com/watch?v=fc9RsmFwyQg).[13]

Lipomastia

Lipomastia is the presence of excessive adipose tissue in typical breast areas before pubertal transition. Its prevalence and epidemiology are unknown, but with increasing obesity, it is often confused for premature thelarche or precocious puberty. Given that lipomastia can mimic premature puberty, careful examination to exclude premature thelarche is important[4]. When encountering the obese patient with concern for possible premature thelarche vs. breast adiposity, the examination should be performed supine. If no palpable glandular breast tissue is under the fat pad of the chest wall, lipomastia can be confirmed.[4] There is no treatment required, and expectant management with anticipatory guidance should be given.

Hypomastia, Amastia, and Athelia

Hypomastia or amastia manifests as congenital absence of breast tissue, and athelia as congenital absence of the nipple (Fig. 14.8). The prevalence is extremely rare. Etiologies are thought to be destruction of the milk line during embryologic formation (Poland syndrome; Fig. 14.9) or chest wall trauma or radiation as a neonate.[1,2] However,

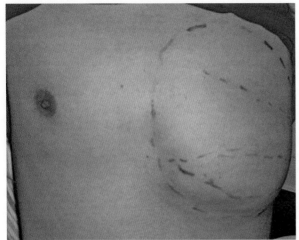

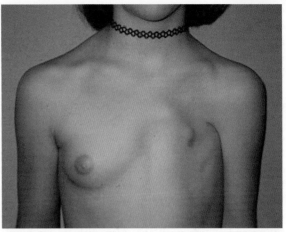

Fig. 14.9 Poland syndrome with absence of pectoralis muscle and absence of ipsilateral breast. (From Atlas of Reconstructive Breast Surgery. Delay, Emmanuel; Meruta, Andreea Carmen. Published January 1, 2020. Pages 281-291. © 2020. Fig 23.3.)

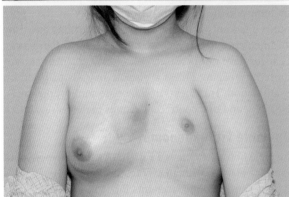

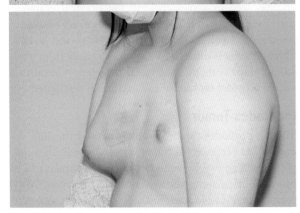

Fig. 14.8 Athelia and amastia. (From Poland Syndrome Associated With Ipsilateral Lipoma and Dextrocardia; The Annals of Thoracic Surgery Volume 92, Issue 6, December 2011, Pages 2250-2252); Amastia (From Plastic Surgery, Volume 3: Craniofacial, Head and Neck Surgery and Pediatric Plastic Surgery Fifth Edition Copyright © 2024 fig 32.4.)

these conditions can also occur with endocrine disorders associated with delayed puberty such as hypothyroidism, ovarian failure, and androgen excess, as well as chronic systemic diseases which can present as delayed puberty. The differential diagnosis should include screening for breast flattening/ironing. This is described as the harmful practice of ironing, pressing, or pounding breasts to delay growth in order to disguise the onset of puberty in a girl, which is often viewed in some communities to shield pubertal development in an attempt to protect the girls from sexual exploitation.[14] Additionally, Poland syndrome, which results from underdevelopment or absence of the pectoralis major muscle on the hypoplastic breast side, should be considered in the differential. Testing for these conditions revolves around historical trauma, pubertal timeline, and clinical examination. Consider screening for hypothyroidism or androgen excess as appropriate. The provider should also inquire about nutritional state and start evaluation for delayed puberty if no breast development by age 13.[15] If there is no underlying pathology, consultation for surgical augmentation may be desired once puberty is complete.

Breast Asymmetry

Breast asymmetry is defined as a discrepancy between the sexual maturity rating of individual breasts. This condition is an exceedingly common complaint at the onset of breast development (thelarche), as it is often asymmetric. Asymmetry is usually more noticeable in early breast development and lessens in appearance at higher sexual maturity rating levels.[3,4]

Resolution often occurs by late adolescence; however, asymmetry may persist in 25% of persons after age 18.[10,12] Though a common and benign condition, the etiology for those with marked discrepancy is thought to be the result of interruption of the milk line during development.[1,10,12] The differential diagnosis includes Poland syndrome, breast mass, and fibrocystic changes. When evaluating, perform a careful breast examination to evaluate for a breast mass, cyst, or abscess in both the sitting and supine positions. Also evaluate for nipple discharge. Consider measuring each breast in the vertical and horizontal planes for comparison with later examinations (i.e., 12 to 6 o'clock; 3 to 9 o'clock).[5,7] If marked discrepancy is noted on examination, consideration of imaging to rule out an underlying mass effect may be warranted with breast ultrasound. If the examination is normal, reassurance with options for a padded bra and periodic examinations until final breast maturation occurs (approximately age 18) are appropriate. If solely an anatomic abnormality, the patient may desire a plastic surgery consultation once reaching sexual maturity rating 4 (https://www.youtube.com/watch?v=Qhel396GkE).

BREAST MASS

The most common mass in this age group are fibroadenomas, followed by fibrocystic changes. Neonates may have hypertrophy in the first weeks to months of life because of exposure to maternal hormones.[16] Primary breast cancer is exceedingly rare.[1,17] When performing an examination, palpate the breast tissue upright and in the supine position. If a palpable mass is noted, discern if there is concern for an infectious etiology. Also assess for bilaterality, the location, lymphadenopathy, pain, mobility vs. fixed, and solid or cystic components. A breast ultrasound is the preferred modality for screening of a palpable mass, as it can distinguish between solid and cystic masses and help delineate abscesses. Mammography is not indicated in patients younger than 25 years, as increased breast tissue density makes for a less sensitive test[18] (Fig. 14.10).

Fibroadenoma

Fibroadenomas are the most common breast mass in adolescence, accounting for 67% to 94% of masses.[1,2,19] These masses are estrogen sensitive and can be bilateral. Often, they present as discrete, rubbery, mobile masses, which are painless, typically at 15 to 17 years of age. If suspected, confirmation of the diagnosis is best seen with breast ultrasound imaging (Fig. 14.11). If less than 5 cm in size and asymptomatic, observation can be performed for 3 to 6 months. If painful or enlarging, excision is the treatment of choice by a skilled breast surgeon.

Fibrocystic Changes

Fibrocystic breast changes are noted in up to 90% of breast tissue.[2] This condition presents as painful nodules or lumpy tissue in the breast, commonly in the upper outer quadrants of the breast, thought to be caused by an imbalance in estrogen and progesterone. Fibrocystic changes have no increased risk of breast cancer and require no imaging unless a discrete mass is palpated on examination. Treatments of choice are comfort measures, NSAIDs, and oral contraceptive pills to decrease pain.

Juvenile Fibroadenoma

Juvenile fibroadenoma is a variant of a fibroadenoma but rapidly enlarges, with an average size of 5 to 10 cm. This type of fibroadenoma accounts for 1% to 8% of fibroadenomas seen in adolescents.[1,2,11] On physical examination, overlying skin changes may be observed because of rapid growth (ulceration, necrosis, stretch), and juvenile fibroadenoma is difficult to distinguish easily from phyllodes tumor without imaging. If detected, referral to a skilled provider for biopsy and excision is warranted.

Phyllodes Tumor

Though phyllodes tumor usually occurs in the 40th decade, it has been seen in young women as well. They may appear benign on ultrasound imaging and similar to a fibroadenoma, making magnetic resonance imaging (MRI) useful to delineate in some instances. Treatment with excision by a skilled breast surgeon is recommended.[1,2,6,7]

Pseudoangiomatous Stromal Hyperplasia

Pseudoangiomatous stromal hyperplasia (PASH) typically presents in premenopausal women; however, it has also been seen in the pediatric population. Presentation is similar to the fibroadenoma as a firm, painless, mobile mass. It is a benign condition that can additionally

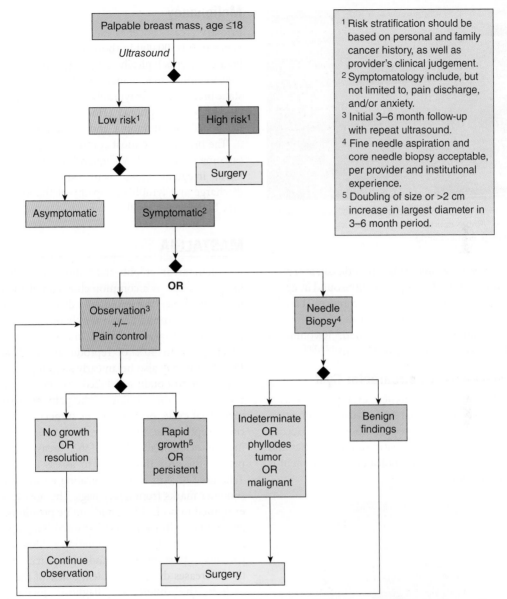

Fig. 14.10 Suggested clinical care algorithm for children presenting with a palpable breast mass. (From McLaughlin CM, Gonzalez-Hernandez J, Bennett M, Piper HG. Pediatric breast masses: an argument for observation. *J Surg Res.* 2018;228:247-252.)

occur in the contralateral breast.[2,20] On imaging, the mass may resemble a fibroadenoma. Histologically, it differs from the fibroadenoma but can mimic low-grade angiosarcomas. Histologic staining on biopsy or excisional specimen is required to differentiate between PASH and malignancy.[20] It is thought to be the result of a hyperproliferative response to progesterone. Treatment

is complete excision, as recurrence could occur if an incomplete resection is performed.

Juvenile Papillomatosis/Intraductal Papilloma

Juvenile papillomatosis/intraductal papilloma is caused by papillary hyperplasia of ductal tissue, leading to a mobile

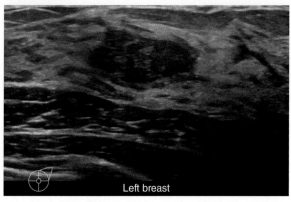

Fig. 14.11 Hypoechoic circumscribed mass located within breast tissue. (Photo courtesy Kristin Porter MD, PhD, University of Alabama, Birmingham.)

cystic mass in dense stroma. This condition can also present with bloody nipple discharge. On ultrasound imaging, it is described as "Swiss cheese" in appearance. These lesions are at risk for later breast cancer development and should be monitored closely in adulthood.[1] Recommend treatment is excision with negative margins.[1,2,4,5,19]

Cyst of Montgomery/Retroareolar Cyst

Cyst of Montgomery/retroareolar cyst presents as a painful, palpable, retroareolar mass caused by obstruction of the Montgomery areolar tubercle (sebaceous gland) (Fig. 14.12). If symptomatic, oral antibiotics and ultrasound for resolution are indicated; no treatment is required if asymptomatic.[2,7,19]

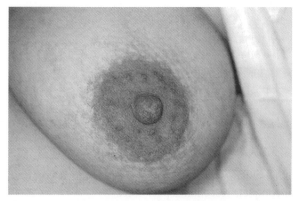

Fig. 14.12 Multiple areolar Montgomery tubercles noted circumferential to the nipple and in areolar space, which, if obstructed, cause cysts of Montgomery. (From Dermatologic diseases of the breast and nipple; Journal of the American Academy of Dermatology Volume 43, Issue 5, Part 1, November 2000, Pages 733-754)

Malignancy

Primary breast cancer is exceedingly rare, with an incidence of 0.1/100,000 in those under age 20.[18] Secondary breast cancer is typically caused by radiation to the chest wall for other malignancies such as lymphoma. Metastatic breast cancer is typically caused by other malignancies such as lymphoma (Hodgkin and non-Hodgkin), hepatocellular carcinoma, and rhabdomyosarcoma.

The breast is the most common site for rhabdomyosarcoma metastasis.[18] Malignancy will present as a hard, fixed, irregular mass, with skin retraction; nipple discharge and lymphadenopathy of the axillary region may be present as well.

MASTALGIA

Although rare in prepubertal children, mastalgia, or pain in the breast(s), is a common chief complaint in the gynecology clinic. The etiology is diverse, including premenstrual hormone/fibrocystic changes, medication use (i.e., oral contraceptive pills), and exercise or trauma, affecting up to 40% of reproductive-aged women.[7,19] Breast pain may also be an early sign of pregnancy. It is imperative to obtain a detailed history, including location and laterality, timing of the pain, association with menstrual cycle, prior injury or surgery, and hormone/contraceptive use. Pregnancy should be ruled out early in the evaluation. During the breast examination, palpate the area thoroughly to assess for any masses. Take note of skin marks indicating an ill-fitting bra or shoulder marks from heavy bags. The breasts should be examined in both sitting and supine positions. A breast and axillary ultrasound is warranted if a palpable mass is identified on breast examination.[21] Most commonly, patients report bilateral and symmetric breast pain that increases during the luteal phase of the menstrual cycle.[22] The differential diagnosis includes benign growth pains, costochondritis, and chest wall trauma. Mastalgia is very rarely a presenting sign of malignancy. The mainstay of management is patient reassurance with instructions to wear a supportive, well-fitting bra. A trial of oral or topical NSAIDs may be considered for treatment. If the patient is taking a combined oral contraceptive pill, consider decreasing the ethinyl estradiol dose. There are also some data to support the use of vitamin E (1200 IU) ± evening primrose oil supplementation.[7]

NIPPLE DISCHARGE

Nipple discharge is the release of any fluid from the nipple-areolar complex and may occur at any age.[5,7] It is uncommon in children and adolescents who are nonpuerperal.[19] This condition is usually benign and self-limiting. However, it warrants evaluation if unilateral, single duct, intermittent, or persistent in nature. Cytologic evaluation of the discharge is unreliable. A quick test for blood with a Hemoccult card can be helpful.[21] If the discharge is milky, pregnancy should be ruled out. The thyroid should be evaluated with a thyroid-stimulating hormone (TSH) level and the pituitary with a prolactin level. A prolactin level in excess of 100 ng/mL is suggestive of a pituitary tumor.[6,21] A thorough history including laterality, timing (spontaneous versus provoked), and appearance of the discharge should be obtained. Carefully review the medication list, as there are many that cause galactorrhea such as antihypertensives, tricyclic antidepressants, antipsychotics, cannabis, and systemic hormone therapy.[5,6] If a palpable mass is identified on examination, a breast ultrasound is warranted.[5] Nipple discharge can be classified as physiologic or pathologic (Table 14.2). On physical examination, thoroughly exmine the breast, palpating for masses. Attempt to reproduce the discharge. If it is reproducible, note if the discharge comes from single or multiple ducts. Be sure to palpate the thyroid gland. The differential diagnosis is largely based on the appearance of the discharge. Galactorrhea—milky discharge—can be caused by pregnancy, drugs (prescription or illicit), thyroid dysfunction, chest trauma, a prolactin-secreting tumor, or chronic renal disease. This milky discharge can also be seen in term neonates resulting from stimulation by transplacental maternal hormone, which is benign and short-lived.[23] Multicolored and sticky discharge suggests ductal ectasia. Montgomery tubercles are located on the areola and can secrete clear to brownish fluid. If serous or serosanguinous, consider intraductal papilloma. Purulent discharge results from an infectious etiology.[19] Nonpathologic discharge usually resolves spontaneously. Discourage manipulation, as this will perpetuate the discharge.[7] Treat the underlying cause if identified. If an intraductal papilloma is present, it should be excised.[6]

KEY POINTS

- Breast concerns such as an abscess, variants of breast/nipple shape and size, and nipple discharge are relatively uncommon, mostly benign, and do not require intervention.
- Ruling out other endocrine and gonadal disorders is warranted, as is evaluating for a mass.
- The most common breast mass in the adolescent is fibroadenoma followed by fibrocystic breast changes. Fortunately, neither is predisposed to breast cancer formation.

TABLE 14.2 Types of Nipple Discharge
Physiologic
• Provoked
• Multiple ducts
• Various colors
Pathologic
• Spontaneous
• Unilateral
• Single duct
• Bloody, serous
• Persistent
Galactorrhea
• Puerperal
• Nonpuerperal
• Persistent
• Provoked
• May be voluminous

Adapted from Micaela Weaver, Ashley Stuckey: Benign Breast Disorders. Obstetrics and Gynecology Clinics of North America, Volume 49, Issue 1, March 2022, Pages 57-72.[21]

REVIEW QUESTIONS

1. When evaluating for a palpable mass, which of the following is considered most concerning for increased future risk of breast cancer?
   a. Juvenile fibroadenoma
   b. Fibrocystic breast change
   c. Retroareolar cyst
   d. Juvenile papillomatosis

2. A patient presents with a complaint of "small breast size." She is 13 years old, breast sexual maturity rating 1, BMI and height at 45th percentile for age. What is the next best step in her evaluation?
   a. Reassurance that this is normal puberty
   b. Re-evaluation in 6 months with repeat physical examination

   c. Referral to endocrine or pediatric gynecology for evaluation

   d. Referral to plastic surgery for augmentation consult

3. A 15-year-old patient presents with unilateral breast discharge that she describes as cloudy and noticed in her undergarments and when she squeezes her nipple to "see if it has gone." After review of history, you see no medications that would illicit discharge, and on physical examination, no masses are noted and you are able to express cloudy, serous discharge bilaterally. Her primary doctor has sent records with a fasting prolactin of 22 ng/mL. What are the next steps in evaluation?

   a. Discourage manual breast expression and/or breast stimulation

   b. Repeat fasting prolactin

   c. Vitamin E supplement

   d. Urine pregnancy test

REFERENCES

1. De Silva NK. Breast development and disorders in the adolescent female. *Best Pract Res Clin Obstet Gynaecol.* 2018;48:40-50. doi:10.1016/j.bpobgyn.2017.08.009
2. Elsedfy H. A clinical approach to benign breast lesions in female adolescents. *Acta Biomed.* 2017;88(2):214-221. doi:10.23750/abm.v88i2.6666
3. Kaplowitz P, Bloch C; Section on Endocrinology, American Academy of Pediatrics. Evaluation and referral of children with signs of early puberty. *Pediatrics.* 2016; 137(1). doi:10.1542/peds.2015-3732
4. Tenedero CB, Oei K, Palmert MR. An approach to the evaluation and management of the obese child with early puberty. *J Endocr Soc.* 2021;6(1):bvab173. doi:10.1210/jendso/bvab173
5. Fallat ME, Ignacio Jr RC. Breast disorders in children and adolescents. *J Pediatr Adolesc Gynecol.* 2008;21(6):311-316. doi:10.1016/j.jpag.2007.10.007
6. Templeman C, Hertweck SP. Breast disorders in the pediatric and adolescent patient. *Obstet Gynecol Clin North Am.* 2000;27(1):19-34. doi:10.1016/s0889-8545(00)80004-2
7. Boone A, Hoover K. Chapter 9 breast disorders. In: Hertweck SP, Dwiggins ML, eds. *Clinical Protocols in Pediatric and Adolescent Gynecology.* 2nd ed. CRC Press; 2022.
8. Lozito A, Vinci V, Talerico E, et al. Review of tuberous breast deformity: developments over the last 20 years. *Plast Reconstr Surg Glob Open.* 2022;10(5):e4355. doi:10.1097/GOX.0000000000004355
9. Nordenström A, Ahmed SF, van den Akker E, et al. Pubertal induction and transition to adult sex hormone replacement in patients with congenital pituitary or gonadal reproductive hormone deficiency: an Endo-ERN clinical practice guideline. *Eur J Endocrinol.* 2022;186(6):G9-G49. doi:10.1530/EJE-22-0073
10. Nuzzi LC, Firriolo JM, Pike CM, Cerrato FE, DiVasta AD, Labow BI. The effect of surgical treatment on the quality of life of young women with breast asymmetry: a longitudinal, cohort study. *Plast Reconstr Surg.* 2020;146(4):400e-408e. doi:10.1097/PRS.0000000000007149
11. Miranda E. Congenital defects of the skin and hands. In: Coran AG, ed. *Pediatric Surgery.* 7th ed. Mosby; 2012:1711-1724.
12. DiVasta AD, Weldon CB, Labow BI. The breast: examination and lesions. In: Emans SJ, Laufer MR, DiVasta AD, eds. *Emans, Laufer, Goldstein's Pediatric & Adolescent Gynecology.* 7th ed. Philadelphia: Wolters Kluwer; 2020:781.
13. Hisham A, Abd Latib M, Basiron N. Juvenile breast hypertrophy: a successful breast reduction of 14.9% body weight without recurrence in a 5-year follow-up. *Case Rep Surg.* 2017;2017:3491012. doi:10.1155/2017/3491012
14. Amahazion F. Breast ironing: a brief overview of an underreported harmful practice. *J Glob Health.* 2021;11:03055. doi:10.7189/jogh.11.03055
15. Blondell RD, Foster MB, Dave KC. Disorders of puberty. *Am Fam Physician.* 1999;60(1):209-218.
16. Banikarim C, De Silva NK. Breast masses in children and adolescents. In: Drutz JE, Middleman AB, Blake D, eds. UpToDate. 2022. https://www.uptodate.com/contents/breast-masses-in-children-and-adolescents
17. McLaughlin CM, Gonzalez-Hernandez J, Bennett M, Piper HG. Pediatric breast masses: an argument for observation. *J Surg Res.* 2018;228:247-252. doi:10.1016/j.jss.2018.03.056
18. Jayasinghe Y. Preventive care and evaluation of the adolescent with a breast mass. *Semin Plast Surg.* 2013;27(1):13-18. doi:10.1055/s-0033-1343990
19. Mareti E, Vatopoulou A, Spyropoulou GA, et al. Breast disorders in adolescence: a review of the literature. *Breast Care (Basel).* 2021;16(2):149-155. doi:10.1159/000511924
20. Shehata BM, Fishman I, Collings MH, et al. Pseudoangiomatous stromal hyperplasia of the breast in pediatric patients: an underrecognized entity. *Pediatr Dev Pathol.* 2009;12(6):450-454. https://doi.org/10.2350/08-09-0528.1
21. Weaver M, Stuckey A. Benign breast disorders. *Obstet Gynecol Clin North Am.* 2022;49(1):57-72. doi:10.1016/j.ogc.2021.11.003
22. Balleyguier C, Arfi-Rouche J, Haddag L, Canale S, Delaloge S, Dromain C. Breast pain and imaging. *Diagn Interv Imaging.* 2015;96(10):1009-1016. doi:10.1016/j.diii.2015.08.002
23. Banikarim C, De Silva NK. Breast disorders in children and adolescents. In: Drutz JE, Middleman AB, Blake D, eds. UpToDate; 2022. https://www.uptodate.com/contents/breast-disorders-in-children-and-adolescents

Pediatric Vulvovaginal Conditions

Jennifer L. Bercaw-Pratt and Ana Luisa Cisneros-Camacho

INTRODUCTION

Pediatric and adolescent patients frequently present to the office with vulvar or vaginal concerns. The most common concerns include prepubertal and postpubertal vulvovaginitis, lichen sclerosus, labial adhesions, and vulvar ulcers (Table 15.1).

PREPUBERTAL VULVOVAGINITIS

Prepubertal vulvovaginitis is a term used to describe vulvar and vaginal inflammation in females before puberty. It is a common complaint causing parents to seek medical attention, but the exact prevalence is not well understood. In one study of 191 premenarchal females surveyed at the time of their well-child visit, 2% reported current vulvovaginal symptoms, with 49% reporting any history of vulvovaginal symptoms not associated with urinary tract infections or trauma.[2]

The most common etiology of prepubertal vulvovaginitis is nonspecific and is thought to be the result of many factors. Prepubertal females have smaller perineal bodies and underdeveloped labia minora with hairless, less fatty labia majora compared with postpubertal females. This difference in anatomy increases the risk of traumatic irritation to the labia and the risk of exposure to enteric bacteria.[3-5] In addition, some females are exposed to contact irritants such as harsh soaps and bubble baths, which can cause genital irritation.[3-5]

Frequently, prepubertal females struggle with personal hygiene. When cleaning after bowel movements, children frequently wipe "back to front" or not as carefully as adults. This can result in exposure of fecal bacteria to the vagina. In addition, prepubertal females may not take the time to void completely or spread their legs far enough apart, which results in the urine refluxing into the vagina. This is termed *vaginal voiding,* and this urine collection in the vagina can act as a medium for bacteria to grow. Other hygiene concerns for prepubertal females include poor handwashing, nose picking, thumb sucking, or scratching, which can introduce oropharyngeal and skin bacteria to the vagina.[3-5] Beyond concerns for poor hygiene, the pH of the prepubertal vagina is alkaline because of the presence of less lactobacilli and hypoestrogenic compared with the postpubertal vagina, which allows pathogenic bacteria to grow.[3-5]

The clinical presentation of prepubertal vulvovaginitis involves genital discomfort (itching, irritation, and/or burning), erythema, and abnormal vaginal discharge. A detailed history can be taken to determine symptoms, the length of time symptoms have been present, questions about hygiene (Table 15.2), and treatments that have already been attempted to relieve symptoms.

A physical examination should be performed to assess pubertal development, any abnormalities of the genital anatomy, skin changes, presence of vaginal discharge, and presence of vaginal voiding. A vaginal culture can be obtained. When collecting the vaginal culture, care should be made to avoid direct contact of the swab with the hymen, causing discomfort. If the vagina cannot be swabbed, a vaginal lavage with normal saline can be used to aid in the collection of vaginal culture. If symptoms are persistent despite treatment or there is concern for a foreign body, further assessment of the vagina with vaginoscopy can be performed. In the setting of pruritus, an evaluation for pinworms can be performed by putting tape around the anus first thing in

TABLE 15.1   Vulvovaginal Concerns

	Etiology	Evaluation
Prepubertal vulvovaginitis	Nonspecific	Exam, possible vaginal culture
Postpubertal vulvovaginitis	Nonspecific	Exam, vaginal cultures
Lichen sclerosus	Unknown	Exam
Labial adhesions	Inflammation of vulvar skin in hypoestrogenic environment	Exam
Aphthous vulvar ulcers[1]	Idiopathic, nonspecific inflammatory response to systemic bacterial, viral, and fungal illnesses	Exam, HSV testing, varies across practices, refer to section below on aphthous ulcers
	Differential Diagnosis	**Treatment**
Prepubertal vulvovaginitis	Foreign body vaginitis, vaginitis caused by chlamydia or gonorrhea, pinworm infection, dermatoses, precocious puberty, urinary pathology	Improved genital hygiene, hypoallergenic vulvar care, topical barrier emollients, estrogen, antibiotics if specific pathogen is found on vaginal culture, evaluation and treatment of constipation
Postpubertal vulvovaginitis	Physiologic leukorrhea, foreign objects, dermatoses, infections (yeast, bacterial vaginosis, sexually transmitted infections)	Improved genital hygiene, hypoallergenic vulvar care, topical emollients, antibiotics if specific pathogen is found on vaginal culture
Lichen sclerosus	Vitiligo, can have subtle and early skin changes, trauma/injury, lichen simplex chronicus	Hypoallergenic vulvar care, topical corticosteroids, topical calcineurin inhibitors
Labial adhesions	Vulvar-vaginal variants such as lower vaginal outlet obstruction	Topical estrogen or topical betamethasone 0.05%
Aphthous vulvar ulcers	HSV ulcers, Behcet disease, inflammatory bowel disease (i.e., Crohn disease), trauma	Symptomatic treatment

HSV, Herpes simplex virus.

TABLE 15.2   Questions to Assess Hygiene

How frequently does the patient take a bath or shower?
What type of soaps are used for bathing? For detergents?
Does the patient take bubble baths?
Is the child toilet trained?
How does the child sit on the toilet when voiding?
How does the patient wipe in the restroom? Front to back? Or back to front?
Does the patient experience urine dribbling or urinary incontinence?
Does the patient wear loose-fitting clothes?

TABLE 15.3   Differential Diagnosis for Prepubertal Vulvovaginitis

Nonspecific Vulvovaginitis	Bacterial Vulvovaginitis
Vaginitis caused by gonorrhea or chlamydia	Psoriasis
Lichen sclerosus	Vaginitis caused by foreign body
Allergic contact dermatitis	Voiding dysfunction
Eczema	Ectopic ureter
Precocious puberty	Pinworms

the morning. Finally, if there is concern for sexual abuse, testing can be performed for gonorrhea and chlamydia.

The differential diagnosis of prepubertal vulvovaginitis includes foreign body vaginitis, vaginitis caused by chlamydia or gonorrhea, pinworm infection, dermatologic conditions, precocious puberty, and urinary pathology (Table 15.3).[3-5] If gonorrhea or chlamydia is detected, a careful evaluation for sexual abuse should be undertaken. Prepubertal vulvovaginitis is frequently treated with yeast medications, but it is important to note that *Candida* is not commonly found in the vagina of prepubertal females.[6,7] *Candida* is a common cause of diaper dermatitis but is rarely found on vaginal culture of prepubertal females with vulvovaginitis unless risk factors are present, including immunosuppression, diabetes, or recent antibiotic use.[6,7]

Studies have shown that the majority of prepubertal vulvovaginitis is nonspecific with no specific pathogen found. In only about 25% to 40% of cultures, a pathogen can be found associated with symptoms of vulvovaginitis.[3,6,7] As a result, the vaginal culture should only be treated if the bacteria are isolated and growing extensively on culture.[6] Because of hygiene factors in prepubertal females, the most common pathogens found on vaginal culture are from enteric and respiratory organisms (Table 15.4).

Nonspecific prepubertal vulvovaginitis is treated by encouraging improved hygiene measures (Table 15.5). Topical emollients can provide symptomatic relief. In

TABLE 15.4 Common Pathogens Seen on Vaginal Culture of Prepubertal Females

Organism	Treatment
Group A streptococci beta-hemolytic (*S. pyogenes*)	Penicillin family
Group B streptococci beta-hemolytic (*S. agalactiae*)	Penicillin family
Staphylococcus coagulase positive (*S. aureus*)	Penicillin family
Haemophilus influenza	Penicillin family
Escherichia coli	Azithromycin
Enterococcus faecalis	Penicillin family
Enterobiasis vermicularis	Mebendazole or pyrantel pamoate

From References 5.

TABLE 15.5 Prepubertal Hygiene Recommendations

Bathe every day with warm water for a short period
Eliminate bubble baths
Avoid contact irritants by using fragrance-free soaps and detergents
Wipe from front to back when using the restroom
When using the restroom to void, sit with legs wide on the toilet seat and lean forward to avoid vaginal voiding; sitting backward on the toilet may make spreading the legs easier
Wear loose-fitting underwear and clothes
Avoid sitting in wet, tight underwear or bathing suits for long periods

severe cases of prepubertal vulvovaginitis where the patient has vulvar inflammation and irritation, a low-potency topical steroid such as triamcinolone acetonide ointment 1% can be applied to the affected area, such as the labia majora, twice a day until symptoms improve.[3-5] If a specific pathogen is found on vaginal culture, a susceptible antibiotic should be used.

POSTPUBERTAL VULVOVAGINITIS

Postpubertal vulvovaginitis is a term used to describe vulvar and vaginal inflammation in females after puberty. Postpubertal vulvovaginitis is a common complaint in adolescents. This section will focus on nonsexually acquired postpubertal vulvovaginitis, as sexually transmitted infections are discussed in Chapter 20.

After puberty, the epithelium in postpubertal adolescents is more resistant to infection compared with that of the prepubertal female. This is because of increasing estrogen levels and a decrease in vaginal pH, caused in part by the increased presence of lactobacilli.[5] Two of the most common nonsexually acquired causes of postpubertal vulvovaginitis are yeast infections and bacterial vaginosis. The majority of women (75%) will experience at least one vaginal yeast infection and almost half will have two or more infections.[4] Vaginal yeast infections are typically associated with *Candida albicans,* although recurrent infections can be caused by *Candida glabrata.*[5] There is a greater risk of vaginal yeast infection after treatment with broad-spectrum antibiotics and in the presence of immunodeficiency such as human immunodeficiency virus (HIV) and diabetes mellitus.[5]

Bacterial vaginosis is considered the most common cause of vaginal irritation and discharge in women, and prevalence among adolescents ages 14 to 19 has been reported at 23%.[5] Bacterial vaginosis is caused by a shift in vaginal flora, with a decrease in peroxidase-producing *Lactobacillus* and an increase in the presence of anaerobic gram-negative rods, particularly *Gardnerella vaginalis.*[5] This shift causes the vaginal pH to rise.

Postpubertal vulvovaginitis presents with vulvovaginal complaints such as genital discomfort (itching, irritation, and/or burning), erythema, and abnormal vaginal discharge. Vaginal yeast infections are typically associated with a thick, white, odorless vaginal discharge associated with genital discomfort. Bacterial vaginosis is not a vaginitis but is a vaginosis, so signs of inflammation are typically absent, but it does present with a thin white/gray discharge that is adherent to the vagina.

A detailed history should assess for hygiene, possible foreign objects such as tampons/condoms, use of over-the-counter feminine products such as douches, symptoms of genital discomfort and features of any vaginal discharge (color, odor, association with menses), the length of the time the symptoms have been present, and treatments that have already been attempted to relieve symptoms.

Specific features on physical examination to assess include any skin changes, presence of vaginal discharge, vulvar itching, and/or presence of vaginal voiding. If a pelvic examination is performed, the cervix should be examined for inflammation, lesions, and any cervical motion or adnexal tenderness. Swabs can be obtained of vaginal fluid and, if needed, of the endocervix. If the patient is not sexually active, the physical examination can be limited to an external genital examination with only blind vaginal swab collection if discharge is seen.

A wet preparation of any vaginal discharge can be made using saline and 10% potassium hydroxide (KOH) on two separate samples. Vaginal yeast infections can be diagnosed on KOH wet preparation when either budding yeast, hyphae, or pseudohyphae are seen (Fig. 15.1). A yeast culture is not recommended unless the infection is recurrent.

Bacterial vaginosis is diagnosed based on a wet preparation (Fig. 15.2) using the Amsel criteria (Table 15.6).

Gram staining of the vaginal fluid has been considered the gold standard of diagnosing bacterial vaginosis

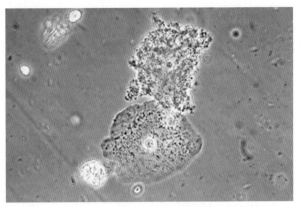

Fig. 15.2 Microscopy showing clue cell *(top)* and normal epithelial cell. (From Rein M. [1978]. Image #14574. CDC Public Health Image Library. https://phil.cdc.gov/Details.aspx?pid=14574)

TABLE 15.6	**Amsel Criteria**
1.	Thin white/gray vaginal discharge
2.	More than 20% of clue cells seen on saline wet preparation (vaginal epithelial cells coated with *coccobacilli*)
3.	Positive amine "fishy" odor on addition of KOH to the specimen
4.	Vaginal pH >4.5

but is rarely done clinically.[8] Newer commercial testing for both vaginal yeast infections and bacterial vaginosis is available with high sensitivity and specificity compared with traditional wet preparation but has not been well studied in the adolescent population.[9]

The differential diagnosis of postpubertal vulvovaginitis includes physiologic leukorrhea, foreign objects, dermatoses, and vaginal infections (caused by yeast, bacterial vaginosis, and sexually transmitted infections).[4,5] The management options for these patients depends on the diagnosis. Patients with physiologic leukorrhea, an asymptomatic clear to white vaginal discharge, can be reassured that the discharge is normal. Patients with retained foreign objects such as tampons and condoms will often present with a foul-smelling vaginal discharge, with symptoms resolving with removal of the foreign object. Vulvar inflammation and irritation can result from chemical irritants found in feminine hygiene products, soaps, detergents, perfumed products, and bubble baths.[8] Sitz baths and barrier

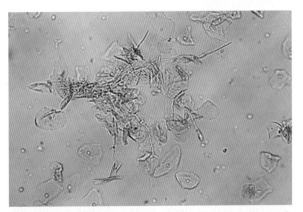

Fig. 15.1 Vaginal wet mount showing *Candida*. (From Brown S. [1976]. Image 15676. CDC Public Health Image Library. https://phil.cdc.gov/Details.aspx?pid=15675)

TABLE 15.7 Postpubertal Hygiene Recommendations
Consistent condom use
Avoid the use of feminine hygiene products such as douches
Wear loose cotton underwear
Use mild and unscented soaps and detergents
Avoid bubble baths
Wipe front to back when using the restroom
Avoid tight-fitting clothes

emollients can be useful in reducing symptoms along with counseling patients on good genital hygiene (Table 15.7). Similar to nonspecific prepubertal vulvovaginitis, in severe cases of vulvar inflammation and irritation, a low-potency topical steroid such as triamcinolone acetonide ointment 1% can be applied to the affected area twice a day until symptoms improve.

Vaginal yeast infections can be treated with either over-the-counter intravaginal creams or suppositories such as clotrimazole, miconazole, terconazole, and tioconazole. Dosing is based on the formulation and strength. Oral fluconazole is also used in the treatment of vaginal yeast infections. Patients can elect for either option, as topical or oral treatment of vaginal yeast infections is equally effective.[8] Bacterial vaginosis is treated with either oral metronidazole or vaginal preparations of metronidazole or clindamycin. Treatment of sexual partners is not recommended.[8]

VULVAR LICHEN SCLEROSUS

Lichen sclerosus is an inflammatory dermatologic condition causing hypopigmentation that commonly affects the anogenital region. The exact prevalence of lichen sclerosus is not known, but a report from a general adult gynecology practice estimated a prevalence of 1.7%.[10] Vulvar lichen sclerosus can be diagnosed at any age but is typically diagnosed either in prepubertal or menopausal females. Pediatric vulvar lichen sclerosus accounts for ~7% to 15% of all cases diagnosed.[11] The average age of diagnosis of pediatric vulvar lichen sclerosus is 6 to 7 years.[12,13]

The etiology of lichen sclerosus is unknown. Patients with the condition are more likely to suffer from autoimmune conditions and have higher levels of autoantibodies compared with controls; however, this does not confirm it is an autoimmune disease.[11] Lichen sclerosus can run in families, which has led to research on human leukocyte antigen (HLA) association but further studies are needed.[11]

The most common symptoms of lichen sclerosus at presentation are pruritus, vulvar pain, dysuria, constipation, and bleeding.[14] The classic feature of vulvar lichen sclerosus is a well-defined plaque of hypopigmentation with sclerosus in a figure of eight configuration (surrounding the vulva, perineum, and perianal skin)[11,14] (Fig. 15.3). It is rare for lichen sclerosus to occur in the proper vagina (superior to the hymen).[11] Other skin changes can occur such as ecchymoses, petechiae, fissures, erosions, and hemorrhagic blisters.[14] As most adults are not familiar with this skin condition, children can be mistakenly referred to child protective services because of the ecchymoses of lichen sclerosus.[15] Vulvar vitiligo is another inflammatory dermatologic condition that causes hypopigmentation that can also occur in patients with lichen sclerosus, which can make diagnosis challenging.[14]

Lichen sclerosus can progress to vulvar structural distortion, resulting in atrophy of the labia minora,

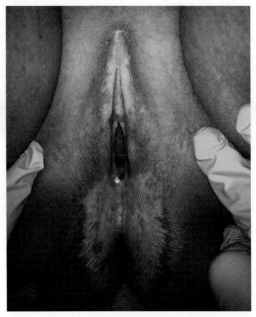

Fig. 15.3 Typical appearance of lichen sclerosus. (From Bercaw-Pratt JL, Boardman LA, Simms-Cendan JS; North American Society for Pediatric and Adolescent Gynecology. Clinical recommendation: pediatric lichen sclerosus. *J Pediatr Adolesc Gynecol.* 2014;27[2]:111-116. doi:10.1016/j.jpag.2013.11.004)

adhesions of the clitoral hood, and/or introital stenosis, all of which may be permanent and require surgical correction.[16] A recent study found 25% of pediatric patients with lichen sclerosus had vulvar structural distortion.[16]

Unlike in adults, vulvar biopsy is not typically performed in the diagnosis of pediatric vulvar lichen sclerosus. It should be reserved for cases with uncertain diagnosis or lack of response to treatment. If biopsy is undertaken, it should be from the most hypopigmented area affected, and the histopathology is distinctive, occurring in all age groups.[11]

Most clinical recommendations divide the treatment of lichen sclerosus into two phases: induction of remission and maintenance[11] (Table 15.8). Since 1991, the gold standard of treatment of lichen sclerosus has been topical corticosteroids.[11,13] No single regimen exists for induction of remission, but the mainstays of therapy include topical high-potency corticosteroids such as clobetasol propionate, mometasone furoate, and betamethasone dipropionate.[11,13,17] Ointments are the preferred vehicle because they have a low rate of contact dermatitis and good penetration.[11,17] After improvement in symptoms and skin changes, patients can be transitioned to lower-potency corticosteroids such as triamcinolone acetonide, methylprednisolone aceponate, or hydrocortisone.[11,13,17] Maintenance treatment should be continued and decreased in potency until the patient has long-term control of the disease with no symptoms and normal skin findings.[11] Patients should be followed closely initially then can be moved to less frequent follow-up if the disease is well controlled.[11] If the disease worsens, the potency of corticosteroid can be retitrated as needed.[11] The most common side effects of the use of topical corticosteroids include superimposed *Candida* infection, erythema, and stinging from application of the steroid (see Table 15.8). Prolonged use of topical steroids can be associated with thinning of the dermis and, rarely, hypothalamic-pituitary-adrenal axis suppression, though this has not been reported in long-term studies of corticosteroid treatment of lichen sclerosus.[11,18]

Topical calcineurin inhibitors such as tacrolimus and pimecrolimus can also be used in the management of lichen sclerosus.[11,17] A randomized controlled trial compared the use of pimecrolimus with clobetasol in adults and found a similar reduction in symptoms such as itching and burning; however, the pimecrolimus was felt to be less effective in terms of overall treatment.[19] A possible benefit of these options is a reduced risk of skin atrophy, but the options are more expensive than topical steroids, and there is a possible causal association with lymphoma and skin cancer associated with their use.[10,17] The primary side effect of topical calcineurin inhibitors is a burning sensation during application when first initiating treatment that tends to resolve with continued use.[17] Some authors have suggested using topical calcineurin inhibitors in the maintenance stage of lichen sclerosus.[20,21]

Compliance with medical management of lichen sclerosus is very important, as the risk of developing vulvar structural distortion is greatly increased in the setting of noncompliance.[16] The vulvar structural distortion can be seen with atrophy of the labia minora, adhesions of the clitoral hood, and/or introital stenosis, though in children adhesions of the clitoris are most common.[16,22] The vulvar structural distortion can lead to symptoms affecting reproductive and sexual health such as urinary tract outflow obstruction, retention pseudocysts, and dyspareunia.[22] Medical management is not always effective in resolving the vulvar structural distortion of lichen sclerosus, so surgical management may be required but should only be undertaken in patients with symptoms.[11,16] Surgical management is typically with sharp adhesiolysis or fractional ablative carbon dioxide laser.[16] Both require anesthesia and do not prevent recurrence.[16]

TABLE 15.8 **Treatment of Vulvar Lichen Sclerosus in Children**	
Induction of Remission	Clobetasol propionate
	Betamethasone dipropionate
	Mometasone furoate
Maintenance	Triamcinolone acetonide
	Methylprednisolone aceponate
	Hydrocortisone
Common Side Effects	Candidiasis – treat with antifungals
	Erythema – decrease potency of steroid
	Vulvar irritation – typically resolves with continued treatment

Vulvar lichen sclerosus is a lifelong disease and will typically recur. Parents should be educated on the importance of long-term follow-up to reduce the risk of developing vulvar structural distortion.[11,16] The link between adult-onset lichen sclerosus with squamous cell carcinoma of the vulva is well known, but only case reports have linked pediatric lichen sclerosus with vulvar melanoma and earlier development of squamous cell carcinoma in adulthood.[11,13,23]

VULVAR APHTHOUS ULCERS

Nonsexually transmissible vulvar ulcers are referred to as *aphthous ulcers, Lipschütz ulcers,* and *nonsexually acquired genital ulcerations* (NSGUs) in the literature. They are a rare occurrence in nonsexually active girls. The exact prevalence is largely unknown. Rosman and colleagues identified a total of 74 cases in the literature of acute genital ulcers in nonsexually active girls from 2004 to 2009.[24] A few smaller case series have noted a seasonal trend but findings have not been consistent.[25,26]

Vulvar aphthous ulcers are mostly thought to be idiopathic, secondary to a nonspecific, reactive immune response.[27] There are, however, cases of vulvar ulcers associated with infectious agents, autoimmune disorders, inflammatory diseases, malignancy, and medication exposures (Table 15.9). Of these, viral syndromes have been most frequently identified as a likely trigger.[24] Huppert and colleagues reported four cases of acute cytomegalovirus (CMV) or Epstein-Barr virus (EBV) in a review of 20 aphthous ulcers, and Farhi and colleagues identified four cases of acute EBV in 13 patients.[26,28] Most recently, there have been new reports of vulvar ulcers associated with COVID-19 infection and seen in response to the Pfizer COVID-19 vaccine.[27,29]

It is important to highlight that vulvar ulcers have also been cited as cutaneous manifestations of Crohn's disease in young girls.[30] Interestingly, the labia majora is the most common location for cutaneous Crohn's disease and often precedes gastrointestinal symptoms, which can pose a diagnostic dilemma in recurrent or persistent lesions.[30]

There is no standardized workup for vulvar ulcers in nonsexually active young girls. The diagnosis is clinical and requires exclusion of other conditions based on a thorough history and detailed examination. Herpes simplex virus (HSV) should be ruled out when applicable. Additionally, a bacterial culture can help rule out

a bacterial superinfection, especially in patients with increased risk (i.e., immunosuppression) or those with significant systemic symptoms.[24] Retrospective studies have shown an overall low yield of completing long panels of viral serologies for cases of vulvar ulcers in young girls. Some providers suggest using criteria to guide their practice (Table 15.10).[24]

TABLE 15.9 Differential Diagnosis of Vulvar Ulcers in Nonsexually Active Girls

Idiopathic	
Autoimmune/ Inflammatory	Behcet disease
	Inflammatory bowel disease (i.e., Crohn disease)
	Mouth and genital ulcers with inflamed cartilage (MAGIC syndrome)
	Bullous pemphigoid
	Pemphigus vulgaris
	Pyoderma gangrenosum
	Stevens-Johnson syndrome/ toxic epidermolytic necrosis (SJS/TEN)
	Autoimmune progesterone dermatitis
	Periodic fever, aphthous stomatitis, pharyngitis, adenitis (PFAPA)
Infectious	Epstein-Barr virus (BPV)
	Cytomegalovirus (CMV)
	Parvovirus B19
	Mycoplasma
	Influenza A
	Salmonella
	Paratyphoid
	Mumps
	COVID-19
Malignancy	Leukemia
Medical Exposures	Nonsteroidal antiinflammatory drugs
	Pfizer COVID-19 vaccine

From References 24–29.

TABLE 15.10   Criteria to Guide Further Viral Workup

History of exposure to infected contacts
Persistent fevers
Lymphadenopathy
Pharyngitis
Persistent fatigue

TABLE 15.11   Symptoms Suggestive of an Underlying Disease

Joint symptoms
GI complaints
Ocular changes
Oral lesions (recurrent)
Other dermatologic features and spread beyond vulva

GI, Gastrointestinal.

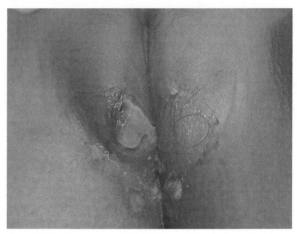

Fig. 15.4 Labial ulcers. (From Deitch HR, Huppert J, Adams Hillard PJ. Unusual vulvar ulcerations in young adolescent females. *J Pediatr Adolesc Gynecol.* 2004;17[1]:13-6. doi: 10.1016/j. jpag.2003.11.015)

Given the association of vulvar ulcers with other underlying conditions, it is important to keep a broad differential (see Table 15.9). Recurrent or persistent cases of vulvar ulcers associated with certain symptoms (Table 15.11) should trigger a referral to either rheumatology, ophthalmology, gastroenterology, or dermatology for further investigation. Biopsies of ulcerative lesions are not recommended in this patient population and are only suggested if there is a recurrence or a concern for a specific dermatologic condition (i.e., autoimmune bullous diseases).[24,31]

Vulvar aphthous ulcers have a sudden onset. They can present as a single unroofed crater or as multiple lesions distributed throughout the labia majora, minora, perineum, and even clitoris (Fig. 15.4). In one case series of 62 patients, 50% of nonsexually active girls with vulvar ulcers also had a history of oral ulcers, but only 4 had a workup concerning for Behcet disease.[24,25] Retrospective studies have consistently shown that patients with vulvar aphthous ulcers often experience prodromal symptoms including low-grade fever, fatigue, and headaches before the appearance of ulcerative lesions.[24] Patients will present with exquisite tenderness to touch, making sitting and ambulation difficult. They will also complain of dysuria, which can contribute to a delay in diagnosis, as the workup focuses on urinary tract infection. In more severe cases, the fear of exacerbating symptoms with voiding can lead to urinary retention.

A concern for vulvar ulcers in young girls is often a cause for anxiety in parents because of the need of screening for sexually transmitted causes.

Overall, vulvar aphthous ulcers tender to be larger in size than those for HSV, often ≥1.0 cm in diameter.[26] They have been described as white spots or blood blisters that rupture revealing a necrotic base. They are most often shallow lesions (~2 mm deep) with well-demarcated edges.[26] They can be associated with vulvar cellulitis and a superficial exudate.[24-26] Some patients will present with "kissing lesions," which are ulcers that are mirror images of each other on both sides of the involved vulva. If a bedside examination is limited from poor pain control, an examination under anesthesia should be considered.

The focus of treatment of vulvar aphthous ulcers is symptomatic relief and prevention of scarring. Vulvar aphthous ulcers are self-limited. In a prospective study of 20 young girls with vulvar aphthous ulcers, pain symptoms lasted on average 10 days, and 75% of cases healed within 1 to 3 weeks.[26] Conservative management options to consider are listed in Table 15.12.[32] Surrounding cellulitis and superimposed bacterial infections are treated with antibiotics based on culture sensitivities. In cases of urinary retention or poor pain management with oral

TABLE 15.12 Conservative Measures for Symptom Relief of Vulvar Aphthous Ulcers

At least twice-daily plain water sitz baths
Void in a bathtub or use a squirt bottle filled with water to help dilute urine
Oral analgesia with acetaminophen, NSAIDS ± narcotics (parenteral if needed)[a]
Topical anesthetics (i.e., lidocaine jelly)
Bland emollients (i.e., zinc oxide, petrolatum)
Limit shaving, especially the use of razors, as microtrauma can facilitate seeding of an infection
Bladder drainage with Foley catheter for urinary retention

[a]It is important to recognize that there is literature to suggest limiting NSAID use because of a concern for medication-exposure oro-genital ulcer formation even though a link has not been proven.[23,25]

NSAID, Nonsteroidal antiinflammatory drug.

analgesia and topical agents, inpatient hospital care should be considered.

There are no standardized recommendations for optimal treatment regimens, particularly in the case of prolonged ulcers or recurrence. Systemic and topical corticosteroids have been beneficial in treating oral aphthous ulcers, leading many to extrapolate these results for vulvar aphthae. Small case series have commented on the use of oral and topical steroids with mixed results. Several oral regimens have been used including oral prednisone with doses ranging from 10 to 60 mg/day, most often starting at 10 to 25 mg for recurrent mild or moderate aphthae and at 40 to 50 mg for severe cases.[24,33] The duration varies widely from 5 to 7 days to 14 to 16 days, with larger doses requiring time for titration as ulcers heal.[33]

Recurrence is expected in about one-third of patients with milder symptoms, smaller lesions, and shorter durations.[26] Careful evaluation of other systemic illnesses should follow (see Table 15.11).[24] The antiinflammatory properties of doxycycline have led some to consider it as prophylactic treatment for recurrent disease. In one retrospective study of 26 girls and women with vulvar aphthous ulcers, 14 patients (8 with moderate to severe ulceration and 6 with mild lesions) received doxycycline prophylaxis (50–100 mg per day) and reported no recurrences during a mean follow-up of 18.3 months.[33]

LABIAL ADHESIONS

Labial adhesions describe the midline fusion of the labia minora and may involve the region of the clitoral hood (Fig. 15.5). They are also referred to as *labial fusion, labial agglutination,* or *labial synechiae* in the literature.[34]

Adhesions of the labia minora are a common finding in prepubertal females between ages 3 months and 6 years.[35] The prevalence is estimated to range between 0.6% and 5% within this population, with peak incidence between ages 13 and 23 months of age.[35-38] This is likely an underestimation of the true prevalence because many cases are asymptomatic, are mild, and go unnoticed. Cases have also been reported in adolescents, adults, and older women, all in a hypoestrogenic state.[38]

Labial adhesions are considered an acquired condition, often found in the absence of any other upper genital tract pathology.[38] The exact cause remains unclear. One prevailing theory is that labial adhesions form secondary to inflammation along the labial minora in the setting of a low-estrogen vulvar environment.[35] Local irritation along the labia causes sloughing of epithelial cells, leaving denuded edges in proximity. These adhere along the midline and remain fused as re-epithelialization occurs, a process thought to be mediated by overactive macrophages and predilection for fibrosis in a low estrogenic state.[37,39] This theory supports why labial adhesions are most often found in prepubertal females and rarely in newborns or women of reproductive age.

Isolated cases of labial adhesions have been well documented without clear evidence of an active inflammatory process and without presenting symptoms.[37]

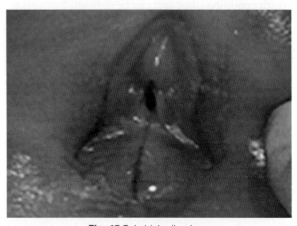

Fig. 15.5 Labial adhesions.

TABLE 15.13 Etiology of Inflammation Causing Labial Adhesions

Poor Perineal Hygiene

  Stool contamination
  Vaginal voiding
  Diaper rash

Vaginal Infection

  Candida
  Group A streptococcus
  Neisseria gonorrhea
  Gardnerella vaginalis
  Chlamydia trachomata
  Trichomonas vaginalis

Trauma

  Sexual abuse
  Female circumcision
  Straddle injury
  Excessive perineal cleaning

Vulvar Dermatoses

  Lichen sclerosis
  Graft vs. host disease
  Bechet disease
  Steven-Johnson syndrome

However, labial adhesions can also be found in association with local inflammation. Different infectious and noninfectious causes can activate an inflammatory response (Table 15.13). It is important to recognize that labial adhesions themselves can be a nidus for irritation and inflammation of the vulvovaginal area from trapped urine and vaginal secretions. Therefore determining which condition came first can be difficult.

Two key risk factors among prepubertal infants and young children are diaper dependence and the transition out of diaper use.[38] In some more rare cases, it is also important to consider labial adhesions as a complication found secondary to a noninfectious vulvar dermatopathology or even systemic disease.

Most cases of labial adhesions are asymptomatic and identified on routine genital examination by a pediatrician or during diaper changing by the observant parent. No further testing is indicated unless there are concerns for systemic, urinary, or vulvar symptoms.

The extent of labial adhesions can vary on presentation. Adhesions can be thin and translucent or thick. They can form anywhere along the edge of the labia and be of varying lengths. Complete agglutination refers to the fusion of the entire length of the labia minora, from the level of the clitoris to the posterior fourchette, typically with a small pinhole opening that serves as a means for urine to exit (see Fig. 15.5).

In symptomatic patients, common signs and symptoms include a pulling sensation, difficulty with urination, postvoid urinary dribbling, vaginal discharge, vulvar pain, or recurrent urinary tract/vaginal infections.[38] In severe cases of agglutination without an orifice for urine exit, the child may present with urinary retention.

In general, reports of discharge, odor, pruritus, pain, dysuria, or erythema should raise the concern for a superimposed infectious process. Concurrent pediatric vulvovaginitis should be considered. Poor hygiene can cause or exacerbate vulvar disease; therefore obtaining an in-depth history of hygiene practices (see Table 15.2) can effectively help clarify risk factors, guide counseling, and determine management options. Also, given the role of trauma in the pathophysiology of labial adhesions, one must screen for abuse and clarify any other source of genital injury. Traumatic genital injury is discussed in detail in Chapter 17.

Three features of labial adhesions to document and use as a guide for surveillance include length of fusion, thickness of adhesions, and list of obstructed anatomic structures (Table 15.14). Recently, there have been efforts to establish a classification system for labial adhesions to then help standardize treatment based on specific clinical findings, reducing use of trial-and-error strategies; however, more studies are needed.[34,40]

TABLE 15.14 Features of Labial Adhesions

Length of Fusion	Use percentage value to describe length (e.g., 100% being complete fusion along entire length of labia minora).
Thickness of Adhesions	Differentiate between thick (dense) and thin (translucent) midline raphe.
Obstructed Anatomic Structures	Comment on vulvar/vaginal structures not visualized because of obstruction from adhesions. Important landmarks include clitoris, urethra, introitus, and posterior fourchette.

Sometimes adhesions can also be multifocal and have a fenestrated appearance. A simple anatomic drawing showing the location and length of adhesions is also an effective way of documenting findings.[41] If a careful genital examination is not possible, the patient may require sedation.

It is important to be familiar with the female genital anatomy to differentiate labial adhesions from other causes of vulvar-vaginal variants, including those resulting in lower vagina outlet obstruction (i.e., imperforate hymen and vaginal agenesis).

The management of labial adhesions is determined by the presence and severity of urinary and vulvar symptoms. We provide a management algorithm to consider in Fig. 15.6. Overall, optimizing hygiene practices is a valuable tool for long-term vulvar health (see Table 15.5). We emphasize the use of conservative measures and trials of topical therapies before considering surgical interventions unless the patient has urinary retention.

Asymptomatic patients with labial adhesions without risk for urinary retention or infection can be managed conservatively. For most prepubertal girls, spontaneous resolution occurs once endogenous estrogen production begins.[38,42] A study by Pokorny in 1992 revealed rates of spontaneous resolution as high as 80% within 1 year.[43] Optimizing hygiene practices during this time can help prevent further progression of agglutination.

The following are suggested cases for which medical management is indicated:
- Patients reporting urinary or vulvar symptoms
- Asymptomatic patients with extensive labial fusion causing a change in urinary stream
- Patients with recurrent febrile illness for which collecting a clean urine sample is difficult[38]

Which agent to start with requires shared decision making with review of potential side effects. Topical estrogen therapy is the most common agent used for the medical management of labial adhesions.[37,38] Apply the cream once or twice daily using a fingertip or a cotton

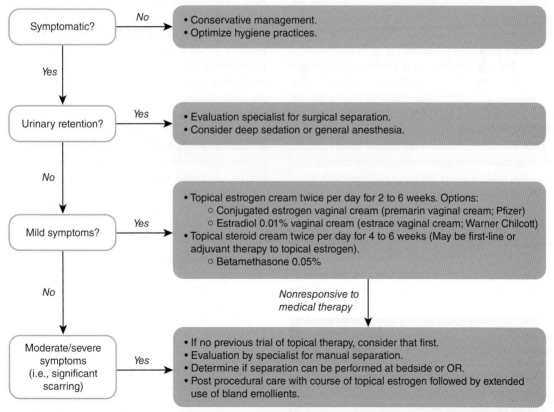

Fig. 15.6 Suggested management algorithm for prepubertal girls with labial adhesions. *OR,* Operating room.

swab along the midline raphe. No internal vaginal application is needed. Care should be taken to avoid any force that could result in tearing. Thinner adhesions may separate with gentle traction used during application. The duration most often ranges from 2 to 6 weeks.[35,38] Estrogen is thought to help mature the vulvar epithelium and aid with healing of microtrauma. Education on correct placement of cream and the quantity of cream to use can help reduce medical therapy failure.

Given concerns for systemic absorption and subsequent side effects, the goal should be to ensure correct technique and discontinue therapy once labial adhesions are completely resolved within a reasonable time frame.[37,38] Prolonged use of estrogen beyond 3 months has been associated with local irritation, vulvar hyperpigmentation, breast bud formation, and even small vaginal bleeding in more severe cases.[35,38,39] These side effects are transient and typically resolve once therapy is discontinued. If no improvement is noted after adherence to a topical regimen, steroids should be considered.

Topical betamethasone 0.05% is an alternative agent. Steroids are thought to decrease inflammation; however, prolonged use can have side effects of erythema, pruritus, folliculitis, and skin atrophy.[37,38] Topical steroids are applied twice per day with plans for re-evaluation in 2 to 6 weeks. It appears to have similar efficacy to estrogen creams and as such could be used as an option for primary, secondary, or adjunctive therapy.[35,37] If a patient fails the initial estrogen regimen, betamethasone is a reasonable next choice.

If after excellent adherence to topical treatment, the patient fails medical management, consider manual separation. This is often a rare situation but seen with thick, nontranslucent raphe or even in more severe cases of significant obstruction to urinary flow. Manual separation is rarely performed in the office because of discomfort (Table 15.15). Use of topical anesthetic agents should be considered before the attempt. Care should be taken to dose these agents based on age and weight in kilograms. For institutions with outpatient medical sedation

TABLE 15.15 **Criteria for In-Office Manual Separation**
Access to topical anesthesia with or without adjunctive sedation
Cooperative patient
Thin, translucent labial adhesions

as an option, this should be offered. There is no specific technique to guide separation; however, most providers agree on the use of a lubricated cotton swab or probe, which is inserted behind the labia minora and then gently pulled forward along the midline raphe.[35,38]

Emergent surgical management for labial adhesions is reserved for cases of urinary obstruction that require fast action and as such rely on the use of deep sedation or general anesthesia. For cases involving thicker adhesions, making an initial incision with a sharp blade may help create a plane for further blunt dissection.[38] Magnification with surgical loupes can aid in ensuring all strokes are within the avascular plane of the midline raphe, therefore minimizing bleeding risk.[38] Postoperative care involving the use of topical estrogen cream for 1 to 2 weeks followed by a bland barrier emollient for at least 6 months has been recommended.[38] Once complete resolution is reached, intermittent use of barrier creams with maintenance of effective vulvar hygiene measures is recommended.

Recurrence of adhesions during the prepubertal period is common, with known risk factors cited as diaper dependence, poor perineal hygiene, recurrent genital infection, or persistent medical or dermatologic disorders.[35,44] Observation, medical management, or surgical intervention are all management options in the setting of recurrence. Determining which option is better requires an individualized plan based on clinical presentation, risk stratification, and a discussion of the limitations and benefits of medical vs. procedural interventions. There are data to suggest that retreatment of persistent or recurrent labial adhesions with topical estrogen therapy can be successful in at least 35% of cases.[45] In general, optimizing perineal care will help improve outcomes; hence taking time to reassess home practices at every follow-up visit will often have great yield.

RESEARCH GAPS

- A better understanding of the vaginal flora of asymptomatic prepubertal females is needed along with the pathogenic bacteria that causes bacterial vulvovaginitis in these patients.
- The optimal treatment of recurrent vaginal yeast infections and recurrent bacterial vaginosis infection.
- More information is needed between the association of bacterial vaginosis and other sexually transmitted infections.

- Continued research is needed to better understand the etiology of vulvar lichen sclerosus and the optimal treatment plan for relief of symptoms, resolution of skin changes associated with lichen sclerosus, and prevention of vulvar structure distortion.

KEY POINTS

- Nonspecific prepubertal vulvovaginitis is treated by encouraging improved hygiene measures.
- Lichen sclerosus is treated with high-potency topical corticosteroids that are used to achieve remission of symptoms and skin changes with long-term maintenance with either lower-potency corticosteroids or topical calcineurin inhibitors.
- Vulvar aphthous ulcers are mostly thought to be idiopathic but can be caused by infection, autoimmune disorders, malignancy, and medication exposures.
- Labial adhesions are often asymptomatic and can be managed with conservative therapy.

REVIEW QUESTIONS

1. A happy 3-year-old girl with no medical history presents to the clinic with her family concerned that the entrance to the vagina seems more closed than before. She still wears pullups to go to bed but otherwise is potty-trained. There have been no concerns for fever, vulvar rash, or complaints of pulling, itching, or pain. On examination the urethral meatus is normal in appearance and nonobstructed despite 75% of labial agglutination without any evidence of irritation or active rash. What is the next best step?
   a. Estradiol cream therapy trial
   b. Trial of oral antibiotics
   c. Immediate surgery for manual separation
   d. Conservative management with surveillance
2. A 9-year-old, previously healthy patient presents to the emergency room with vulvar pain, burning with urination, and difficulty with ambulation for the past 2 days. On examination there are bilateral 3-cm ulcers on the labia majora, each with raised edges and a necrotic base without any exudates. There is no concern for sexual abuse or foul play. The patient denies any other symptoms or medical history. What is the most likely causative agent?
   a. Hidradenitis suppurativa
   b. Bechet disease

   c. *Escherichia coli*
   d. Epstein-Barr virus
3. A 4-year-old presents with acute onset of vulvar pruritus and vaginal discharge without evidence of any bleeding. Her older sister had a cold last week. What is the most likely cause?
   a. Pinworms
   b. Viral infections
   c. Foreign object in the vagina
   d. Respiratory organism

REFERENCES

1. Sartor RA, Lawson A, Moncada-Madrazo M, Altchek C, Vash-Margita A, Cron J. Vulvar Aphthous Ulcers in Perimenarchal Adolescents after COVID-19 Vaccination: A Multicenter Case Series. *J Pediatr Adolesc Gynecol.* 2023;36(3):268-272. doi:10.1016/j.jpag.2023.01.003
2. Delago C, Finkel MA, Deblinger E. Urogenital symptoms in premenarchal girls: parents' and girls' perceptions and associations with irritants. *J Pediatr Adolesc Gynecol.* 2012;25(1):67-73. doi:10.1016/j.jpag.2011.08.002
3. Romano ME. Prepubertal vulvovaginitis. *Clin Obstet Gynecol.* 2020;63(3):479-485. doi:10.1097/GRF.0000000000000536
4. Loveless M, Myint O. Vulvovaginitis – presentation of more common problems in pediatric and adolescent gynecology. *Best Pract Res Clin Obstet Gynaecol.* 2018;48: 14-27. doi:10.1016/j.bpobgyn.2017.08.014
5. Zuckerman A, Romano M. Clinical recommendation: vulvovaginitis. *J Pediatr Adolesc Gynecol.* 2016;29(6):673-679. doi:10.1016/j.jpag.2016.08.002
6. Jarienė K, Drejerienė E, Jaras A, Kabašinskienė A, Čelkienė I, Urbonavičienė N. Clinical and microbiological findings of vulvovaginitis in prepubertal girls. *J Pediatr Adolesc Gynecol.* 2019;32(6):574-578. doi:10.1016/j.jpag.2019.08.009
7. Alaniz VI, Kobernik EK, George JS, Smith YR, Quint EH. Comparison of short-duration and chronic premenarchal vulvar complaints. *J Pediatr Adolesc Gynecol.* 2021;34(2):130-134. doi:10.1016/j.jpag.2020.11.016
8. Itriyeva K. Evaluation of vulvovaginitis in the adolescent patient. *Curr Probl Pediatr Adolesc Health Care.* 2020;50(7):100836. doi:10.1016/j.cppeds.2020.100836
9. Schwebke JR, Taylor SN, Ackerman R, et al. Clinical validation of the Aptima bacterial vaginosis and Aptima *Candida/Trichomonas* vaginitis assays: results from a prospective multicenter clinical study. *J Clin Microbiol.* 2020;58(2):e01643-19. doi:10.1128/JCM.01643-19
10. Goldstein AT, Marinoff SC, Christopher K, Srodon M. Prevalence of vulvar lichen sclerosus in a general

gynecology practice. *J Reprod Med.* 2005;50(7): 477-480.

11. Lee A, Fischer G. Diagnosis and treatment of vulvar lichen sclerosus: an update for dermatologists. *Am J Clin Dermatol.* 2018;19(5):695-706. doi:10.1007/s40257-018-0364-7

12. Powell J, Wojnarowska F. Childhood vulvar lichen sclerosus: an increasingly common problem. *J Am Acad Dermatol.* 2001;44(5):803-806. doi:10.1067/mjd.2001.113474

13. Ellis E, Fischer G. Prepubertal-onset vulvar lichen sclerosus: the importance of maintenance therapy in long-term outcomes. *Pediatr Dermatol.* 2015;32(4):461-467. doi:10.1111/pde.12597

14. Veronesi G, Virdi A, Leuzzi M, et al. Vulvar vitiligo and lichen sclerosus in children: a clinical challenge. *Pediatr Dermatol.* 2021;38(5):1012-1019. doi:10.1111/pde.14771

15. Wood PL, Bevan T. Lesson of the week: child sexual abuse enquiries and unrecognised vulval lichen sclerosus et atrophicus. *BMJ.* 1999;319(7214):899-900. doi:10.1136/bmj.319.7214.899

16. Kherlopian A, Fischer G. Does compliance to topical corticosteroid therapy reduce the risk of development of permanent vulvar structural abnormalities in pediatric vulvar lichen sclerosus? A retrospective cohort study. *Pediatr Dermatol.* 2022;39(1):22-30. doi:10.1111/pde.14840

17. Tong LX, Sun GS, Teng JM. Pediatric lichen sclerosus: a review of the epidemiology and treatment options. *Pediatr Dermatol.* 2015;32(5):593-599. doi:10.1111/pde.12615

18. Smith YR, Quint EH. Clobetasol propionate in the treatment of premenarchal vulvar lichen sclerosus. *Obstet Gynecol.* 2001;98(4):588-591. doi:10.1016/s0029-7844(01) 01496-x

19. Goldstein AT, Creasey A, Pfau R, Phillips D, Burrows LJ. A double-blind, randomized controlled trial of clobetasol versus pimecrolimus in patients with vulvar lichen sclerosus. *J Am Acad Dermatol.* 2011;64(6):e99-e104. doi:10.1016/j.jaad.2010.06.011

20. Anderson K, Ascanio NM, Kinney MA, Krowchuk DP, Jorizzo JL. A retrospective analysis of pediatric patients with lichen sclerosus treated with a standard protocol of class I topical corticosteroid and topical calcineurin inhibitor. *J Dermatolog Treat.* 2016;27(1):64-66.

21. Dinh H, Purcell SM, Chung C, Zaenglein AL. Pediatric lichen sclerosus: a review of the literature and management recommendations. *J Clin Aesthet Dermatol.* 2016;9(9):49-54.

22. Bercaw-Pratt JL, Boardman LA, Simms-Cendan JS, North American Society for Pediatric and Adolescent Gynecology. Clinical recommendation: pediatric lichen sclerosus. *J Pediatr Adolesc Gynecol.* 2014;27(2):111-116. doi:10.1016/j.jpag.2013.11.004

23. La Spina M, Meli MC, De Pasquale R, et al. Vulvar melanoma associated with lichen sclerosus in a child: case report and literature review. *Pediatr Dermatol.* 2016;33(3):e190-e194. doi:10.1111/pde.12838

24. Rosman IS, Berk DR, Bayliss SJ, White AJ, Merritt DF. Acute genital ulcers in nonsexually active young girls: case series, review of the literature, and evaluation and management recommendations. *Pediatr Dermatol.* 2012;29(2):147-153. doi:10.1111/j.1525-1470.2011.01589.x

25. Deitch HR, Huppert J, Adams Hillard PJ. Unusual vulvar ulcerations in young adolescent females. *J Pediatr Adolesc Gynecol.* 2004;17(1):13-16. doi:10.1016/j. jpag.2003.11.015

26. Huppert JS, Gerber MA, Deitch HR, Mortensen JE, Staat MA, Adams Hillard PJ. Vulvar ulcers in young females: a manifestation of aphthosis. *J Pediatr Adolesc Gynecol.* 2006;19(3):195-204. doi:10.1016/j.jpag.2006.02.006

27. Christl J, Alaniz VI, Appiah L, Buyers E, Scott S, Huguelet PS. Vulvar aphthous ulcer in an adolescent with COVID-19. *J Pediatr Adolesc Gynecol.* 2021;34(3): 418-420. doi:10.1016/j.jpag.2021.02.098

28. Farhi D, Wendling J, Molinari E, et al. Non-sexually related acute genital ulcers in 13 pubertal girls: a clinical and microbiological study. *Arch Dermatol.* 2009;145(1): 38-45. doi:10.1001/archdermatol.2008.519

29. Wojcicki AV, O'Flynn O'Brien KL. Vulvar aphthous ulcer in an adolescent after Pfizer-BioNTech (BNT162b2) COVID-19 vaccination. *J Pediatr Adolesc Gynecol.* 2022;35(2):167-170. doi:10.1016/j.jpag.2021.10.005

30. Schneider SL, Foster K, Patel D, Shwayder T. Cutaneous manifestations of metastatic Crohn's disease. *Pediatr Dermatol.* 2018;35(5):566-574. doi:10.1111/pde.13565

31. Lehman JS, Bruce AJ, Wetter DA, Ferguson SB, Rogers RS III. Reactive nonsexually related acute genital ulcers: review of cases evaluated at Mayo Clinic. *J Am Acad Dermatol.* 2010;63(1):44-51. doi:10.1016/j.jaad.2009.08.038

32. Cizek SM, Tyson N. Pediatric and adolescent gynecologic emergencies. *Obstet Gynecol Clin North Am.* 2022;49(3):521-536. doi:10.1016/j.ogc.2022.02.017

33. Dixit S, Bradford J, Fischer G. Management of nonsexually acquired genital ulceration using oral and topical corticosteroids followed by doxycycline prophylaxis. *J Am Acad Dermatol.* 2013;68(5):797-802. doi:10.1016/j. jaad.2012.10.014

34. Huseynov M, Hakalmaz AE. Labial adhesion: new classification and treatment protocol. *J Pediatr Adolesc Gynecol.* 2020;33(4):343-348. doi:10.1016/j.jpag.2020.03.005

35. Muram D. Treatment of prepubertal girls with labial adhesions. *J Pediatr Adolesc Gynecol.* 1999;12(2):67-70. doi:10.1016/s1083-3188(00)86629-2

36. Myers JB, Sorensen CM, Wisner BP, Furness PD III, Passamaneck M, Koyle MA. Betamethasone cream for the treatment of pre-pubertal labial adhesions. *J Pediatr Adolesc Gynecol.* 2006;19(6):407-411. doi:10.1016/j.jpag.2006.09.005

37. Mayoglou L, Dulabon L, Martin-Alguacil N, Pfaff D, Schober J. Success of treatment modalities for labial fusion: a retrospective evaluation of topical and surgical treatments. *J Pediatr Adolesc Gynecol.* 2009;22(4): 247-250. doi:10.1016/j.jpag.2008.09.003

38. Bacon JL, Romano ME, Quint EH. Clinical recommendation: labial adhesions. *J Pediatr Adolesc Gynecol.* 2015;28(5):405-409. doi:10.1016/j.jpag.2015.04.010

39. Eroğlu E, Yip M, Oktar T, Kayiran SM, Mocan H. How should we treat prepubertal labial adhesions? retrospective comparison of topical treatments: estrogen only, betamethasone only, and combination estrogen and betamethasone. *J Pediatr Adolesc Gynecol.* 2011;24(6): 389-391. doi:10.1016/j.jpag.2011.07.015

40. Dowlut-McElroy T, Higgins J, Williams KB, Strickland JL. Treatment of prepubertal labial adhesions: a randomized controlled trial. *J Pediatr Adolesc Gynecol.* 2019;32(3):259-263. doi:10.1016/j.jpag.2018.10.006

41. Hillard PJA. *Practical Pediatric and Adolescent Gynecology.* Wiley-Blackwell; 2013.

42. Norris JE, Elder CV, Dunford AM, Rampal D, Cheung C, Grover SR. Spontaneous resolution of labial adhesions in pre-pubertal girls. *J Paediatr Child Health.* 2018;54(7):748-753. doi:10.1111/jpc.13847

43. Pokorny SF. Prepubertal vulvovaginopathies. *Obstet Gynecol Clin North Am.* 1992;19(1):39-58.

44. Diagnosis and management of vulvar skin disorders: ACOG practice bulletin summary, number 224. *Obstet Gynecol.* 2020;136(1):222-225. doi:10.1097/AOG.0000000000003945

45. Kumetz LM, Quint EH, Fisseha S, Smith YR. Estrogen treatment success in recurrent and persistent labial agglutination. *J Pediatr Adolesc Gynecol.* 2006;19(6): 381-384. doi:10.1016/j.jpag.2006.09.008

Adolescent Labial Concerns: Labial Hypertrophy, Asymmetry, and Genital Dissatisfaction

Lauren Damle and Rachel Kastl Casey

INTRODUCTION

Puberty is a time of both cognitive and physical change. Pubertal hormones influence the growth and development of breasts and genitalia. The external appearance of the vulva changes significantly; pubic hair begins to grow, the labia minora elongate and protrude compared with the prepubertal state, the clitoris and clitoral hood enlarge, and the labia majora become fuller in appearance. Although breast growth is often expected, many adolescents and their families are unaware of pubertal changes to the labia. The previously small and barely noticeable labia minora become more prominent and may even protrude from outside of the labia majora, prompting a young teen to feel self-conscious and wonder if their body is normal (Table 16.1). Furthermore, if there is evidence of asymmetry or notable vulvar discomfort; this may result in distress or dissatisfaction in both labial appearance and function.[1]

Adolescents may have concerns about the comfort of their external genitalia related to wearing certain clothing styles, bathing suits, or exercising. Most adolescents do not have any frame of reference for the wide range of normal size and appearance of genitalia other than media, family, or in some cases, personal sexual experiences. Similarly, caretakers may have limited experience to appreciate the vast range of normal genital appearances. Media and online representation of genitalia often provide limited examples of genitalia and promote an unrealistic "ideal vulva" that trends toward smaller, less visible labia minora akin to prepubertal labia. Media images may be digitally altered or include images of people who have had cosmetic surgery.

Physicians may also fail to appreciate the diversity in genital appearance, as most medical textbooks use simplified artistic renderings of anatomy rather than photographs to represent the true range of anatomic variation.[2] Sexual maturity rating, known most commonly as *Tanner staging*, describes pubic hair and stages of breast development but does not include any description of changes and development of the vulva and vagina.

DISEASE DEFINITION

Labial hypertrophy refers to the enlargement of the labia minora, typically beyond the labia majora.[3] However, there is no standard diagnostic criteria for labial hypertrophy, and wide ranges of normal sizes for labia are reported in the literature. Labia minora vary greatly in terms of size (length and width), pigmentation, texture, and symmetry. There is no agreed upon measurement of the labia minora that is classified as pathologic. Various labia minora width measurements have been proposed as a cut-off for hypertrophy, ranging between >3 and 5 cm.[4-6] Labial hypertrophy is subjective; labial

TABLE 16.1	**Vulvar Changes in Puberty**
Labia majora	Fuller in appearance
Clitoris and clitoral hood	Enlarge in tandem
Labia minora	Elongate and may protrude
	May be asymmetric
	May grow asynchronously

size that one person considers too large may be considered normal by another.[7]

Labial asymmetry refers to a discrepancy between the width of the labia minora, although the degree of discrepancy is not defined. One study cites a discrepancy of >20 mm as significant.[4]

Genital dissatisfaction is a newer term that refers to distress about the appearance of the vulva in the absence of any known endocrine or anatomic abnormality.[8] Societal influence, through online images of digitally altered or surgically modified vulvas accessed through social media or pornography, may contribute to genital dissatisfaction by promoting an unrealistic standard for "normal" genitalia.[9,10]

Prevalence and Epidemiology

Vulvar appearance and labial size are highly variable (Fig. 16.1). The width of the labia minora varies from 1 to 70 mm,[11-15] and reported average labia minora widths in adolescents range between 20 and 36 mm.[4,11] Asymmetry of labia minora width is common among adolescents.[11] Labia minora lengths range from 10 to 100 mm,[11,14,15] with a reported average of 31 mm in adolescents.[11] The majority of adolescent labia minora demonstrate color variation between the base and the tip of the labia and variation in texture (keratinized versus smooth).[11]

There are no published epidemiologic data about the prevalence of genital dissatisfaction among adolescents.

However, adolescent patients seeking care in regard to concerns about labial size, appearance, and function are common in pediatric and adolescent clinics.[4,13] Additionally, current trends suggest that requests for vulva and labia surgery are on the rise[16] and are not uncommon among adolescents. Data from 2016 to 2019 indicate that 18.9% of labiaplasties in the United States were performed on patients under age 18.[17]

Etiology and Pathophysiology

Labial growth and change begin with puberty. Sex hormone stimulation results in enlargement of the clitoris and labia and changes to the hymen appearance and vaginal epithelium. Androgens promote the development of pubic hair on the mons, labia majora, and inner thighs. Little is known about labia minora development in regard to rate of growth, what degree of asymmetry is normal or will persist into adulthood, and when labial development can be considered complete.[4] Individual genital anatomy is varied in appearance and is independent of sexual maturity rating, race, or exogenous hormone exposure (such as hormonal contraceptives).[11]

Clinical Presentation

Patients and their caregivers may present with concerns regarding appearance of the pubertal labia or physical symptoms. Pediatricians, family practitioners,

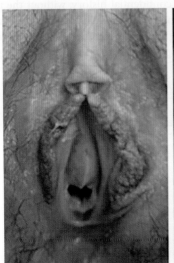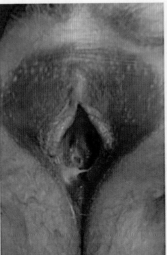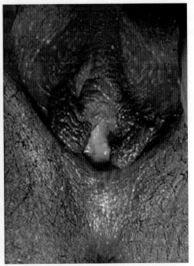

Fig. 16.1 Diversity of vulvar appearance in adolescents. (From Brodie K, Alaniz V, Buyers E, et al. A study of adolescent female genitalia: what is normal? *J Pediatr Adolesc Gynecol.* 2019;32[1]:27-31.)

and gynecologists will frequently encounter patients with questions about their genital appearance and function.

Adolescents may have concerns about how their vulva appears either undressed or with certain form-fitting clothing such as bathing suits, leggings, or sportswear (leotards for dance or ballet, for example). Teens or their caregivers may express worry about the appearance or function of their labia during sexual intimacy.

Common physical symptoms include pain, pruritus, skin changes, and vulvar discomfort in tight-fitting clothing or during participation in sports and exercise. Adolescents may report pain or irritation from friction of the labia on their clothing or the labia becoming caught in their clothing. They may report a sensation of the labia twisting or pinching during certain activities. Menstrual hygiene concerns may include irritation of labia during menstruation or difficulty with tampon or menstrual cup placement.

EVALUATION

A comprehensive medical history with a focus on puberty and genital symptoms should be obtained. It is important to speak directly to the adolescent when taking the history. This helps decipher if the concern is primarily from the adolescent or their caregiver. Including caregivers during history taking remains important to ensure a supportive and inclusive experience during the evaluation, but a separate confidential discussion is imperative to allow a teen time to share information that is personal or private. Appropriate questions regarding this concern include the following:

1. When did puberty begin?
2. When did you notice the labial changes?
3. Do the labia cause any discomfort? If yes, what are the symptoms (pain, pruritus, skin changes)?
4. When do you notice this discomfort (sports, exercise, wearing certain clothing, tampon placement, intimacy)?
5. Does anything improve or worsen with these symptoms?
6. Do you have challenges with menstrual hygiene related to your labia? Can you use tampons or a menstrual cup if you want to?
7. Are you concerned about the appearance of your genitalia?
8. Consider using the Female Genital Self-Image Scale (FGSIS) as an objective measure of genital self-image (Fig. 16.2).[18]

In addition to these questions, it may be helpful to understand hygiene practices, such as bathing, showering, and what type of soap, washcloths, or loofahs are being used. Ask about any over-the-counter products that a patient may have tried. Pubic hair trimming or removal practices and types of clothing/underwear may also be helpful information while formulating a differential diagnosis and plan.

Gender identity and sexuality are important considerations during confidential history taking. If gender identity differs from sex assigned at birth, this may affect a patient's feelings about their genital appearance and function. Adolescents considering or engaging in sexual intimacy may express concerns regarding both appearance and function. A confidential history, without the parent or caregiver, is necessary to fully explore the patient's concerns. During the confidential history, it is important to ask about any prior history of abuse or trauma and to

Please mark an "X" in the box to indicate how strongly you agree or disagree with each statement.

	Strongly disagree	Disagree	Agree	Strongly agree
I feel positively about my genitals.				
I am satisfied with the appearance of my genitals.				
I would feel comfortable letting a sexual partner look at my genitals.				
I think my genitals smell fine.				
I think my genitals work the way they are supposed to work.				
I feel comfortable letting a healthcare provider examine my genitals.				
I am not embarrassed about my genitals.				

Fig. 16.2 Female Genital Self Image Scale. This seven-item self-assessment is scored on a 4-point scale (strongly disagree =1, strongly agree = 4) for a total sum score ranging from 7 to 28; higher scores indicate a more positive genital self-image. (From Herbenick D, Reece M. Development and validation of the female genital self-image scale. *J Sex Med.* 2010;7[5]:1822-30. doi:10.1111/j.1743-6109.2010.01728.x)

take a detailed history about body image, depression, anxiety, and past or current self-harm behaviors.

All patients presenting with genital dissatisfaction related to vulvar appearance and/or function should be screened for body dysmorphic disorder (BDD).[1] The Body Dysmorphic Disorder Questionnaire (BDDQ, https://www.lifespan.org/sites/default/files/lifespan-files/documents/centers/body-dysmorphic/bddq.pdf) for adolescents is a self-report screening instrument with high sensitivity and specificity for body dysmorphia.[8] Patients suspected of having BDD should be referred to a mental health professional.

PHYSICAL EXAMINATION

Physical examination of the external genitalia requires sensitive preparation. Patients may prefer to be examined without their adult caretaker present or may prefer their company during the examination. Always ask the patient their preference for who they would like to have present in the room (the confidential interview can be a good time to ask this).

When performing the external genital examination, always obtain consent before touching the patient's body. Use the examination as an opportunity to counsel about personal body safety. The patient should undress waist down and be provided a gown or drape to cover their body. The legs can be positioned in frog-leg (butterfly) position or in typical gynecologic stirrups. Offering the patient a handheld mirror so that they can watch the examination can help alleviate anxiety and aid in active discussion about examination findings. The patient should be prompted to point to or identify areas of personal concern.[8]

The external genitalia is examined and Tanner stage of pubic hair noted along with any evidence of hair removal. The skin is evaluated for erythema, rashes, pigmentation changes, and lesions such as ulcers, condyloma, hemangiomas, or nevi. The labia may be gently separated to fully assess the labia majora and minora and perform measurements. For patients with specific concerns about the size of the labia, measurements are very helpful (Fig. 16.3). The labia length is the measurement of the labia minora from the superior to inferior

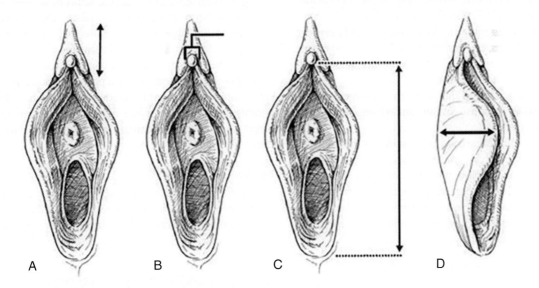

A. clitoral hood length
B. clitoral diameter
C. length of labia minora
D. width of labia minora

Fig. 16.3 Measurements of vulvar anatomy: (A) clitoral length, (B) clitoral width, (C) labia minora length, and (D) labia minora width. (From Brodie K, Alaniz V, Buyers E, et al. A study of adolescent female genitalia: what is normal? *J Pediatr Adolesc Gynecol.* 2019;32[1]:27-31.)

aspect. The labia width is the measurement from the base of the labia minora at the junction with the labia majora to the farthest projection of the tissue. The labia width can be measured at rest and on stretch and both measurements documented. Measurements of the clitoris may be helpful to include.

Additionally, it can be helpful to assess for pain and hyperalgesia of the genitalia. A cotton swab test can be performed to assess sensation of the labia majora and minora, clitoral hood, perineum, and vaginal vestibule.

Differential Diagnosis

When evaluating a teenage patient for concerns about labial size, appearance, or function, it is imperative that a comprehensive differential diagnosis be considered. In addition to labia minora hypertrophy, asymmetry, or genital dissatisfaction, other diagnoses to consider and rule out include:

1. Vulvodynia: pain of the vulva lasting 3 months or more without any other identifiable cause such as infection or skin condition
2. Vestibulodynia: pain of the vaginal vestibule lasting 3 months or more without any other identifiable cause such as infection or skin condition
3. Childhood asymmetric labia majora enlargement (CALME): painless, nontender, unilateral enlargement of the labia majora with normal overlying skin in prepuberty and early puberty
4. Clitoromegaly/hyperandrogenism: enlargement of the clitoris because of an underlying androgen-related condition
5. Other dermatologic conditions: skin tags, fibroepithelial polyps, condylomas, nevus, hemangioma, lipoma
6. BDD: preoccupation with one or more perceived defects or flaws in physical appearance causing clinically significant distress or impairment (a *Diagnostic and Statistical Manual of Mental Disorders, Fifth Edition* [DSM-5] diagnosis)

Management/Treatment Options

For any adolescent presenting with concerns about size, shape, color, or appearance of the vulva, the most important first step is reassurance and education. Counseling should be performed from a perspective of body positivity. Emphasizing the vast diversity of genital appearances in the population is important. Everyone is aware of the diversity in appearance of visible body parts such as our eyes, nose, mouth, ears, height, skin, and hair color but most people are unaware of the variety of appearance of private parts of human bodies. It is often helpful to use this comparison when counseling teens and their caregivers. Use of books and online resources that demonstrate images of natural vulvas are educational for patients and their caregivers and can have a positive impact on genital self-image.[19] Education is sufficient to reassure the majority of adolescents who present with concerns about the appearance and function of their labia.[20] Several options for educational resources are included at the end of this chapter. Some sites that are web based and can be helpful to patients include: https://www.thegreatwallofvulva.com/ https://labialibrary.org.au/

Nonsurgical Management

The primary management of labial hypertrophy and associated genital dissatisfaction is nonsurgical. In addition to education and reassurance regarding their anatomy, adolescents should be counseled about hygiene and lifestyle modifications that may help with comfort. These include the use of unscented soaps (or washing the genitalia with water alone) and wearing loose-fitting, natural fiber clothing and appropriate-size underwear to cover and protect the labia. Application of Vaseline to the labia before exercise may help prevent chafing (just as many athletes do this for other parts of their bodies). While acknowledging that decisions about pubic hair grooming are a personal choice, health care professionals should provide education about how complete removal of this hair exposes the labia to more direct contact with clothing and may increase irritation.[21] See Table 16.2.

Surgical Management

Labiaplasty is a surgical procedure to remove a portion of one or both labia minora in order to reduce the size or change the appearance of the labia. Surgical management of labial hypertrophy and dysphoria should be

TABLE 16.2 Vulvar Hygiene Modifications
• Cleanse with water only
• Avoid scented soaps
• Wear loose-fitting clothing
• Wear natural fiber clothing
• Use appropriately sized underwear
• Apply emollient before exercise
• Minimize pubic hair removal, which may protect the labia

reserved for patients who have completed pubertal development and have persistent symptoms not responsive to the nonmedical interventions.[1] If labiaplasty is considered, it should be delayed until the age of full pubertal maturation,[22] as the labia minora may grow and develop at discordant times. Labiaplasty at a young age before completion of pubertal development runs the risk of future requests for additional surgery if the labia continue to grow.[23]

There are several described surgical approaches to labiaplasty (Fig. 16.4). The most common methods are the edge resection (also called *labial trim*) and the wedge resection. The edge resection involves resection of the outer edge of the labia minora along the entire length of the labia with interrupted suture to reapproximate the resected edge. There is also a sutureless technique using a laser to perform edge resection.[24] This technique often results in removal of the pigmented edge of the labia minora, which may or may not be desirable to the patient. The wedge resection uses removal of a wedge of tissue with anastomosis of the labia minora to preserve the original pigmentation and texture of the edge of the labia minora. This technique carries the risk of tissue necrosis of the anastomosed tissue. Other described surgical approaches are Z-plasty and W-plasty and de-epithelialization.[5] No one procedure is superior to another; the procedure that the surgeon feels more confident performing is the one that should be recommended.

When considering surgical modification of the labia, preoperative counseling to set appropriate expectations for postoperative experience and possible outcomes is critical. Patients must be aware that there will be postoperative pain in this sensitive area and that many physical activities will be limited for several weeks or longer including exercise, activities with direct perineal pressure or contact (bike riding or horseback riding), swimming, and possible interference with menstrual hygiene. Patients must abstain from sexual intimacy until fully healed. Variable cosmetic outcomes are inevitable, and patients should be fully aware that the final cosmetic outcome may not be exactly what they imagined.

After a labiaplasty, a teen will need to manage postoperative pain at home with a combination of nonsteroidal antiinflammatory medications and acetaminophen. Narcotics should be avoided. Perineal ice packs are helpful. Meticulous hygiene with a peri bottle to rinse the labia frequently with water or daily sitz baths is recommended. There is no consensus regarding use of topical or oral antibiotics.[5] Swelling is common in the postoperative period and can last up to 3 to 6 months.[25] More than one postoperative visit may be needed to reassess healing and provide reassurance, especially in the adolescent population.

Common complications from labiaplasty include dehiscence of the surgical suture line, labial hematoma,

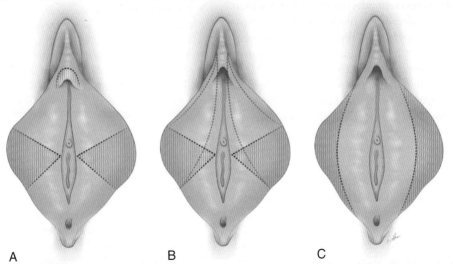

Fig. 16.4 Common surgical techniques for labiaplasty: (A) Wedge resection (B) De-epithelialization (C) Edge resection (or trim). (From Chang SY, Kao SW, Shih YC, Huang JJ. Labiaplasty in Asian women: Motivation, technique feasibility, and patient reported outcomes. *J Plast Reconstr Aesthet Surg.* 2023;85:217-225. https://doi.org/10.1016/j.bjps.2023.07.002.)

flap necrosis (when the wedge resection technique is used), surgical site infection, surgical site pain, and associated urinary retention. Long-term complications include persistent genital pain, altered sensation of the labia minora, dyspareunia, or undesired cosmetic outcome. Some patients may feel too much labial tissue was resected, and others feel like more should have been removed. Removal of a portion of the labia minora may change the appearance of the clitoris and clitoral hood skin in its relationship to the rest of the vulva.[5]

SPECIAL CONSIDERATIONS FOR THIS POPULATION

 Genital surgery in minors involves inherent ethical considerations. Decision for surgery requires both adolescent involvement and consent from the parent or legal guardian. The adolescent must be able to freely assent for labiaplasty, without influence from family members or caretakers. In addition to physical pubertal development, assessment of adolescent emotional maturity and readiness is necessary.

Labial surgery should not be performed for solely cosmetic reasons in minors, and in some states such practice is in violation of federal law.[26] Many major medical societies have issued position statements regarding genital surgery in minors. The Society of Obstetrician and Gynaecologists of Canada (SOGC) discourages genital surgery in adolescents but states that surgery may be considered after mature genital development when there is persistent functional impairment documented on repeat assessments and with appropriate counseling and psychological assessment and ethical considerations.[22] The American College of Obstetrics and Gynecology (ACOG) states that surgical correction (labiaplasty) should be considered only when there is significant congenital malformation or persistent physical symptoms thought to be caused directly by genital anatomic variation.[1]

Adolescence is a time of physical, psychological, and emotional development. It is normal for adolescents to feel self-conscious and wonder if their body is normal. Many teens may be exploring their sexuality and gender identity. It is imperative to allow separate time for a patient to ask questions or share concerns about their physical development, gender identity, and sexuality. Health care professionals should provide evidence-based, age-appropriate evaluation and counseling to support teens and their families in bolstering body awareness and assist them in making age-conscious informed decisions.

RESEARCH GAPS

The medical literature lacks large studies of genital anatomy across diverse populations.[12-15] The few studies of vulvar anatomy variation performed specifically in adolescents are of majority-White-race patient populations.[4,11] Tools for genital self-image, such as the FGSIS, are not validated in the adolescent population, and some questions may be irrelevant to those who are not sexually active. A modified version of FGSIS could be useful in assessing adolescents, but this has not yet been studied.[8] Reasons why some adolescents pursue surgery when the majority are satisfied with reassurance and nonmedical interventions is also unknown. One small descriptive study revealed that the majority of adolescents presenting with concerns about physical discomfort related to labial size were reassured after counseling, and only 9.8% of patients chose surgery.[20] Although the literature suggests that the majority of adults who undergo labiaplasty are satisfied with their outcome,[6] there is a lack of objective outcome data for labiaplasty, especially among adolescents.

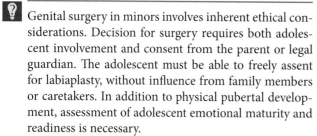

KEY POINTS

- A careful history and examination should involve both a full understanding of symptoms and objective measurements of the labial length and width bilaterally.
- A confidential interview with an adolescent is critical and may allow for identification of BDD.
- Education about genital anatomic diversity and reassurance about normal pubertal development are essential components of treatment and support a body positivity framework.
- First-line therapy for genital dissatisfaction and perceived labial hypertrophy is nonsurgical: reconsider hair removal, apply emollients, avoid fragranced soaps, and wear loose-fitting cotton clothing.
- Surgical intervention is reserved for persistent and refractory cases of labial hypertrophy causing physical symptoms after the completion of puberty; cosmetic labial surgery in minors is never appropriate.
- Labiaplasty can be considered when the patient is emotionally mature and able to make an informed decision with support of a consenting parent or legal guardian.

REVIEW QUESTIONS

1. A 13-year-old cisgender female seeks consultation regarding perceived enlarged labia. The patient reports concerns about the normality of her genitalia and some discomfort when she exercises or wears tight leggings. She recently started combined oral contraceptive pills for management of heavy and painful menses. On examination you note Tanner 3 pubic hair and labia minora that are asymmetric, with a left labia minora width of 35 mm and right labia minora of 25 mm. Her mother is concerned that her own labia look nothing like her daughter's labia. What is the next best step in management?
   a. Explain that her labia are abnormally asymmetric and this may get worse as she gets older.
   b. Counsel the patient and her mother regarding vulvar anatomic diversity, providing visual educational tools and reassurance.
   c. Recommend consultation with a gynecologist for surgical correction of her labia.
   d. Discontinue combined hormonal contraception, as estrogen may promote abnormal labial growth.

2. Which of the following is true regarding labiaplasty?
   a. Labiaplasty can prevent recurrent yeast infections.
   b. Labiaplasty has been proven to improve sexual function.
   c. A complication of wedge resection labiaplasty is flap necrosis.
   d. Edge resection labiaplasty preserves the natural pigmentation and texture of the labia minora.

3. Why is nonsurgical treatment considered first-line treatment for labial hypertrophy, asymmetry, or labial dissatisfaction in adolescents?
   a. This age group may be under stress regarding body appearance and conforming to social or media norms.
   b. Adolescents may lack the emotional maturity to freely assent for the procedure.
   c. Labiaplasty performed solely for cosmetic reasons in patients under the age of 18 is illegal in some jurisdictions.
   d. All of the above.

LINKED RESOURCES

Websites:

https://www.thegreatwallofvulva.com/ An art exhibition and online collection of casts of vulvas celebrating the diversity of anatomy by artist Jamie McCartney.

https://labialibrary.org.au/ An initiative of Women's Health Victoria website to show the natural diversity of women's genitals. This website is part of a bigger project that aims to make sure women who are thinking about female genital cosmetic surgery are properly informed and receive care that is safe and based on proper evidence.

Book:

Petals by Karras, Nick. 2nd edition (2017). Photo collection of 48 different vulvas representing anatomic diversity.

Patient Resources:

NASPAG patient education handout: https://www.naspag.org/assets/docs/labial_hypertrophy_2020.pdf

BritsPAG online publication "So what is a vulva anyway": https://britspag.org/wp-content/uploads/2019/06/So_what_is_a_vulva_anyway_final_booklet.pdf

REFERENCES

1. Committee opinion no. 686: breast and labial surgery in adolescents. *Obstet Gynecol.* 2017;129(1):e17-e19. doi:10.1097/AOG.0000000000001862
2. Andrikopoulou M, Michala L, Creighton SM, Liao LM. The normal vulva in medical textbooks. *J Obstet Gynaecol.* 2013;33(7):648-650. doi:10.3109/01443615.2013.807782
3. Reddy J, Laufer MR. Hypertrophic labia minora. *J Pediatr Adolesc Gynecol.* 2010;23(1):3-6. doi:10.1016/j.jpag.2009.01.071
4. Michala L, Koliantzaki S, Antsaklis A. Protruding labia minora: abnormal or just uncool? *J Psychosom Obstet Gynaecol.* 2011;32(3):154-156. doi:10.3109/0167482X.2011.585726
5. Motakef S, Rodriguez-Feliz J, Chung MT, Ingargiola MJ, Wong VW, Patel A. Vaginal labiaplasty: current practices and a simplified classification system for labial protrusion. *Plast Reconstr Surg.* 2015;135(3):774-788. doi:10.1097/PRS.0000000000001000
6. Rouzier R, Louis-Sylvestre C, Paniel BJ, Haddad B. Hypertrophy of labia minora: experience with 163 reductions. *Am J Obstet Gynecol.* 2000;182(1 Pt 1):35-40. doi:10.1016/s0002-9378(00)70488-1
7. Kalampalikis A, Michala L. Cosmetic labiaplasty on minors: a review of current trends and evidence. *Int J Impot Res.* 2021;18:1-4. doi:10.1038/s41443-021-00480-1
8. Michala L. The adolescent and genital dissatisfaction. *Clin Obstet Gynecol.* 2020;63(3):528-535. doi:10.1097/GRF.0000000000000522
9. Moran C, Lee C. What's normal? Influencing women's perceptions of normal genitalia: an experiment involving exposure to modified and nonmodified images. *BJOG.* 2014;121(6):761-766. doi:10.1111/1471-0528.12578
10. Mowat H, McDonald K, Dobson AS, Fisher J, Kirkman M. The contribution of online content to the promotion and normalisation of female genital cosmetic surgery:

a systematic review of the literature. *BMC Womens Health.* 2015;15:110. doi:10.1186/s12905-015-0271-5

11. Brodie K, Alaniz V, Buyers E, et al. A study of adolescent female genitalia: what is normal? *J Pediatr Adolesc Gynecol.* 2019;32(1):27-31. doi:10.1016/j.jpag.2018.09.007

12. Cao Y, Li Q, Zhou C, Li F, Li S, Zhou Y. Measurements of female genital appearance in Chinese adults seeking genital cosmetic surgery: a preliminary report from a gynecological center. *Int Urogynecol J.* 2015;26(5):729-735. doi:10.1007/s00192-014-2584-6

13. Crouch NS, Deans R, Michala L, Liao LM, Creighton SM. Clinical characteristics of well women seeking labial reduction surgery: a prospective study. *BJOG.* 2011;118(12):1507-1510. doi:10.1111/j.1471-0528.2011.03088.x

14. Kreklau A, Vâz I, Oehme F, et al. Measurements of a 'normal vulva' in women aged 15-84: a cross-sectional prospective single-centre study. *BJOG.* 2018;125(13):1656-1661. doi:10.1111/1471-0528.15387

15. Lloyd J, Crouch NS, Minto CL, Liao LM, Creighton SM. Female genital appearance: "normality" unfolds. *BJOG.* 2005;112(5):643-646. doi:10.1111/j.1471-0528.2004.00517.x

16. The American Society for Aesthetic Plastic Surgery's Cosmetic Surgery National Data Bank: statistics 2018. *Aesthet Surg J.* 2019;39(suppl 4):1-27. doi:10.1093/asj/sjz164

17. Luchristt D, Sheyn D, Bretschneider CE. National estimates of labiaplasty performance in the United States from 2016 to 2019. *Obstet Gynecol.* 2022;140(2):271-274. doi:10.1097/AOG.0000000000004853

18. Herbenick D, Reece M. Development and validation of the female genital self-image scale. *J Sex Med.* 2010;7(5):1822-1830. doi:10.1111/j.1743-6109.2010.01728.x

19. Laan E, Martoredjo DK, Hesselink S, Snijders N, van Lunsen RHW. Young women's genital self-image and effects of exposure to pictures of natural vulvas. *J Psychosom Obstet Gynaecol.* 2017;38(4):249-255. doi:10.1080/0167482X.2016.1233172

20. McQuillan SK, Jayasinghe Y, Grover SR. Audit of referrals for concern regarding labial appearance at the Royal Children's Hospital: 2000-2012. *J Paediatr Child Health.* 2018;54(4):439-442. doi:10.1111/jpc.13819

21. Runacres SA, Wood PL. Cosmetic labiaplasty in an adolescent population. *J Pediatr Adolesc Gynecol.* 2016;29(3):218-222. doi:10.1016/j.jpag.2015.09.010

22. Shaw D, Allen L, Chan C, et al. Guideline no. 423: female genital cosmetic surgery and procedures. *J Obstet Gynaecol Can.* 2022;44(2):204-214.e1. doi:10.1016/j.jogc.2021.11.001

23. Lynch A, Marulaiah M, Samarakkody U. Reduction labioplasty in adolescents. *J Pediatr Adolesc Gynecol.* 2008;21(3):147-149. doi:10.1016/j.jpag.2007.03.100

24. Bizjak-Ogrinc U, Senčar S. Sutureless laser labiaplasty of labia minora. *Sex Med.* 2021;9(5):100406. doi:10.1016/j.esxm.2021.100406

25. Furnas HJ. Trim labiaplasty. *Plast Reconstr Surg Glob Open.* 2017;5(5):e1349. doi:10.1097/GOX.0000000000001349

26. Female Genital Mutilation. 18 U.S.C §116 (2018 Edition, Supplement 3, Title 18).

Traumatic Genital Injury

Jennie Yoost and Courtney Crain

In pediatric and adolescent patients, genital trauma can be from accidental injury or intentional assault. Genital trauma can range by the mechanism of trauma and by the severity and type of injury.[1,2] Types of trauma include blunt, penetrating, insufflation, burns, or coital injuries from consensual sex or sexual assault. Genital trauma can also be in the context of multiple injuries, such as a patient involved in a motor vehicle accident with a pelvic fracture. Genital injuries can be lacerations, hematomas, contusions, burns, bites, abrasions, and crushing injuries from pelvic fractures.[3,4]

Straddle injuries are the most common mechanism of genital trauma in the pediatric population and typically involve blunt trauma. This injury results when a subject straddles an object forcefully, which commonly includes bicycle crossbars, playground equipment, bathtub ledges, or furniture.[1,5] Most straddle injury cases occur under 10 years of age and are more common in the summer months. As most straddle injuries are the result of blunt trauma with objects not capable of penetrating above the pelvic floor, they are generally amenable to nonoperative management.[5,6]

Although straddle injuries are the most common, any genital trauma in children can cause anxiety to guardians and caregivers because of the location of the injury and potential concerns for future gynecologic and psychosexual development.[7,8] In any patient with a history of genital trauma, thorough history and examination is needed. It is imperative to always consider sexual assault or abuse in any child presenting with a genital injury so that interventions can be implemented to reduce long-term sequelae.

PREVALENCE

Pediatric genital injuries account for 0.2% to 0.8% of all reported childhood trauma and can be classified by mechanism, location, and intention.[9,10] The prevalence of accidental genital trauma is best described by three cohort studies evaluating pediatric patients presenting to the emergency department, excluding cases of intentional injury and abuse (Table 17.1). In the cohorts by Spitzer, Iqbal, and Dowlut-McElroy and their colleagues, straddle injures were the most frequently encountered mechanism of injury, accounting for 70.5% to 82% of cases.[7,11,12] Accidental penetrating injuries were less prevalent, accounting for 4.7% to 6% of cases in two cohorts[7,11] and 11% of cases in another.[12] Trauma classified as other forms of injury, including motor vehicle accidents, was reported occurring in 12% of cases in one cohort.[11]

Iqbal and Dowlut-McElroy and their colleagues reported injury prevalence to specific genital structures among 167 and 359 patients, respectively, with accidental genital trauma. Both reported that the labia was the most frequent site of injury (63%–64%), followed by the perineum (21.5%–23%), the vagina (5.9%), and then the rectum and anus (2.9%–5%). Hymen disruption was observed in 8.4% to 10% of cases.[11,12] Spitzer and colleagues reported among 105 pediatric patients that 37% had anterior injuries (defined as the 9 o'clock to 3 o'clock positions on the vulva) and 62% had injuries to the posterior region of the vulva. In this cohort, only 4.7% of injuries involved the hymen [7]

Lacerations are the most common type of injury, reported in up to 86% of accidental trauma, followed by

TABLE 17.1   **Type, Location, and Management of Unintentional Genital Injuries Among Three Large Cohorts**

Study	N	Age (mean)	Type of Injury	Location of Injury	Management
Spitzer et al.	105	5.6	81.9% Straddle injury 4.7% Accidental penetrating 12.4% Other (including motor vehicle)	37.6% Anterior injuries (9 o'clock to 3 o'clock) 62.4% Posterior injuries 4.7% Involving hymen	79.05% Expectant 20.05% Surgical repair
Iqbal et al.	167	6.9	70.5% Straddle injury 23.5% Nonstraddle blunt injury 6.0% Accidental penetrating	64% Labia 21.5% Perineum 8.9% Vulva 7.8% Posterior fourchette 5.9% Vagina 2.9% Rectum 8.4% Involving hymen	87.9% Expectant 12.1% Surgical repair
Dowlut-McElroy et al.	359	6.0	73% Straddle 16% Nonstraddle blunt injury 11% Accidental penetrating	63% Labia 23% Perineum 10% Hymen/vagina 5% Urethra/anus	82% Expectant 18% Surgical repair

abrasions/contusions (9%) and hematomas (4%).[12] Complete injuries through the rectum are more likely to occur with penetrating trauma compared with straddle or blunt injuries.[11]

Sexual Activity and Abuse

Intentional injury from abuse or assault can cause genital trauma, and the examination should be performed by a provider with expertise in child sexual abuse. The prevalence of genital injury from sexual abuse can vary depending on the methodology employed for examination and time since assault.[13] In one study among 14- to 19-year-old patients reporting sexual assault, 19% had hymenal injury and 36% had tears in the posterior fourchette.[14] In another study of 1500 pubertal and prepubertal females examined acutely after assault, diagnostic findings were 12.5 times higher for children reporting genital penetration compared with those reporting only contact.[15] In children, even though it is uncommon, an acute laceration of the hymen of any depth or complete transection below 3 and 9 o'clock is suggestive of sexual abuse.[16] Perineal trauma in children under age 4 also raises suspicion of abuse.[6]

It is also known that with consensual sexual activity, genital trauma can result, although this is not well studied. One study evaluating patients with a history of assault and a comparison group of patients with recent consensual sex found that the posterior fourchette was the genital area most likely injured in both groups.[13] A study among 51 adolescents after consensual sexual activity found that lacerations at the 6 o'clock position were seen in approximately 60% and hymenal lesions, often bruises, in 50%.[17]

ETIOLOGY AND PATHOPHYSIOLOGY

The impact of rising estrogen levels in puberty has a protective effect on genital tissue against minor trauma. In younger, prepubertal patients who are unestrogenized, the genital tissues are relatively fragile and lack significant distensibility. Minor trauma can expose underlying capillary beds, and bleeding can appear excessive relative to the degree of injury.[3] At puberty, with increasing estrogen concentrations, the vagina and hymen become more distensible and less likely to tear with gentle distention such as with tampon use. However, blunt or forceful trauma can still result in lacerations or other injury.[1]

The vulva and pelvic structures have a rich blood supply, and vulvar hematomas develop when the labial

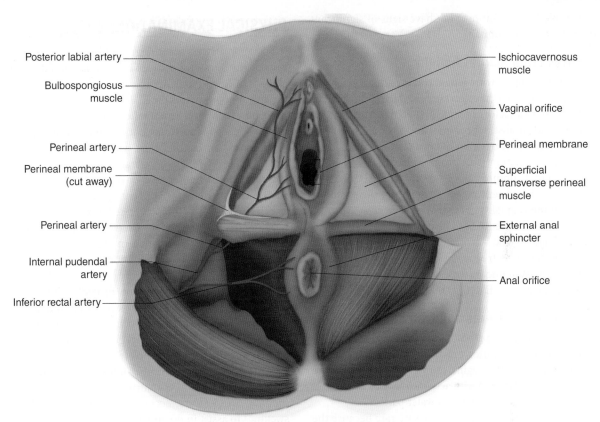

Posterior labial artery

Bulbospongiosus muscle

Perineal artery

Perineal membrane (cut away)

Perineal artery

Internal pudendal artery

Inferior rectal artery

Ischiocavernosus muscle

Vaginal orifice

Perineal membrane

Superficial transverse perineal muscle

External anal sphincter

Anal orifice

Fig. 17.1 Arterial blood supply of the vulva.

branches of the internal pudendal artery are injured. Injury to these vessels occurs when soft tissue and pelvic fascia compress against the pelvic bones during blunt impact (Fig. 17.1). Hematomas can be extensive, as bleeding will track along the planes of the subcutaneous pelvic fascia.[18,19] Pressure from an expanding hematoma can affect a patient's ability to void, can cause necrosis of the skin overlying the hematoma, and can result in tissue sloughing.[20]

CLINICAL PRESENTATION/EVALUATION

Blunt Straddle Injury

Genital pain and bleeding are the most common presenting symptoms after blunt, nonpenetrating genital trauma, such as a straddle injury. In one series 89% of the cohort presented with pain and bleeding, and other presenting complaints included the inability to void or complaints of dysuria.[2,7,12]

Crush or Penetrating Injuries

More severe penetrating injuries can present with gross hematuria or rectal bleeding.[21]

Vulvar and vaginal bleeding from lacerations or hematomas can be profuse because of the rich blood supply of the pelvic structures.[1,7]

Motor vehicle accidents are a common mechanism of injury resulting in pelvic fracture, which can involve bone shards that cause vaginal lacerations.[22] One study found that 17% of children with pelvic fractures sustained genitourinary injuries.[23]

Penetrating injuries are defined as a piercing injury of the genitourinary or anorectal tissues. These injuries are usually more extensive, more commonly involve trauma to the hymen and vagina, and in rare cases cause visceral injury.[5,23] Deep internal vaginal injuries can potentially damage the uterine artery or other branches of the internal iliac artery. These deep injuries can lead to bleeding and accumulation of blood in the perivaginal space, and the patient may not have signs of significant external genital trauma.[24]

Injuries From Sexual Activity

Patients presenting with genital trauma after consensual sexual activity may have certain risk factors for laceration. These risk factors include first coitus, coitus after a long period of abstinence, insertion of foreign objects during activity, congenital vaginal abnormalities, and coitus in association with drug or alcohol use.[1] In rare cases, vaginal rupture can occur. This is described as a laceration several centimeters in length in the posterior aspect of the vaginal wall involving the posterior fornix. In case reports, bleeding can be profuse and even lead to hemorrhagic shock.[25] It is suggested that vaginal rupture may be more frequent after pelvic surgery, pelvic disease, or systemic diseases such as inflammatory bowel syndrome or Ehlers-Danlos syndrome.[25]

Other Injuries: Burns and Insufflation

Other less common presentations of genital trauma include insufflation injuries, burns, and animal bites. Insufflation injuries to the vagina can be from high-pressure water jets in association with activities such as riding a jet ski, water skiing, or playing in a water park.[7,26]

Genital injuries caused by burns are rare because the thighs provide protection to the genital area, unless the burns are very extensive. Burns to the genital region can be the result of accidental immersion burns or abuse. In children less than 5 years of age the most common causative agent was immersion in hot bath water.[27,28] Patients can have animal bites to the genitals, but also could have human bites as the result of rough play, fighting, or sexual activity. Patients with bites can present with cellulitis resulting from microorganisms in human saliva that can cause infection.[24]

With any accidental or intentional genital trauma, the history given by the child, guardians, and any witnesses is the most important element in the initial evaluation. Ideally the patient and other present adults should be questioned separately for corroboration. A verbal child who is injured is typically forthcoming in telling the story of their accident. Clues of sexual abuse include a nonambulatory child; perineal, vaginal, or hymen injury without history of penetrating trauma; extensive or severe trauma; presence of nongenital trauma; and lack of correlation between the history and findings on physical examination.[5,7,23]

PHYSICAL EXAMINATION

Vital signs, airway, breathing, circulation, and evaluation of the sites and sources of trauma should be included in the initial approach. The severity of the trauma, amount of bleeding, and patient stability determine how a physical examination should be performed. In a stable, cooperative patient without severe injuries, an examination can be done without sedation.[4] Children may be reticent to cooperate with a genital examination because of either fear or pain. Force or coercion should never be employed to complete an examination, and in many cases, the use of sedation will allow the provider to get a more thorough evaluation.[20] Examination alone cannot distinguish intentional versus accidental injury, and the examination in an abused child may be normal or nonspecific.[2,29]

During the examination, the provider should systematically examine the genital structures, and any injury should be described in detail, including appearance, location, and size. Normal genital anatomy should also be documented. A complete physical examination also allows inspection for other injuries (inflicted or accidental). Description of injuries can employ the pneumonic TEARS (tears, ecchymosis, abrasions, redness, swelling) to assist in documentation, with each element defined as follows[1,25]:

- Tears: Any breaks in tissue integrity, including fissures, cracks, lacerations, cuts gashes, or rips.
- Ecchymosis: Skin or mucous membrane discolorations caused by damage to small blood vessels beneath the skin or mucosal surface bruising. Extravasation of blood in tissues below an intact epidermis.
- Abrasions: Skin excoriations caused by removal of the epidermal layer with a defined edge. Exposure of the lower epidermis or upper dermis. Most commonly caused by lateral rubbing or sliding against the skin in a tangential manner. The outermost layer of skin is scraped away from the deeper layers.
- Redness: Erythematous skin which is abnormally inflamed because of irritation or injury without a defined edge or border.
- Swelling: Edematous or transient engorgement of tissues.

There are various ways to optimize a genital examination in younger patients. Young patients can be examined in the supine position with downward outward traction of the labia, with gentle separation of the labia, or in the prone knee-chest position (see Chapter 1). One study reported that combining methods demonstrated a greater chance of identifying additional signs of trauma than when only using one examination technique.[30] Application of topical analgesic such as 2% to 5% lidocaine gel over the injury and use of 30- to 60-cc syringes or bulb syringe with warm water or saline irrigation can also help achieve a better examination. Likewise, compression with towels or moist cloths can also be helpful to slow bleeding.[4] Patient comfort can also be aided by child life specialists or distraction.

The examination of a genital laceration includes visualizing the full extent of the injury. Lacerations of the vagina may extend into the fornix, and in prepubertal patients lacerations beyond the hymen are difficult to visualize with external genital examination alone. In these cases, vaginoscopy with a small hysteroscope or cystoscope can be beneficial to visualize the vaginal walls, fornices, and cervix. This tool can also identify the rare cases where vaginal laceration extends into the peritoneal cavity.[31] In the rare instance where the peritoneal cavity is involved in the injury, an exploratory laparotomy or laparoscopy should be performed to determine the full extent of the injuries.[24]

Burn injuries are classified as first, second, and third degree based on whether the burn is limited to the epidermis, involves both epidermis and dermis, or shows more extensive involvement of the epidermis, dermis, and underlying tissue, respectively.[1] For patients with burn injuries, accidental burns are nonuniform in depth and have irregular borders. These burns can be patchy and superficial as the child quickly withdraws from the hot object or liquid. Inflicted burns, as in the case of child abuse, will have well-demarcated lines and uniform depth.[32]

Thorough examination in children is important, as missed genital injuries can result in chronic vulvovaginal concerns such as discomfort, stenosis, and chronic fissures.[6] Furthermore, in patients with intentional assault resulting in genital trauma, missed injuries on examination can delay involvement in psychological support, which is important in long-term management.[8]

IMAGING TECHNIQUES

Imaging studies are determined by the overall degree of trauma. Diagnostic imaging in one analysis did not aid in medical decision making in patients with blunt genital trauma, and examination under anesthesia remained the standard of care.[33] In the setting of an expanding hematoma, or to appreciate the extent of a hematoma, transperineal ultrasonography can be used.[34] Major injuries that include extension into the urinary tract, rectum, or peritoneal cavity will need multidisciplinary consultation. For urinary tract injuries, voiding cystourethrogram or computed tomography imaging can be used.[35]

DIFFERENTIAL DIAGNOSIS

Although a history of accidental or intentional trauma narrows the diagnosis, there are other conditions that can present with genital pain and bleeding in the pediatric population. Lichen sclerosus is a unique dermatologic condition in the pediatric population that can present with acute vaginal bleeding from subepithelial hemorrhages.[36] This dermatologic condition can be misinterpreted as trauma, as these subepithelial hemorrhages can look similar to abrasions or contusions. Acute vulvovaginitis in prepubertal patients or the presence of a foreign body can present with pain and vaginal bleeding.[37] Patients with vulvovaginitis on examination will have erythema and swelling of vulvar structures.[38] These patients will not have a history consistent with trauma.

MANAGEMENT AND TREATMENT

An overview of the management approach for patients with genital injury is detailed in Fig. 17.2. The need for surgical intervention in pediatric and adolescent genital trauma is low, and 79% to 87% of genital injuries in this population have been reported to be managed expectantly.[7,11,12] The highest risks associated with the need for examination under anesthesia include those with penetrating injuries; injuries larger than 3 to 4 cm in size; injuries involving the hymen, vagina, urethra, and anus; injuries that extend beyond the labia; a patient who is unable to tolerate an examination; inability to see the full extent of the injury; and bleeding that cannot be localized.[4,11] Other reviews found that penetrating injuries, a diagnosis of sexual assault, and injuries from motor vehicle accidents also conveyed higher risk of needing assessment under anesthesia.[2,6,7] Older children may also convey an increased need for sedation after genital trauma. It is thought that older children may be

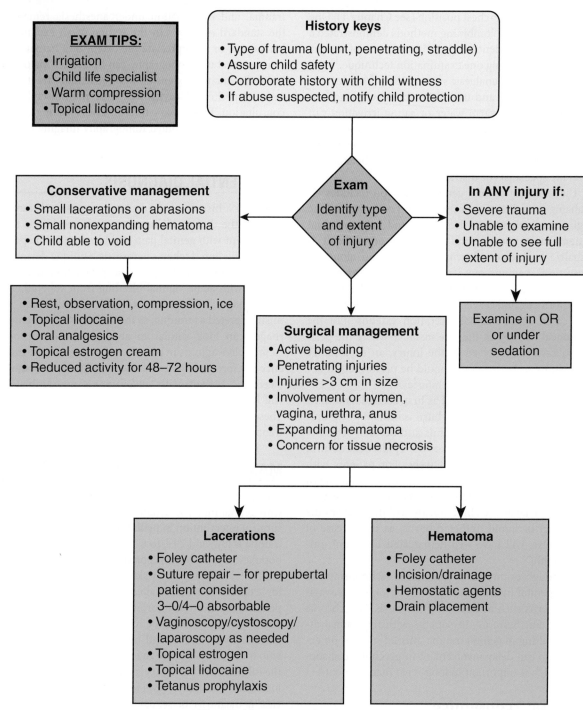

Fig. 17.2 Management of genital trauma.

more active and sustain more forceful injuries. They also may be more difficult to examine in the emergency department or have a higher degree of anxiety about their injuries than younger children.[7]

Conservative Management

Minor bleeding from small lacerations, abrasions, and small nonexpanding hematomas can be managed conservatively. This includes barrier ointments, ice, oral and topical analgesics, instructions for decreased activity, and reassurance.[4] Topical analgesics include 2% to 5% lidocaine gel or ointment. Topical estrogen cream can also be used on small lacerations to promote healing. A prerequisite for conservative management is that the child is able to void spontaneously. Patients and caregivers should be counseled about reduction in physical activity during the critical healing phases, especially for the first 48 to 72 hours. A reduction in activity level helps to ensure that the area is not reinjured before considerable healing has taken place. Most vulvar hematomas will spontaneously resolve over 1 to 5 days with conservative management.[4] Most superficial lacerations or abrasions will resolve within 2 to 3 days.[39]

Surgical Management

Although most pediatric genital trauma can be managed expectantly, 10% to 25% of injuries require operative intervention in the emergency room or operating room.[12] Operative management can be performed in the emergency department if the provider has appropriate surgical tools, lighting, patient positioning, and providers familiar with pediatric sedation in the emergency room setting. When injuries are more extensive, or if the emergency department does not have the capability for pediatric sedation, surgical intervention with general anesthesia in the operating room is needed.

Lacerations

Clean wounds may undergo primary repair. Before closure, the wound should be irrigated well. Indications for secondary closure include deep stab or puncture wounds, contaminated wounds, or presentation after significant delay. Lacerations should be repaired with absorbable suture. In younger prepubertal patients, suture such as 3-0 or 4-0 Monocryl or Vicryl on a small half (SH) needle can be used. Lacerations to the labia, vagina, perineum, and anal sphincter are repaired in a similar fashion to episiotomy repairs in adult patients. A simulation of this type of repair and tools used on a 3D printed pediatric model is shown in Fig. 17.3 and Video 17.1.

Lacerations to the periurethral space can be deep and may require a Foley catheter and meticulous suturing with a small-caliber suture. For vaginal lacerations that are difficult to suture in prepubertal girls, vaginal packing moistened with saline or estrogen cream can be placed and then removed at a later time to assess for hemostasis.[24] Prepubertal girls may also benefit from application of a small amount of estrogen cream twice daily to injured tissue. Estrogen cream may help with healing by promoting granulation tissue and reducing

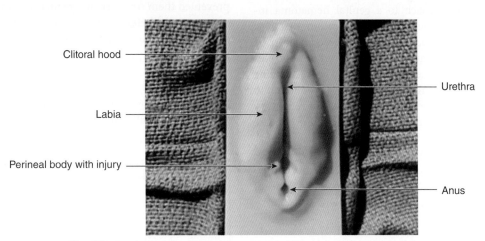

Fig. 17.3 Surgical repair of perineal trauma on a 3D printed pediatric model.

inflammation.[40] Although no published guidance is available, twice-daily estrogen cream to laceration repairs for up to 7 days is frequently used depending on the extent of the injury. Tetanus prophylaxis should be considered if lacerations or penetrating injury was from an unknown object or metal device.[24] Most acute genital injuries heal quickly, with abrasions and superficial lacerations resolving in 2 to 3 days and deeper lacerations recovering similar to episiotomies with a healing time of 6 weeks.[4]

In an operative setting, the use of vaginoscopy or cystoscopy can be employed depending on the extent of the injury and structures involved. As noted previously, lacerations extending to and involving the peritoneal cavity require laparoscopy or laparotomy. Although gynecologists have familiarity with episiotomy repair and vaginal lacerations, more extensive involvement of the urinary system or large rectovaginal injuries may require general surgery, urology, or colorectal surgery consultation.

Hematomas

Surgical intervention for hematomas is recommended when there is progressive growth, pain that is unrelieved, or concern for overlying tissue necrosis because of hematoma expansion.[19] If hematoma formation is near the urethra, the patient's ability to urinate may be compromised, and a catheter should be placed until the swelling resolves. If the hematoma becomes progressively larger, serial hematocrits should be checked. In the majority of cases, observation and cold compresses are all that is indicated; however, with falling hematocrit or patient instability, surgery is necessary.[18]

The surgical approach to a genital hematoma involves an incision over the point of maximum bulge. Blood clots can be evacuated, active bleeding can be localized, and hemostasis can be achieved by suture ligation of bleeding vessels.[41] Generalized venous oozing is common, as the source of bleeding is often difficult to identify. The use of fibrin sealant in a case of refractory bleeding has been described.[42] Packing and a penrose drain can be placed at the inferior region of the hematoma.[4] The use of a Word catheter has also been described.[43] Drains can be removed after 24 hours, and no published evidence supports the concomitant use of antibiotics for short-term drain placement.

Bites and Burns

Genital bite wounds should be thoroughly cleaned, irrigated, and not closed primarily. Antibiotic therapy is recommended with extended-spectrum penicillin with beta-lactamase inhibitors (amoxicillin/clavulanate) for 3 to 5 days. Antibiotics are recommended for human bites and genital bites, as these carry higher risks of infection leading to cellulitis. Tetanus immunization should also be reviewed, and a booster given if necessary.[44]

For minor burns, cooling the area with compresses can reduce swelling and pain. Silver sulfadiazine cream can be used on burns to minimize risks of wound infection. A mixture of topical antibiotic cream and estrogen cream can also be used to minimize scarring.[24] More extensive genital burns may involve surgical management and grafting.

SPECIAL CONSIDERATIONS

The management of patients with genital trauma may be determined by the type of institution. Larger metropolitan institutions that are level 1 trauma centers may have designated pediatric emergency medicine physicians who are credentialed for sedation. Other hospitals may not have the availability to offer adequate procedural sedation in the emergency department, and therefore may rely more heavily on examination under anesthesia in the operating room. Child life specialists may be not available in some institutions to assist with the examination process.

It is unknown if there are long-term sequelae from accidental genital trauma. Adults with a history of childhood sexual assault have fears related to common medical procedures, especially gynecologic examination procedures, and two-thirds reported their fears prevented them from seeking regular health care.[45] It is not reported whether patients with a history of accidental genital trauma may have difficulty with the approach to gynecologic procedures in the future. Providers should consider patients' previous experiences with trauma and work to create interactions where patients feel emotionally and physically safe, so that they have a sense of control and empowerment.

> **KEY POINTS**
> - Always corroborate the history with witnesses and consider screening for sexual assault.
> - Avoid use of coercion or force to facilitate examinations. Instead, optimize emergency department anesthesia if available and child life specialists and maintain a low threshold to proceed to the operating room.

REVIEW QUESTIONS

1. The most common location of genital injury after consensual intercourse or sexual assault is:
   a. The labia
   b. The posterior fourchette
   c. The vaginal side wall
   d. The hymen

2. Which suture is most appropriate for repair of a pediatric perineal laceration?
   a. 3-0 Polydioxanone suture
   b. 2-0 Silk suture
   c. 4-0 Polyglactin suture
   d. 1-0 Monocryl suture

3. Which of the following statements is true?
   a. Antibiotics should be not given after bite injury.
   b. Most straddle injuries require surgical intervention.
   c. Vulvar dermatoses can be mistaken for genital trauma.
   d. Topical estrogen does not aid in perineal wound healing.

REFERENCES

1. Merritt DF. Genital trauma in prepubertal girls and adolescents. *Curr Opin Obstet Gynecol.* 2011;23:307-314.
2. Hoshi R, Uehara S, Hashimoto M, et al. Diagnosis and management of genital injuries in girls: 14-year experience. *Pediatr Int.* 2021;63:523-528.
3. Pokorny SF. Genital trauma. *Clin Obstet Gynecol.* 1997;40:219-225.
4. Cizek SM, Tyson N. Pediatric and adolescent gynecologic emergencies. *Obstet Gynecol Clin North Am.* 2022;49:521-536.
5. Dowd MD, Fitzmaurice L, Knapp JF, Mooney D. The interpretation of urogenital findings in children with straddle injuries. *J Pediatr Surg.* 1994;29:7-10.
6. Scheidler MG, Schultz BL, Schall L, Ford HR. Mechanisms of blunt perineal injury in female pediatric patients. *J Pediatr Surg.* 2000;35:1317-1319.
7. Spitzer RF, Kives S, Caccia N, Ornstein M, Goia C, Allen LM. Retrospective review of unintentional female genital trauma at a pediatric referral center. *Pediatr Emerg Care.* 2008;24:831-835.
8. Petrone P, Rodriguez Velandia W, Dziakova J, Marini CP. Treatment of complex perineal trauma: a review of the literature. *Cir Esp.* 2016;94:313-322.
9. Shnorhavorian M, Hidalgo-Tamola J, Koyle MA, Wessells H, Larison C, Goldin A. Unintentional and sexual abuse-related pediatric female genital trauma: a multiinstitutional study of free-standing pediatric hospitals in the United States. *Urology.* 2012;80:417-422.
10. Casey JT, Bjurlin MA, Cheng EY. Pediatric genital injury: an analysis of the National Electronic Injury Surveillance System. *Urology.* 2013;82:1125-1130.
11. Iqbal CW, Jrebi NY, Zielinski MD, et al. Patterns of accidental genital trauma in young girls and indications for operative management. *J Pediatr Surg.* 2010;45:930-933.
12. Dowlut-McElroy T, Higgins J, Williams KB, Strickland JL. Patterns of treatment of accidental genital trauma in girls. *J Pediatr Adolesc Gynecol.* 2018;31:19-22.
13. McLean I, Roberts SA, White C, Paul S. Female genital injuries resulting from consensual and non-consensual vaginal intercourse. *Forensic Sci Int.* 2011;204:27-33.
14. Adams JA, Girardin B, Faugno D. Signs of genital trauma in adolescent rape victims examined acutely. *J Pediatr Adolesc Gynecol.* 2000;13:88.
15. Gallion HR, Milam LJ, Littrell LL. Genital findings in cases of child sexual abuse: genital vs vaginal penetration. *J Pediatr Adolesc Gynecol.* 2016;29:604-611.
16. Adams JA, Farst KJ, Kellogg ND. Interpretation of medical findings in suspected child sexual abuse: an update for 2018. *J Pediatr Adolesc Gynecol.* 2018;31:225-231.
17. Jones JS, Rossman L, Hartman M, Alexander CC. Anogenital injuries in adolescents after consensual sexual intercourse. *Acad Emerg Med.* 2003;10:1378-1383.
18. Papoutsis D, Haefner HK. Large vulvar haematoma of traumatic origin. *J Clin Diagnostic Res.* 2017;11:QJ01-QJ02.
19. O'Brien K, Fei F, Quint E, Dendrinos M. Non-obstetric traumatic vulvar hematomas in premenarchal and postmenarchal girls. *J Pediatr Adolesc Gynecol.* 2022;35:546-551.
20. Lopez HN, Focseneanu MA, Merritt DF. Genital injuries acute evaluation and management. *Best Pract Res Clin Obstet Gynaecol.* 2018;48:28-39.

21. Abou-Jaoude WA, Sugarman JM, Fallat ME, Casale AJ. Indicators of genitourinary tract injury or anomaly in cases of pediatric blunt trauma. *J Pediatr Surg.* 1996;31:86-89; discussion 90.

22. Bjurlin MA, Fantus RJ, Mellett MM, Goble SM. Genitourinary injuries in pelvic fracture morbidity and mortality using the National Trauma Data Bank. *J Trauma.* 2009;67:1033-1039.

23. Merritt DF. Vulvar and genital trauma in pediatric and adolescent gynecology. *Curr Opin Obstet Gynecol.* 2004;16:371-381.

24. Emans SJ, Laufer MR, DiVasta AD. *Pediatric and Adolescent Gynecology.* 7th ed. Wolters Kluwer; 2020.

25. Schmidt Astrup B, Lykkebo AW. Post-coital genital injury in healthy women: a review. *Clin Anat.* 2015;28:331-338.

26. Berkenbaum C, Balu L, Sauvat F, Montbrun A, Harper L. Severe vaginal laceration in a 5-year-old girl caused by sudden hydro-distention. *J Pediatr Adolesc Gynecol.* 2013;26:e131-e132.

27. Rimmer RB, Weigand S, Foster KN, et al. Scald burns in young children – a review of Arizona burn center pediatric patients and a proposal for prevention in the Hispanic community. *J Burn Care Res.* 2008;29:595-605.

28. Tresh A, Baradaran N, Gaither TW, et al. Genital burns in the United States: disproportionate prevalence in the pediatric population. *Burns.* 2018;44:1366-1371.

29. Heger AH, Ticson L, Guerra L, et al. Appearance of the genitalia in girls selected for nonabuse: review of hymenal morphology and nonspecific findings. *J Pediatr Adolesc Gynecol.* 2002;15:27-35.

30. Boyle C, McCann J, Miyamoto S, Rogers K. Comparison of examination methods used in the evaluation of prepubertal and pubertal female genitalia: a descriptive study. *Child Abuse Negl.* 2008;32:229-243.

31. Golan A, Lurie S, Sagiv R, Glezerman M. Continuous-flow vaginoscopy in children and adolescents. *J Am Assoc Gynecol Laparosc.* 2000;7:526-528.

32. Michielsen DP, Lafaire C. Management of genital burns: a review. *Int J Urol.* 2010;17:755-758.

33. McLaughlin CJ, Martin KL. Radiologic imaging does not add value for female pediatric patients with isolated blunt straddle mechanisms. *J Pediatr Adolesc Gynecol.* 2022;35:541-545.

34. Sherer DM, Stimphil R, Hellmann M, Abdelmalek E, Zinn H, Abulafia O. Transperineal sonography of a large vulvar hematoma following blunt perineal trauma. *J Clin Ultrasound.* 2006;34:309-312.

35. Ramchandani P, Buckler PM. Imaging of genitourinary trauma. *Am J Roentgenol.* 2009;192:1514-1523.

36. Simms-Cendan J, Hoover K, Marathe K, Tyler K. NASPAG clinical opinion: diagnosis and management of lichen sclerosis in pediatric and adolescent patients. *J Pediatr Adolesc Gynecol.* 2022;35:112-120.

37. Sanfilippo JS, Wakim NG. Bleeding and vulvovaginitis in the pediatric age group. *Clin Obstet Gynecol.* 1987;30:653-661.

38. Romano ME. Prepubertal vulvovaginitis. *Clin Obstet Gynecol.* 2020;63:479-485.

39. McCann J, Miyamoto S, Boyle C, Rogers K. Healing of nonhymenal genital injuries in prepubertal and adolescent girls: a descriptive study. *Pediatrics.* 2007;120:1000-1011.

40. Horng HC, Chang WH, Yeh CC, et al. Estrogen effects on wound healing. *Int J Mol Sci.* 2017;18(11):2325.

41. Ernest A, Knapp G. Severe traumatic vulva hematoma in teenage girl. *Clin Case Rep.* 2015;3:975-978.

42. Whiteside JL, Asif RB, Novello RJ. Fibrin sealant for management of complicated obstetric lacerations. *Obstet Gynecol.* 2010;115:403-404.

43. Mok-Lin EY, Laufer MR. Management of vulvar hematomas: use of a Word catheter. *J Pediatr Adolesc Gynecol.* 2009;22:e156-e158.

44. Stevens DL, Bisno AL, Chambers HF, et al; Infectious Diseases Society of America. Practice guidelines for the diagnosis and management of skin and soft tissue infections: 2014 update by the Infectious Diseases Society of America. *Clin Infect Dis.* 2014;59:e10-e52.

45. McGregor K, Julich S, Glover M, Gautam J. Health professionals' responses to disclosure of child sexual abuse history: female child sexual abuse survivors' experiences. *J Child Sex Abus.* 2010;19:239-254.

18

Primary Ovarian Insufficiency and Turner Syndrome*

Rama D. Kastury and Tazim Dowlut-McElroy

INTRODUCTION

Primary ovarian insufficiency (POI) refers to the decline of ovarian function before age 40 years. Also known as *hypergonadotropic hypogonadism*, POI has previously been referred to as *premature ovarian failure* or *premature menopause*. It can manifest at variable developmental stages, from early childhood through adulthood. Postmenarchal individuals experience oligomenorrhea or amenorrhea for ≥4 months in conjunction with elevations in follicle-stimulating hormone (FSH). However, normal variations in the length of menstruals cycle during early adolescence can lead to a delay in diagnosis. Early detection and a low threshold for clinical suspicion are essential. Once POI has been diagnosed, it is important to determine the etiology and begin appropriate evaluations, referrals, and management to properly counsel the patient and family.[1,2]

Disease

- Primary ovarian insufficiency
- Turner syndrome (TS)

Definition

Primary ovarian insufficiency:
- Oligomenorrhea/amenorrhea for at least 3–4 months
- Elevated FSH >25 IU/L on two occasions 1 month apart[1]

Turner syndrome:
- Missing or structurally altered X chromosome and one or more typical clinical manifestations affecting development, growth, or multiple organ systems

---

*Parts of this chapter are presented in concise and easy-to-grasp bullets.

- Missing X-chromosome material can occur in all cells (monosomic TS) or a percentage of cells (mosaic TS)

PREVALENCE AND EPIDEMIOLOGY

Primary ovarian insufficiency:
- 0.01% <20 years old[3]
- 0.1% <30 years[3]
- 1% <40 years[4]
- Factors affecting age at natural menopause:
  - Ethnicity: The prevalence of POI in the United States is higher in Black and Hispanic women compared with White women and lower in women with Chinese and Japanese ancestry.[5,6]
  - Lifestyle: Smoking is a risk factor for earlier onset of menopause.[1]
  - Socioeconomic factors: Higher socioeconomic status was associated with later onset of menopause. Lower cognitive scores in childhood were associated with earlier menopause.[1]

Turner syndrome:
- Prevalence: 1/2000 to 2500[7,8]
- Epidemiology: Median age of diagnosis is 15.1 years[9]

ETIOLOGY AND PATHOPHYSIOLOGY

POI consists of a continuum of diminishing ovarian function associated with elevated FSH and decreased anti-müllerian hormone (AMH) levels. The etiology includes autoimmune disease, infectious causes, exposure to radiation and chemotherapy, and genetic causes including chromosome abnormalities and a growing list of single-gene disorders (Table 18.1). However, the majority (75%–90%) of POI remains idiopathic.[10]

TABLE 18.1	**Differential Diagnosis of POI**
Category	**Diagnosis**
Genetic Causes	**Sex Chromosome Abnormalities:**
	Turner syndrome (45,X)
	Mosaic Turner syndrome (45,X/46,XX; 45,X/46,XY)
	Fragile X premutation carriers
	Trisomy X with or without mosaicism
	46,XX or 46,XY gonadal dysgenesis
	Trisomy 21
	Single-Gene Abnormalities:
	Galactosemia (*GALT* gene)
	Congenital adrenal hyperplasia (*CYP17A1* gene)
	Bloom syndrome (*BLM* gene)
	Fanconi anemia (*FANCA, FANCB, FANCC,* and other genes)
	Ataxia telangiectasia (*ATM* gene, biallelic variants)
	Werner syndrome (*RECQL2* gene)
	Blepharophimosis, ptosis, epicanthus inversus syndrome (*FOXL2* gene)
	FSH receptor mutation (FSHR gene)
	Aromatase deficiency (*CYP19A1* gene)
	NR5A1 gene
	BMP15 gene
	BMPR1B gene
Autoimmune	Autoimmune lymphocytic oophoritis
	Autoimmune polyglandular syndrome
Infectious	Mumps oophoritis
	HIV, tuberculosis, varicella, shigella, malaria, Cytomegalovirus (CMV)
Iatrogenic	Radiation therapy
	Chemotherapy with gonadotoxic agents
	Bilateral oophorectomy/gonadectomy
Environmental	Phthalates
	Bisphenol-A smoking (tobacco)

AMH levels increase in an inconsistent manner during adolescence and reach their highest point in the early 20s. As a result, interpreting serum AMH levels in adolescents can be challenging. Additionally, AMH levels are typically suppressed during chemotherapy, rendering them less useful in individuals receiving treatment. Lastly, although an ultrasound can directly measure antral follicles (2–10 mm), there are no established normal ranges for this measurement in adolescents (Fig. 18.1).[11]

MANIFESTATIONS OF DISEASE

Primary Ovarian Insufficiency

Individuals present with delayed puberty, primary or secondary amenorrhea, irregular menses ≥ 4 months apart, infertility, vasomotor symptoms (hot flashes, night sweats), vaginal dryness, or mood changes. Intermittent remission and return of ovarian function can occur in 5%–10% of cases.[2,12]

Long-term manifestations include:
- Lack of development of secondary sexual characteristics
- Metabolic disorders
- Osteopenia/osteoporosis
- Cardiovascular disease
- Infertility
- Vulvovaginal atrophy

Turner Syndrome

In individuals with TS, it is also important to consider the following clinical manifestations:
- Growth failure (short stature)
- Congenital heart anomalies
- Hypertension
- Thyroid dysfunction
- Impaired glucose function
- Hyperlipidemia
- Celiac disease
- Hearing loss
- Strabismus, nearsightedness, ptosis
- Dental complications
- Renal anomaly (e.g., horseshoe kidney)
- Neuropsychological/behavioral issues (anxiety, nonverbal learning difficulty)
- Skeletal abnormalities

Recommended referrals for patients with TS include pediatric endocrinology, pediatric cardiology, pediatric and adolescent gynecology (with expertise in fertility preservation), genetics, psychology, audiology, ophthalmology, and dentistry.[13]

CLINICAL PRESENTATION AND EVALUATION

Very young children with TS may present with short stature (Table 18.2). Older children and adolescents

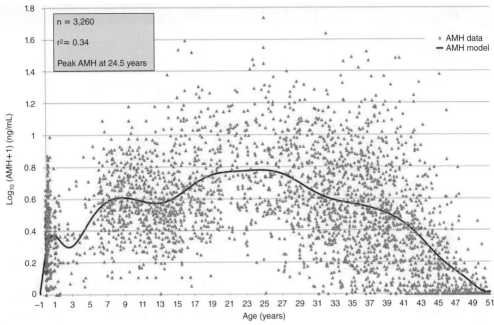

Fig. 18.1 Serum Anti-Mullerian Hormone levels from Conception to Menopause. Kelsey TW, Wright P, Nelson SM, Anderson RA, Wallace WH. A validated model of serum anti-müllerian hormone from conception to menopause. PLoS One. 2011;6(7):e22024. doi:10.1371/journal.pone.0022024

TABLE 18.2	Recommended Imaging Studies in Individuals with POI or TS
Imaging	**Comments**
Pelvic ultrasound	To evaluate for presence of a uterus, bilateral ovaries, müllerian anomalies, or pelvic masses.
Renal ultrasound	Individuals with TS often can have renal anomalies such as pelvic kidney or horseshoe kidney.
Dual energy x-ray absorptiometry (DXA)	POI increases the risk of low bone mineral density (BMD) or osteoporosis, as also seen in individuals with TS. Start DXA screening to monitor BMD once adult HRT dosing is achieved. Screen every 5 years, or sooner as clinically indicated.
Echocardiography	Individuals with TS have a high incidence of congenital heart disease such as bicuspid aortic valve, coarctation of the aorta, and aortopathy.[13]

HRT, Hormone replacement therapy; *POI,* primary ovarian insufficiency; *TS,* Turner syndrome.

with POI present with delayed or arrested pubertal development and primary or secondary amenorrhea. Young adults may present with infertility, hot flashes, night sweats, vaginal dryness, and dyspareunia.

TESTING RELEVANT TO THE CONDITION

The clinician should consider ordering the following (Table 18.3):
- Beta-human chorionic gonadotropin (HCG)
- Prolactin
- Thyroid function tests
- FSH, luteinizing hormone (LH), estradiol, AMH
- Chromosome analysis (karyotype)
- Fragile X testing (FMR1 polymerase chain reaction [PCR]/Southern blot repeat analysis)
- Adrenal antibodies (21-hydroxylase antibodies)
- Thyroid antibodies (thyroid peroxidase antibodies)
- Not recommended: Anti-ovarian antibodies and inhibin B[14]
  Additional recommendations for TS:
- Twenty-cell karyotype of peripheral blood with consideration for second tissue (buccal)
- Renal ultrasound

TABLE 18.3	**Classic Signs and Physical Examination**	
	POI	**Turner Syndrome**
Classic signs	Primary or secondary amenorrhea Delayed or arrested puberty Infertility Vasomotor symptoms	Short stature, growth failure Congenital heart anomalies: bicuspid aorta, coarctation of aorta Webbed neck Hearing loss POI

Physical
  examination
	Height and weight percentiles on growth curve
	Tanner staging: breast and pubic hair
	Genitourinary exam: Assess for signs of
	  hypoestrogenization[2]
		Blood pressure
		Short stature, webbed neck, widely spaced
		  nipples (phenotypic features of Turner syndrome
		  are variable)

POI, Primary ovarian insufficiency.

- Thyroid studies
- Hemoglobin A1c
- Fasting lipid
- Liver function tests
- 25-Hydroxyvitamin D
- Celiac screen
- Hearing examination
- Ophthalmologic examination[13]

MANAGEMENT/TREATMENT OPTIONS

Hormone Therapy

Hormone therapy (HT) promotes the development and maintenance of secondary sexual characteristics (breast and uterine growth in cis-females) and promotes bone, cardiovascular, and sexual health. Estrogen and progestin therapy are tailored to the individual's specific level of pubertal progression.

In prepubertal patients, a stepwise approach that mirrors typical ovarian function is recommended (Table 18.4):

1. **Phase 1:** Induction of breast development and puberty. Initiation of low-dose transdermal or oral 17-β estradiol (transdermal is preferred) at age 11 to 12 years, with a gradual increase every 6 months.
2. **Phase 2:** Establishment of normal menses and achieving normal bone mineralization. Addition of progesterone once breakthrough bleeding occurs or after 18 to 24 months of estrogen therapy.
3. **Phase 3:** Long-term management. Once breast development is complete, continuation of adult dose of estrogen and progestin.[2,13-15]

Dosing of estrogen and progesterone therapy is adjusted if POI is diagnosed after pubertal development.

It is important to remember that pregnancies can occur in patients diagnosed with POI, as up to 10% of patients with the condition can ovulate and conceive spontaneously. Therefore contraceptive counseling is highly recommended for adolescents with POI. Hormonal contraception, such as combination (estrogen and progesterone) oral contraceptive pills (cOCPs),

TABLE 18.4	**Selected Hormone Replacement Therapy Regimen for Primary Ovarian Insufficiency[12]**	
Medication	**Puberty Initiation Dosing**	**Adult Dosing**
Micronized 17-β estradiol (oral, E2)	0.03 mg/day	2–4 mg daily
Micronized 17-β estradiol (transdermal)	3–7 μg/day	50–100 μg 2×/wk
Progestin Therapy		
Medroxyprogesterone acetate		10 mg daily × 12 days or 5 mg daily
Micronized progesterone (e.g., Prometrium)		200 mg daily × 12 days or 100 mg daily
Levonorgestrel-releasing intrauterine system		52 mg (~20 mcg/day)

can also play a crucial role in adolescents. Many teens with POI may feel more comfortable taking cOCPs like their peers, and these drugs can help normalize their treatment. Utilizing combined hormonal contraceptive methods exceeds hormone replacement therapy doses of estrogen and progesterone. While providing contraception and a more age associated regimen, there have been no long term studies assessing risk and benefits of hormonal contraception over hormone therapy in adolescents with POI. It is important for health care providers to discuss the available options with their patients and their families, taking into account individual preferences, values, and medical history.[16]

SPECIAL CONSIDERATIONS FOR THIS POPULATION

Fertility Considerations

1. Long-term fertility implications should be discussed with individuals with POI and TS and their families. Some individuals may be candidates for fertility preservation. Counseling about options for building a family and referral to an expert in fertility preservation in children and adolescents is recommended.
2. Fertility preservation via ovarian tissue cryopreservation (OTC) or controlled ovarian stimulation and oocyte cryopreservation may be available for select individuals with POI and TS.

Pregnancy and TS

1. Individuals with TS contemplating pregnancy should be counseled about the increased risk of spontaneous abortion, hypertensive disorders of pregnancy, and cardiovascular complications including aortic dissection and death.
2. Preconceptual, antepartum, and postpartum monitoring by providers with expertise in TS decreases the risk of pregnancy complications.[17]
3. Echocardiography and cardiac magnetic resonance imaging (MRI) are recommended within 2 years before planned pregnancy or assisted reproductive technology (ART). ART or spontaneous pregnancy should be avoided in cases of ascending aortic size index (ASI) of ≥ 2.5 cm/m^2 or ASI of 2 to 2.5 cm/m^2 and associated risk factors for aortic dissection (bicuspid aortic valve, elongation of transverse aorta, coarctation of aorta, and hypertension). During pregnancy, an echocardiogram should be repeated at around 20 weeks of gestation if no risk factors for aortic dissection exist and at 4- to 6-week intervals and during the first 6 months postpartum if ASI ≥ 2.0 or any risk factors for aortic dissection exist.[13]
4. A multidisciplinary approach to care is imperative for patients with TS. This includes psychological support and peer support in addition to pediatric and adolescent gynecology, endocrinology, cardiology, and medical genetics.

Bone Mineral Density

1. Given short stature and small bone size in individuals with TS, BMD may be falsely reduced. It is important to adjust measurements for height when interpreting DXA scan results in this population.

Thyroid Function Monitoring

1. Thyroid function testing is recommended annually for individuals with POI and/or TS.
2. Annual screening for diabetes is recommended in patient with POI on HRT, and TS patients (starting at age 10).[12]

RESEARCH GAPS

- Identification of genetic causes in individuals with idiopathic POI
- Outcomes of fertility preservation in individuals with TS
- Genotype/phenotype correlation in individuals with TS and mosaic TS

KEY POINTS

- POI is defined as oligomenorrhea/amenorrhea ≥ 4 months and elevated FSH >25 IU/L on two occasions 1 month apart before age 40.
- POI can present variably as delayed puberty, primary or secondary amenorrhea, oligomenorrhea, infertility, vasomotor symptoms, vaginal dryness, or mood changes.
- Initial evaluation for POI includes beta-HCG, prolactin, thyroid function studies, FSH, LH, estradiol, AMH, chromosome analysis (karyotype), fragile X testing, 21-hydroxylase antibodies, and thyroid peroxidase antibodies.
- In TS it is important to consider other comorbidities, screen accordingly, and include the appropriate referrals.
- HRT is recommended for individuals with POI (Table 18.4).

SUPPLEMENTAL MATERIAL FOR CHAPTER

European Society for Human Reproduction and Embryology (ESHRE) Guideline Group on POI, Webber L, Davies M, et al. ESHRE guideline: management of women with premature ovarian insufficiency. *Hum Reprod.* 2016;31(5):926-937.

Emans SJ, Laufer MR, DiVasta AD, eds. *Pediatric & Adolescent Gynecology.* 7th ed. Wolters-Kluwer; 2020.

Gravholt CH, Andersen NH, Conway GS, et al. Clinical practice guidelines for the care of girls and women with Turner syndrome: proceedings from the 2016 Cincinnati International Turner Syndrome Meeting. *Eur J Endocrinol.* 2017;177(3):G1-G70. doi:10.1530/EJE-17-0430

REVIEW QUESTIONS

1. A 16-year-old female presents with a 6-month history of irregular and lighter menses. LMP was 35 days ago and consisted of spotting for 1 day. Thelarche and pubarche were at age 11 and menarche at age 12 years. She previously had 28-day menstrual cycles with menstrual bleeding for 5 days. Her mother has a history of Hashimoto thyroiditis. Laboratory tests: Urine human chorionic gonadotropin (hCG): negative; TSH: 1.62 (ref: 0.50–4.30); FSH: 118; Prolactin: normal. What is your next best step in evaluating her for POI?
   a. Pelvic ultrasound
   b. Consult rheumatology
   c. Start OCPs
   d. Order repeat laboratory tests, including FSH, LH, and estradiol

2. A 16-year-old female is referred from her pediatrician for secondary amenorrhea. She has a remote history of growth failure as a newborn but has remained in the seventh percentile for height. She has no other health concerns. She had menarche at age 12 years, which were initially irregular but became regular by age 13, occurring monthly with bleeding lasting for 5 days. Beginning 1 year ago, her menses became shorter, lighter, and eventually stopped 8 months ago. Laboratory tests from the pediatrician: Urine human chorionic gonadotropin (hCG): negative; TSH: 3.12 mIU/L (0.50–4.30 mIU/L), FSH: 36 mIU/L; prolactin: normal. You recommended

repeating the laboratory tests before the office visit and receive the following: serum hCG <5, FSH 59 mIU/L, estradiol <5 pg/mL, TSH 2.95 mIU/L; prolactin: normal. On physical examination you note that the patient's height is 148.1 cm (less than third percentile). Breasts and pubic hair are Tanner stage 4. Mid-parental height is 165 cm. What is your next best step?
   a. Consult endocrinology
   b. Start OCPs
   c. Chromosome analysis
   d. Repeat FSH and add LH and estradiol

3. A 17-year-old female with galactosemia presents with known history of POI since age 10 years. She has been on hormone replacement therapy (HRT) for puberty induction and is now on maintenance adult-dose HRT. She reports a recent radial head fracture after falling on an outstretched arm at standing height. What additional testing would you perform?
   a. Check estradiol level
   b. Dual energy x-ray absorptiometry (DXA) scan
   c. Check FSH level
   d. Start her on vitamin D supplementation

REFERENCES

1. European Society for Human Reproduction and Embryology (ESHRE) Guideline Group on POI, Webber L, Davies M, et al. ESHRE guideline: management of women with premature ovarian insufficiency. *Hum Reprod.* 2016;31(5):926-937.
2. Emans SJ, Laufer MR, DiVasta AD, eds. *Pediatric & Adolescent Gynecology.* 7th ed. Wolters-Kluwer; 2020.
3. Sadeghi MR. New hopes for the treatment of primary ovarian insufficiency/premature ovarian failure. *J Reprod Infertil.* 2013;14(1):1-2.
4. Coulam CB, Adamson SC, Annegers JF. Incidence of premature ovarian failure. *Obstet Gynecol.* 1986;67:604-606.
5. Luborsky JL, Meyer P, Sowers MF, Gold EB, Santoro N. Premature menopause in a multi-ethnic population study of the menopause transition. *Hum Reprod.* 2003;18:199-206.
6. Wu X, Cai H, Kallianpur A, et al. Impact of premature ovarian failure on mortality and morbidity among Chinese women. *PLoS One.* 2014;9(3):e89597. doi:10.1371/journal.pone.0089597
7. Bondy CA, Turner Syndrome Study Group. Care of girls and women with Turner syndrome: a guideline of the Turner Syndrome Study Group. *J Clin Endocrinol Metab.* 2007;92(1):10-25. doi:10.1210/jc.2006-1374

8. Nielsen J, Wohlert M. Chromosome abnormalities found among 34,910 newborn children: results from a 13-year incidence study in Arhus, Denmark. *Hum Genet.* 1991;87(1):81-83. doi:10.1007/BF01213097

9. Berglund A, Stochholm K, Gravholt CH. The epidemiology of sex chromosome abnormalities. *Am J Med Genet C Semin Med Genet.* 2020;184(2):202-215. doi:10.1002/ajmg.c.31805

10. Nelson LM. Clinical practice: primary ovarian insufficiency. *N Engl J Med.* 2009;360(6):606-614. doi:10.1056/NEJMcp0808697

11. Sanfilippo JS, Lara-Torre E, Gomez-Lobo V. *Sanfilippo's Textbook of Pediatric and Adolescent Gynecology.* 2nd ed. CRC Press; 2020.

12. van Kasteren YM, Schoemaker J. Premature Ovarian Failure: a systematic review on therapeutic interventions to restore ovarian function and achieve pregnancy. *Hum Reprod Update.* 1999;5(5):483-492.

13. Gravholt CH, Andersen NH, Conway GS, et al. Clinical practice guidelines for the care of girls and women with Turner syndrome: proceedings from the 2016 Cincinnati International Turner Syndrome Meeting. *Eur J Endocrinol.* 2017;177(3):G1-G70. doi:10.1530/EJE-17-0430

14. Primary ovarian insufficiency in adolescents and young women. Committee opinion no. 605: American College of Obstetricians and Gynecologists. *Obstet Gynecol.* 2014;124(1):193-197.

15. Davis-Kankanamge CN, Vash-Margita A. Premature/primary ovarian insufficiency (POI). In: Hertweck SP, Dwiggins ML, eds. *Clinical Protocols in Pediatric and Adolescent Gynecology.* 2nd ed. CRC Press; 2022.

16. Bidet M, Bachelot A, Bissauge E, et al. Resumption of ovarian function and pregnancies in 358 patients with premature ovarian failure. *J Clin Endocrinol Metab.* 2011; 96(12):3864-3872.

17. Cadoret F, Parinaud J, Bettiol C, et al. Pregnancy outcome in Turner syndrome: a French multi-center study after the 2009 guidelines. *Eur J Obstet Gynecol Reprod Biol.* 2018;229:20-25.

PCOS and Common Androgen Abnormalities in Adolescents

Tania S. Burgert and Emily Paprocki

INTRODUCTION

Androgen excess in females can manifest clinically as hirsutism, severe acne, male-pattern balding, deepening of the voice, and enlargement of the clitoris. Biochemical correlates may include elevated levels of androgenic steroids stemming either from the ovaries or adrenals. The degree of association between clinical features of androgen excess and biochemical hyperandrogenism varies greatly between individuals and depends on the sensitivity of the pilosebaceous unit.[1] When hirsutism does not correlate with androgenic steroid levels, it is deemed idiopathic.[2] The most common etiology for mild to moderate androgen excess in adults and adolescents is PCOS. Late-onset congenital adrenal hyperplasia (CAH) and severe insulin resistance syndromes are other conditions that may present with symptoms of androgen excess during adolescence. Virilizing features such as clitoral enlargement, voice deepening, and rapidly worsening hirsutism should be evaluated for androgen-producing tumors.

CLINICAL FEATURES OF ANDROGEN EXCESS

Hirsutism is defined as the presence of excessive coarse terminal hair in areas of the body that are responsive to the effect of androgens. A commonly used clinical tool for assessing hirsutism is the modified Ferriman-Gallwey (F-G), a pictogram that allows for visual grading in nine body areas (upper lip, chin, chest, lower and upper abdomen, lower and upper back, upper arms, and thighs). Each area is scored separately from 0 (absent) to 4 (extensive) hair growth. In adults, a summation score of ≥4 to 6 has been suggested to indicate clinically

relevant hirsutism by the 2023 International PCOS Guidelines[3] (Fig. 19.1). Clinically, these cut-off scores also guide the assessment of hirsutism in adolescents.

Although the F-G scoring system can help quantify clinical features of hair in androgen-sensitive areas, scoring remains observer dependent and may be inaccurate if cosmetic hair removal has occurred in these areas.

Hirsutism must be differentiated from hypertrichosis, which denotes hair growth in androgen-independent body areas such as the forearms and lower legs. Hypertrichosis is not associated with hyperandrogenism, and hair is usually vellus and noncoarse. Hypertrichosis may be hereditary among teens of Middle Eastern or Mediterranean descent. Hypertrichosis can be observed in states of malnutrition,[4] but can also be medication induced (e.g., diazoxide or phenytoin).

Acne may indicate androgen excess in adults, but in adolescents is a common manifestation of puberty. Androgen excess contributes to acne through stimulating sebum production, but other factors such as bacterial colonization also play a role, explaining the poor correspondence between severity of acne and androgen levels.[5] Still, severe, cystic acne should prompt a search for biochemical correlates in adolescence.

Hidradenitis suppurativa refers to inflamed painful nodules and abscesses involving the pilosebaceous units of the axillae, groin, perineum, and breast region and should prompt further consideration of androgen excess.[6]

Androgenic alopecia is diffuse thinning of crown hair with the frontal hairline preserved. It is uncommon in adolescents, yet when present should be evaluated for biochemical hyperandrogenism.

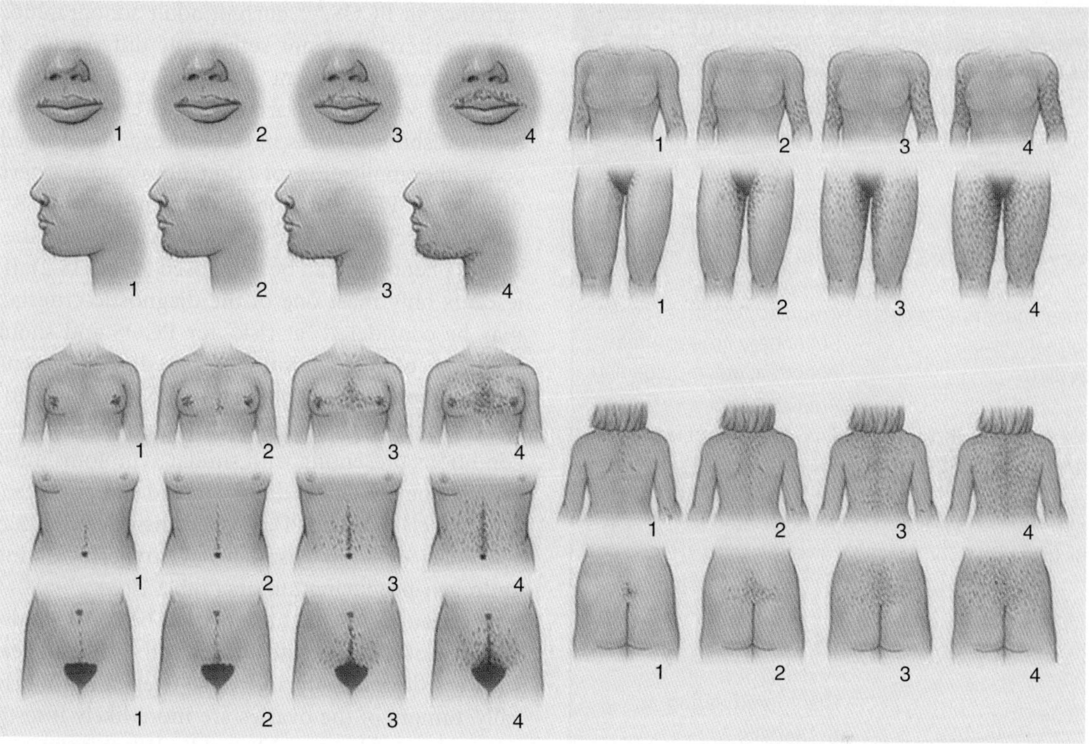

Fig. 19.1 Modified Ferriman-Gallwey visual pictogram for grading terminal hair in nine androgen-sensitive body areas. A score of 0 should be given if there is no hair in the assessed body region. A total score of ≥4 to 6 is considered a clinical sign of hirsutism.[82]

PCOS

PCOS is a heterogeneous condition where the severity of clinical expression is compounded by environmental, nutritional, lifestyle, and transgenerational factors. PCOS in terms of nomenclature originated as an acronym standing for Polycystic Ovary Syndrome. However, ovarian cysts are not part of the PCOS diagnosis and therefore the origins of the acronym are misleading. PCOS more accurately affects ovarian function and morphology, manifesting in a tendency toward ovulation dysregulation and hormonal imbalance that favors ovarian testosterone production. Minor upregulation of adrenal androgens can also be seen, but modest elevations in dehydroepiandrosterone sulfate or androstenedione provide limited additional information in the diagnosis of PCOS. Prominent elevation of adrenal hormones should direct the clinician toward considering adrenal pathologies instead of PCOS.

Short- and long-term consequences of menstrual dysfunction and hormonal imbalance may include hirsutism and treatment-resistant/cystic acne, hidradenitis suppurativa, insulin resistance, weight gain, type 2 diabetes, metabolic dysfunction-associated steatotic liver disease (MASLD), endometrial hyperplasia, subfertility, depression/anxiety, and in adults disordered eating (Table 19.1).

In adolescents, the diagnosis can be challenging because key clinical features of PCOS such as irregular menstrual cycles are also physiologically present in this age group.

Diagnosis

Currently, the international PCOS guidelines endorse application of the Rotterdam Criteria for diagnosing PCOS in adults and recommend the National Institutes of Health Criteria (menstrual irregularity and hyperandrogenism) for adolescents.[7,3] Both sets of criteria overlap in the diagnostic features of menstrual dysregulation and clinical and/or biochemical hyperandrogenism. However, the Rotterdam Criteria allow for sonographic evidence of polycystic ovarian morphology (not the same as ovarian cysts) to substitute for either menstrual dysregulation or hyperandrogenism. In adults this has led to the diagnosability of a broader clinical spectrum, which also includes an ovulatory

TABLE 19.1 PCOS Co-Associated Signs, Symptoms, and Morbidities

Short Term	Long Term
Treatment-resistant acne	Androgenic alopecia
Hirsutism/hidradenitis suppurativa	Adult acne
	Hirsutism/hidradenitis suppurativa
Primary and secondary amenorrhea	Anovulatory but regular menstrual cycles
Irregular menstrual cycles	Irregular menstrual cycles
Abnormal uterine bleeding	Secondary amenorrhea
	Abnormal uterine bleeding
Prediabetes	Prediabetes
Type 2 diabetes mellitus	Type 2 diabetes mellitus
Metabolic syndrome	Metabolic syndrome
Metabolic dysfunction-asssociated steatotic liver disease	Metabolic dysfunction-asssociated steatotic liver disease
	Cardiovascular disease
	Sleep apnea
Depression	Depression
	Anxiety
	Disordered eating
	Subfertility
	Miscarriage
	Gestational diabetes
	Preeclampsia

and nonandrogenic PCOS phenotype. In support of phenotypic distinctions, the recent 2023 update of the international PCOS guidelines has furthermore endorses Anti-Muellerian Hormone level in the diagnostic consideration of adult PCOS.[3] Genome-wide association studies validate the expression of similar genetic underpinnings for classical and nonclassical phenotypes of PCOS, further supporting the variability in expression of the condition.[8]

In adolescents, although some ovarian sonographic features may reflect the severity of the reproductive disturbance in PCOS,[9,10] current adult sonographic diagnostic criteria may not sufficiently differentiate PCOS from normal adolescent ovarian morphology.[11] Therefore until normative ovarian features and specific PCOS distinguishing features have been examined in adolescents, the application of adult ultrasound criteria for diagnosing PCOS is not recommended until 8 years post menarche.[7] Therefore in adolescents only the classical B phenotype can be diagnosed (Table 19.2). If adolescents only meet one of the diagnostic criteria, they may be considered "at risk" for PCOS and should be followed and offered symptom-based management.[3]

It is important to note that PCOS in adults and adolescents is a diagnosis of exclusion and therefore other conditions presenting with similar symptoms must first be ruled out. Such conditions include adrenal disorders (i.e., nonclassical CAH), thyroid disorders, primary or secondary ovarian insufficiency, hyperprolactinemia, androgen-producing tumors (Table 19.3).

Ovarian or adrenal tumors must be considered when the presentation is acute and/or with virilizing features such as clitoromegaly and voice deepening. Biochemically, tumors of the ovaries are more likely if testosterone is elevated beyond 200 ng/dL. When examining for tumors of the adrenal glands, concern should arise if dehydroepiandrosterone-sulfate rises above 700 µg/dL. When there is concern for either adrenal or ovarian tumors, imaging studies should be pursued. Although transabdominal ultrasound would be the first step in imaging evaluation, if negative, magnetic resonance imaging (MRI) should be considered.[12] Nonclassical CAH is differentiated from PCOS by a morning 17-hydroxyprogesterone value of >200 ng/dL.

In general, any chronic illness or form of malnutrition may also lead to irregular menstrual cycles. Under this premise, irregular menstrual cycles in type 1 diabetes have long been attributed to chronic disease and poor metabolic control. However, in recent years the

TABLE 19.2 Adult PCOS Phenotypes A–D

Phenotypes	Menstrual Dysfunction	Clinical or Biochemical Hyperandrogenism	Sonographic Ovarian Features of PCOS
A: complete	X	X	X
B: classical[a]	X	X	
C: ovulatory		X	X
D: nonandrogenic	X		X

[a]Only phenotype B can be diagnosed in adolescents and is based on National Institutes of Health criteria.
(Adapted from Lubna P, Seifer D. *Current and Emerging Concepts in PCOS.* 2nd ed. Springer; 2022.)

TABLE 19.3 Non-PCOS Etiologies of Menstrual Dysfunction and/or Hyperandrogenism

Etiologies	Clinical Findings	Evaluation
Hypothyroidism	Menstrual irregularity, possible hypertrichosis, possible weight gain	Elevated TSH
Disordered eating (anorexia/bulimia)	Menstrual irregularity, hypertrichosis	Low/prepubertal LH, FSH, low estradiol
Hyperprolactinemia	Menstrual irregularity, possible acne, mild hirsutism (prolactin stimulates adrenal androgens), galactorrhea	Fasting elevated prolactin; differential: pituitary mass or drug induced: antipsychotic, SSRI, methyl-dopa; other cause: prominent elevation of TSH, renal disease
Type 1 diabetes	Secondary PCOS, menstrual irregularity, hirsutism, acne	Elevated total and/or free testosterone in the setting of T1DM
Nonclassical CAH	Irregular menstrual cycles, acne, hirsutism	Morning 17-hydroxyprogesterone >200 ng/dL (>6.05 nmol/L)
Androgen-producing tumors	Signs of virilization: voice deepening/clitoromegaly, acute onset, rapidly progressing hirsutism	Testosterone >200 ng/dL (>6.94 nmol/L) consider ovarian tumor: perform ultrasound and/or MRI DHEA-S >700 µg/dL (18.9 µmol/L) Consider adrenal tumor: perform ultrasound and/or CT
Cushing syndrome	Irregular menstrual cycles, hirsutism, central weight gain, hypertension Plethora, violaceous striae	Elevated afternoon serum cortisol or elevated late night salivary cortisol or elevated urinary free cortisol Failed morning cortisol suppression after dexamethasone the night before

CT, Computed tomography; *DHEA-S,* dehydroepiandrosterone sulfate; *FSH,* follicle-stimulating hormone; *LH,* luteinizing hormone; *MRI,* magnetic resonance imaging; *PCOS,* polycystic ovary syndrome; *SSRI,* selective serotonin reuptake inhibitor; *T1DM,* type 1 diabetes mellitus; *TSH,* thyroid-stimulating hormone.

notion of "secondary" PCOS has emerged, attributed to the effect of intensive insulin therapy on the ovaries, leading to anovulation with a rise in testosterone.[13-15]

Pathophysiology

PCOS pathophysiology does not have a definable origin, but rather follows a circular pattern that snowballs into a self-perpetuating vicious cycle. The cycle is fed by environmental, metabolic, genetic, epigenetic, and neuroendocrine factors.[16]

Independent of obesity but exaggerated by the degree of adiposity, insulin resistance is a central finding in adults and adolescents with PCOS.[17-19] However, despite whole-body insulin resistance, steroidogenic organs like the ovaries remain insulin-sensitive, allowing for high circulating insulin levels to exert their effect.[20] Insulin directly promotes testosterone production from ovarian theca cells and acts as a co-gonadotropin by enhancing luteinizing hormone (LH) effect on the ovaries.[21] Even without the effect of insulin, there is intrinsic upregulation of ovarian testosterone production in PCOS. The elevated testosterone, in a circular fashion, further augments insulin resistance and perpetuates the ovarian effect of hyperinsulinemia. Insulin resistance itself also lowers hepatic sex hormone–binding globulin

(SHBG) production, which leaves more testosterone in the unbound and free/biochemically active form.

In addition to the effects of insulin, there is dysregulation of the hypothalamic-pituitary-ovarian axis with enhanced LH drive, which promotes testosterone production. Further perpetuating the LH drive is a reduced sensitivity of LH to negative feedback from estrogen and progesterone. It has been suggested that elevated testosterone levels enhance LH resistance to feedback inhibition by progesterone and estrogen.[22,23]

Genome-wide association studies seem to further support the circular premise, with genetic PCOS loci found in areas of gonadotropin signaling, ovarian cellular signaling, and regions associated with energy metabolism/insulin resistance and type 2 diabetes mellitus (Fig. 19.2).

Assessment
Ovulatory Dysfunction

Pathologic ovulatory dysregulation can be difficult to determine in adolescents, as cycles are commonly irregular the first 2 to 3 years post menarche, until the hypothalamic-pituitary-ovarian axis has physiologically matured.[24-26] Given that normal cycle intervals vary from year to year post menarche, irregularity is defined differently from the first to the fourth year post menarche (Table 19.4).

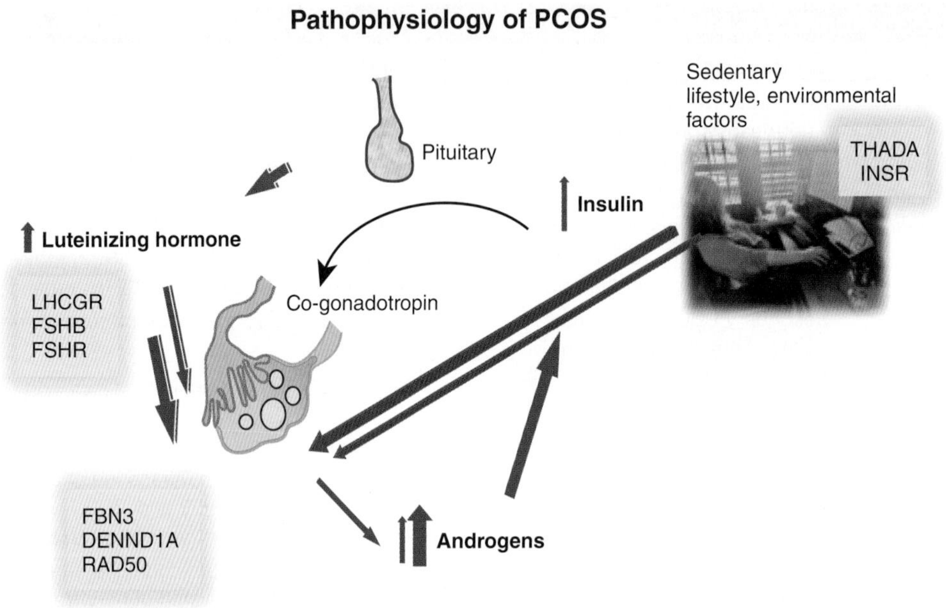

Pathophysiology of PCOS

Fig. 19.2 Vicious cycle of PCOS. Hyperandrogenism perpetuating insulin resistance, which enhances go-nadotropin (LH) drive. There is also intrinsic dysregulation of the hypothalamic-pituitary-ovarian feedback loop as well as intrinsic upregulation of androgen production in steroidogenic tissues like the ovaries. Genome-wide association studies (rose squares) found genetic association in all areas of the cycle.

TABLE 19.4 Abnormal Menstrual Patterns in Adolescents Based on Years Post Menarche

	First Year Post Menarche	Second Year Post Menarche	Third Year Post Menarche	Fourth Year Post Menarche
Menstrual pattern	Any menstrual pattern, including stretches of amenorrhea, are considered normal during the first year post menarche.	Irregular cycles and skipping of cycles are still considered normal.	Cycles should now be more regular (every 21–45 days) between menstrual periods.	Adult menstrual cycle with intervals of 21–35 days (at least eight cycles a year) should be established.
Interpretation	PCOS cannot be considered.	If periods are >90 days apart, the adolescent should be evaluated for PCOS.	If periods are >45 days apart or <21 days, the adolescent should be evaluated for PCOS.	If periods are >35 days apart or <21 days, the adolescent should be evaluated for PCOS.

(Adapted from Lubna P, Seifer D. *Current and Emerging Concepts in PCOS.* 2nd ed. Springer; 2022.)

Biochemical Hyperandrogenism

Although adrenal androgens can be upregulated in PCOS, most androgen production stems from the ovaries in the form of testosterone. Therefore the diagnosis of PCOS relies on total and/or free testosterone elevation. Because of the low SHBG in PCOS, the most sensitive determinant of hyperandrogenism is free testosterone, most accurately measured by equilibrium dialysis.[27] Alternatively, the free androgen index can be calculated from measures of SHBG and total testosterone and can serve as a substitute assessment of free testosterone. Total testosterone should be measured using tandem

BOX 19.1 Biochemical Hyperandrogenism in PCOS

Total and Free Testosterone

- More sensitive than other androgens
- High-quality assays such as liquid chromatography-tandem mass spectrometry
- No actual cut-offs recommended – should be based on lab reference range and normal values derived from well-characterized populations
  - Total Testosterone > 40-50 ng/dL
  - Free Testosterone > 1.4-1.7 nmol/L
- More important than a one-time value is persistent elevation
  - Diurnal/menstrual cycle variability
  - If a patient was on hormone therapy (i.e., combined oral contraceptive pills), a 3-month washout period is recommended before testing
- Other androgen elevations provide limited additional information in diagnosing PCOS but may be of use in ruling out other conditions

PCOS, Polycystic ovarian syndrome.

mass spectrometry.[28] Because of diurnal hormone variability, it is recommended to not rule in or rule out PCOS based on a one-time measure.[29] Peak testosterone levels occur in the morning, which is the best time to measure levels. Before testing for hyperandrogenism a 3-month washout period from any hormone treatment, such as oral contraceptive pills, is advised[3] (Box 19.1).

Comorbidities

Prediabetes and Type 2 Diabetes

Even though insulin resistance does not factor into defining and diagnosing PCOS, insulin resistance is tightly linked to the pathophysiology and perpetuation of the clinical phenotype, leading to a higher incidence and earlier onset of prediabetes and type 2 diabetes in mostly obese adults and adolescents with PCOS.[30,31] Data on prediabetes and type 2 diabetes in lean adolescents with PCOS are difficult to extrapolate because of the common comorbidity of obesity. Still, prediabetes as assessed by an oral glucose tolerance test may be present across the body mass index (BMI) spectrum.[32,33]

Metabolic dysfunction-asssociated steatotic liver disease: MASLD

MASLD, previously knows as NAFLD (non-alcoholic fatty liver disease)[34] is closely tied to insulin resistance

and deteriorating glucose metabolism and more commonly occurs in the male sex.[35] In adults with PCOS, NAFLD risk is independently associated with high serum androgens.[36] In adolescents and adults with PCOS, NAFLD may occur across all BMI categories.[37] Therefore screening liver functions should be obtained at the time of PCOS diagnosis, independently of BMI, and if persistently elevated greater than two times the upper limit, a referral to hepatology for further diagnostics and management is indicated.[38]

Obesity/Metabolic Syndrome

General and central obesity are greatly increased in adults with PCOS[39] and may start in childhood.[40] The degree of obesity is strongly tied to metabolic syndrome in adolescents of both sexes[41] and in adolescents with PCOS.[42] Metabolic syndrome is a constellation of metabolic disturbances that are known to enhance cardiovascular risk in adults. The most common definition requires any three of the following five criteria to be present: impaired glucose metabolism, central obesity, hypertension, and dyslipidemia related to either high-density lipoprotein (HDL) or triglycerides (Box 19.2). In adults with PCOS, the hyperandrogenic phenotype has the highest risk prevalence of dyslipidemia[43] and an overall higher prevalence of metabolic syndrome.[44] In adolescents with PCOS, the risk of metabolic syndrome is 2.5-fold higher than for those without PCOS[45] and more common in the classical (hyperandrogenic) phenotype.[42]

Emotional/Behavioral

In recent years, a greater understanding of the psychological burden associated with PCOS has emerged. In adults, health-related quality of life is diminished,[46] and incidence and prevalence of depressive and anxiety symptoms are high.[47,48] Body image distress may contribute to the depression and anxiety seen in this condition,[49] and the odds of disordered eating are increased.[50]

BOX 19.2 Metabolic Syndrome: Any Three of the Listed Metabolic Features

≥ 3 of the following criteria:
- Abnormal glucose metabolism
- Central obesity
- Hypertriglyceridemia
- Low HDL Cholesterol
- Elevated blood pressure

HDL, High-density lipoprotein.

For adolescents, data are still emerging, but a small study out of Turkey found that clinical manifestations of hyperandrogenism were associated with low self-concept, high level of anxiety, and high level of depressive symptoms.[51] However, during a recent meta-analysis of adolescent data as part of the 2023 international PCOS guideline, only depression was more prevalent in teens with PCOS. Therefore, screeening for depression with health asssessment questionnaires is recommended and short forms are readily available online.[3] Clinicians should be aware of the heightened risk of mood disorder in PCOS and take new comorbidities and life events into consideration.

Treatment

The three interrelated targets of treatment are menstrual dysregulation, hyperandrogenism, and insulin resistance/obesity with the goal of symptom control and metabolic risk reduction. Lifestyle counseling should therefore accompany all management recommendations. Common pharmacotherapies include combined oral contraceptives, antiandrogens, and metformin. Given the lack of evidence for superiority of one treatment modality over another, individualized, patient-centered, and culturally sensitive[52] approaches are recommended.

Lifestyle

Obesity compounds all symptoms of PCOS, and studies in adolescents have shown that intensive lifestyle modification can improve menstrual cycle regularity and androgen levels.[53,54] Currently, no specific dietary approach has proven superior for weight management in adolescents with PCOS, and therefore multicomponent intervention, including diet, exercise, and behavioral strategies, are recommended.[3]

Hormone Treatment

Combined hormonal contraceptives (CHCs; can be pills, patch, or ring) should be offered if clinical features of hyperandrogenism and menstrual dysregulation are the main concern, especially if there is also a need for reliable contraception. The estrogen component in the CHCs increases hepatic production of SHBG, thereby lowering circulating free/bioavailable testosterone. All CHCs contain the same type of estrogen—ethinyl estradiol—with only the dose varying in different formulations. The progestin component in CHCs ensures endometrial decidualization and therefore protects against endometrial

hyperplasia, a potential risk of prolonged anovulation. Progestins also reduce LH-driven ovarian androgen production via negative gonadotropin feedback. Many types of progestins are available, classified by generation or degree of androgenicity. Fourth-generation progestins such as drospirenone have the added benefit of androgen receptor blockade and may more effectively alleviate clinical signs of hyperandrogenism.[55] However, CHCs containing drospirenone were found to have a slightly higher thrombogenic risk than those with a similar ethinyl estradiol dose and third-generation progestins.[56,57]

There is no specific recommendation when choosing CHCs for adolescents with PCOS, though the choice should be guided by an understanding of not only the dose-related impact of ethinyl estradiol but also by an appreciation of the varying effects of different types of progesterones (see https://pedsendo.org/wp-content/uploads/2021/04/PCOS_Provider_Toolkit-4.2021.pdf).

If there is a contraindication for estrogen use or if daily medications are not desired, cyclic medroxyprogesterone acetate (5–10 mg/10 days) every 3 to 4 months can be used to prevent endometrial hyperplasia in those without need for contraception.[16] If contraception is desired, the levonorgestrel intrauterine device (IUD) is another option that prevents endometrial hyperplasia while reducing the discomfort of intermittent menstrual cycles.

Metformin

Metformin is an insulin sensitizer that is commonly used in the management of obese, insulin-resistant adolescents and may have beneficial cardiometabolic effects.[58] In PCOS, a metformin-induced decrease of circulating insulin additionally lowers androgen production. Metformin also directly (insulin independently) reduces steroidogenic enzyme activity in ovarian theca cells.[59] This may explain metformin treatment regularizing menstrual cycles in not only overweight but also normal-weight adults.[60] Metformin is not approved by the Food and Drug Administration (FDA) for use in adolescent PCOS but is widely used off-label, as it is cost-effective and has a good safety profile for long-term use. Metformin can cause mild to moderate gastrointestinal side effects that are commonly short-lived and can be reduced by taking metformin with food and starting at a low dose of 500 mg daily and increasing as tolerated to 1500 to 2000 mg daily divided BID. Long-term metformin use may lower vitamin B_{12} levels, and therefore yearly monitoring and supplementation are recommended.

For some adolescents, the use of extended-release metformin can be considered due to the benefit of once daily dosing and the potential decrease in gastrointestinal side effects which may lead to improved adherence.

Combination of CHCs and Metformin

An important consideration when treating overweight adolescents with CHCs for their contraceptive and cosmetic benefits is that additive treatment with metformin may ameliorate some of the negative cardiometabolic effects of CHCs.[7,61]

Antiandrogens

Spironolactone is a potassium-sparing diuretic that exerts an antiandrogenic effect through androgen receptor blockade and is the most frequently used antiandrogen to treat hirsutism and acne in the United States.[62] The combination of spironolactone with a CHC improves hirsutism better than a CHC alone.[63] Spironolactone slows and thins new hair growth without affecting hair that is already present. Therefore the impact of therapy is not noticeable until 6 to 9 months into treatment. If pregnancy is a risk, secure contraception is recommended because of the potential antiandrogenic effect of spironolactone on a male conceptus. The usual dose is 100 to 200 mg divided BID, and potassium monitoring is recommended 1 to 2 months into therapy. The risk of postural hypotension with poor hydration habits should be discussed. For a comparison of treatment effects see Table 19.5.

Additional Therapies

Vitamin D deficiency is common in adults and adolescents[64] with PCOS and contributes to menstrual dysregulation, insulin resistance, and hyperandrogenism. In adults, vitamin D supplementation improves most aspects of PCOS symptomatology and therefore should be considered a safe and cost-effective adjunct treatment in PCOS management.[65]

Myo-inositol is found in unprocessed grains and beans and fresh citrus fruits. It is sold as a supplement and has an insulin-sensitizing effect. D-chiro-inositol is derived from myo-inositol via insulin-stimulated epimerase and has a physiologic ratio of 40:1 A myo/di-chiro-inositol ratio is ideal for restoring ovarian function and improving insulin sensitivity, decreasing BMI, and lowering androgen levels.[66] Similarly to metformin, when myo-inositol was added to the treatment with CHCs, the negative impact of CHCs on weight and metabolic profile improved.[67] The recommended dose of 40:1 myo/di-chiro inositol is 4 g divided BID, and although side effects are gastrointestinal in nature, they are less common than with metformin treatment.

CONGENITAL ADRENAL HYPERPLASIA

CAH is a group of autosomal recessive disorders affecting cortisol biosynthesis. Reduced activity of an enzyme required for cortisol production leads to chronic overstimulation of the adrenal cortex and accumulation of precursors proximal to the blocked enzymatic step.[68] Defective adrenal steroidogenesis caused by mutations in the 21-hydroxylase gene *(CYP21A2)* constitutes the most frequent cause of CAH.[69] Around 300 *CYP21A2* gene mutations have been reported, and based on the severity of the phenotype, there are two forms—classical and nonclassical (NCCAH)—with classical being divided further into salt wasting and simple virilizing (Table 19.6).

NCCAH represents a mild form of CAH. Patients are not born with ambiguous genitalia, and they are not typically cortisol deficient. They usually present with clinical symptoms in late childhood, adolescence, or

TABLE 19.5 **Efficacy of Commonly Used Therapeutic Options for Managing PCOS-Related Problems in Adolescents**			
Treatment	**Menstrual Dysfunction**	**Hyperandrogenism**	**Metabolic Benefit**
Metformin	±	±	+
Oral contraceptive pill (OCP)	+	+	−
Cyclic progesterone	+	−	−
OCP + metformin	+	+	+
Antiandrogen	±	+	±

(Adapted from Lubna P, Seifer D. *Current and Emerging Concepts in PCOS.* 2nd ed. Springer; 2022.)

TABLE 19.6   Types of CAH Caused by 21-Hydroxylase Deficiency

	Classic Salt Wasting		Classic Simple Virilizing		Nonclassic	
	Males	Females	Males	Females	Males	Females
Age at dx	Birth-6 mo	Birth-1 mo	2-4 yr	Birth-2 yr	Child to adult	
External genitalia	Normal	Ambiguous	Normal	Ambiguous	Normal	Usually normal; may have clitoromegaly
Aldosterone	Low		Normal		Normal	
Cortisol	Low		Low		Normal	
17-OHP	Basal >20,000 ng/dL		Basal >10,000–20,000 ng/dL		ACTH stimulated 1,500–10,000 ng/dL	
% of normal 21-OH activity	0		1-2		20-50	

adulthood; however, some may remain asymptomatic. NCCAH accounts for 6% of children and adolescents presenting with androgen excess.[70] Its overall incidence ranges from 1:100 to 1:1000 and varies by ethnicity.[69]

Pathophysiology

The most common form of CAH is caused by a lack of the 21-hydroxylase enzyme, which converts 17-hydroxyprogesterone to 11-deoxycortisol and progesterone to deoxycorticosterone. These products are then precursors for cortisol and aldosterone production. The 21-hydroxylase enzyme deficiency leads to the blockage of cortisol synthesis. The result is corticotropin stimulation of the adrenal cortex and accumulation of cortisol precursors, which are diverted to sex hormone biosynthesis[71] (Fig. 19.3). Mutations in the *CYP21A2* gene cause varying degrees of 21-hydroxylase activity loss. Patients with a residual enzymatic activity in the range of 20% to 60% have a mild NCCAH phenotype, whereas no enzymatic activity leads to a classical CAH phenotype.[72]

Diagnosis

In childhood, NCCAH commonly presents with premature adrenarche. Clinical findings in girls with NCCAH include labial adhesions, premature pubarche, clitoromegaly, advanced bone age, early body odor and acne, and a short adult height prediction compared with midparental height.[73] In adolescent and adult women, NCCAH presents with hirsutism (59%–78%), anovulatory menstrual dysfunction (55%), acne (33%), decreased fertility (12%), and androgenic alopecia.[74]

NCCAH is an important exclusion criterion for PCOS. Alterations in hypothalamic-pituitary-ovarian function with androgen excess and the appearance of a polycystic ovary–like phenotype may be present in women with CAH.[74] Up to 63% of patients with NC-CAH meet criteria for PCOS, with hyperandrogenism and menstrual irregularity.[69] Assessment for biochemical hyperandrogenism shows that patients with NC-CAH have significantly higher levels of total and free testosterone compared with other etiologies of hyperandrogenism, including PCOS.[75] The distinction between this hereditary defect and other hyperandrogenemic entities is crucial not only for therapeutic reasons but also for genetic counseling. For this reason, a screening 17-hydroxyprogesterone level should be obtained in all patients being evaluated for hyperandrogenism.

Assessment

NCCAH cannot usually be diagnosed on the newborn screen done at birth.[76] These patients are not typically diagnosed until they become symptomatic later on in childhood or adulthood. First-line screening for NC-CAH is done with a serum 17-hydroxyprogesterone level. This should be drawn at 8:00 am in the follicular phase of the menstrual cycle, if possible. Afternoon 17-hydroxyprogesterone level measurements can yield false-negative results.[77] Azziz and Zacur suggest that 17-hydroxyprogesterone values below 200 ng/dL (6 nmol/L) should rule out NCCAH (95% specificity and sensitivity).[78] Serum 17-hydroxyprogesterone levels greater than 1500 ng/dL (45 nmol/L) have been described as diagnostic of NCCAH.[74] Livadas and colleagues assessed 280 fully genotyped individuals with NCCAH and suggested that a basal 17-hydroxyprogesterone level of >200 ng/dL (6 nmol/L) was diagnostic of

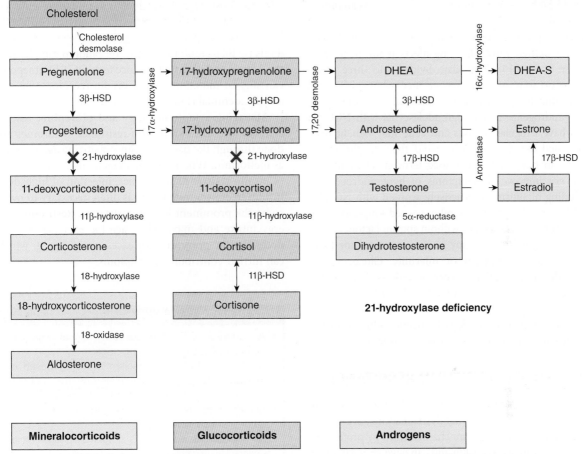

Fig. 19.3 The 21-hydroxylase enzyme converts 17-hydroxyprogesterone to 11-deoxycortisol and progesterone to deoxycorticosterone. These products are then precursors for cortisol and aldosterone production. 21-Hydroxylase enzyme deficiency leads to the blockage of cortisol synthesis. The result is corticotropin stimulation of the adrenal cortex and accumulation of cortisol precursors, which are diverted to sex hormone biosynthesis. In the schematic DHEA stands for Dehydroepiandrosterone and the S in DHEA-S stands for sulfate.

NCCAH, whereas a value between 130 and 200 ng/dL (4 and 6 nmol/L) required an adrenocorticotropic hormone (ACTH) stimulation test. They suggest that a 17-hydroxyprogesterone value post-cosyntropin (synthetic ACTH) of >1000 ng/dL (30 nmol/L) is diagnostic of NCCAH.[69] The Endocrine Society Clinical Practice Guideline on CAH caused by 21-hydroxylase deficiency recommends an ACTH stimulation test be performed if basal 17-hydroxyprogesterone is between 200 and 1000 ng/dL (6 and 30 nmol/L). 17-Hydroxyprogesterone levels should be drawn before and 60 minutes after cosyntropin 250 μg intravenous (IV) is given. ACTH-stimulated 17-hydroxyprogesterone levels greater than 1000 ng/dL (30 nmol/L) confirm NCCAH,

although lower levels do not completely exclude NCCAH (or carrier status for classical CAH).[71] Genetic testing may be useful if ACTH stimulation testing results are indeterminate.

Treatment

Because clinical presentation can vary, patients with NCCAH are treated according to their individual symptoms. Glucocorticoids are used to treat girls with NCCAH if they have early and rapid progression of pubarche with advanced bone age that will adversely affect adult height. They are also treated if they develop symptoms of virilization that suggest a more severe enzymatic dysfunction.[71] Early initiation of glucocorticoids (i.e., 1 year before puberty, bone age <9 years) can protect genetically determined height potential.[79] Hydrocortisone, which is preferred over prednisone or dexamethasone because of their growth-limiting effects, is administered at a dose of 6 to 15 mg/m²/day, divided into three doses. Hydrocortisone may be discontinued when girls reach their adult height, especially if there are no findings of hyperandrogenism. Although adolescents with NCCAH who have irregular menses and acne may benefit from continued low-dose glucocorticoid therapy, glucocorticoids can have undesirable long-term effects, and they may not improve all symptoms of hyperandrogenism, including hirsutism. Alternatively, women with NCCAH and hyperandrogenism are often treated long-term with oral contraceptives with or without spironolactone. Long-term glucocorticoid therapy is often reserved for treatment-resistant symptoms or infertility. Glucocorticoid stress dosing for major surgery or serious illness is not required for patients with NCCAH unless ACTH stimulation testing results in cortisol level less than 14 to 18 µg/dL or if the patient develops iatrogenic adrenal insufficiency from chronic glucocorticoid treatment.[71]

SYNDROMES OF INSULIN RESISTANCE

In adolescents, insulin resistance syndromes can present with hirsutism and menstrual dysregulation. Severe insulin resistance syndromes are characterized by profoundly reduced sensitivity to insulin and can have varied etiology and presentation. Often, insulin resistance is clinically expressed in the context of obesity. However, in some patients, insulin resistance can develop without obesity or in association with generalized or regional lack of adipose tissue. These patients may have pathogenic single-gene mutations. Severe insulin resistance syndromes can be grouped into those affecting insulin signaling and those affecting adipocyte development and function.[80]

Clinical features of severe insulin resistance include abnormal glucose homeostasis, ovarian dysfunction causing menstrual irregularity, hyperandrogenism, acanthosis nigricans, dyslipidemia and hepatic steatosis, lipodystrophy, and growth disorders.[80] Severe insulin resistance leads to beta-cell decompensation, but the timing of this can vary. Diabetes may develop in the neonatal period in the most severe cases but not until the fourth decade or beyond in mild cases.

Most commonly, insulin receptor gene defects present peripubertally with oligomenorrhea, hyperandrogenism,

and acanthosis nigricans, which is a similar presentation to PCOS. Often, hyperglycemia or a diagnosis of diabetes has yet to develop. However, significantly elevated insulin levels (>1000–1500 mcIU/mL) on random sample or at the 2-hour oral glucose tolerance test (OGTT) timepoint can suggest mutations in the insulin receptor gene and may be identifiable on genetic testing.[80,81]

Managing symptomatology and preventing associated comorbidities of insulin resistance syndromes are done through the use of insulin-sensitizing agents, such as metformin. When treating diabetes as a consequence of insulin resistance syndromes, injection of high-dose insulin in concentrated form is often necessary to overcome the prominent insulin resistance. Restricting energy intake and maximizing aerobic exercise are also necessary for prevention of excess weight gain, which can further contribute to symptoms.

> ### KEY POINTS
>
> - A diagnosis of PCOS requires menstrual dysregulation as defined by gynecologic age.
> - Biochemical hyperandrogenism is mainly based on elevated total and/or free testosterone. The best time to capture elevated levels is in the morning.
> - Screening for depression/anxiety and metabolic conditions is recommended.
> - All adolescents with PCOS should be counseled on healthy lifestyle practices, and pharmacologic treatment should be symptom and patient preference driven, with an understanding of specific drug effects in PCOS.
> - NCCAH is a mild form of CAH caused by a mutation in the *CYP21A2* gene that can present similarly to PCOS and should be ruled out in the evaluation for PCOS.
> - Severe insulin resistance syndromes can present like PCOS in adolescents. A highly elevated insulin level, especially in a nonobese adolescent, should prompt furter evaluation for insulin resistance syndromes.

▌ REVIEW QUESTIONS

1. Which of the following is a diagnostic criterion for PCOS in adolescents?
   a. Elevated LH/FSH ratio
   b. Oligomenorrhea
   c. Polycystic ovaries on ultrasound
   d. Premature adrenarche

2. Which of the following comorbidities are adolescents with PCOS *not* at increased risk for?
   a. Anxiety
   b. Type 1 diabetes mellitus
   c. Metabolic dysfunction-associated steatotic liver disease
   d. Metabolic syndrome
3. What is the best approach to screening for nonclassical CAH?
   a. ACTH stimulation test
   b. Genetic testing for *CYP21A2* mutation
   c. Morning serum 17-hydroxyprogesterone level
   d. Clinical examination assessing for clitoromegaly

REFERENCES

1. Rosenfield RL. Hirsutism and the variable response of the pilosebaceous unit to androgen. *J Investig Dermatol Symp Proc.* 2005;10(3):205-208.
2. Escobar-Morreale HF, Carmina E, Dewailly D, et al. Epidemiology, diagnosis and management of hirsutism: a consensus statement by the Androgen Excess and Polycystic Ovary Syndrome Society. *Hum Reprod Update.* 2012;18(2):146-170.
3. Teede HJ, Tay CT, Laven J, et al. International PCOS Network. Recommendations from the 2023 international evidence-based guideline for the assessment and management of polycystic ovary syndrome. *Fertil Steril.* 2023;120(4):767-793. doi:10.1016.
4. Schulze UM, Pettke-Rank CV, Kreienkamp M, et al. Dermatologic findings in anorexia and bulimia nervosa of childhood and adolescence. *Pediatr Dermatol.* 1999;16(2):90-94.
5. Karrer-Voegeli S, Rey F, Reymond MJ, Meuwly JY, Gaillard RC, Gomez F. Androgen dependence of hirsutism, acne, and alopecia in women: retrospective analysis of 228 patients investigated for hyperandrogenism. *Medicine (Baltimore).* 2009;88(1):32-45.
6. Garg A, Neuren E, Strunk A. Hidradenitis suppurativa is associated with polycystic ovary syndrome: a population-based analysis in the United States. *J Invest Dermatol.* 2018;138(6):1288-1292. doi:10.1016/j.jid.2018.01.009.
7. Pena AS, Witchel SF, Hoeger KM, et al. Adolescent polycystic ovary syndrome according to the international evidence-based guideline. *BMC Med.* 2020;18(1):72.
8. Day F, Karaderi T, Jones MR, et al. Large-scale genome-wide meta-analysis of polycystic ovary syndrome suggests shared genetic architecture for different diagnosis criteria. *PLoS Genet.* 2018;14(12):e1007813.
9. Youngster M, Ward VL, Blood EA, Barnewolt CE, Emans SJ, Divasta AD. Utility of ultrasound in the diagnosis of

polycystic ovary syndrome in adolescents. *Fertil Steril.* 2014;102(5):1432-1438.
10. Rackow BW, Vanden Brink H, Hammers L, Flannery CA, Lujan ME, Burgert TS. Ovarian morphology by transabdominal ultrasound correlates with reproductive and metabolic disturbance in adolescents with PCOS. *J Adolesc Health.* 2018;62(3):288-293.
11. Fulghesu AM, Canu E, Casula L, Melis F, Gambineri A. Polycystic ovarian morphology in normocyclic non-hyperandrogenic adolescents. *J Pediatr Adolesc Gynecol.* 2021;34(5):610-616.
12. Bruggeman BS, Bernier A. Hirsutism and menstrual irregularity in a 16-year-old girl. *Pediatr Rev.* 2021;42(8):449-452.
13. Codner E, Soto N, Lopez P, et al. Diagnostic criteria for polycystic ovary syndrome and ovarian morphology in women with type 1 diabetes mellitus. *J Clin Endocrinol Metab.* 2006;91(6):2250-2256.
14. Busiah K, Colmenares A, Bidet M, et al. High prevalence of polycystic ovary syndrome in type 1 diabetes mellitus adolescents: is there a difference depending on the NIH and Rotterdam criteria? *Horm Res Paediatr.* 2017;87(5):333-341.
15. Thong EP, Codner E, Laven JSE, Teede H. Diabetes: a metabolic and reproductive disorder in women. *Lancet Diabetes Endocrinol.* 2020;8(2):134-149.
16. Witchel SF, Oberfield SE, Pena AS. Polycystic ovary syndrome: pathophysiology, presentation, and treatment with emphasis on adolescent girls. *J Endocr Soc.* 2019;3(8):1545-1573.
17. Dunaif A, Segal KR, Futterweit W, Dobrjansky A. Profound peripheral insulin resistance, independent of obesity, in polycystic ovary syndrome. *Diabetes.* 1989;38(9):1165-1174.
18. Cree-Green M, Rahat H, Newcomer BR, et al. Insulin resistance, hyperinsulinemia, and mitochondria dysfunction in nonobese girls with polycystic ovarian syndrome. *J Endocr Soc.* 2017;1(7):931-944.
19. Stepto NK, Cassar S, Joham AE, et al. Women with polycystic ovary syndrome have intrinsic insulin resistance on euglycaemic-hyperinsulaemic clamp. *Hum Reprod.* 2013;28(3):777-784.
20. Wu S, Divall S, Wondisford F, Wolfe A. Reproductive tissues maintain insulin sensitivity in diet-induced obesity. *Diabetes.* 2012;61(1):114-123.
21. Diamanti-Kandarakis E, Dunaif A. Insulin resistance and the polycystic ovary syndrome revisited: an update on mechanisms and implications. *Endocr Rev.* 2012;33(6):981-1030.
22. Eagleson CA, Gingrich MB, Pastor CL, et al. Polycystic ovarian syndrome: evidence that flutamide restores sensitivity of the gonadotropin-releasing hormone pulse

generator to inhibition by estradiol and progesterone. *J Clin Endocrinol Metab.* 2000;85(11):4047-4052.

23. Stener-Victorin E, Padmanabhan V, Walters KA, et al. Animal models to understand the etiology and pathophysiology of polycystic ovary syndrome. *Endocr Rev.* 2020;41(4):bnaa010.

24. Legro RS, Lin HM, Demers LM, Lloyd T. Rapid maturation of the reproductive axis during perimenarche independent of body composition. *J Clin Endocrinol Metab.* 2000;85(3):1021-1025.

25. Assens M, Dyre L, Henriksen LS, et al. Menstrual pattern, reproductive hormones, and transabdominal 3D ultrasound in 317 adolescent girls. *J Clin Endocrinol Metab.* 2020;105(9):dgaa355.

26. Pena AS, Doherty DA, Atkinson HC, Hickey M, Norman RJ, Hart R. The majority of irregular menstrual cycles in adolescence are ovulatory: results of a prospective study. *Arch Dis Child.* 2018;103(3):235-239.

27. Azziz R, Carmina E, Dewailly D, et al. The Androgen Excess and PCOS Society criteria for the polycystic ovary syndrome: the complete task force report. *Fertil Steril.* 2009;91(2):456-488.

28. Salameh WA, Redor-Goldman MM, Clarke NJ, Mathur R, Azziz R, Reitz RE. Specificity and predictive value of circulating testosterone assessed by tandem mass spectrometry for the diagnosis of polycystic ovary syndrome by the National Institutes of Health 1990 criteria. *Fertil Steril.* 2014;101(4):1135-1141.e2.

29. Witchel SF, Oberfield S, Rosenfield RL, et al. The diagnosis of polycystic ovary syndrome during adolescence. *Horm Res Paediatr.* 2015.

30. Kakoly NS, Khomami MB, Joham AE, et al. Ethnicity, obesity and the prevalence of impaired glucose tolerance and type 2 diabetes in PCOS: a systematic review and meta-regression. *Hum Reprod Update.* 2018;24(4):455-467.

31. Hudnut-Beumler J, Kaar JL, Taylor A, et al. Development of type 2 diabetes in adolescent girls with polycystic ovary syndrome and obesity. *Pediatr Diabetes.* 2021;22(5):699-706.

32. Flannery CA, Rackow B, Cong X, Duran E, Selen DJ, Burgert TS. Polycystic ovary syndrome in adolescence: impaired glucose tolerance occurs across the spectrum of BMI. *Pediatr Diabetes.* 2013;14(1):42-49.

33. Li L, Chen X, He Z, Zhao X, Huang L, Yang D. Clinical and metabolic features of polycystic ovary syndrome among Chinese adolescents. *J Pediatr Adolesc Gynecol.* 2012;25(6):390-395.

34. Rinella ME, Lazarus JV, Ratziu V, Francque SM, Sanyal AJ, Kanwal F, Romero D, Abdelmalek MF, Anstee QM, Arab JP, Arrese M, Bataller R, Beuers U, Boursier J, Bugianesi E, Byrne CD, Narro GEC, Chowdhury A, Cortez-Pinto H, Cryer DR, Cusi K, El-Kassas M, Klein S, Eskridge W, Fan J, Gawrieh S, Guy CD, Harrison SA, Kim SU, Koot BG, Korenjak M, Kowdley KV, Lacaille F, Loomba R, Mitchell-Thain R, Morgan TR, Powell EE, Roden M, Romero-Gómez M, Silva M, Singh SP, Sookoian SC, Spearman CW, Tiniakos D, Valenti L, Vos MB, Wong VW, Xanthakos S, Yilmaz Y, Younossi Z, Hobbs A, Villota-Rivas M, Newsome PN; NAFLD Nomenclature consensus group. A multisociety Delphi consensus statement on new fatty liver disease nomenclature. *Ann Hepatol.* 2024 Jan-Feb;29(1):101133. doi:10.1016/j.aohep.2023.101133. Epub 2023 Jun 24. PMID: 37364816.

35. Burgert TS, Taksali SE, Dziura J, et al. Alanine aminotransferase levels and fatty liver in childhood obesity: associations with insulin resistance, adiponectin, and visceral fat. *J Clin Endocrinol Metab.* 2006;91(11):4287-4294.

36. Rocha ALL, Faria LC, Guimaraes TCM, et al. Nonalcoholic fatty liver disease in women with polycystic ovary syndrome: systematic review and meta-analysis. *J Endocrinol Invest.* 2017;40(12):1279-1288.

37. Falzarano C, Lofton T, Osei-Ntansah A, et al. Nonalcoholic fatty liver disease in women and girls with polycystic ovary syndrome. *J Clin Endocrinol Metab.* 2022;107(1):258-272.

38. Vos MB, Abrams SH, Barlow SE, et al. NASPGHAN clinical practice guideline for the diagnosis and treatment of nonalcoholic fatty liver disease in children: recommendations from the Expert Committee on NAFLD (ECON) and the North American Society of Pediatric Gastroenterology, Hepatology and Nutrition (NASPGHAN). *J Pediatr Gastroenterol Nutr.* 2017;64(2):319-334.

39. Lim SS, Davies MJ, Norman RJ, Moran LJ. Overweight, obesity and central obesity in women with polycystic ovary syndrome: a systematic review and meta-analysis. *Hum Reprod Update.* 2012;18(6):618-637.

40. Koivuaho E, Laru J, Ojaniemi M, et al. Age at adiposity rebound in childhood is associated with PCOS diagnosis and obesity in adulthood-longitudinal analysis of BMI data from birth to age 46 in cases of PCOS. *Int J Obes (Lond).* 2019;43(7):1370-1379.

41. Weiss R, Dziura J, Burgert TS, et al. Obesity and the metabolic syndrome in children and adolescents. *N Engl J Med.* 2004;350(23):2362-2374.

42. Hart R, Doherty DA, Mori T, et al. Extent of metabolic risk in adolescent girls with features of polycystic ovary syndrome. *Fertil Steril.* 2011;95(7):2347-2353.e1.

43. Pinola P, Puukka K, Piltonen TT, et al. Normo- and hyperandrogenic women with polycystic ovary syndrome exhibit an adverse metabolic profile through life. *Fertil Steril.* 2017;107(3):788-795.e2.

44. Yang R, Yang S, Li R, Liu P, Qiao J, Zhang Y. Effects of hyperandrogenism on metabolic abnormalities in

patients with polycystic ovary syndrome: a meta-analysis. *Reprod Biol Endocrinol.* 2016;14(1):67.

45. Fazleen NE, Whittaker M, Mamun A. Risk of metabolic syndrome in adolescents with polycystic ovarian syndrome: a systematic review and meta-analysis. *Diabetes Metab Syndr.* 2018;12(6):1083-1090.

46. Coffey S, Bano G, Mason HD. Health-related quality of life in women with polycystic ovary syndrome: a comparison with the general population using the Polycystic Ovary Syndrome Questionnaire (PCOSQ) and the Short Form-36 (SF-36). *Gynecol Endocrinol.* 2006;22(2):80-86.

47. Hung JH, Hu LY, Tsai SJ, et al. Risk of psychiatric disorders following polycystic ovary syndrome: a nationwide population-based cohort study. *PLoS One.* 2014;9(5):e97041.

48. Cooney LG, Lee I, Sammel MD, Dokras A. High prevalence of moderate and severe depressive and anxiety symptoms in polycystic ovary syndrome: a systematic review and meta-analysis. *Hum Reprod.* 2017;32(5):1075-1091.

49. Alur-Gupta S, Chemerinski A, Liu C, et al. Body-image distress is increased in women with polycystic ovary syndrome and mediates depression and anxiety. *Fertil Steril.* 2019;112(5):930-938.e1.

50. Lee I, Cooney LG, Saini S, Sammel MD, Allison KC, Dokras A. Increased odds of disordered eating in polycystic ovary syndrome: a systematic review and meta-analysis. *Eat Weight Disord.* 2019;24(5):787-797.

51. Almis H, Orhon FS, Bolu S, Almis BH. Self-concept, depression, and anxiety levels of adolescents with polycystic ovary syndrome. *J Pediatr Adolesc Gynecol.* 2021;34(3):311-316.

52. Schweisberger CL, Hornberger L, Barral R, et al. Gender diversity in adolescents with polycystic ovary syndrome. *J Pediatr Endocrinol Metab.* 2022;35(11):1422-1428.

53. Hoeger K, Davidson K, Kochman L, Cherry T, Kopin L, Guzick DS. The impact of metformin, oral contraceptives, and lifestyle modification on polycystic ovary syndrome in obese adolescent women in two randomized, placebo-controlled clinical trials. *J Clin Endocrinol Metab.* 2008;93(11):4299-4306.

54. Lass N, Kleber M, Winkel K, Wunsch R, Reinehr T. Effect of lifestyle intervention on features of polycystic ovarian syndrome, metabolic syndrome, and intima-media thickness in obese adolescent girls. *J Clin Endocrinol Metab.* 2011;96(11):3533-3540.

55. Kriplani A, Periyasamy AJ, Agarwal N, Kulshrestha V, Kumar A, Ammini AC. Effect of oral contraceptive containing ethinyl estradiol combined with drospirenone vs. desogestrel on clinical and biochemical parameters in patients with polycystic ovary syndrome. *Contraception.* 2010;82(2):139-146.

56. Jick SS, Hernandez RK. Risk of non-fatal venous thromboembolism in women using oral contraceptives containing drospirenone compared with women using oral contraceptives containing levonorgestrel: case-control study using United States claims data. *BMJ.* 2011;342:d2151.

57. Parkin L, Sharples K, Hernandez RK, Jick SS. Risk of venous thromboembolism in users of oral contraceptives containing drospirenone or levonorgestrel: nested case-control study based on UK General Practice Research Database. *BMJ.* 2011;342:d2139.

58. Burgert TS, Duran EJ, Goldberg-Gell R, et al. Short-term metabolic and cardiovascular effects of metformin in markedly obese adolescents with normal glucose tolerance. *Pediatr Diabetes.* 2008;9(6):567-576.

59. Diamanti-Kandarakis E, Christakou CD, Kandaraki E, Economou FN. Metformin: an old medication of new fashion: evolving new molecular mechanisms and clinical implications in polycystic ovary syndrome. *Eur J Endocrinol.* 2010;162(2):193-212.

60. Yang PK, Hsu CY, Chen MJ, et al. The efficacy of 24-month metformin for improving menses, hormones, and metabolic profiles in polycystic ovary syndrome. *J Clin Endocrinol Metab.* 2018;103(3):890-899.

61. Al Khalifah RA, Florez ID, Dennis B, Thabane L, Bassilious E. Metformin or oral contraceptives for adolescents with polycystic ovarian syndrome: a meta-analysis. *Pediatrics.* 2016;137(5):e20154089.

62. Somani N, Turvy D. Hirsutism: an evidence-based treatment update. *Am J Clin Dermatol.* 2014;15(3):247-266.

63. Ezeh U, Huang A, Landay M, Azziz R. Long-term response of hirsutism and other hyperandrogenic symptoms to combination therapy in polycystic ovary syndrome. *J Womens Health (Larchmt).* 2018;27(7):892-902.

64. Simpson S, Seifer DB, Shabanova V, et al. The association between anti-Mullerian hormone and vitamin 25(OH)D serum levels and polycystic ovarian syndrome in adolescent females. *Reprod Biol Endocrinol.* 2020;18(1):118.

65. Morgante G, Darino I, Spano A, et al. PCOS physiopathology and vitamin D deficiency: biological insights and perspectives for treatment. *J Clin Med.* 2022;11(15):4509.

66. Kamenov Z, Gateva A. Inositols in PCOS. *Molecules.* 2020;25(23):5566.

67. Pkhaladze L, Barbakadze L, Kvashilava N. Myo-inositol in the treatment of teenagers affected by PCOS. *Int J Endocrinol.* 2016;2016:1473612.

68. Caglayan S, Takagi-Niidome S, Liao F, et al. Lysosomal sorting of amyloid-beta by the SORLA receptor is impaired by a familial Alzheimer's disease mutation. *Sci Transl Med.* 2014;6(223):223ra20.

69. Livadas S, Dracopoulou M, Dastamani A, et al. The spectrum of clinical, hormonal and molecular findings in 280

individuals with nonclassical congenital adrenal hyperplasia caused by mutations of the CYP21A2 gene. *Clin Endocrinol (Oxf)*. 2015;82(4):543-549.

70. Idkowiak J, Elhassan YS, Mannion P, et al. Causes, patterns and severity of androgen excess in 487 consecutively recruited pre- and post-pubertal children. *Eur J Endocrinol*. 2019;180(3):213-221.

71. Speiser PW, Arlt W, Auchus RJ, et al. Congenital adrenal hyperplasia due to steroid 21-hydroxylase deficiency: An Endocrine Society clinical practice guideline. *J Clin Endocrinol Metab*. 2018;103(11):4043-4088.

72. Simonetti L, Bruque CD, Fernandez CS, et al. CYP21A2 mutation update: comprehensive analysis of databases and published genetic variants. *Hum Mutat*. 2018;39(1): 5-22.

73. Witchel SF. Nonclassic congenital adrenal hyperplasia. *Curr Opin Endocrinol Diabetes Obes*. 2012;19(3):151-158.

74. Witchel SF. Non-classic congenital adrenal hyperplasia. *Steroids*. 2013;78(8):747-750.

75. Carmina E, Rosato F, Janni A, Rizzo M, Longo RA. Extensive clinical experience: relative prevalence of different androgen excess disorders in 950 women referred because of clinical hyperandrogenism. *J Clin Endocrinol Metab*. 2006;91(1):2-6.

76. Held PK, Shapira SK, Hinton CF, Jones E, Hannon WH, Ojodu J. Congenital adrenal hyperplasia cases identified by newborn screening in one- and two-screen states. *Mol Genet Metab*. 2015;116(3):133-138.

77. Esquivel-Zuniga MR, Kirschner CK, McCartney CR, Burt Solorzano CM. Non-PCOS hyperandrogenic disorders in adolescents. *Semin Reprod Med*. 2022;40(1-02):42-52.

78. Azziz R, Zacur HA. 21-Hydroxylase deficiency in female hyperandrogenism: screening and diagnosis. *J Clin Endocrinol Metab*. 1989;69(3):577-584.

79. Azziz R, Hincapie LA, Knochenhauer ES, Dewailly D, Fox L, Boots LR. Screening for 21-hydroxylase-deficient nonclassic adrenal hyperplasia among hyperandrogenic women: a prospective study. *Fertil Steril*. 1999;72(5): 915-925.

80. Semple RK, Savage DB, Cochran EK, Gorden P, O'Rahilly S. Genetic syndromes of severe insulin resistance. *Endocr Rev*. 2011;32(4):498-514.

81. Paprocki E, Barral RL, Vanden Brink H, Lujan M, Burgert TS. GnRH agonist improves hyperandrogenism in an adolescent girl with an insulin receptor gene mutation. *J Endocr Soc*. 2019;3(6):1196-1200.

82. Rosenfield RL. Clinical practice. Hirsutism. *N Engl J Med*. 2005;353(24):2578-2588.

Sexually Transmitted Infections, HIV Pre-exposure Prophylaxis, and Expedited Partner Therapy

Cynthia Holland-Hall and Lauren Matera

INTRODUCTION

Over one-third of high school students report having ever had sexual intercourse, with over half of high school seniors stating that they have had sex. Almost one-fifth (16%) of high school seniors report having had four or more sex partners. Of students who are sexually active, only 54% report using a condom with their last sexual encounter.[1]

Although sexually transmitted infections (STIs) affect people of all ages, adolescents are at increased risk. Inconsistent condom use, early sexual debut, and increased numbers of partners increase the chances of contracting an STI. Rates of reported *Chlamydia trachomatis* infections, though decreasing slightly in recent years, remain highest in adolescents and young adults (AYAs) ages 15 to 24 years, with almost two-thirds of these infections reported in this age group in 2020. Other STIs, including *Neisseria gonorrhoeae* and syphilis, have seen increased prevalence in recent years.[1]

Transmission of STIs is through sexual contact, and STIs can only be definitively prevented by abstaining from sexual activity. Risk can be decreased by consistent, correct condom use and by ensuring that partners have been tested and are negative for STIs. Vaccination against hepatitis B and human papillomavirus (HPV) dramatically lowers the risk of these viral STIs. The risk of contracting an STI increases with increasing number of partners. STIs are endemic in some communities, and this may confer a greater risk than individual sexual practices. Black and Indigenous populations have the highest rates of STI, highlighting the racial and ethnic health disparities and barriers to care that can affect these populations.

Providers who care for adolescents must have comfort and experience screening, recognizing, testing, and treating these infections given their high prevalence. A free, easy-to-navigate, and self-paced STI online curriculum is available at https://www.std.uw.edu/.[2]

CONSENT AND CONFIDENTIALITY

A comprehensive and inclusive sexual history is key to understanding what screening and care an adolescent needs (Fig. 20.1, also see Chapter 2 for more information

Partners
- How many partners have you had in your lifetime? In the last six months?
- Are your partners men, women, both? Are your partners cisgender, transgender, nonbinary?

Practices
- What types of sex do you have?
- Do you have vaginal sex? Oral sex? Anal sex?

Protection from STIs
- Do you use condoms if your partner has a penis? How do you use them?
- Do you use dental dams when engaging in oral-vaginal sex?

Past history of STIs
- Have you ever been diagnosed with an STI?
- If you have had an STI, were you treated and completed your treatment?

Pregnancy intention
- Do you have a desire to become pregnant?
- How are you preventing pregnancy if not? Would you like to talk about options for preventing pregnancy

Fig. 20.1 How to take a sexual history. *STIs,* Sexually transmitted infections.

on confidential interview). All major professional organizations, including the American Academy of Pediatrics[3] and the American College of Obstetricians and Gynecologists,[4] recommend that developmentally appropriate confidential care be provided to all adolescents. (See Chapter 2 for more information on confidentiality for adolescents.) The opportunity to have a private discussion with their provider is vital to allowing adolescents to take increased responsibility for their own health care. This is especially important when it comes to sexual and reproductive health. Adolescents are more likely to seek necessary reproductive health services when they believe these services will be provided confidentially.[5] Providers must remain nonjudgmental and engage in shared decision making in order to establish an effective therapeutic relationship with their patients. The Centers for Disease Control and Prevention (CDC) has a video that highlights some patient perspectives on the importance of these conversations in the medical visit.[6]

There is a shift in conversations with adolescents about STIs, moving away from shame and stigma, as highlighted by Dr. Teodora Elvira Wi, a World Health Organization leader, in her outstanding TED Talk. She emphasizes the importance of reframing these discussions with our patients. (See https://www.ted.com/talks/teodora_elvira_wi_how_talking_about_sex_could_end_stis.)

Currently, all 50 states and the District of Columbia allow minors to consent to STI testing and treatment; certain states require a minor to be of a certain age to provide consent. Some states include protection of a minor's confidentiality in their legislation, whereas others allow for parental notification. The right to human immunodeficiency virus (HIV) testing and treatment is explicitly included as part of this in 32 states. State-specific laws regarding confidentiality and parental notification can be accessed at the Guttmacher Institute (www.guttmacher.org).[7]

SCREENING GUIDELINES[8]

Sexually active cisgender women younger than 25 years should be screened at least yearly for *N. gonorrhoeae* and *C. trachomatis* using a provider- or patient-collected vaginal swab; both modalities have equal sensitivity and specificity. First-catch urine screening can also be employed, though swabs are preferred in patients with a vagina because of somewhat higher sensitivity.[9] In populations with a high prevalence of *Trichomonas vaginalis* infections (e.g., sexual health clinics, teen clinics, detention facilities), screening for this organism is also recommended.

Patients who engage in receptive anal or oral intercourse may be screened at these sites as well; the Food and Drug Administration cleared two brands of nucleic acid amplification tests (NAATs) for extragenital screening in 2019. Before this clearance, many large academic and commercial laboratories performed internal validation studies, enabling providers to use these tests on extragenital specimens.[10]

Syphilis screening should be offered to patients with increased risk of infection or in areas of high prevalence. Although a diagnosis of infection requires a two-step laboratory process, screening can be done first with a nontreponemal test, either Venereal Disease Research Laboratory (VRDL) or rapid plasma reagin (RPR). If this test is positive, additional treponemal tests such as the fluorescent treponemal antibody absorbed (FTA-ABS) test or the *Treponema pallidum* passive particle agglutination (TP-PA) assay are necessary for confirmation. Screening with a treponemal test first, followed by a nontreponemal test (reverse-sequence algorithm) is also acceptable.

Screening in the transgender and gender diverse (TGD) AYA population should be approached based on anatomy and specific sexual practices. TGD people who have a vagina, uterus, or cervix should receive screening equivalent to cisgender women (i.e., annual gonorrhea and chlamydia screening, Pap smears starting at age 21). If a TGD person has had gender-affirming surgery, screening guidelines may differ based on their anatomy.

Screening recommendations are summarized in Table 20.1. Treatment options for positive screening tests are included in Table 20.2.

SEXUALLY TRANSMITTED INFECTIONS

Bacterial Infections

Chlamydia and gonorrhea are both spread by sexual contact (genital, anal, or oral). Detection of these infections with regular screening is important because untreated infections can lead to complications including pelvic inflammatory disease, tubal scarring, and infertility, as well as increased risk of ectopic pregnancy and chronic pelvic pain.[8] Both infections can also be transmitted vertically from a pregnant person to an infant during childbirth. As reinfection among adolescents is common, counseling on adherence to treatment and techniques to prevent reinfection are paramount.

Chlamydia

C. trachomatis (Box 20.1), a gram-negative intracellular pathogen, is the most common reportable bacterial

TABLE 20.1   Screening Recommendations for STIs

Infection	Population	Specimen	Testing Modality
Chlamydia trachomatis	Sexually active persons with a vagina/cervix <25 years old	Vaginal swab or first-catch urine	NAAT
Neisseria gonorrhoeae	Sexually active persons with a vagina/cervix <25 years old	Vaginal swab or first-catch urine	NAAT
Trichomonas vaginalis	Consider in high-prevalence populations	Vaginal swab or first-catch urine	NAAT Culture Point-of-care test Microscopy/wet prep
Syphilis (Treponema pallidum)	Consider in high-prevalence populations (current HIV or other STI, history of incarceration or sex work, sex with MSM, living in area with higher rate of syphilis)	Serum	Nontreponemal tests: VRDL or RPR Treponemal tests: FTA-ABS, TP-PA, others
Human papilloma virus	Persons 21 years or older with a cervix	Cervical cells	Pap smear
HIV	Screen all sexually active persons aged 13–64 years at least once in lifetime[a]	Serum	Combined immunoassay for HIV-1/HIV-2 antigen/antibody

FTA-ABS, Fluorescent treponemal antibody absorbed; HIV, human immunodeficiency virus; MSM, men who have sex with men; NAAT, nucleic acid amplification test; RPR, rapid plasma reagin; STI, sexually transmitted infection; TP-PA, T. pallidum passive particle agglutination; VRDL, Venereal Disease Research Laboratory.

[a]In addition, screen periodically based on (1) personal risk factors: >1 sex partner since most recent HIV test, sex work, and injection drug use and (2) sex partner(s) risk factors: injection drug use, HIV infection, sex with MSM.

(From Papp J, Schachter J, Gaydos C, der Van Pol B Recommendations for the laboratory-based detection of Chlamydia trachomatis and Neisseria gonorrhoeae–2014. MMWR Reccom Rep. 2014;63(RR02):1–19; American College of Obstetricians and Gynecologists. Committee opinion no. 596. Obstet Gynecol. 2014;123:1137-1139.)

TABLE 20.2   Common Sexually Transmitted Infections: A Summary[8]

Infection	Type of Organism	Possible Signs and Symptoms	Treatment
Chlamydia (uncomplicated urogenital infection)	Gram-negative bacterium	Vaginal discharge Cervicitis Irregular bleeding Dysuria Pelvic pain	Recommended: Doxycycline 100 mg PO BID × 7 days Alternative: Azithromycin 1 g PO once
Gonorrhea (uncomplicated urogenital infection)	Gram-negative bacterium	Vaginal discharge Cervicitis Irregular bleeding Pelvic pain	Ceftriaxone 500 mg IM once if <150 kg Ceftriaxone 1000 mg IM once if >150 kg
Trichomonas	Parasite	Vaginal discharge	Recommended: Metronidazole 500 mg PO BID × 7 days Alternative: Tinidazole 2 g PO once
Syphilis (primary, secondary, or early latent)	Bacterium (Spirochete)	Primary: Painless genital ulcer Secondary: Skin rashes; systemic symptoms Tertiary: Variable symptoms Refer to Table 20.3 for more detail	Benzathine penicillin G 2.4 million units IM once

Continued

TABLE 20.2   **Common Sexually Transmitted Infections: A Summary[8]—cont'd**

Infection	Type of Organism	Possible Signs and Symptoms	Treatment
Genital warts (external: vulva, perineum, external anus)	Virus	Papular, flat, or verrucous warts	Patient applied: Imiquimod 3.75% or 5% cream OR Podofilox 0.5% solution or gel Provider administered: Cryotherapy; surgical removal OR Trichloroacetic acid (TCA) 80%–90% solution
HSV (genital herpes)	Virus	Genital vesicles progressing to ulcerations Systemic symptoms (fever, chills, swollen lymph nodes)	Initial outbreak: Acyclovir 400 mg PO TID × 7–10 days OR Valacyclovir 1 g PO BID × 7–10 days Recurrent outbreaks: Acyclovir 800 mg PO BID × 5 days OR Valacyclovir 1 g PO daily × 5 days Daily suppressive therapy: Acyclovir 400 mg PO BID OR Valacyclovir 500 mg or 1 g PO daily

BID, Twice a day; *IM,* intramuscular; *PO,* orally; *TID,* three times a day.

BOX 20.1   Chlamydia and Gonorrhea in the Adolescent

- Spread by sexual contact (genital, anal, or oral).
- Can be transmitted vertically from a pregnant person to infant during childbirth.
- Transmission can only be definitively prevented by abstaining from sexual activities.
- Risk can be decreased by consistent, correct condom use, and by ensuring that partners have been tested and are negative.
- Infections must be reported to the health department.
- Sexual partners should be empirically treated.

infection in the United States. The highest prevalence is in AYA females (ages 15–24 years). Although most chlamydial infections are asymptomatic,[11] patients can present with vaginal discharge, abnormal vaginal spotting, bleeding (particularly postcoital bleeding), dysuria, or pelvic pain. On examination, the cervix may appear normal, or there may be evidence of mucopurulent cervicitis such as pus from the os or cervical friability.

There is increasing evidence of rectal chlamydia infections among cisgender women presenting to sexual health clinics, even in the absence of reported receptive anal intercourse. Like genitourinary (GU) chlamydia infections, most rectal infections are asymptomatic. Some experts have hypothesized that inadequately treated or untreated rectal chlamydia may lead to autoinoculation of the urogenital tract, leading to recurrent chlamydial infections.[12] Current treatment of chlamydia is with oral doxycycline for 7 days. Treatment with a single dose of azithromycin is an alternative, but this is less effective at eradicating the organism, particularly in the rectal tissue (see Table 20.2). Partners also should be treated.

Gonorrhea

N. gonorrhoeae (Box 20.1) is a gram-negative bacterium and is the second most common reportable bacterial infection in the United States. Like chlamydial infections, gonococcal infections in people with a cervix are often asymptomatic. If signs or symptoms are present, they can include mucopurulent cervicitis, vaginal discharge, abnormal vaginal bleeding, or pelvic pain.

N. gonorrhoeae has developed resistance to most antibiotics, and parenteral ceftriaxone is the only first-line treatment currently recommended by the CDC (see Table 20.2). If the recommended treatment regimen is not used, test of cure is recommended 3 to 4 weeks after completing therapy. Patients with suspected antimicrobial-resistant gonorrhea should be evaluated with culture and antimicrobial susceptibility testing. Suspected treatment failures should be reported to the CDC using a form or through the CDC website (see Table 20.2). Partners also should be treated.

Trichomoniasis

T. vaginalis is a protozoan infection that is sexually transmitted and is most commonly diagnosed in patients with a cervix. Routine screening is not recommended for asymptomatic, HIV-negative people, except in at-risk populations. *Trichomonas* infections may be asymptomatic or may present with a frothy vaginal discharge, dysuria, pruritus, and possibly pelvic pain/lower abdominal pain. The characteristic "strawberry cervix" (Fig. 20.2) of trichomoniasis is seen in a minority of infected patients but is highly specific to this infection. *T. vaginalis* infection is associated with increased risk of HIV transmission and adverse pregnancy outcomes such as premature rupture of the membranes.[8]

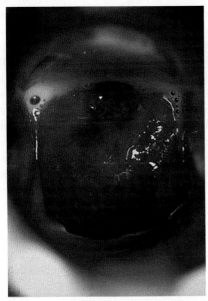

Fig. 20.2 Strawberry cervix with punctuate hemorrhages as a result of *Trichomonas vaginalis* infection. (From Lewis DA. Trichomoniasis. *Medicine*. 2010;38(6):291-293.)

Trichomonas can be transmitted via sexual contact with a partner who has the infection. Transmission via anal or oral intercourse has not been well described. Recommended treatment of trichomoniasis is oral metronidazole for 7 days, though alternative regimens are available. Topical antiinfective agents (such as metronidazole vaginal gel) do not reliably eradicate the infection and should not be used. Sexual partners should be treated.

Syphilis

Syphilis, caused by the spirochetal bacteria *T. pallidum*, is an STI with manifestations that depend on the stage of the disease. Patients with primary syphilis may present with a painless ulcer (chancre), which often begins as a papule and may progress to an ulcer. This lesion resolves within days to weeks. If undetected and untreated, the infection may proceed to latent syphilis, where there are no visible signs or symptoms of the disease, or to secondary or tertiary syphilis. The stages of syphilis infection are highlighted in Table 20.3.

Syphilis infections are increasing in the United States, with increasing numbers of cases being identified in cisgender women. Syphilis can be transmitted via unprotected sexual intercourse and can cause significant complications in pregnancy, including congenital infection. Although syphilis infections are most common in men, the rate of syphilis infections in women nearly tripled between 2015 and 2019, which was then followed by a significant increase in cases of congenital syphilis in 2020.[8] Adolescents who are most at risk include those who engage in transactional sex or are victims of sex trafficking, who engage in substance use (especially methamphetamine or heroin use), who experience homelessness, or who have been incarcerated. Adolescents in areas where syphilis is highly prevalent (most recently, the West and Southeast of the United States) are also at risk; it is important to be aware of local trends in your area of practice.[13]

Treatment for primary, secondary, or early-latent syphilis is with a single dose of intramuscular (IM) benzathine penicillin (see Table 20.2). In penicillin-allergic patients, desensitization and treatment with penicillin are recommended. Patients with tertiary syphilis require multiple doses of penicillin. A complete discussion of the evaluation and management of late-latent or tertiary syphilis is beyond the scope of this text; this condition should be managed in consultation with an experienced provider.

TABLE 20.3   Summary of the Various Stages of Syphilis Infection With Common Symptoms[8]

Early Syphilis	Late Syphilis	Neurosyphilis	Latent Syphilis

• **Primary Syphilis**
  • Characterized by painless chancre (ulcer)
  • Lasts 3-6 weeks
  • Serologic testing may be negative
  • Diagnosis can be made by darkfield microscopy of a lesion exudate
• **Secondary Syphilis**
  • Characterized by skin rash, mucus membrane lesions, systemic symptoms (fever, lymphadenopathy, malaise)
  • Appears during primary chancre healing or weeks later
	• **Tertiary Syphilis**
	  • Can appear years after initial infection if not treated earlier
	  • Manifestations depend on involved organ systems
	• **Cardiovascular**
	  • Aortitis involving the ascending thoracic aorta, characterized by aortic dilation and aortic valve regurgitation
	• **Gummatous**
	  • Characterized by "gummas"-heaped up granulatmous lesions
		• May present at any time after initial infection
		• Seen most commonly in patients with HIV
		• Manifestations vary based on organs affected
		• **Early Neurosyphilis**
		  • Asymptomatic
		  • Meningitis
		  • Ocular syphilis
		  • Otosyphilis
		• **Late Neurosyphilis**
		  • Paresis
		  • Tabes dorsalis
			• Asymptomatic
			• *T. pallidum* persists without appropriate treatment
			• **Early**
			  • Infection occured within previous 12 month
			  • Affected persons are still infectious
			• **Late**
			  • Infection occured >12 months previous
			  • Affected persons are not considered infectious

Human Papillomavirus and Genital Warts

HPV (Box 20.2) is the most common STI in AYA, though most remain asymptomatic and may never be aware that they have been infected.

Anogenital warts (condyloma acuminatum) are most commonly caused by HPV serotypes 6 and 11, which are transmitted via contact with infected skin or mucosa. Warts are typically found on the perineum, vulva, perianal or anal skin, or suprapubic skin. Lesions vary in appearance and size. They may be flat, papular, or verrucous and may be solitary or clustered. Warts can also be found on the vaginal walls, cervix, or urethra. They are rarely painful or pruritic but may cause some discomfort depending on their location.

Diagnosis of genital warts is typically by visual inspection. Without treatment, lesions may spontaneously regress or may persist. The treatment of external warts may be patient-applied (imiquimod, podofilox) or provider-applied medication (trichloroacetic acid), cryotherapy, or surgical removal. Most patients respond within 3 months of topical treatment. Mucosal warts of the vagina, cervix, anus, or urethral meatus should be treated by an experienced professional, typically with cryotherapy or surgical treatment. The goal of treatment is elimination of the warts and resolution of symptoms. Despite the treatment of visible lesions, the patient may continue to spread HPV to sexual partners indefinitely.

Oncogenic strains of HPV, most commonly types 16 and 18, are associated with cervical, anal, vulvovaginal, and head and neck cancers. Screening for cervical cancer should be performed using a Papanicolaou smear (Pap) starting at age 21 years in immunocompetent hosts.

Routine administration of the nonavalent HPV vaccine is recommended for all adolescents. The vaccine confers significant protection against nononcogenic

---

BOX 20.2   HPV in the Adolescent

• Anogenital warts most commonly caused by HPV 6 or 11
• The most common oncogenic strains are HPV 16 and 18
• Diagnosed by visualization of warts on examination
  • Pap smear starting at age 21
• Treatment options for warts:
  • Self-applied: imiquimod, podofilox
  • Provider applied:
  Trichloroacetic acid (TCA) or Bichloroacetic acid (BCA) 80%–90% solution
  Cryotherapy
  Surgical removal
• Risk reduction:
  • Vaccination with nonavalent HPV vaccine
  • Delay onset of sexual activity and limit number of sexual partners

strains 6 and 11 as well as seven oncogenic strains that together are associated with the majority of cervical cancers. The vaccine is recommended at age 11 to 12 years but can be administered as early as age 9. Adolescents under age 15 at the start of the vaccine series need two doses (at 0 and 6–12 months), whereas those beginning the series after the 15th birthday need three doses (at 0, 1–2, and 6 months). The the HPV vaccine is approved through age 26 if not vaccinate already.

Genital Herpes

In North America, herpes simplex virus (HSV) is the most common cause of genital ulcers, with both HSV-1 and HSV-2 commonly implicated. HSV-1 is most commonly transmitted via oral contact and may cause oral or cutaneous lesions, though it is increasingly recognized as a cause of genital ulcers, especially in AYA. HSV-2 is primarily sexually transmitted and may cause genital ulcers.[14]

Primary infection with HSV can vary in clinical presentation, though outbreaks caused by HSV-1 and HSV-2 are indistinguishable in their clinical presentations. Some patients are asymptomatic or present with mild symptoms that may be overlooked. If symptomatic, patients may initially have groupings of painful, small (2–4 mm) vesicles with erythematous base. These vesicles progress to ulcerations and erosions, which are more likely to be seen a few days into the outbreak. Systemic symptoms, including fever, malaise, and lymphadenopathy, may accompany the primary outbreak. Primary lesions can last several weeks and often appear within 2 weeks of exposure to the virus.

HSV infection is not curable. After primary genital infection, HSV remains latent in the sacral ganglia and can cause recurrence of symptoms. HSV-2 is more commonly associated with frequent, recurrent outbreaks than HSV-1. Duration of symptoms during recurrent outbreaks is shorter than during primary outbreaks and often less severe. Many patients experience a prodrome before eruption of recurrent lesions, characterized by tingling, itching, burning, or shooting pain in the genital area. Initiation of treatment during this prodromal phase may limit the severity of the outbreak.

Although there is risk of sexual transmission of HSV in the presence of obvious ulcers, asymptomatic viral shedding is seen in both patients who have had primary genital infection and patients who have never exhibited symptoms of HSV. Patients with known HSV should be

> **BOX 20.3 Possible Indications for Serologic HSV Testing[8]**
>
> - Recurrent genital lesions/symptoms with negative polymerase chain reaction (PCR) testing
> - To obtain a confirmed diagnosis of genital herpes—clinical finding consistent with HSV without laboratory confirmation
> - Testing to determine the patient's infection status when a partner is diagnosed with HSV

counseled on the risk of transmission and the importance of consistent, correct condom use to decrease the risk. There is evidence that daily suppressive treatment with antivirals can decrease the risk of HSV-2 transmission between sexual partners, and it should therefore be offered to all patients diagnosed with HSV-2.[15] At this time there is no evidence regarding daily suppressive treatment and HSV-1 transmission.

The approach to treatment of HSV infection may include episodic treatment of outbreaks or daily suppressive treatment (see Table 20.2). Episodic treatment of primary HSV outbreaks is with acyclovir or valacyclovir, typically for 7 to 10 days or until resolution of symptoms. Recurrent outbreaks can be treated similarly, though the duration of treatment is shorter. Daily suppressive treatment for patients with recurrent or frequent HSV outbreaks can help prevent these symptomatic episodes. Pain management should not be overlooked and may include nonsteroidal antiinflammatory drugs (NSAIDs) and topical analgesics.

Routine screening for HSV is not recommended, though in a patient with concerning symptoms, HSV polymerase chain reaction (PCR) testing (scraping the base of an active lesion) is recommended. PCR may distinguish between HSV-1 and HSV-2, and this may be useful when counseling on natural history and the consideration of daily suppressive therapy. Serologic antibody testing for HSV-1 and HSV-2 is available and should be based on the HSV-specific glycoprotein G1 or G2. Possible indications for serologic testing are in Box 20.3. If serologic testing is performed, care should be taken when interpreting results because overinterpretation of indeterminant findings can have significant psychological ramifications on the patient.

Pelvic Inflammatory Disease

Pelvic inflammatory disease (PID) is an infection of the upper genital tract that may involve the endometrium, fallopian tubes, and/or ovaries. PID increases the risk of infertility, ectopic pregnancy, and chronic pelvic pain, and thus is associated with extremely high morbidity and cost. Prompt recognition and appropriate treatment are therefore critical.

The majority of PID has historically been attributed to *N. gonorrhoeae* and *C. trachomatis*. More recent studies, however, identify these organisms in only 25% to 50% of cases. PID is typically a polymicrobial infection, with anaerobic organisms, bacterial vaginosis–associated bacterium (BVAB), and even respiratory and enteric pathogens potentially playing a role in pathogenesis. *Mycoplasma genitalium* is also prevalent in persons with PID, though its precise role as a pathogen has yet to be fully elucidated.[16]

The primary presenting symptom of PID is typically lower abdominal or pelvic pain. Other symptoms may include vaginal discharge, abnormal vaginal bleeding, or urinary symptoms. Systemic symptoms such as fever occasionally are present. Mild gastrointestinal symptoms such as vomiting may be present but usually do not predominate the clinical picture. Symptoms may be subtle or even absent, and providers need to maintain a high index of suspicion for this diagnosis in sexually active adolescents with abdominal or pelvic pain.

PID is a clinical diagnosis, characterized by cervical motion tenderness, uterine tenderness, or adnexal tenderness on bimanual examination. The speculum examination may reveal mucopurulent cervicitis with cervical discharge and/or friability. White blood cells may be present on microscopic evaluation of cervicovaginal discharge. If there is no evidence of lower genital infection, alternative diagnoses should be considered. Other than STI testing and a urine pregnancy test, laboratory evaluation may not be necessary. If performed, laboratory tests may be normal or may be notable for leukocytosis or elevated inflammatory markers such as C-reactive protein (CRP). A fever over 101°F also supports the diagnosis of PID.

Most patients with PID can be successfully treated in the outpatient setting. Hospitalization may be considered for certain situations (Table 20.4), including failure to respond to outpatient therapy within 48 hours or difficulty taking oral medications due to nausea and vomiting. Antimicrobial therapy must cover *N. gonorrhoeae*, *C. trachomatis*, and anaerobic pathogens. Current recommended inpatient and outpatient treatment regimens are included in Table 20.5. Alternative treatment regimens may be found in the *CDC STI Treatment Guidelines, 2021*. Patients treated in the outpatient setting

---

TABLE 20.4   Criteria to Consider Hospitalization for PID Treatment[8]

Ill-appearing patient or unstable vital signs (e.g., hypotension, tachycardia)
Unable to tolerate oral medications
Tubo-ovarian abscess
No clinical response to outpatient treatment
Cannot exclude a surgical emergency (e.g., appendicitis)

TABLE 20.5   Pelvic Inflammatory Disease Treatment Regimens[8]

Outpatient Regimens (14 days)	Inpatient Regimens
Ceftriaxone 500 mg IM, single dose* PLUS Doxycycline 100 mg PO twice daily PLUS Metronidazole 500 mg PO twice daily	Cefoxitin 2 g IV every 6 hours PLUS Doxycycline 100 mg PO every 12 hours
Cefoxitin 2 g IM, single dose WITH Probenecid 1 g orally PLUS Doxycycline 100 mg PO twice daily PLUS Metronidazole 500 mg PO twice daily	Ceftriaxone 1 g IV every 12 hours PLUS Doxycycline 100 mg PO every 12 hours PLUS Metronidazole 500 mg PO or IV every 12 hours

IM, Intramuscular; *IV*, intravenous; *PO*, oral.
*Patients weighing >150 kg should receive Ceftriaxone 1 g IM

---

should be reevaluated 48 to 72 hours after initiation of treatment to ensure improvement. Patients treated in the inpatient setting can usually be transitioned to an oral regimen 24 to 48 hours after significant clinical improvement. They should complete a 14-day course of treatment with doxycycline and metronidazole.

Special Considerations in PID

Tubo-ovarian abscess. Tubo-ovarian abscess (TOA) is a serious complication of PID characterized by the presence of a complex inflammatory mass of the adnexa, often with associated peritonitis. Rupture of a TOA is rare but is a surgical emergency that can lead to sepsis. Patients who have been diagnosed with PID and are acutely ill-appearing, are febrile, have an adnexal mass felt on examination, or do not respond as expected to initial antibiotic therapy should be evaluated for TOA. Pelvic ultrasound is the preferred imaging modality. Most TOAs can be conservatively managed with parenteral PID regimens (see Table 20.5); interventional radiology may optimize therapy through localized drainage of the abscess. Surgery is rarely indicated but may be required for more extensive or recurrent disease.[17]

Patients with intrauterine device. If a pelvic infection is suspected or diagnosed at the time of planned intrauterine device (IUD) insertion, the insertion of the device should be delayed until the infection has completely resolved. If a patient develops PID with an IUD already in place, the device need not be removed (unless the patient requests removal) because most infections can be successfully treated with the IUD in place. Currently, the CDC does not provide specific guidelines for managing tubo-ovarian abscesses in women with IUDs. However, common protocols involve inpatient treatment with intravenous antibiotics, and the consideration of IUD removal if there is no observed clinical improvement.[18]

Mycoplasma genitalium[19]

M. genitalium, once considered an emerging infection, is recognized now as a genital pathogen that is likely sexually transmitted. *M. genitalium* has been identified in patients with cervicitis and PID at higher rates than in asymptomatic women, suggesting it may play a role in these conditions. Asymptomatic infection with *M. genitalium,* which may represent colonization, is also common, and the consequences are unknown.

Routine screening for *M. genitalium* is not recommended. In patients with persistent or recurrent cervicitis or PID that is refractory to treatment, endocervical NAAT for *M. genitalium* should be considered. If available, testing for macrolide resistance should be conducted given the high rate of treatment failures caused by macrolide resistance. Treatment is not recommended for asymptomatic patients. Symptomatic patients with positive testing should be treated with a two-step regimen including oral doxycycline for 7 days followed by either oral moxifloxacin for 7 days (if macrolide resistant or resistance is not known) or azithromycin for 4 days (if not macrolide resistant).

Chancroid[20]

Chancroid (caused by *Haemophilus ducreyi*) is very rarely diagnosed in North America in recent decades. The clinical

syndrome is characterized by painful ulcers (contrasted to the *painless* ulcer of syphilis), which appear within a week after initial infection, classically accompanied by suppurative inguinal adenopathy. Ulcers may be present on the vulvovaginal area or, less commonly, on the cervix.

Chancroid has been shown to enhance transmission of HIV-1. It is important to evaluate for HIV coinfection if a diagnosis of chancroid is made.

Diagnosis of chancroid is technically difficult, as there are no widely available tests for this organism. HSV can sometimes be mistaken for chancroid, and so testing of suspect lesions for both HSV and *H. ducreyi* is recommended if chancroid is suspected. Syphilis should also be ruled out. Treatment is with macrolides, fluoroquinolones, or cephalosporins.[10]

TREATMENT OF STIs

Prompt treatment of STIs is important to reduce the risk of complications and to limit transmission to sexual partners. Patients should be counseled to abstain from sexual intercourse for 7 days after treatment and that their partners should be notified and treated as well. Patients with a diagnosis of one STI should be tested for other STIs and HIV if this has not recently been done.

Test of cure immediately after treatment is not necessary if a recommended treatment regimen is used and symptoms (if any) have resolved. Patients with a diagnosis of chlamydia, gonorrhea, or trichomoniasis should return for repeat testing (test of reinfection) in 3 months because reinfection with the same or another organism is common in the months after treatment.

Treatment options for common STIs are included in Table 20.2. Up-to-date treatment guidelines for STIs, including more alternative regimens, may be found in the *CDC STI Treatment Guidelines, 2021.* The CDC also maintains a smartphone application that includes easy-to-search menus with the most recent treatment guidelines.

PREEXPOSURE PROPHYLAXIS FOR HIV

Preexposure prophylaxis (PrEP) is a medication regimen that can help prevent acquisition of HIV in people at risk for contracting the virus. PrEP is highly effective, reducing the risk of getting HIV from sex by about 99% when taken as prescribed. Adolescents may be candidates for PrEP if they have had anal or vaginal sex within the last 6 months and any of the following conditions: an HIV-positive

TABLE 20.6	**Follow-Up Recommendations for PrEP**[21]
Visit Interval	**Recommended Interventions**
Every 3 months	• HIV antigen/antibody tests; HIV-1 RNA assay • Assess medication adherence
Every 6 months	• Assess renal function in patients with CrCl <90 mL/min • Bacterial STI screening (gonorrhea, chlamydia, syphilis)
Yearly	• Assess renal function in all patients • Lipid panel

CrCl, Creatinine clearance.

sexual partner, a bacterial STI (specifically gonorrhea or syphilis in patients with a cervix), or inconsistent condom use during intercourse. It is appropriate to discuss and offer PrEP to any adolescent who wishes to reduce their risk of contracting HIV.[21]

Before starting PrEP, adolescents must have a documented negative HIV antigen/antibody test within 1 week and no signs and symptoms of acute HIV infection. For adolescents whose risk for HIV is through receptive vaginal intercourse, emtricitabine 200 mg/tenofovir disoproxil fumarate 300 mg (Truvada; Gilead) is the only approved medication. Other formulations of PrEP have not been evaluated in this population. The initial prescription is for daily medication, with up to a 90-day supply.

After the initial prescription of PrEP, patients need to be followed closely (Table 20.6). Some literature suggests that adolescents may need closer follow-up than adults to facilitate adherence to therapy.

Full prescribing information may be found in the CDC Clinical Practice Guideline[21] for PrEP. A brief informational video about PrEP for patients is also available.

PARTNER TREATMENT

Partner treatment is a critical component of management for all curable STIs. Partner notification of an STI diagnosis can be challenging for adolescents who are still learning to navigate and negotiate their sexual relationships. Health departments may provide assistance for persons with HIV or syphilis infection, but few have the resources to provide notification services for other STIs. Providers may help their patients by role-playing the conversation

with them or directing them to one of several online services that generate anonymous text messages to partners informing them of the diagnosis and need for treatment.

Ideally, partners will follow up with their own health care providers or at a local sexual health clinic for treatment as well as comprehensive assessment for other STIs and HIV. If a patient feels that their partner is unwilling or unlikely to pursue these services, expedited partner therapy (EPT) may be an option. With EPT, the provider prescribes medication for their patient's recent sex partners (typically defined as all partners within the past 2–3 months), and the patient delivers the medication (or prescription) to their partners along with written information about the STI diagnosis and prescribed treatment. There is evidence suggesting that the use of EPT may result in lower reinfection rates with chlamydia and gonorrhea compared with standard partner referral.[22,23]

The CDC supports the use of EPT as one option to facilitate partner treatment for gonorrhea and chlamydia. EPT is now permissible in most states, but legislation surrounding its implementation varies. Some states permit treatment for *Trichomoniasis* infections as well as gonorrhea and chlamydia. Some require the partner's name to be provided on the prescription; others do not. The CDC provides information on the use of EPT, including the legal status of EPT in each state, on its website (www.cdc.gov/std/ept). Providers must adhere to state law when providing EPT to their patients, including proper documentation of EPT provision.

Table 20.7 includes treatment regimens for EPT for partners with gonorrhea, chlamydia, or *Trichomoniasis*. Cismale partners may be treated for *Trichomoniasis* with a single dose of metronidazole. For gonococcal infections, every effort should be made to have the partner treated with IM ceftriaxone. If this is impossible, the use of oral cefixime may be considered.

KEY POINTS

- STIs are highly prevalent in AYAs.
- A comprehensive sexual history is key to understanding what screening a patient needs for STIs.
- Sexually active AYAs should be screened regularly for common STIs, including chlamydia and gonorrhea.
- PrEP is highly effective for the prevention of HIV in persons at risk for this infection.
- EPT is a valuable tool to facilitate timely treatment of sexual partners after diagnosis of a curable STI.

TABLE 20.7   Providing Expedited Partner Therapy

Partners must be provided with written information on the STI diagnosis, treatment prescribed (including use, risks, and side effects), and recommendation to seek comprehensive reproductive healthcare.

Infection	Treatment for Male Partners[a]	Treatment for Female Partners[b]
Neisseria gonorrhoeae	Cefixime 800 mg once[c]	Cefixime 800 mg once[c]
Chlamydia trachomatis	Doxycycline 100 mg twice daily × 7 days[d]	Doxycycline 100 mg twice daily × 7 days[d]
Trichomonas vaginalis	Metronidazole 2 g once	Metronidazole 500 mg twice daily × 7 days

All treatments listed are administered orally.
[a]Or any partner without a vagina/cervix.
[b]Or any partner with a vagina/cervix.
[c]Only if partner is unable to obtain treatment with ceftriaxone 500 mg intramuscular.
[d]Azithromycin 1 g orally × 1 may be considered if adherence to doxycycline therapy is considered unlikely.

REVIEW QUESTIONS

1. A healthy 15-year-old states that she would like to speak with you today about contraception and sexual health. She asks to speak with you alone, as she has not yet told her parents that she is sexually active. She asks if she needs her parents' permission to start birth control and to be tested for sexually transmitted infections. You inform her that:
   a. She may consent to STI services without her parents' permission.
   b. She may consent to birth control without her parents' permission.
   c. She needs her parents' consent for all sexual health services.

2. A sexually active patient asks what STI screening tests she needs today. She was first sexually active 6 months ago at age 15 and has had one cisgender male partner. They have oral sex and vaginal sex, and she reports they use condoms every single time. She has never had STI screening and would like to know what tests you recommend for her today. Which of the following should you order?
   a. Vaginal swab for gonorrhea and chlamydia using a NAAT
   b. Vaginal swab for HPV using PCR
   c. Serum for HIV
   d. Serum for HSV

3. A 16-year-old cisgender female presents with 3 days of pelvic pain and irregular vaginal bleeding. Her last period was 2 weeks ago. She is sexually active with a cisgender male partner for 6 months. They do not use condoms. On examination, she is uncomfortable but not ill-appearing, with significant bilateral lower quadrant tenderness. You perform a bimanual examination and speculum examination, which is notable for a friable cervix, white vaginal discharge, and bilateral adnexal tenderness. She denies nausea and reports she can return to the clinic within a few days for a follow-up visit. Which of the following treatments do you prescribe?
   a. Ceftriaxone IM once and oral doxycycline for 14 days
   b. Ciprofloxacin orally for 14 days
   c. Ceftriaxone IM once, oral doxycycline for 14 days, and oral metronidazole for 14 days
   d. Ceftriaxone IM only

STI Resources

1. Online STI Training Opportunities
   A. National STD Curriculum (uw.edu)
      i. A free educational website from the University of Washington STD Prevention Training Center
      ii. Includes quick references, self-study modules, and question bank
   B. STD Clinical Slides: Download clinical images to be used for self-study or other education purposes (https://www.cdc.gov/std/products/infographics.htm)
2. Online support for patient care
   A. STI Treatment Guidelines, 2021
      i STI Treatment Guidelines – Pocket Card
   B. A Guide to Taking a Sexual History
      1. Video: Let's Talk About Sexual Health for providers and young adults
      2. Brief sexual behavior questions for all patients

C. Minors' consent laws by state

D. STD Clinical Consultation Network – Course consultative services for providers with challenging STI clinical questions

3. PrEP Resources

A. CDC PrEP Basics

   i. https://www.cdc.gov/hiv/basics/prep.html

   ii. https://www.youtube.com/watch?time_continue=3&v=1_eo17YahCo&feature=emb_title

   iii. Clinicians' Quick Guide: Preexposure Prophylaxis for the Prevention of HIV Infection in the United States – 2021 Update

B. Comprehensive Prescribing Resources

   i. Preexposure Prophylaxis for the Prevention of HIV Infection in the United States – 2021 Update

   ii. Clinical Provider Supplement for PrEP

4. EPT Resources

A. CDC State Guidelines (https://www.cdc.gov/std/ept/legal/default.htm)

5. Patient-Facing Education

A. Amaze.org: Brief, medically accurate educational videos for adolescents on STI and HIV

B. CDC – STD Fact Sheets

6. Podcasts

A. National STD Curriculum podcast reviews and updates on a variety of clinical STI topics

B. STI podcast on Apple Podcasts and BMJ podcast discussing STI issues, including clinical and more global topics

REFERENCES

1. Centers for Disease Control and Prevention. *2019 Youth Risk Behavior Survey Data*. CDC.gov; Updated November 22, 2022. Accessed April 4, 2023. www.cdc.gov/yrbs

2. Barbee L, Blain M, Cannon C, et al. *National STD Curriculum*. 2nd ed. University of Washington; Updated October 5, 2021. Accessed October 26, 2022. https://www.std.uw.edu/

3. Maslyanskaya S, Alderman E. Confidentiality and consent in the care of the adolescent patient. *Pediatr Rev*. 2019; 40(10):508-516. https://doi.org/10.1542/pir.2018-0040

4. Committee on Adolescent Health Care. ACOG committee opinion no. 803: confidentiality in adolescent health care. *Obstet Gynecol*. 2020;135(4):171-177.

5. Grilo S, Catallozzi M, Santelli JS, et al. Confidentiality discussions and private time with a health-care provider for youth. *J Adolesc Health*. 2019;64(3):311-318. https://doi.org/10.1016/j.jadohealth.2018.10.301

6. Centers for Disease Control and Prevention. *Let's Talk About Sexual Health*. YouTube; Published November 30, 2012. Accessed November 29, 2022. https://www.youtube.com/watch?v=dvmb9eUu0p4&feature=emb_title

7. Public Policy Office. *Minors' Access to STI Services*. Guttmacher Institute; Updated March 1, 2023. Accessed April 4, 2023. https://www.guttmacher.org/state-policy/explore/minors-access-sti-services

8. Workowski KA, Bachmann L, Chan P, et al. Sexually transmitted infections, 2021. *MMWR Recomm Rep*. 2021;70(No. RR-04):1-187.

9. Papp J, Schachter J, Gaydos C, Van der Pol B. Recommendations for the laboratory-based detection of Chlamydia trachomatis and Neisseria gonorrhoeae–2014. *MMWR Reccom Rep*. 2014;63(RR02):1-19.

10. *FDA Clears First Diagnostic Tests for Extragenital Testing for Chlamydia and Gonorrhea*. United States Food and Drug Administration; Published May 23, 2019. Accessed October 25, 2022. https://www.fda.gov/news-events/press-announcements/fda-clears-first-diagnostic-tests-extragenital-testing-chlamydia-and-gonorrhea

11. Mosure DJ, Berman S, Fine D, DeLisle S, Cates W Jr, Boring JR III. Genital Chlamydia infections in sexually active female adolescents: do we really need to screen everyone? *J Adolesc Health*. 1997;20(1):6-13.

12. Khosropour CM, Dombrowski JC, Vojtech L, et al. Rectal Chlamydia trachomatis infection: a narrative review of the state of the science and research priorities. *Sex Transm Dis*. 2021;48(12):e223-e227. doi:10.1097/OLQ.000000000000154

13. US Preventive Services Task Force. Screening for syphilis infection in nonpregnant adolescents and adults: US Preventive Services Task Force reaffirmation recommendation statement. *JAMA*. 2022;328(12):1243-1249.

14. Bernstein D, Bellamy A, Hookill E, et al. Epidemiology, clinical presentation, and antibody response to primary infection with herpes simplex virus type 1 and type 2 in young women. *Clin Infect Dis*. 2013;56(3):344-351. doi:10.1093/cid/cis891

15. Wald A, Zeh J, Selke S, et al. Reactivation of genital herpes simplex virus type 2 infection in asymptomatic seropositive persons. *N Engl J Med*. 2000;342(12):844-850. https://doi.org/10.1056/NEJM200003233421203

16. Mitchell CM, Anyalechi GE, Cohen CR, Haggerty CL, Manhart LE, Hillier SL. Etiology and diagnosis of pelvic inflammatory disease: looking beyond gonorrhea and chlamydia. *J Infect Dis*. 2021;224(12 suppl 2):S29-S35. doi:10.1093/infdis/jiab067

17. Lareau S, Biegi R. Pelvic inflammatory disease and tubo-ovarian abscess. *Infect Dis Clin North Am.* 2008;22(4):693-708. doi:10.1016/j.idc.2008.05.008

18. Curtis K, Jatlaoui T, Tepper N, et al. US selected practice recommendations for contraceptive use, 2016. *MMWR Recomm Rep.* 2016;65(4):1-66.

19. DiMarco DE, Urban MA, McGowan JP, et al. *Mycoplasma Genitalium Management in Adults.* NYSDOH AIDS Institute: Clinical Guidelines Program; Published September 2020. https://www.ncbi.nlm.nih.gov/books/NBK583532/

20. Lewis D. Epidemiology, clinical features, diagnosis and treatment of Haemophilus ducreyi – a disappearing pathogen? *Expert Rev Anti Infect Ther.* 2014;12(6):687-696. doi:10.1586/14787210.2014.892414

21. US Public Health Service. *Preexposure Prophylaxis for the Prevention of HIV Infection in the United States – 2021 Update Clinical Practice Guideline.* Centers for Disease Control and Prevention; Published 2021. Accessed October 22, 2022. https://www.cdc.gov/hiv/pdf/risk/prep/cdc-hiv-prep-guidelines-2021.pdf

22. Schillinger JA, Kissinger P, Calvet H, et al. Patient-delivered partner treatment with azithromycin to prevent repeated Chlamydia trachomatis infection among women: a randomized, controlled trial. *Sex Transm Dis.* 2003;30(1):49-56. doi:10.1097/00007435-200301000-00011

23. Golden MR, Whittington WL, Handsfield HH, et al. Effect of expedited treatment of sex partners on recurrent or persistent gonorrhea or chlamydial infection. *N Engl J Med.* 2005;352(7):676-685. doi:10.1056/NEJMoa041681

Contraception

Amanda V. French

INTRODUCTION AND BACKGROUND

Why Is Contraception Important?

Contraception is the practice that allows a person to prevent pregnancy. Between 2015 and 2017, approximately 40% of never-married teenagers ages 15 to 19 years had had sexual intercourse.[1] Although the percentage has trended slightly downward since 2002, the proportion is still significant.

In 2010, there were 57 pregnancies per 1000 females ages 15 to 19 years in the United States,[2] which translates to 600,000 teen pregnancies annually.[3] For those ages 10 to 14 years, there were 1.08 pregnancies per 1000 females in 2010. Despite the declining birth rate—17.4 births per 1000 adolescents in 2018[4]—teens ages 15 to 19 still have the highest rate of unintended pregnancy of all age groups.[5]

Teens are at risk for sexually transmitted infections (STIs). The Centers for Disease Control and Prevention (CDC) data show that those ages 15 to 24 acquire half of all new STIs. In 2018, the rate of reported chlamydia was 3306 cases per 100,000 females ages 15 to 19, which was 1.3% higher than the 2017 reported rate. For this age group, reported gonorrhea cases in 2018 were 548.1 per 100,000 females—also higher than the 2017 rate[6] (see Chapter 20). Dual contraceptive method use (barrier plus another contraceptive) is therefore especially important for adolescents.

According to the National Center for Health Statistics (NCHS) Data Brief in 2015, sexually active adolescent females most commonly choose external condoms, withdrawal, and oral contraceptive pills for contraception.[1] These short-acting methods have more opportunity for human error, and therefore higher failure rates. Fewer teens choose long-acting reversible methods, which have lower failure rates (perfect and typical use rates are the same, with efficacy >99%). For those who choose short-acting methods, there are many apps and reminder alarms to help remember when the next dose is due or to trigger refill notifications.

The Pearl Index: What Is It?

The Pearl Index (PI), expressed as number of contraceptive failures per 100 woman-years (HWY) of use, estimates contraceptive efficacy (Table 21.1). The PI is calculated two ways: "actual" or "typical" use includes all pregnancies that occur in all months of exposure to the contraception method in a study, and "perfect" use includes only pregnancies in subjects who use the contraceptive method correctly and only during the period in which perfect use occurred. The PI is calculated by dividing the number of unintended pregnancies by the number of months the contraception was used.[7]

$$PI = (\text{number of pregnancies} \times 12) \times 100 / (\text{number of women in the study} \times \text{duration of the study in months})$$

If no contraception is used, the PI is 85 for both perfect and typical use. Counseling should be based on typical use. Life table methods are also used to calculate the probability of a contraceptive failure, but unlike PI, do not assume a constant failure over time, and thus attempt to eliminate the time-related bias of the PI calculation.

SPECIAL CONSIDERATIONS IN TEENS: CONTRACEPTIVE COUNSELING

Contraception Counseling

Contraception counseling is an important interaction between patient and health care provider. Care must be

TABLE 21.1 Pearl Index Stratified by Efficacy of Commonly Used Contraceptive Methods

Method	Estimated Pearl Index for Typical Use (Ranked by Lowest to Highest Failure Rate)
Etonogestrel implant	0.1 (most effective)
Levonorgestrel IUD	0.7
Copper IUD	0.8
Depot medroxyprogesterone	4
Combined estrogen/progesterone oral contraceptives	7
Progesterone-only oral contraceptives	7
Estrogen/progesterone patches	7
Estrogen/progesterone vaginal ring	7
Diaphragm	12
Condoms (external/internal)	13 for external condoms, 21 for internal condoms
Withdrawal	20
Cervical cap	23
Spermicide	28
Gel	28 (least effective)

IUD, Intrauterine device.
Remember: A higher PI means more frequent contraceptive failure!

taken to avoid coercion and influence of personal or institutional bias and to intentionally keep in mind the patient's values and background, as there is a long history of reproductive mistreatment, in particular for marginalized persons.[8] Cost, time constraints or inability to go to a clinic, legal restrictions, lack of knowledge or misinformation, social or cultural concerns, and health care provider or parental attitudes are additional examples of barriers teens face when seeking contraception.

A Guttmacher report estimates that 21 million women were in need of publicly funded contraception supplies or services in 2016 because of being under the age of 20 or because of an income level below 250% of the poverty level. For the privately insured, the Affordable Care Act

(outlined in the Health Resources and Services Administration Women's Preventative Services Guidelines), as well as some state laws, require most private health plans to cover Food and Drug Administration (FDA)–approved contraceptive methods and counseling. [9]

By removing financial and access barriers, the Contraceptive CHOICE Project[10] promoted long-acting reversible contraceptives (LARCs) to reduce unintended pregnancy. Although both the American Academy of Pediatrics (AAP) and the American College of Obstetricians and Gynecologists (ACOG) recommend LARC (see Table 21.5) as safe and effective first-line contraception for teens, they are not often used.[11] In the CHOICE study, 14- to 17-year-olds choosing LARC preferred the subdermal implant; 18- to 20-year-olds preferred the intrauterine device (IUD). Among the 14- to 19-year-olds, 82% of LARC users were still using their method at 12 months, compared with 49% of non-LARC contraceptive users. There was no significant change in number of sexual partners in any of the groups at 12 months. However, the overall numbers of pregnancy, birth, and abortion among CHOICE teen participants were significantly lower, illustrating that when comprehensive counseling is provided and barriers are removed, more teens choose LARC and continue to use it.[12]

Consent and confidentiality for adolescents must be considered. Adolescents have the right to confidentiality; however, many factors, including electronic medical records and laws, pose challenges.[13] The Guttmacher Institute has a chart that shows current state laws[14] and policies that are helpful when navigating confidentiality and consent questions (Table 21.2).[15] (See Chapter 2.) Education is also important. Comprehensive sex education (CSE) has been shown to increase communication between teens and parents or medical providers and improve media literacy,[16] which is valuable as many adolescents use the Internet as a primary information source. The Title X family planning program is a federal grant program to provide comprehensive and confidential reproductive health counseling and services; in 2019, 17% of patients seen at a Title X clinic were younger than age 20.[17] School-based health centers may also provide convenient services for teens, but unfortunately many do not provide contraception.[18]

Shared decision making is a process to ensure teens pick a contraceptive option that works best for them (Table 21.3 and Box 21.1 provide information on how

TABLE 21.2   Quick Resources for Patients and Providers

Organization	Link
HealthyChildren, section on Teen, Dating & Sex, American Academy of Pediatrics	HealthyChildren.org
CDC US Medical Eligibility Criteria for Contraceptive Use, available on the CDC website or as a free app	App: US MEC and US SPR Website: cdc.gov
For Patients, Healthy Teens, American College of Obstetricians and Gynecologists	Acog.org
Resources for Adolescents and Parents, Society for Adolescent Health and Medicine	Adolescenthealth.org
For Patients, Patient Handouts and Resources for Patients, North American Society for Pediatric and Adolescent Gynecology	Naspag.org
Birth Control, Planned Parenthood	Plannedparenthood.org
An Overview of Consent to Reproductive Health Services by Young People, Guttmacher Institute	Guttmacher.org

TABLE 21.3   Tips for Adolescent Contraceptive Counseling[35]

How to begin	• Use language that is understandable for teens. • Provide age-appropriate handouts and information sources. • Maintain confidentiality and know your state laws. • Ensure decision making is shared and reflects the goals and wishes of the patient.
What to address during the visit	• What are the patient's goals? Contraception? Menstrual suppression? Medical benefits of contraception (acne, for example)? Gender-related concerns? • What does the patient already know? • A complete history, including personal and family history and any medications. • Pay close attention for any contraindications to types of contraception. • Sexual history—is sexually transmitted infection (STI) screening indicated? • Cost of method and can they do the method consistently? • Any questions or concerns?
Information to provide	• What are the options, the risks and benefits, the instructions for use? • How to start using the chosen method, and how long it takes to "work." • What kinds of things to seek medical attention for. • When to come back for a follow-up visit.
Things to consider	• Acknowledge reproductive mistreatment of marginalized individuals. • Be cognizant of bias (yours and those around you). • Prioritize the patient's values, preferences and lived experiences.[8]

Adapted from Todd N, Black A. Contraception for Adolescents. J Clin Res Pediatr Endocrinol. 2020;12(Suppl 1):28-40. doi:10.4274/jcrpe.galenos.2019.2019.S0003.[22]
Remember: Dispelling myths and sharing benefits are key features of birth control counseling.

to start a conversation about contraception). The ACOG recommends an initial reproductive health visit between the ages of 13 and 15,[19] which is an opportunity to establish rapport, answer questions, and provide education. *Of note, a pelvic examination is not required for initiation of contraception.* To easily review contraceptive methods, medical conditions, side effects, and contraindications, the US Medical Eligibility Criteria (MEC) for Contraceptive Use has a free mobile application (see Table 21.2).[20] *It should be noted that none of the reversible contraceptive choices impair long-term fertility potential.*[21]

Adolescents may or may not choose to have relationships that include sexual activity. They may use terms like *outercourse* and *abstinence*, which have varied meanings to different people, but generally include sexual activities with the exception of penis-in-vagina intercourse. Providers can and should discuss healthy

"I want you to achieve your personal goals, complete your education, and live your best life, and part of that is avoiding pregnancy before you are ready. I would like to be a part of that conversation with you."

relationships and educate teens that oral sex, anal sex, and manual stimulation all carry a small risk of introducing semen into the vagina and could result in pregnancy and/or STI (see Table 21.3). Best practices for adolescent health care include taking a sexual health history, screening for STI, counseling, and providing contraception access. Medical offices can provide explicit descriptions of confidential services rendered. Sensitive topics are best discussed with the adolescent alone in an honest, nonjudgmental, supportive environment, keeping in mind the patient's age.

The overall risk of developing cancer over a lifetime is similar among women who have used birth control and women who have not used birth control. In fact, newer studies are showing birth control users may have a lower chance of developing cancer. Using birth control pills may have an estimated net increase of life expectancy of 1 to 2 months, in addition to effects from preventing unwanted pregnancy.[23]

What Are the Choices for Contraception?

The choices are briefly outlined in Tables 21.4 and 21.5. There are hormonal and nonhormonal as well as short- and long-acting options. Surgical sterilization and fertility awareness methods (charting temperature, ovulation, and cervical mucus) are not generally used by adolescents.

Pills, Patches, and Rings

Oral contraceptive pills (OCs) are used by approximately one-fourth of women between the ages of 15 and 44. Combination OCs (COCs), as well as hormonal patches and rings, are a combination of estrogen and progestin. The mechanism of action is the result of multiple factors. Progestin feeds back to the hypothalamus and decreases gonadotropin-releasing hormone (GnRH) pulse frequency, which reduces follicle-stimulating hormone (FSH) and luteinizing hormone (LH) secretion, which in turn inhibits ovarian follicle development and prevents ovulation. Progestin also thickens cervical mucus, preventing sperm from advancing to the upper genital tract.[24] Effects on fallopian tube motility and receptivity of the endometrium may also affect fertilization and implantation. Adding estrogen increases the potency of the progestin effects. Estrogen weakly inhibits FSH and stabilizes the endometrium, which minimizes irregular bleeding.[25] OCs, patches, and rings must be prescribed in the United States but are easy to initiate and discontinue and can manage excess menstrual bleeding, pain, menstrual migraines, premenstrual dysphoric disorder, irregular menstrual bleeding, endometriosis, hirsutism, and acne. They have been shown to decrease the risk of endometrial cancer, ovarian cancer, and colon cancer.[26-28]

Progestin-only methods include pills (POP), which contain either norethindrone or drospirenone. In addition to the progestational effects, drospirenone has antimineralocorticoid activity, which could lessen complaints of fluid retention. Different synthetic progestins are used in IUDs, which contain levonorgestrel (LNG), and the contraceptive implant, which contains etonogestrel (see Table 21.5).

COCs include varying doses of estrogen and various types and doses of progestin. The estrogen component is either estradiol, ethinyl estradiol (EE), or estetrol. The majority of COCs currently available contain between 10 and 35 µg EE.

The various options for starting and continuing OCs are tailored to patient preference (Box 21.2, Box 21.3 and Box 21.5). The "quick start" method may improve compliance without significant side effects.[29]

When initiating contraception, discuss possible side effects Box 21.6 and what to expect and when to call for advice to impart realistic expectations. Taking pills at night or with food may mitigate nausea, or antiemetics may be considered for those with severe initial symptoms. Teens may have different schedules on weekends and weekdays; navigating new medicine or side effects during school may be an issue. If unscheduled bleeding occurs when taking pills continuously, options for management include taking a 4-day pill-free interval then restarting active pills or taking two pills a day for several days until bleeding stops. If more than one pill is taken in a single day, side effects like nausea are more common; antiemetic medication can be helpful. Taking pills with food can also help curb nausea. Common practice is to see an adolescent in the office for a visit that includes a blood pressure check and addressing concerns or questions about 3 months after newly starting an OC,

TABLE 21.4 What Are the Choices for Contraception?

What Is the Name of the Contraception Method?	How Do You Use It?	Why Would You Pick This?	Myths and Common Concerns	Why Would You Avoid It (see US MEC for Comprehensive Information)?
The pill (combined oral contraceptive, or COC)	Take once daily at the same time; usually taking it after dinner is the easiest way to stay consistent and avoid nausea. Choices for how to start taking pills? See Box 21.4	Easy to start, easy to stop. Can help with heavy bleeding, cramps, acne, ovarian cysts, mood changes associated with cycles, and irregular periods	Does COC cause weight gain? There are no data to support that this is true. What if family members have breast cancer? COC users do not appear to have an increased risk for breast cancer. What if I cannot swallow pills? Chewable pills are available. Is a lighter period normal when taking COCs? Yes, because the lining of the uterus is less thick when on COC.	Side effects are usually mild: headaches, nausea, breast tenderness. If any history or increased risk for venous thromboembolism (VTE), you should not take COCs. If you cannot remember to take a pill every day. Will not protect against STI.
Progestin-only pills (POPs)	Same as COC (see above) Norethindrone pills: a 28-day pack without hormone-free pills Drospirenone: 28-day packs have four hormone-free pills	If estrogen is contraindicated	Backup contraception recommended if POPs are started more than 5 days from menses onset or if POP is taken more than 3 hours late.	Not as effective for acne. Increased chance of irregular bleeding versus COC. Will not protect against STI. More exact dosing than COC.
The patch There are two types: 1. Ethinyl estradiol 35 mcg and norelgestromin 150 mcg (EE/N) 2. Ethinyl estradiol 30 mcg and levonorgestrel 120 mcg (EE/LNG)	Apply and replace a patch once a week to a clean, dry area of skin on the abdomen, buttocks, or back. EE/N patch can also be applied to the upper arm. Do not put patch on the breast. Rotate location to avoid skin irritation. Patches are changed once a week for 3 weeks, followed by a patch-free week when menses occur. If a patch is placed late (>48 h) or peels or falls off for more than 24 hours, a backup method is needed for 1 week	Only need to change the patch once a week. Good option if ingesting oral medicine is difficult or causes side effects	Will it stick? The patch becoming unstuck and skin irritation are uncommon. Patch is good for up to 9 days even though instructions say to change it at 7 days of use. Can you see it? The patch is visible on the skin and only comes in one color. You can put the patch on your body in a place that is not visible to others.	Patches have similar systemic side effects, contraindications, and benefit profiles as COCs. The average serum EE concentration is higher with patch versus COC, and there may be a small increased risk for VTE[30], overall risk is still low. There is a "black box warning" for EE/N patch: contraindicated if body mass index (BMI) ≥30 kg/m^2 (increased VTE risk). Patches may be less effective in obese users.[31]

Method	Instructions	Benefits	Common questions	Risks and contraindications
The vaginal ring There are two types: 1. ENG/EE: 120 mcg per day of etonogestrel (ENG) and 15 mcg/day of ethinyl estradiol 2. 150 mcg segesterone acetate and 13 mcg ethinyl estradiol (SA/EE)	1. ENG/EE ring is inserted into the vagina for 21 days, then removed for 7 days and discarded, during which time menstruation occurs, and then a new ring is inserted 2. SA/EE ring is inserted for 21 days and removed for 7 days, but you reinsert and use the *same ring* for thirteen 28-day cycles	Rings are more private than COC Nausea and breast tenderness are less common with rings, compared with COC[32] Both rings are plastic and latex-free	Will it fall out? It generally does not, and if it does, push it back into the vagina. Can I put it in the wrong place? The ring releases hormone so it only needs to be in the vagina and feel comfortable.	Risks and contraindications similar to COC. Both contraceptive rings must be inserted into the vagina by the user. Local irritation is possible; toxic shock syndrome is possible but rare. SA/EE ring is slightly larger than the ENG/EE ring.
The shot (DMPA) There are two versions: 1. Intramuscular, 150 mg of depot medroxyprogesterone 2. Subcutaneous, 104 mg of depot medroxyprogesterone (DMPA-SC)	Start anytime it is reasonably certain that you are not pregnant Shots are given every 11–13 weeks	Privacy, high efficacy, and a convenient dose schedule Can self-inject DMPA-SC *Tends to decrease incidence of seizures; helpful for those with epilepsy*[33]	What if I am late for my shot? Injections can be given up to 2 weeks late (15 weeks from previous shot) without a need for additional contraceptive backup.	Subcutaneous injections are often preferred over intramuscular injection in persons with bleeding disorders to avoid intramuscular hematoma. Irregular bleeding is common. Ovulation may not resume for up to a year after the last shot.
Cervical cap and diaphragm	Prescription only Both are silicone cups Both must be filled with spermicide and inserted into the vagina to cover the cervix Cervical cap is smaller Both must be left in for at least 6 hours after sex	No hormones Devices are reusable	Must use for every episode of sex. Cannot leave a cervical cap in for more than 2 days after sex. Cannot leave a diaphragm in for more than 24 hours after sex.	Cervical caps and diaphragms require advanced planning and can be challenging to insert, messy, and do not protect against STI. Toxic shock syndrome has not been reported with cervical cap use, but has been reported with the diaphragm.[34]
External condom (formerly known as *male condom*)	Latex, plastic, or synthetic worn over the penis	No hormones Protects against sexually transmitted infection (STI) Easy to buy Do not need a prescription, sometimes can get them at school[36]	Single use only. Be aware of latex allergy for condoms made with latex.	Must use correct technique. Check the expiration date. Recommended in addition to hormonal methods for protection against STI.

Continued

TABLE 21.4 What Are the Choices for Contraception?—cont'd

What Is the Name of the Contraception Method?	How Do You Use It?	Why Would You Pick This?	Myths and Common Concerns	Why Would You Avoid It (see US MEC for Comprehensive Information)?
Internal condom (formerly known as *female condom*)	Sheath with a ring at each end—one ring is inserted into the vagina and the other ring hangs out about an inch from the vaginal opening	No hormones Protects against STI Do not need a prescription Easy to buy	Single use only. Be aware of latex allergy for condoms made with latex.	Must use correct technique. Check the expiration date. Recommended in addition to hormonal methods for protection against STI.
Spermicide	Can and should be used with condoms, diaphragms, and cervical caps Available over the counter as cream, gel, foam, suppository, or film Insert deep into vagina at least 10–15 minutes before intercourse	No hormones Do not need a prescription Easy to buy	Must be repeated if more than 1 hour passes before sex or if intercourse is going to happen again.	Higher failure rate compared with other methods if used alone. Must use for every episode of sex. Does not protect against STI. Can be messy or cause local irritation.
Withdrawal ("pulling out")	The penis is withdrawn from the vagina before ejaculation			Higher failure rate compared with other methods. Does not provide STI protection. Widely practiced; providers should proactively ask adolescents about this behavior and encourage them to choose more effective contraception methods.
The sponge	A plastic spermicide-containing sponge Insert into vagina up to 24 hours before sex Works by physically blocking the cervix Sponge must be left in place for 6 hours after sex	No prescription needed	Single use only. Must insert into vagina every episode of sex.	Higher failure rate compared with other methods. Does not protect against STI. Can be messy or cause local irritation. Toxic shock has been reported.[37]
Contraceptive gel	Prescription gel: lactic acid, citric acid, and potassium bitartrate Makes vaginal pH more acidic (inhospitable to sperm) 5 g vaginally via applicator up to 1 hour before sex	Not spermicide and not hormonal Can use with oral contraceptives	Single use only. Must insert into vagina every episode of sex.	Higher failure rate compared with other methods. Does not protect against STI. Cannot use with vaginal ring. Can be messy or cause local irritation.

Adapted from Nichole A. Tyson: Reproductive Health: Options, Strategies, and Empowerment of Women. Obstetrics and Gynecology Clinics of North America Volume 46, Issue 3, September 2019, Pages 409-430.[38]

TABLE 21.5 Long-Acting Reversible Contraceptives (LARCs)

Type of LARC	How Does It Work?	Why Would You Choose It?	Common Myths and Questions	Why Would You Avoid It?
The implant Contains 68 mg of etonogestrel	Matchstick-sized implant, placed in the inner side of the nondominant arm (8–10 cm from medial epicondyle and 3–5 cm below the groove between the biceps and triceps) Releases progestin Local anesthesia for placement and removal Pressure bandage for 24 hours	Very effective for contraception, FDA approved for 3 years of use, but data suggest that it is effective for up to 5 years[39]	Can you feel it? Yes, and you should be able to feel it. The implant can stay in for up to 4 years. How does it come out? Easily removed under local anesthesia. Can I get another one in the same spot? Yes! Will the implant cause weight gain? Implant users do not seem to gain more weight than nonusers.	Persistent irregular bleeding is the most common reason for having an implant removed Lower continuation rates for the implant as compared with IUD or depot medroxyprogesterone, mostly because of irregular bleeding[40] For those who wish to totally suppress menses, the implant may not be the best choice; it is an ideal option for those who experience cramps, as Nexplanon is a treatment for dysmenorrhea Insertion requires trained provider (Nexplanon.com)[41] Implant migration to other parts of the body is very rare
Intrauterine device (IUD) There are five types: 1. 52 mg of levonorgestrel (LNG), up to 8 years of use 2. 19.5 mg LNG, up to 5 years of use 3. 13.5 mg LNG, up to 3 years of use 4. Copper (Cu-IUD), up to 12 years of use	Small, plastic, T-shaped device, inserted into uterus, that works by preventing fertilization LNG IUD also releases progestin, thickens cervical mucus, thins endometrial lining	LNG IUD can treat heavy menstrual bleeding, even in the setting of bleeding disorders,[42] dysmenorrhea, and endometriosis[43,44] IUD has no significant drug interactions with other medications Very effective for contraception Long lasting	Only the Cu-IUD and the 52-mg LNG IUD can be used for emergency contraception (Table 21.6). Can be placed with or without local anesthesia or sedation. Can be placed at any time during the menstrual cycle. 52-mg LNG IUD and Cu-IUD have immediate contraceptive efficacy—other IUDs require backup method for 7 days. Is there a risk for ectopic pregnancy with an IUD in place? The risk of ANY pregnancy is very small, so the overall risk of ectopic pregnancy with an IUD is not increased.	52-mg LNG IUD is most associated with amenorrhea Light bleeding is common, especially in first 3–6 months of use, usually more favorable by 1 year Cu-IUD cannot be used if patient has copper allergy Adolescent consent for LARC is based on state law (see information supplied by the Guttmacher Institute)[14] Complete confidentiality may not be possible when billing for devices and insertion, especially if sedation is used or complications occur Should not place IUD with active pelvic infection, uterine anomaly, or distorted uterine cavity Cu-IUD users may have heavier menses Toxic shock syndrome has been reported[45] Uterine perforation and device expulsion are uncommon

BOX 21.2   Benefits of Hormonal Birth Control

Helps prevent against:
Ovarian cysts
Iron-deficiency anemia
Reduces:
Menstrual cramps
Menstrual bleeding problems
Ovulation pain
Excess hair on face or body
Acne
Symptoms of polycystic ovarian syndrome (irregular bleeding, acne, excess hair on face or body)
Symptoms of endometriosis (pelvic pain, irregular bleeding)
Premenstrual syndrome
Menstrual migraine headaches
Asthma
Ovarian cancer in those with BRCA1 and BRCA2

BOX 21.3   Dispelling Myths

Does not cause a build-up of hormones in a person's body
Birth control users do not need a rest from taking birth control
Does not make people infertile after they stop taking COCs
Does not cause birth defects or multiple births
Does not change sexual behavior or make a young person have their first sexual experience earlier
The birth control pill does not collect in the stomach; instead, the pill dissolves each day
Does not disrupt an existing pregnancy
Does not cause long-term fertility concerns; return to fertility occurs within 2 months after stopping

COC, Combined oral contraceptive.

BOX 21.4   How Do You Take OCs?

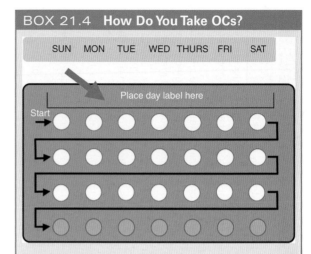

Tip: Set a daily alarm on your phone for the time you take your pill!
Quick start: Start pills immediately on any day of the cycle after a negative pregnancy test. The packs come with stickers to change the days of the week on the top row. You will start every pack on that same day of the week moving forward and take one pill every day at the same time.
Cyclically: Start at the first pill in the pack when your period starts. Take one active pill every day at the same time, in order, for 28 days. The last 7 days of a 28-day pill pack do not contain hormones; this is the week that menstrual bleeding happens. You will have a period every month.
Continuously: Start at the first pill in the pack. Take one active pill every day at the same time, in order, for 21 days. Discard the last week of pills and start a new pack of pills without taking any breaks. You will not have a period.
Extended use: Start at the first pill in the pack. Take only the 21 active pills for two packs, then take all 28 pills for the third pack. You will have a period every 3 months.

the patch, or the ring. The teen is routinely seen annually thereafter or as concerns or issues arise.

Adolescence is a crucial time for bone accrual. In teens, COCs have been associated with smaller gains or loss of bone mass, especially in the first 3 years after menarche, though long-term effects are not well understood. OCs with the lowest doses of EE (20 mcg) seem to provide inadequate sex steroids for optimal bone accrual.[46,47]

BOX 21.5   What Happens If You Are Taking an OC and You Miss One?

If one pill is missed, it is taken as soon as possible, and the next tablet is taken at the usual time. If two pills in a row are missed in the first or second week of a pill pack, backup contraception must be used. The user takes two pills the day the error is realized, then two pills the next day, then returns to one pill per day.

BOX 21.6 What Kinds of Risks and Side Effects Are There for Teens Using Hormonal Contraception?

- Irregular bleeding, nausea, breast tenderness, and mild headache usually need no treatment and will self-resolve.
- Weight gain is a common concern, but **people who use birth control and people who do not use birth control gain the same amount of weight over time**.[25]
- Blood clots (venous thromboembolism, or VTE) are **rare** in teens:
  - Baseline risk for VTE is about 1 in 10,000 (nonusers).
  - Risk for VTE for low-dose COC users is about 3–4 in 10,000. **(The risk for VTE in pregnancy and postpartum is about 20 per 10,000.)**
  - Risk for VTE is highest in the first 6 months of OC use and then decreases.
  - **If high risk for VTE, progestin-only contraception is preferred.**
- Signs of VTE: Consider "**ACHES**": **A**, abdominal pain (gallbladder, liver adenoma, pancreatitis); **C**, chest pain (pulmonary embolism); **H**, headache (stroke, migraine); **E**, eye problems (hypertension, stroke); **S**, severe leg pain (VTE).

Injectable Contraceptives

Depot medroxyprogesterone (DMPA) is the only injectable contraceptive available in the United States; there are intramuscular and subcutaneous formulations. Subcutaneous DMPA (DMPA-SC) uses a smaller needle and can be self-administered Box 21.7, which can improve access and increase reproductive autonomy. This formulation should be made available alongside the provider-administered intramuscular version.[48] Intramuscular and subcutaneous formulations are slightly different doses but are given at the same dosing interval and have the same indications for use. Although not specifically FDA approved for self-injection, DMPA-SC has been found to be safe and effective when self-administered.[49]

DMPA has historically been associated with weight gain[51]; however, a 2016 Cochrane review found limited evidence for weight gain with progestin-only contraceptives; most studies show a mean weight gain of less than 2 kg and little difference in weight change over time for DMPA users versus nonusers.[51] Despite the common perception of increased depression with progestin use, a systematic review in 2019 showed inconsistent evidence

TABLE 21.6 Emergency Contraception Options

Method	Dose	Timing	Efficacy	Notes	Approximate Cost
Levonorgestrel pills (LNG)	1.5 mg (either one 1.5-mg pill or two 0.75-mg pills)	Best within 3 days of unprotected intercourse	Lowers chance of pregnancy by 75%–89%	Available over the counter at a pharmacy and online. May work less well if >165 lb.	$11–$45
Ulipristal acetate pills	One 30-mg pill	Within 5 days of unprotected intercourse	Lowers chance of pregnancy by 85%	Needs prescription. May work less well if >195 lb. **After taking ulipristal acetate, hormonal contraception cannot be started for 5 days.**	$50
Copper IUD	(Paragard)	Within 5 days of unprotected intercourse	Lowers chance of pregnancy by 99.9%	Must be placed by medical professional, associated with menorrhagia, can remain in place up to 12 years for contraception	$0–$1300 but often covered by insurance or available through family planning programs
LNG IUD	52-mg–releasing devices (Liletta, Mirena)	Within 5 days of unprotected intercourse	Lowers chance of pregnancy by 99.9%	Must be placed by medical professional, can remain in place up to 8 years for contraception	$0–$1300 but often covered by insurance or available through family planning programs

BOX 21.7   How to Self-Administer DMPA-SC

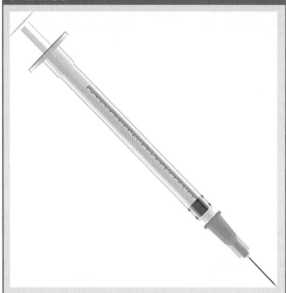

- Gently shake the prefilled syringe a few times, and place the needle on the syringe.
- Clean off the site on your belly or leg with an alcohol swab.
- Remove the cap from the needle and inject DMPA-SC into your belly or thigh at a 45-degree angle.
- Apply pressure to the injection spot.
- Dispose of syringe and needle in a sharps container or empty hard plastic laundry jug.

For an illustrated step-by-step guide from reproductive-access.org, see references 49 and 50.

Adapted from chrome-extension://efaidnbmnnnibpcajpcglclefind-mkaj/https://www.nationalfamilyplanning.org/file/documents—service-delivery-tools/NFPRHA—Depo-SQ-Resource-guide—FINAL-FOR-DISTRIBUTION.pdf

to support the association of DMPA with mood changes,[52] and a systematic review from 2018 showed no evidence to support an association of increased depression with DMPA.[53] A common concern with DMPA use is bone loss. Bone loss may be related to duration of use, but, importantly, the loss is largely or completely reversed when DMPA is discontinued.[54,55] In 2004, the FDA added a black box warning to packaging that cautioned against use >2 years; however, ACOG states that the potential risks to bone must be weighed against

the likelihood of pregnancy and, instead of a hard stop at 2 years of use, recommends individualized care, exercise, calcium and vitamin D supplementation, and education about contraceptive alternatives.[56] In adolescents, DMPA has been associated with smaller gains or loss of bone mass, and though the long-term effects are not well understood, there are no data to show that DMPA changes fracture risk in teens or later in life.[46,56] Routine bone mineral density evaluation is therefore *not* recommended in adolescents, and there is no evidence to support estrogen supplementation for DMPA users. The World Health Organization has concluded that the advantages of DMPA generally outweigh the *theoretical* fracture risk in users younger than 18 years.[57]

All progestin-only contraceptive methods change proliferative endometrium to secretory and eventually suppress endometrial growth; however, all are associated with unscheduled bleeding. In the Contraceptive Choice Project, 26% of those who stopped using DMPA listed bleeding as the main reason for switching methods.[58] Unscheduled bleeding is initially common but usually managed expectantly, as frequency and duration of bleeding decrease over time; about half of DMPA users are amenorrheic by 1 year.[59] Users may dislike irregular bleeding, and repeated injections may be poorly tolerated in some patients. For self-injectors, remembering the timing of DMPA is important.

Long-Acting Reversible Contraceptives

LARCs are supported as safe and effective for adolescents by the ACOG[60] and the AAP.[61] As user error is virtually eliminated, LARCs are the most effective contraception available. There are six available LARCs: five IUDs and one progestin subdermal implant (see Table 21.5). There are many common misconceptions concerning LARCs and fertility, device insertion, infection, pain, and concerns about a device inside the body. Counseling and education improve acceptability and continuation rate of LARC among teens.[12] The IUD is *not* significantly associated with upper genital tract infection.[20] Testing for STI is not required before IUD insertion if there are no risk factors, but routine screening can be done on the same day as device insertion. If STI is diagnosed with an IUD in place, removal of the device is not required while an antibiotic is started. Unless there is an active untreated infection,

BOX 21.8 Managing Unscheduled Bleeding With LARCs[66]

- NSAIDs are effective short-term for IUD users until bleeding profile improves.
- The implant is associated with more persistent bleeding compared with the IUD.
- Combination OC, doxycycline, ulipristal acetate and tamoxifen may help manage bleeding associated with the implant.

KEY POINTS

Contraception counseling:

- Includes a patient-centered, shared decision-making approach.
- Provides unbiased information in a confidential setting, ensuring privacy.
- Addresses each of the contraceptive options that are safe to use, as well as the risks, benefits (including noncontraceptive benefits), alternatives, and indications for use.
- Addresses STI education and prevention.
- Promotes education and resources to optimize healthy sexual experiences.

or if pregnancy cannot be excluded, offering same-day LARC placement to adolescents removes barriers to care and increases use. Concerns about a higher risk of device expulsion and adverse effects on fertility for teens using IUDs are generally unfounded and do not outweigh the benefits.[62] Allergy to LARC components is rare. The 13.5-mg LNG IUD and the 19.5-mg LNG IUD are slightly smaller than the 52-mg LNG IUD and use a 3.8-mm inserter (4.4- to 4.8-mm inserters are used for the higher-dose LNG IUD), which might make insertion easier for nulliparous teens. Cramping is not uncommon for several hours to even weeks after insertion. Unscheduled bleeding with LARCs is common. For IUD users, the bleeding profile usually improves after 90 days, and increased bleeding may be associated with device malposition or expulsion. For implant users, bleeding may persist and lead to dissatisfaction and continuation of the method (see Box 21.8).

Emergency Contraception

Education about emergency contraception (EC) can and should be incorporated into routine contraceptive counseling Box 21.6. Adolescents are more likely to use EC if it is prescribed and/or obtained before need.[63] Adolescents may not know about EC or how to obtain it, and misunderstanding is common.[64] EC is intended as a backup, for occasional use, when the regular form of contraception fails. Levonorgestrel works by delaying or inhibiting ovulation. Ulipristal acetate also prevents ovulation Placement of an IUD[65] within 5 days of unprotected intercourse is highly effective EC, with the advantage of concurrently initiating long-acting contraception. In contrast to oral EC, IUD efficacy is not affected by the weight of the patient.

REVIEW QUESTIONS

1. You are seeing a 14-year-old cisgender female who comes in with a parent today. The parent demands that you place an implant in this patient's arm for contraception, as "I know she won't take a pill every day." You talk to the patient privately about all available options, and she tells you that she wants a prescription for OC. What do you do?
   a. Try to convince the patient to get the implant
   b. Offer the patient an IUD
   c. Write a prescription for OC and go over the instructions for use
   d. Tell the patient it is important to involve the parent in this decision
2. You are discussing contraception options with a 16-year-old in your office. Which of the following statements is false about contraception options?
   a. Unscheduled bleeding is the most common side effect of the contraceptive implant.
   b. The LNG IUD can treat heavy menstrual bleeding and cramping.
   c. Oral contraceptive pills are highly associated with weight gain.
   d. Condoms are the only contraceptive method that also protects against STI transmission.
3. You have a 15-year-old transgender male in your office who is requesting an IUD to be placed. The patient asks if you have to tell his mother that he is getting an IUD. What is the correct response?
   a. You never have to involve the parent or guardian
   b. You always have to involve the parent or guardian
   c. It depends on the laws in your state

REFERENCES

1. Martinez GM, Abma JC. Sexual activity and contraceptive use among teenagers aged 15-19 in the United States, 2015-2017. *NCHS Data Brief.* 2020;(366):1-8.
2. Sedgh G, Finer LB, Bankole A, Eilers MA, Singh S. Adolescent pregnancy, birth, and abortion rates across countries: levels and recent trends. *J Adolesc Health.* 2015;56(2):223-230. doi:10.1016/j.jadohealth.2014.09.007
3. Kost K, Maddow-Zimet I, Arpaia A. *Pregnancies, Births and Abortions Among Adolescents and Young Women in the United States, 2013: National and State Trends by Age, Race and Ethnicity.* Published September 7, 2017. https://www.guttmacher.org/report/us-adolescent-pregnancy-trends-2013. Accessed August 20, 2022.
4. Martin JA, Hamilton BE, Osterman MJK. Births in the United States, 2018. *NCHS Data Brief.* 2019;(346):1-8.
5. Finer LB. Unintended pregnancy among U.S. adolescents: accounting for sexual activity. *J Adolesc Health.* 2010;47(3):312-314. doi:10.1016/j.jadohealth.2010.02.002
6. Centers for Disease Control and Prevention. *Sexually Transmitted Disease Surveillance 2018.* U.S. Department of Health and Human Services; 2019. doi:10.15620/cdc.79370
7. Pearl R. Factors in human fertility and their statistical evaluation. *Lancet.* 1933;222(5741):607-611. doi:10.1016/S0140-6736(01)18648-4
8. Patient-Centered Contraceptive Counseling. https://www.acog.org/en/clinical/clinical-guidance/committee-statement/articles/2022/02/patient-centered-contraceptive-counseling. Accessed February 3, 2023.
9. Guttmacher Institute. Paying for Contraception in the United States. Published January 23, 2020. https://www.guttmacher.org/fact-sheet/paying-contraception-united-states. Accessed August 19, 2022.
10. Secura GM, Madden T, McNicholas C, et al. Provision of no-cost, long-acting contraception and teenage pregnancy. *N Engl J Med.* 2014;371(14):1316-1323. doi:10.1056/NEJMoa1400506
11. Menon S, Committee on Adolescence. Long-acting reversible contraception: specific issues for adolescents. *Pediatrics.* 2020;146(2):e2020007252. doi:10.1542/peds.2020-007252
12. Birgisson NE, Zhao Q, Secura GM, Madden T, Peipert JF. Preventing unintended pregnancy: the contraceptive CHOICE project in review. *J Womens Health.* 2015;24(5):349-353. doi:10.1089/jwh.2015.5191
13. ACOG committee opinion no. 599: committee on adolescent health care: adolescent confidentiality and electronic health records. *Obstet Gynecol.* 2014;123(5):1148-1150. doi:10.1097/01.AOG.0000446825.08715.98
14. Guttmacher Institute. State Policies on Contraception. Published February 1, 2023. https://www.guttmacher.org/united-states/contraception/state-policies-contraception. Accessed February 3, 2023.
15. Guttmacher Institute. An Overview of Consent to Reproductive Health Services by Young People. Published March 14, 2016. https://www.guttmacher.org/state-policy/explore/overview-minors-consent-law. Accessed September 11, 2022.
16. Goldfarb ES, Lieberman LD. Three decades of research: the case for comprehensive sex education. *J Adolesc Health.* 2021;68(1):13-27. doi:10.1016/j.jadohealth.2020.07.036
17. Family Planning Annual Report: 2020 National Summary. Published Online 2020:168. https://opa.hhs.gov/sites/default/files/2021-09/title-x-fpar-2020-national-summary-sep-2021.pdf
18. Guttmacher Institute. Meeting the Sexual and Reproductive Health Needs of Adolescents in School-Based Health Centers. Published April 21, 2015. https://www.guttmacher.org/gpr/2015/04/meeting-sexual-and-reproductive-health-needs-adolescents-school-based-health-centers. Accessed September 12, 2022.
19. American College of Obstetricians and Gynecologists' Committee on Adolescent Health Care. The initial reproductive health visit: ACOG committee opinion, number 811. *Obstet Gynecol.* 2020;136(4):e70-e80. doi:10.1097/AOG.0000000000004094
20. Curtis KM, Tepper NK, Jatlaoui TC, et al. U.S. medical eligibility criteria for contraceptive use, 2016. *MMWR Recomm Rep.* 2016;65(3):1-103. doi:10.15585/mmwr.rr6503a1
21. Yland JJ, Bresnick KA, Hatch EE, et al. Pregravid contraceptive use and fecundability: prospective cohort study. *BMJ.* 2020;371:m3966. doi:10.1136/bmj.m3966
22. Todd N, Black A. Contraception for adolescents. *J Clin Res Pediatr Endocrinol.* 2020;12(suppl 1):28-40. doi:10.4274/jcrpe.galenos.2019.2019.S0003
23. Havrilesky LJ, Gierisch JM, Moorman PG, et al. Oral contraceptive use for the primary prevention of ovarian cancer. *Evid ReportTechnology Assess.* 2013;(212):1-514.
24. Baird DT, Glasier AF. Hormonal contraception. *N Engl J Med.* 1993;328(21):1543-1549. doi:10.1056/NEJM199305273282108
25. Speroff L. The formulation of oral contraceptives: does the amount of estrogen make any clinical difference? *Johns Hopkins Med J.* 1982;150(5):170-176.
26. Maguire K, Westhoff C. The state of hormonal contraception today: established and emerging noncontraceptive health benefits. *Am J Obstet Gynecol.* 2011;205(suppl 4):S4-S8. doi:10.1016/j.ajog.2011.06.056
27. Arowojolu AO, Gallo MF, Lopez LM, Grimes DA, Garner SE. Combined oral contraceptive pills for treatment of acne. *Cochrane Database Syst Rev.* 2009;(3):CD004425. doi:10.1002/14651858.CD004425.pub4

28. Bahamondes L, Valeria Bahamondes M, Shulman LP. Non-contraceptive benefits of hormonal and intrauterine reversible contraceptive methods. *Hum Reprod Update.* 2015;21(5):640-651. doi:10.1093/humupd/dmv023

29. Lara-Torre E. "Quick Start", an innovative approach to the combination oral contraceptive pill in adolescents. Is it time to make the switch? *J Pediatr Adolesc Gynecol.* 2004;17(1):65-67. doi:10.1016/j.jpag.2003.11.005

30. Heit JA, Kobbervig CE, James AH, Petterson TM, Bailey KR, Melton LJ. Trends in the incidence of venous thrombo-embolism during pregnancy or postpartum: a 30-year population-based study. *Ann Intern Med.* 2005;143(10):697-706. doi:10.7326/0003-4819-143-10-200511150-00006

31. Simmons KB, Edelman AB. Hormonal contraception and obesity. *Fertil Steril.* 2016;106(6):1282-1288. doi:10.1016/j.fertnstert.2016.07.1094

32. Ahrendt HJ, Nisand I, Bastianelli C, et al. Efficacy, acceptability and tolerability of the combined contraceptive ring, NuvaRing, compared with an oral contraceptive containing 30 microg of ethinyl estradiol and 3 mg of drospirenone. *Contraception.* 2006;74(6):451-457. doi:10.1016/j.contraception.2006.07.004

33. Najafi M, Sadeghi MM, Mehvari J, Zare M, Akbari M. Progesterone therapy in women with intractable catamenial epilepsy. *Adv Biomed Res.* 2013;2:8. doi:10.4103/2277-9175.107974

34. Wilson CD. Toxic shock syndrome and diaphragm use. *J Adolesc Health Care.* 1983;4(4):290-291. doi:10.1016/s0197-0070(83)80015-1

35. Planned Parenthood. Condoms. How to Put on a Condom Video. https://www.plannedparenthood.org/learn/birth-control/condom. Accessed October 22, 2022.

36. Society for Adolescent Health and Medicine. Condom availability in schools: a practical approach to the prevention of sexually transmitted infection/HIV and unintended pregnancy. *J Adolesc Health.* 2017;60(6):754-757. doi:10.1016/j.jadohealth.2017.03.019

37. Centers for Disease Control (CDC). Toxic-shock syndrome and the vaginal contraceptive sponge. *MMWR Morb Mortal Wkly Rep.* 1984;33(4):43-44, 49.

38. Tyson NA. Reproductive health: options, strategies, and empowerment of women. *Obstet Gynecol Clin North Am.* 2019;46(3):409-430. doi:10.1016/j.ogc.2019.04.002

39. Ali M, Akin A, Bahamondes L, et al. Extended use up to 5 years of the etonogestrel-releasing subdermal contraceptive implant: comparison to levonorgestrel-releasing subdermal implant. *Hum Reprod Oxf Engl.* 2016;31(11):2491-2498. doi:10.1093/humrep/dew222

40. Moray KV, Chaurasia H, Sachin O, Joshi B. A systematic review on clinical effectiveness, side-effect profile and meta-analysis on continuation rate of etonogestrel contraceptive implant. *Reprod Health.* 2021;18(1):4. doi:10.1186/s12978-020-01054-y

41. Request Clinical Training Form – Nexplanon Training. https://nexplanontraining.com/request-clinical-training/in-person-training/. Accessed October 22, 2022.

42. Adeyemi-Fowode OA, Santos XM, Dietrich JE, Srivaths L. Levonorgestrel-releasing intrauterine device use in female adolescents with heavy menstrual bleeding and bleeding disorders: single institution review. *J Pediatr Adolesc Gynecol.* 2017;30(4):479-483. doi:10.1016/j.jpag.2016.04.001

43. Bayer LL, Hillard PJA. Use of levonorgestrel intrauterine system for medical indications in adolescents. *J Adolesc Health.* 2013;52(suppl 4):S54-S58. doi:10.1016/j.jadohealth.2012.09.022

44. ACOG committee opinion no. 760: dysmenorrhea and endometriosis in the adolescent. *Obstet Gynecol.* 2018;132(6): e249-e258. doi:10.1097/AOG.0000000000002978

45. Balayla J, Gil Y, Mattina J, Al-Shehri E, Ziegler C. Streptococcal toxic shock syndrome after insertion of a levonorgestrel intrauterine device. *J Obstet Gynaecol Can.* 2019;41(12):1772-1774. doi:10.1016/j.jogc.2019.02.017

46. Bachrach LK. Hormonal contraception and bone health in adolescents. *Front Endocrinol.* 2020;11:603. doi:10.3389/fendo.2020.00603

47. Agostino H, Di Meglio G. Low-dose oral contraceptives in adolescents: how low can you go? *J Pediatr Adolesc Gynecol.* 2010;23(4):195-201. doi:10.1016/j.jpag.2009.11.001

48. CDC. Injectables. US SPR. Reproductive Health. Published May 20, 2021. https://www.cdc.gov/reproductivehealth/contraception/mmwr/spr/injectables.html. Accessed February 5, 2023.

49. Kohn JE, Berlan ED, Tang JH, Beasley A. Society of Family Planning committee consensus on self-administration of subcutaneous depot medroxyprogesterone acetate (DMPA-SC). *Contraception.* 2022;112:11-13. doi:10.1016/j.contraception.2022.03.023

50. NFPRHA. Depo-SQ Resource Guide. https://www.nationalfamilyplanning.org/file/documents—-service-delivery-tools/NFPRHA—-Depo-SQ-Resource-guide—--FINAL-FOR-DISTRIBUTION.pdf. Accessed February 6, 2023.

51. Lopez LM, Ramesh S, Chen M, et al. Progestin-only contraceptives: effects on weight. *Cochrane Database Syst Rev.* 2016;(8):CD008815. doi:10.1002/14651858.CD008815.pub4

52. Dianat S, Fox E, Ahrens KA, et al. Side effects and health benefits of depot medroxyprogesterone acetate: a systematic review. *Obstet Gynecol.* 2019;133(2):332-341. doi:10.1097/AOG.0000000000003089

53. Worly BL, Gur TL, Schaffir J. The relationship between progestin hormonal contraception and depression: a systematic review. *Contraception.* 2018;97(6):478-489. doi:10.1016/j.contraception.2018.01.010

54. Scholes D, LaCroix AZ, Ichikawa LE, Barlow WE, Ott SM. Change in bone mineral density among adolescent women using and discontinuing depot medroxyprogesterone acetate contraception. *Arch Pediatr Adolesc Med.* 2005;159(2):139-144. doi:10.1001/archpedi.159.2.139

55. Harel Z, Johnson CC, Gold MA, et al. Recovery of bone mineral density in adolescents following the use of depot medroxyprogesterone acetate contraceptive injections. *Contraception.* 2010;81(4):281-291. doi:10.1016/j.contraception.2009.11.003

56. Committee opinion no. 602: depot medroxyprogesterone acetate and bone effects. *Obstet Gynecol.* 2014;123(6):1398-1402. doi:10.1097/01.AOG.0000450758.95422.c8

57. d'Arcangues C. WHO statement on hormonal contraception and bone health. *Contraception.* 2006;73(5):443-444. doi:10.1016/j.contraception.2006.01.002

58. Diedrich JT, Zhao Q, Madden T, Secura GM, Peipert JF. Three-year continuation of reversible contraception. *Am J Obstet Gynecol.* 2015;213(5):662.e1-e8. doi:10.1016/j.ajog.2015.08.001

59. Hubacher D, Lopez L, Steiner MJ, Dorflinger L. Menstrual pattern changes from levonorgestrel subdermal implants and DMPA: systematic review and evidence-based comparisons. *Contraception.* 2009;80(2):113-118. doi:10.1016/j.contraception.2009.02.008

60. Adolescents and Long-Acting Reversible Contraception: Implants and Intrauterine Devices. https://www.acog.org/en/clinical/clinical-guidance/committee-opinion/articles/2018/05/adolescents-and-long-acting-reversible-contraception-implants-and-intrauterine-devices. Accessed February 7, 2023.

61. Ott MA, Sucato GS, Committee on Adolescence. Contraception for adolescents. *Pediatrics.* 2014;134(4):e1257-e1281. doi:10.1542/peds.2014-2300

62. Foran T, Butcher BE, Kovacs G, Bateson D, O'Connor V. Safety of insertion of the copper IUD and LNG-IUS in nulliparous women: a systematic review. *Eur J Contracept Reprod Health Care.* 2018;23(5):379-386. doi:10.1080/13625187.2018.1526898

63. Committee on Adolescence. Emergency contraception. *Pediatrics.* 2012;130(6):1174-1182. doi:10.1542/peds.2012-2962

64. Williams BN, Jauk VC, Szychowski JM, Arbuckle JL. Adolescent emergency contraception usage, knowledge, and perception. *Contraception.* 2021;103(5):361-366. doi:10.1016/j.contraception.2021.01.003

65. Turok DK, Gero A, Simmons RG, et al. Levonorgestrel vs. copper intrauterine devices for emergency contraception. *N Engl J Med.* 2021;384(4):335-344. doi:10.1056/NEJMoa2022141

66. Henkel A, Goldthwaite LM. Management of bothersome bleeding associated with progestin-based long-acting reversible contraception: a review. *Curr Opin Obstet Gynecol.* 2020;32(6):408-415. doi:10.1097/GCO.0000000000000664

Contraception for Adolescents With Medical Complexities

Ashley M Ebersole, Serena Margaret Liu, Elise D Berlan, and Nichole Tyson

INTRODUCTION

Contraception counseling is recommended to be a routine part of preventive health care visits. The American Academy of Pediatrics (AAP) recommends that pediatricians have a working knowledge of contraception to help adolescents reduce the risks and negative consequences of unintended pregnancy.[1] Similarly, the American College of Obstetricians and Gynecologists (ACOG) recommends that all obstetrician-gynecologists routinely address the contraceptive needs of patients regardless of age.[2] Contraception counseling should be nonjudgmental, comprehensive, and inclusive. This includes offering counseling to all adolescents regardless of medical conditions, including physical or intellectual disabilities. Adolescents and young adults with mild to moderate intellectual or developmental disability are just as likely to be sexually active as are their peers without disability.[3] Most adolescents with disabilities do not receive the appropriate reproductive health counseling that they need.[3]

The focus of this chapter is contraception provision for adolescents with medical complexities, as the benefits and risks of contraceptive use for adolescents with certain conditions may be different from those of healthy adolescents. Although the chapter is thorough, it is not comprehensive of all medical conditions. In addition to the standard elements of providing contraception care described in detail elsewhere,[4] we recommend the reader adopt a standardized approach to assessing contraceptive needs for adolescents with medical complexity (Box 22.1).

The US Medical Eligibility Criteria (US MEC) for Contraceptive Use from the Centers for Disease Control

> **BOX 22.1 Standardized Approach to Assessing Contraceptive Needs for Adolescents With Medical Complexity**
>
> 1. Review the pregnancy-related risks associated with the medical condition and related medications.
> 2. Review the contraindications to any contraceptive methods related to the medical condition.
> 3. Consider the benefits of contraceptives for the underlying medical condition.

> **BOX 22.2 The US Medical Eligibility Criteria (US MEC) for Contraceptive Use**
>
> US MEC categorizes medical eligibility for contraceptive use into four categories:
> 1. A condition for which there is no restriction for the use of the contraceptive method
> 2. A condition for which the advantages of using the method generally outweigh the theoretical or proven risks
> 3. A condition for which the theoretical or proven risks usually outweigh the advantages of using the method
> 4. A condition that represents an unacceptable health risk if the contraceptive method is used
>
> Categories are applied to method initiation and continuation, as the guidance may vary if the medical condition worsened while using the contraceptive method.

and Prevention (CDC) provide evidence-based guidance on medical eligibility for the initiation and continuation of contraceptive methods among people with various characteristics and medical conditions (Box 22.2).[5] This resource is also available for free online and in an app.

The World Health Organization (WHO) also provides an evidence-based guideline for the provision of contraception.[6] When considering the CDC and WHO guidelines for contraceptive counseling, one must recognize that adolescents and teenagers are generally a healthier population than adults. There are limited available data on hormonal contraceptive effects in the teenage and adolescent population; however, the negative effects associated with hormonal contraception (i.e., risk of venous thromboembolism [VTE]) increase with increasing age.

UNIQUE CONSIDERATIONS FOR ADOLESCENTS

The provision of contraception for adolescents requires unique considerations (Box 22.3).

All efforts should be made to provide and maintain confidentiality to adolescents seeking contraception. The AAP states that protecting adolescent confidentiality during contraception care is in the best interest of the adolescent.[1] Consider steps that may improve the discreetness of contraception when clinically appropriate. For example, adolescents needing to conceal the method from family or partners wanting a highly effective contraception may be interested in intrauterine devices (IUDs) or the implant, as those methods do not require trips to the pharmacy and require little maintenance. Additionally, cutting IUD strings flush to the level of the external os may provide privacy, as sexual partners cannot feel them.

When providing contraception counseling for adolescents, the provider is encouraged to use shared decision making to help the adolescent find the method that is right for them. In this approach, it is important to understand the patient's preferences and priorities about contraception. Asking a question such as, "What are you looking for in a birth control method?" may help guide

the conversation. Shared decision making should consider menstrual symptoms and methods, which may provide improvement in those symptoms in addition to contraception. If contraceptive effectiveness is the patient's priority, tiered counseling or effectiveness counseling is appropriate.[1] However, it is important to consider cultural and historical perspectives that may affect a person's contraceptive choice. Historical and contemporary eugenic and racist practices may make people of color or in poverty wary of long-acting reversible contraceptives (LARCs). In addition, certain adolescents may prefer a method that they are more in control of that does not require a visit to their provider for discontinuation.[7]

Ultimately, the provider's role is to help the adolescent initiate the contraceptive method that best fits their preferences and priorities and is safe to use in the context of medical complexity (Box 22.4). When considering medical comorbidities and their interaction with hormonal contraception, the provider must weigh these risks with the risk of pregnancy, which would expose the patient to higher levels of estrogen and progestogen than any available hormonal contraception

LONG-ACTING REVERSIBLE CONTRACEPTIVES IN ADOLESCENTS

LARCs (IUD and subdermal implants) are safe and effective in the adolescent population. It should be noted that IUDs can be safely inserted in adolescents as both a form of contraception and emergency contraception (see section on "Use of Emergency Contraception" on page 238),[8] contrary to some of the misconceptions associated with IUD insertion in this population[9] (Box 22.5).

Expulsion in adolescents and young adults may be more common in patients with abnormal uterine bleeding

BOX 22.5   **Truths About Intrauterine Devices in Adolescents**

1. IUDs are safe and effective for adolescents and young adults.
2. IUDs can be used as contraception and emergency contraception.
3. Expulsion is more common in adolescents in comparison to the adult population; however, this should not deter placement.
4. Anticipatory guidance can relieve pain experienced with IUD insertion and break down barriers to IUD placement.
5. A paracervical block for IUD insertion is effective for reducing pain in adolescents.

or heavy menstrual bleeding.[10] Studies have demonstrated a range of expulsion rates in this population; however, a systematic review found a higher expulsion rate among adolescents and young adults in comparison with adults, with an expulsion rate of 8%.[11] Despite the higher expulsion rate, it should be noted that postplacental IUD insertion has been found to have even higher expulsion rates,[12] yet are cost-effective nonetheless[13]; therefore the 8% expulsion rate should not deter a provider from placing an IUD.

Despite its effectiveness, a barrier to IUD insertion in the adolescent population appears to be fear of pain with insertion. An association between anticipated pain and experienced pain has been demonstrated,[14] which can be relieved with anticipatory counseling.[15] Pain with IUD insertion in adolescents is similar to adults.[16,17] On the visual analogue scale, adolescents rate their pain from 30 to 70 mm, depending on whether a paracervical block is used.[16] Pain reduction can be accomplished using a paracervical block in the adolescent population, similar to the adult population.[16,17]

The frames of the IUD come in different sizes, with the copper IUD measuring 32 × 36 mm, levonorgestrel (LNG) 52 mg measuring 32 × 32 mm, and the LNG 19.5 and 13.5 measuring 30 × 28 mm. Although data are limited in adolescent populations, they suggest that people receiving smaller IUDs are more likely to report "no to mild pain" with insertion.[18] Newer data suggest that smaller-framed IUDs may be associated with decreased expulsion in the nulliparous population.[18] It should be noted that these data include two copper IUDs, one of which is not yet available on the market in the United States.[19]

MEDICAL COMPLEXITIES

RHEUMATOLOGIC CONDITIONS

Pregnancy in patients with rheumatologic conditions, which can affect adolescents and young adults, may lead to serious maternal or fetal adverse outcomes.[20] Adverse maternal events include worsening of preexisting proteinuria, increased thrombosis risk, and worsening of osteoporosis; fetal adverse outcomes may be fetal growth restriction or teratogenic effects resulting from medication.[20] Reproductive health counseling is crucial for patients with rheumatologic diseases to optimize personal health. Shared decision making is a vital component of contraception counseling that considers the patient a unique individual with their own reproductive goals.

Both the CDC and the American College of Rheumatology (ACR) have evidence-based recommendations about best practices for contraception in patients with rheumatologic diseases but differ in a couple recommendations discussed further in Table 22.1.[5,20]

Special considerations should be made for patients on mycophenolate mofetil/mycophenolic acid (MMF) taking contraception.[20] MMF may reduce the serum concentrations of estrogen and progestins, rendering them less effective. IUDs, barrier methods paired with combined contraceptive pills, or the etonogestrel implant are preferred in patients with MMF.

NEUROLOGIC CONDITIONS

Epilepsy

Epilepsy is often diagnosed and managed during childhood, and so providers should be aware of how to counsel these patients on hormonal contraception and be familiar with hormonal interactions with antiepileptic medication. Patients with seizure disorders may experience a higher rate of anovulation, amenorrhea, and irregular menses.[21] Although ACOG does not recommend initiating hormonal contraception before puberty, it recommends physicians discuss a plan for when menarche arrives.[21]

For patients with epilepsy, pregnancy may increase their risk for seizure.[22] Complications in the fetuses and children of mothers with epilepsy may include fetal loss and perinatal death, congenital malformations, neonatal hemorrhage, low birth weight, developmental delay, and childhood epilepsy.[22] Additionally, certain anticonvulsant medications are known to be teratogenic (Box 22.6).[23-25]

TABLE 22.1   **CDC Versus ACR Recommendations on Contraception for Rheumatoid Conditions**

	CDC	ACR	Additional Information
SLE With Negative aPL (Mild)	• All hormonal and nonhormonal forms acceptable	• All hormonal and nonhormonal forms acceptable EXCEPT for patch	
SLE With Negative aPL (Moderate to Severe)	• All hormonal and nonhormonal forms acceptable *Except for thrombocytopenia – MEC 3 for Cu IUD and DMPA initiation; MEC 2 for continuation	• Nonhormonal and progestin-only contraception acceptable • Avoid estrogen	
SLE With Positive aPL	• Nonhormonal contraception acceptable • MEC 3 for all progestin-based contraception • MEC 4 for estrogen	• Nonhormonal, progestin-only pills and LNG IUD acceptable • No estrogen-based contraception	• Must weigh risks and benefits when considering MEC 3 contraception (see text)

When reviewing the guidelines, note that MEC 3 does not reflect an absolute contraindication. Rather, medical professionals should weigh the risks associated with pregnancy in adolescent patients in addition to the risks associated with rheumatoid conditions. For example, an adolescent patient with SLE and positive aPL who prioritizes avoiding pregnancy and is counseled about the elevated risks associated with progestin-based contraception may opt for the progestin-based method with the least systemic progestin, LNG IUD.

ACR, American College of Rheumatology; *aPL*, antiphospholipid antibody; *CDC*, Centers for Disease Control and Prevention; *CHC*, combined hormonal contraception; *DMPA*, depot medroxyprogesterone acetate; *IUD*, intrauterine device; *LNG*, levonorgestrel; *MEC*, Medical Eligibility Criteria; *SLE*, systemic lupus erythematosus.

BOX 22.6   Teratogenic Anticonvulsant Medications

1. Valproic acid
2. Pregabalin
3. Topiramate
4. Phenobarbital
5. Phenytoin
6. Carbamazepine

BOX 22.7   Anticonvulsants That Decrease Effectiveness of Hormonal Contraception

1. Phenytoin
2. Carbamazepine
3. Barbiturates
4. Primidone
5. Topiramate
6. Oxcarbazepine

For people using hormonal contraception, the provider should consider their interactions with anticonvulsants. Certain anticonvulsants may decrease the effectiveness of hormonal contraception (Box 22.7). If a combined estrogen-progestin oral contraceptive (COC) is used, the minimum suggested estrogen dose for adolescents and teenagers is 30 μg.[5] Contrarily, serum levels of lamotrigine are decreased when used in combination with combined hormonal contraceptives (CHCs).[5] For patients using lamotrigine for treatment of seizures, this may lower their seizure threshold and worsen control of their epilepsy (CDC US MEC category 3).[5] Therefore when prescribing or changing contraceptive methods, care should be coordinated with the patient's neurologist to adjust antiepileptic medication to ensure therapeutic levels.

Finally, contraception may provide benefit to patients with epilepsy. There is a positive correlation between seizure frequency and mean estrogen/progesterone ratios, with fewer reported seizures when progesterone levels are elevated.[26] Although the data are limited by small studies, depo medroxyprogesterone acetate (DMPA) has been shown to reduce seizure frequency.[27] However, not all progestins have the same impact. A 2016 Cochrane review found very low-certainty evidence of no difference between norethindrone and placebo and moderate to low certainty evidence of no difference between progesterone and placebo for the treatment of catamenial epilepsy.[28]

For patients who are using hormonal contraception to prevent pregnancy and who have refractory seizures on polytherapy with enzyme-inducing anticonvulsants, it is prudent to recommend barrier contraception in addition to their hormonal contraception because of the increased likelihood of drug-drug interactions.[21] All forms of emergency contraception are safe in patients with seizure disorders who are on anticonvulsants.[29]

Migraine With Aura

People with a history of headaches should be evaluated for migraine with aura at the time of contraception counseling.[30] Auras are complex neurologic symptoms, which most commonly manifest in visual symptoms but also include sensory, speech, language, motor, brainstem, or retinal symptoms.[31] Patients with migraine with aura who use CHCs are at increased risk for stroke. If an adolescent is describing symptoms consistent with migraines with aura, a neurologic examination with a professional should be completed before making the formal diagnosis. CHCs should be avoided (CDC US MEC category 4); however, the absolute risk of stroke is low even in the presence of migraine with aura. Additionally, the risk of pregnancy particularly for the adolescent population, including the risk of stroke and the additional risks that come with pregnancy in this population, far outweigh the risk caused by hormonal contraception in the setting of migraines with aura. It is important to always individualize assessment of harms and benefits and practice shared decision making.

HEMATOLOGIC CONDITIONS

Thromboembolism/Stroke

Thromboembolisms and strokes are not common in the adolescent population, as the risk of VTE increases with age and comorbidities that come with aging. With that said, special consideration should be taken in patients with history of deep vein thrombosis (DVT), history of pulmonary embolism (PE), current DVT/PE, history of stroke, or otherwise at risk for thrombosis when prescribing hormonal contraception.

Estrogen in CHCs increases hepatic production of serum coagulation factors and fibrinogen, thereby increasing the risk of thromboembolism.[70] The CDC MEC recommends that CHCs be avoided in all patients with acute DVT/PE or those with a history of DVT/PE (CDC US MEC category 3-4).[32] According to a 2014 Cochrane review, the relative risk of VTE in women using COCs with ethinyl estradiol is 2.5 to 5.5 times the risk of VTE in women without COC use.[33] Evidence suggests that hormonal contraception with <50 μg ethinyl estradiol has a reduced risk of VTE compared with pills containing 50 μg ethinyl estradiol,[34] an elevated dose no longer prescribed in hormonal contraception available today. A novel oral contraceptive pill containing 14.2 mg of estetrol and 3 mg of drospirenone (Nextstellis in the United States and Drovelis or Lydisilka in the European Union) was recently developed. Whereas most COCs use ethinyl estradiol, the new pill contains estetrol, a naturally occurring estrogen. A phase 3 clinical trial containing 1674 women demonstrated that estetrol 14.2 mg/drospirenone 3 mg was efficacious, and no participants had a thrombotic event.[35] The estetrol 14.2 mg/drospirenone 3 mg COC may have lower rates of thrombosis compared with traditional COCs, though commercial availability may be limited because of lack of insurance coverage.

Although the CDC considers the benefits of DMPA to outweigh the risks in someone with DVT/PE (CDC US MEC category 2), this risk is considered unacceptable in someone with a history of stroke (CDC US MEC category 3).[5] The data are not strong, but there is some evidence for increased risk of VTE associated with the use of DMPA.[36,37] Data do not demonstrate similar effects with other progestin-only methods; however, the CDC also recommends against continuing progestin-only pills, LNG-IUDs, and the etonogestrel implant in those with a stroke (CDC US MEC category 3).[5] It is acceptable to initiate a new, non-DMPA, progestin-only method (progestin-only pills, LNG-IUDs, and the etonogestrel implant) in patients with stroke history as long as the thrombotic event did not occur while using the method.[5] Similar to DVT/PE, estrogen-based contraception should not be used in anyone with a history of stroke (CDC US MEC category 4).

Other Risk Factors for Thrombosis

Thrombosis is rare, with a baseline risk of 1 to 5/10,000 women-years versus 3 to 15/10,000 women-years for users of hormonal contraception. In pregnancy, the risk increases fivefold, which is even higher than on hormonal contraception. These rates are based on the general population and are even lower in younger populations.[38-40]

Although there are no contraindications for people with first-degree relatives with a history of DVT/PE, it is not recommended that a person with a known thrombogenic mutation (e.g., factor V Leiden mutation, prothrombin

G20210A mutation, protein C, protein S, or antithrombin deficiency) use estrogen-based contraception (CDC US MEC category 4).[5] Progestins are acceptable for patients with a history of thrombosis and outweigh the higher VTE risks associated with pregnancy.[38] It should be noted that the majority of adolescents report engaging in sexual activity before completing high school with limited use of contraception.[38] Routine thrombophilia testing is not recommended before initiating hormonal contraception, unless the patient has symptoms that would warrant thrombophilia testing.[41]

There is increased risk for VTE among patients undergoing major surgery with prolonged immobilization; therefore CHCs should be avoided (CDC US MEC category 4).[5,42] All progestin-only methods are acceptable alternatives in this population (CDC US MEC category 2).

Heavy Menstrual Bleeding

Heavy menstrual bleeding (HMB) is defined qualitatively as "excessive menstrual blood loss which interferes with the woman's physical, emotional, social and material quality of life, and which can occur alone or in combination with other symptoms" and objectively as 80 mL or more of menstrual blood loss per month.[43] LNG-IUD is considered a first-line treatment for people with nonacute HMB.[44] The Mirena 52-mg LNG-IUD is Food and Drug Administration (FDA) approved for treatment of HMB.[45] In fact, two recent studies of LNG use in adolescents found that 39.8% to 51% of users of an LNG-IUD reported amenorrhea.[46,47] Among adolescents with bleeding diatheses, use of the 52-mg LNG-IUD led to amenorrhea or spotting in approximately 60% of users.[48,49] Therefore in adolescents with HMB who desire contraception, LNG-IUD should be considered a first-line method given its contraceptive efficacy and benefits for the treatment of HMB.[50]

CHCs are another contraceptive for adolescents with HMB that may provide the dual benefit of contraception and treatment of their HMB.[51] CHCs with 30 to 35 µg of ethinyl estradiol are preferred in patients with HMB compared with COCs with ultralow-dose pills (10 µg ethinyl estradiol or less). Ultralow-dose pills may be less effective at controlling bleeding.[52,53] Triphasic pills have not been found to be more effective than monophasic pills in controlling vaginal bleeding.[54] Additionally, extended cycling of COCs (skipping placebo pills) may also reduce the frequency of menstrual bleeding and thereby provide treatment for HMB. This may be done by counseling the patient about skipping placebo pills and by prescribing a prepackaged extended-cycle monophasic COC.[55]

Finally, patients may also achieve a reduction in HMB with DMPA, with up to 46% of users experiencing amenorrhea at 1 year.[56] ACOG offers clinical guidance of how to use hormonal contraception for menstrual suppression[55] (Table 22.2).

CONTRACEPTION IN OVERWEIGHT TEENS

The impact of obesity on contraceptive effectiveness has not been well studied because clinical trials exclude populations with body mass index (BMI) >30 kg/m^2, with even less data among the adolescent population. Some contraceptives may be less effective in overweight adolescents. Data on contraceptive patch users weighing ≥90 kg (≥198 lb) experienced more contraceptive failures compared with those users weighing <90 kg.[57] A 2016 Cochrane review found that there is no significant

TABLE 22.2	Hormonal Options for Menstrual Suppression	
Medication	**Dose**	**Amenorrhea**
COC	Monophasic skipping placebo pills or prescribed extended cycle	88% at 12 months
Patch	Continuously or extended cycle	Moderate
Ring	Continuously or extended cycle (exchange ring every 4 weeks, avoiding hormonal-free interval)	Excellent
Oral progestin	Varies by progestin	Irregular bleeding, but improves with prolonged use
DMPA	150 mg IM; 104 mg SQ	68%–72% at 2 years
Implant	Etonogestrel 68 mg	22% at 1 year, improves with prolonged use
LNG-IUD	LNG 52 mg	50% at 1 year; 60% at 2 years

Adapted from ACOG.[54]

difference in the efficacy of *most* hormonal contraceptives based on the user's weight.[30]

Weight gain is a common reported reason for contraception discontinuation.[58] There is no evidence that weight gain is caused by hormonal contraception, including oral pills, patches, rings, implants, or IUDs.[58] DMPA use in the adolescent population has been evaluated with different outcomes around weight gain. A prospective study of 450 adolescents over 18 months found that DMPA was associated with higher weight gain in comparison to CHC pills and nonusers (9.4 kg vs. 0.2 kg vs. 3.1 kg, P <0.001).[59] However, this was particularly true in patients with a BMI >30 kg/m^2, but not with BMI >30 kg/m^2. Another study on DMPA in adolescents suggests that a subset of patients may be more susceptible to weight gain early on.[60] People who experienced more than 5% weight gain over 6 months were more likely to experience excessive weight gain after 36 months.[60] Overall, DMPA is still an acceptable method in overweight adolescents, and given the known data, weight gain should be evaluated for the first 6 months to guide management.

Use of Emergency Contraception

Emergency contraception for adolescents comes in the same form as for adults: LNG pill, ulipristal acetate (UPA), LNG-IUD, and copper IUD. The IUDs, both progesterone and copper, are the most effective form of emergency contraception, regardless of BMI, and should be considered in adolescents.[61] Of note, recent research suggests that the LNG-IUD is noninferior to the copper IUD for emergency contraception.[8] While the use of the LNG-IUD for emergency contraception is recommended by the Society for Family Planning, there are critics who suggest additional rigorous research is needed prior to a universal recommendation of the practice.[62-64] Emergency contraceptive pills (ECPs) may be less effective in people with BMI ≥30 kg/m^2 compared with BMI <30 kg/m^2.[65] One study demonstrated a 4.4-fold increase in risk of pregnancy in participants with obesity using the LNG ECP compared with normal/underweight people.[66] For the UPA ECP, studies demonstrated a twofold increase in risk of pregnancy in participants with obesity compared with normal/underweight people; however, this was not statistically significant.[66,67] In fact, the limit of contraceptive efficacy appears to be at a weight of 70 kg for LNG ECP users and 88 kg for UPA ECP users.[66] Therefore the Society for Family Planning recommends clinicians counsel patients that the UPA ECP is more effective than LNG ECPs in overweight and obese persons

and those with body weight 70 kg or greater (Grade 1C recommendation).[62]

EATING DISORDERS AND HORMONAL CONTRACEPTION

Eating disorders commonly arise during adolescent years.[68] This population may present with irregular menses or amenorrhea. ACOG recommends against the use of CHC for the treatment of amenorrhea in patients with eating disorders, as it has not shown to improve BMD and can mask progression of improvement with the presence of withdrawal bleeding.[69]

For sexually active patients, this population is at risk of pregnancy, and counseling on contraception should be provided. Although eating disorders are not listed as a condition in the CDC US MEC, all hormonal contraceptive methods can be safely recommended to patients in this population.[70] Caution should be used when considering DMPA, given its association with low bone mineral density (BMD)[70]; however, shared decision making should be made with the patient, as the risks of pregnancy may outweigh the benefit.

Teens With Cancer

Adolescent patients with cancer or undergoing treatment may be at risk of abnormal uterine bleeding because of their underlying malignancy or treatment.[71] Collaboration with the adolescent's oncologist when choosing a treatment plan for menstrual suppression or for acute uterine bleeding is highly recommended (Box 22.8).[72]

Adolescents in this population are at risk of pregnancy if sexually active, and so contraception counseling is important. Based on the CDC US MEC guidelines, cancer patients can safely use all hormonal contraception (category 1 or 2), unless they have hormonally

---

BOX 22.8 Considerations When Choosing Treatment for Menstrual Suppression or Acute Bleeding

1. Mental status
2. Hemoglobin and platelet level (and expected nadirs)
3. Planned cancer treatment
4. VTE risk
5. Contraception desires
6. End goal/desires for future to be achieved
7. Contraceptive desires

VTE, Venous thromboembolism.

sensitive breast cancer. An exception is also made for the initiation of the IUD in cervical and endometrial cancer because of concern for seeding. When considering estrogen-based contraception, physicians must consider the patient's baseline risk of VTE, which can be increased in this population because of fast-growing cancers, hematologic cancers, need for surgery/central venous catheters, and comorbidities associated with cancer.[72] The risk of pregnancy may outweigh these risks, however, and shared decision making should be made.

SOLID ORGAN TRANSPLANT

Many adolescents and young adults who have received solid organ transplants do not feel well informed about sexual health and desire more guidance.[73] Transplant practitioners also feel unequipped to counsel this population on contraceptive options.[73] Patients who have received a solid organ transplant and are sexually active should be informed that they are at risk of becoming pregnant and should be on effective contraception, especially if they are on teratogenic medication.[73]

Patients who have undergone solid organ transplantation without complications may use any contraceptive method, including hormonal and nonhormonal types (CDC US MEC category 2). However, those with complications including graft failure (acute or chronic), rejection, and cardiac allograft vasculopathy should avoid estrogen-based contraception because of the risk of elevated blood pressure (CDC US MEC category 4).[5] This recommendation comes from the risk of VTE, hypertension, and coronary artery disease among transplant patients.[74-76] Uncomplicated solid organ transplant recipients started on CHC should have their blood pressure monitored to detect new-onset hypertension.

All progestin-based forms of contraception, including DMPA, are listed as CDC US MEC category 2. Consideration should be made with adolescents on chronic corticosteroids or those with renal-mediated bone disease because of the reversible low BMD associated with DMPA and the minimal data on this population.[77] Both copper and LNG-IUDs are safe in recipients with uncomplicated solid organ transplant. Historically, there have been concerns regarding placement of IUDs in immunocompromised patients; however, data do not support an increase in pelvic inflammatory disease in this population.[73] Neither Cu-IUDs or LNG-IUDs should be initiated in patients with complications from

solid organ transplant (CDC US MEC category 3) given case reports of contraceptive failures using Cu-IUD post-transplant.[5,78,79] However, if the IUD is already in place, the benefits of continuing the method outweigh the risks (CDC US MEC category 2).[5] If the priority is pregnancy prevention, another LARC (implant) is still a safe and acceptable method to use in this setting.

GASTROINTESTINAL DISORDERS

Inflammatory Bowel Disease

Most patients with irritable bowel disease (IBD) may safely use all contraceptive methods. Contraceptives do not increase the risk for IBD progression or relapse.[80] Some patients with IBD may have malabsorption, decreasing the efficacy of COCs, but the benefits of the contraceptives are still considered to outweigh the risks (CDC US MEC category 2).[5,80,81] Adolescents with IBD are less likely to have increased risk for VTE, unless they have active or extensive disease, surgery, immobilization, corticosteroid use, vitamin deficiencies, or fluid depletion. If they do have these risk factors, they should avoid CHC use (CDC US MEC category 3).[5] In this setting, all other forms of hormonal and nonhormonal contraception are still safe and acceptable for use (CDC US MEC category 2).

HYPERTENSION

Patients with hypertension (HTN) are at increased risk for stroke and myocardial infarction, and this risk increases among those using CHCs.[82] This risk is multifactorial, as the estrogen component of the CHC increases angiotensin levels, and both estrogen and progesterone increase aldosterone. Both influences may contribute to HTN.[83]

Like most medical conditions in adolescents, there are not specific contraception guidelines for adolescents with HTN. For HTN, we use the CDC MEC for guidance. HTN in pediatrics is defined as average systolic blood pressure (SBP) and/or diastolic blood pressure (DBP) that is ≥95th percentile for gender, age, and height on three or more occasions.[84] In adults, HTN is defined by two or more absolute blood pressure readings with SBP ≥130 or DBP ≥80 obtained on two or more occasions.[85] This definition of HTN is different for adults versus pediatrics, and the existing guidelines for contraception in those with HTN use the adult definitions.

Even for patients with well-controlled HTN, CHCs are a CDC MEC category 3, as the HTN may be more difficult to manage while on CHCs.[80] CHCs should be avoided in those with SBP ≥140 and DBP ≥90 (CDC MEC category 3). For those with SBP ≥160 and DBP ≥100 or vascular disease secondary to HTN, CHCs become a category 4 and DMPA becomes a category 3.[5]

BONE HEALTH

The adolescent years are a crucial time for bone growth, as over 50% of the skeleton is laid down during adolescence.[86] Risk factors for diminished bone density include, among others, restrictive eating disorders, chronic corticosteroid use, and sickle cell disease. Patients at increased risk for diminished BMD should use caution when starting DMPA or low-dose CHCs (≤20 mcg). Estrogen promotes bone growth and mineralization, and DMPA suppresses ovarian production of estradiol.[87] Both DMPA and CHCs containing 20 mcg ethinyl estradiol have been shown to decrease BMD in adolescents.[88] Fortunately, studies have shown that this decrease in BMD is reversible in adolescents and returns to baseline levels after discontinuation of DMPA.[89] This recovery in BMD may occur as early as 24 weeks after discontinuing DMPA therapy.[90]

KEY POINTS

- Contraception counseling should be offered to all adolescents regardless of medical complexities or disabilities.
- In additional to the standard elements of providing contraception care described in detail elsewhere, we recommend the reader adopt a general approach to assessing contraceptive needs for adolescents with medical complexity as follows: (1) review the pregnancy-related risks associated with the medical condition and related medications, (2) review the contraindications to any contraceptive methods related to the medical condition, and (3) consider the benefits of contraceptives for the underlying medical condition.
- Providers should familiarize themselves with the US MEC for Contraceptive Use, which provides guidance about the use of contraceptive methods for pregnancy prevention by people who have certain characteristics or medical conditions. This resource is also available for free online and in an app.

▌ REVIEW QUESTIONS

1. A 16-year-old adolescent with female sex assigned at birth who identifies as male recently suffered a DVT and has been on anticoagulant therapy for 4 months. A thrombophilia workup identified the cause of the thromboembolism was a protein C deficiency. Since starting the anticoagulation, the patient reports heavy menstrual bleeding. Periods last for 10 days, and they are changing pads every 30 minutes. The patient desires effective contraception but would like something that also helps with his heavy menstrual bleeding. Which method is reasonable to prescribe to treat heavy menstrual bleeding?
   a. Etonogestrel implant
   b. 52 mg LNG-IUD
   c. Combined hormonal pill
   d. Progestin-only pill
   e. A, B, and D

2. A 19-year-old female adolescent with migraines with aura presents to your office for contraception counseling. She has been taking topiramate for the past 2 years and feels that her migraines are under better control. How would you counsel her about contraceptive methods?
   a. Because she has migraines with aura, she is at increased risk for stroke if she takes a CHC. This risk is minimal and is considered acceptable by the CDC US MEC (category 2).
   b. She should discontinue the topiramate before starting contraception.
   c. Topiramate may induce the metabolism of CHCs and therefore make them less effective.
   d. DMPA may induce the metabolism of topiramate, and her migraines may worsen.

3. A 17-year-old patient who is >99th percentile in her weight presents to your office for a well-child check. They disclose that they are sexually active and want to start birth control, and you provide contraception counseling. Their weight is 91.1 kg and height is 5′4″. Which of the following statements about contraception for this patient is TRUE?
   a. The levonorgestrel emergency contraceptive pill may be less effective.
   b. The levonorgestrel intrauterine device would be an effective option.
   c. She has an elevated risk for thromboembolism.
   d. She may be more likely to experience a contraceptive failure if she uses progestin-only pills.
   e. A, B, and C

REFERENCES

1. Committee on Adolescence. Contraception for adolescents. *Pediatrics.* 2014;134(4):e1244-e1256.
2. Committee opinion no. 710 summary: counseling adolescents about contraception. *Obstet Gynecol.* 2017;130(2):486-487.
3. Roden RC, Schmidt EK, Holland-Hall C. Sexual health education for adolescents and young adults with intellectual and developmental disabilities: recommendations for accessible sexual and reproductive health information. *Lancet Child Adolesc Health.* 2020;4(9):699-708.
4. Gavin L, Pazol K. Update: providing quality family planning services – recommendations from CDC and the U.S. Office of Population Affairs, 2015. *MMWR Morb Mortal Wkly Rep.* 2016;65(9):231-234.
5. Curtis KM, Tepper NK, Jatlaoui TC, et al. U.S. Medical Eligibility Criteria for Contraceptive Use, 2016. *MMWR Recomm Rep.* 2016;65(3):1-103.
6. World Health Organization. *Medical Eligibility Criteria for Contraceptive Use.* World Health Organization; 2015.
7. Higgins JA. Celebration meets caution: LARC's boons, potential busts, and the benefits of a reproductive justice approach. *Contraception.* 2014;89(4):237-241.
8. Turok DK, Gero A, Simmons RG, et al. Levonorgestrel vs. copper intrauterine devices for emergency contraception. *N Engl J Med.* 2021;384(4):335-344. doi:10.1056/NEJMoa2022141
9. Stanwood NL, Garrett JM, Konrad TR. Obstetrician-gynecologists and the intrauterine device: a survey of attitudes and practice. *Obstet Gynecol.* 2002;99(2):275-280. doi:10.1016/s0029-7844(01)01726-4
10. Keenahan L, Bercaw-Pratt JL, Adeyemi O, Hakim J, Sangi-Haghpeykar H, Dietrich JE. Rates of intrauterine device expulsion among adolescents and young women. *J Pediatr Adolesc Gynecol.* 2021;34(3):362-365. doi:10.1016/j.jpag.2020.11.003
11. Diedrich JT, Klein DA, Peipert JF. Long-acting reversible contraception in adolescents: a systematic review and meta-analysis. *Am J Obstet Gynecol.* 2017;216(4):364.e1-364.e12. doi:10.1016/j.ajog.2016.12.024
12. Averbach SH, Ermias Y, Jeng G, et al. Expulsion of intrauterine devices after postpartum placement by timing of placement, delivery type, and intrauterine device type: a systematic review and meta-analysis. *Am J Obstet Gynecol.* 2020;223(2):177-188. doi:10.1016/j.ajog.2020.02.045
13. Washington CI, Jamshidi R, Thung SF, Nayeri UA, Caughey AB, Werner EF. Timing of postpartum intrauterine device placement: a cost-effectiveness analysis. *Fertil Steril.* 2015;103(1):131-137. doi:10.1016/j.fertnstert.2014.09.032
14. Dina B, Peipert LJ, Zhao Q, Peipert JF. Anticipated pain as a predictor of discomfort with intrauterine device placement. *Am J Obstet Gynecol.* 2018;218(2):236.e1-236.e9. doi:10.1016/j.ajog.2017.10.017
15. Newton JR, Reading AE. The effects of psychological preparation on pain at intrauterine device insertion. *Contraception.* 1977;16(5):523-532. doi:10.1016/0010-7824(77)90075-0
16. Akers AY, Steinway C, Sonalkar S, et al. Reducing pain during intrauterine device insertion: a randomized controlled trial in adolescents and young women. *Obstet Gynecol.* 2017;130(4):795-802. doi:10.1097/AOG.0000000000002242
17. Mody SK, Kiley J, Rademaker A, Gawron L, Stika C, Hammond C. Pain control for intrauterine device insertion: a randomized trial of 1% lidocaine paracervical block. *Contraception.* 2012;86(6):704-709. doi:10.1016/j.contraception.2012.06.004
18. Gemzell-Danielsson K, Schellschmidt I, Apter D. A randomized, phase II study describing the efficacy, bleeding profile, and safety of two low-dose levonorgestrel-releasing intrauterine contraceptive systems and Mirena. *Fertil Steril.* 2012;97(3):616-622.e1-e3. doi:10.1016/j.fertnstert.2011.12.003
19. Hubacher D, Schreiber CA, Turok DK, et al. Continuation rates of two different-sized copper intrauterine devices among nulliparous women: interim 12-month results of a single-blind, randomized, multicentre trial. *EclinicalMedicine.* 2022;51:101554. doi:10.1016/j.eclinm.2022.101554
20. Sammaritano LR, Bermas BL, Chakravaty EE, et al. 2020 American College of Rheumatology guideline for the management of reproductive health in rheumatic and musculoskeletal diseases. *Arthritis Rheumatol.* 2020;72(4):529-556.
21. Gynecologic management of adolescents and young women with seizure disorders: ACOG committee opinion number 806. *Obstet Gynecol.* 2020;135(5):e213-e220. doi:10.1097/AOG.0000000000003827
22. Yerby MS, Kaplan P, Tran T. Risks and management of pregnancy in women with epilepsy. *Cleve Clin J Med.* 2004;71(suppl 2):S25-S37.
23. Tomson T, Battino D, Bonizzoni E, et al. Comparative risk of major congenital malformations with eight different antiepileptic drugs: a prospective cohort study of the EURAP registry. *Lancet Neurol.* 2018;17(6):530-538.
24. Kirkpatrick L, Van Cott AC, Kazmerski TM, Bravender T. Contraception and reproductive health care for adolescent and young adult women with epilepsy. *J Pediatr.* 2022;241:229-236.
25. Coste J, Blotier PO, Mirand S, et al. Risk of early neurodevelopmental disorders associated with in utero exposure to valproate and other antiepileptic drugs: a nationwide cohort study in France. *Sci Rep.* 2020;10(1):17362.
26. Backstrom T. Epileptic seizures in women related to plasma estrogen and progesterone during the menstrual cycle. *Acta Neurol Scand.* 1976;54(4):321-347.

27. Mattson RH, Cramer JA, Caldwell BV, Siconolfi BC. Treatment of seizures with medroxyprogesterone acetate: preliminary report. *Neurology*. 1984;34(9):1255-1258.

28. Maguire MJ, Nevitt SJ. Treatments for seizures in catamenial (menstrual-related) epilepsy. *Cochrane Database Syst Rev*. 2019;10(10):CD013225.

29. Gynecologic Management of Adolescents and Young Women With Seizure Disorders: ACOG Committee Opinion, Number 806. *Obstet Gynecol*. 2020;135(5): e213-e220. doi:10.1097/AOG.0000000000003827.

30. Lopez LM, Bernholc A, Chenet M, et al. Hormonal contraceptives for contraception in overweight or obese women. *Cochrane Database Syst Rev*. 2016;(8): CD008452.

31. Headache Classification Committee of the International Headache Society (I). The International Classification of headache disorders, 3rd ed. *Cephalalgia*. 2018;38(1):1-211.

32. Curtis KM, Jatlaoui TC, Tepper NK, et al. U.S. Selected Practice Recommendations for Contraceptive Use, 2016. *MMWR Recomm Rep*. 2016;65(4):1-66.

33. de Bastos M, Stegeman BH, Rosendaal FR, et al. Combined oral contraceptives: venous thrombosis. *Cochrane Database Syst Rev*. 2014;(3):CD010813.

34. Gerstman BB, Piper JM, Tomita DK, Ferguson WJ, Stadel BV, Lundin FE. Oral contraceptive estrogen dose and the risk of deep venous thromboembolic disease. *Am J Epidemiol*. 1991;133(1):32-37.

35. Creinin MD, Westhoff CL, Bouchard C, et al. Estetrol-drospirenone combination oral contraceptive: North American phase 3 efficacy and safety results. *Contraception*. 2021;104(3):222-228.

36. Mantha S, Karp R, Raghavan V, et al. Assessing the risk of venous thromboembolic events in women taking progestin-only contraception: a meta-analysis. *BMJ*. 2012;345: e4944.

37. van Hylckama Vlieg A, Helmerhorst FM, Rosendaal FR. The risk of deep venous thrombosis associated with injectable depot-medroxyprogesterone acetate contraceptives or a levonorgestrel intrauterine device. *Arterioscler Thromb Vasc Biol*. 2010;30(11):2297-2300.

38. Dietrich JE, Srivaths L. Navigating hormones and gynecologic concerns among female adolescents in the settings of thrombophilia and anticoagulation. *J Pediatr Adolesc Gynecol*. 2015;28(6):549-553. doi:10.1016/j. jpag.2015.05.005

39. American College of Obstetricians and Gynecologists' Committee on Practice Bulletins—Obstetrics. ACOG practice bulletin no. 196: thromboembolism in pregnancy. *Obstet Gynecol*. 2018;132(1):e1-e17. doi:10.1097/AOG.0000000000002706. Erratum in: *Obstet Gynecol*. 2018;132(4):1068.

40. Practice Committee of the American Society for Reproductive Medicine. Combined hormonal contraception

and the risk of venous thromboembolism: a guideline. *Fertil Steril*. 2017;107(1):43-51. doi:10.1016/j.fertnstert.2016.09.027

41. Middeldorp S. Is Thrombophilia Testing Useful? Hematology. 2011. https://bhs.be/storage/app/media/ uploaded-files/4.%20Middeldorp-2011-Is%20 thrombophilia%20testing%20useful.pdf

42. Douillet D, Chapelle C, Ollier E, Mismetti P, Roy PM, Laporte S. Prevention of venous thromboembolic events in patients with lower leg immobilization after trauma: systematic review and network meta-analysis with meta-epidemiological approach. *PLoS Med*. 2022;19(7): e1004059.

43. Prentice A. Fortnightly review. Medical management of menorrhagia. *BMJ*. 1999;319(7221):1343-1345.

44. Zia A, Kouides P, Khodyakov D, et al. Standardizing care to manage bleeding disorders in adolescents with heavy menses – a joint project from the ISTH pediatric/neonatal and women's health SSCs. *J Thromb Haemost*. 2020; 18(10):2759-2774.

45. Mirena (levonorgestrel) [prescribing information]. Bayer HealthCare Pharmaceuticals Inc.; 2022.

46. Schwartz BI, Alexander M, Breech LL. Levonorgestrel intrauterine device use for medical indications in nulliparous adolescents and young adults. *J Adolesc Health*. 2021; 68(2):357-363.

47. Parks MA, Zwayne N, Temkit M. Bleeding patterns among adolescents using the levonorgestrel intrauterine device: a single institution review. *J Pediatr Adolesc Gynecol*. 2020;33(5):555-558.

48. Hernandez AMC, Dietrich JE. Gynecologic management of pediatric and adolescent patients with Ehlers-Danlos syndrome. *J Pediatr Adolesc Gynecol*. 2020;33(3):291-295.

49. Huguelet PS, Laurin JL, Thornhill D, Moyer G. Use of the levonorgestrel intrauterine system to treat heavy menstrual bleeding in adolescents and young adults with inherited bleeding disorders and Ehlers-Danlos syndrome. *J Pediatr Adolesc Gynecol*. 2022;35(2): 147-152.e1.

50. National Institute for Health and Care Excellence (NICE). *Heavy Menstrual Bleeding: Assessment and Management*. London: NICE; 2021.

51. Borzutzky C, Jaffray J. Diagnosis and management of heavy menstrual bleeding and bleeding disorders in adolescents. *JAMA Pediatr*. 2020;174(2):186-194.

52. Archer DF, Nakajima ST, Sawyer AT, et al. Norethindrone acetate 1.0 milligram and ethinyl estradiol 10 micrograms as an ultra low-dose oral contraceptive. *Obstet Gynecol*. 2013;122(3):601-607.

53. Altshuler AL, Hillard PJ. Menstrual suppression for adolescents. *Curr Opin Obstet Gynecol*. 2014;26(5):323-331.

54. Van Vliet HA, Grimes DA, Lopez LM, Schulz KF, Helmerhorst FM. Triphasic versus monophasic oral

contraceptives for contraception. *Cochrane Database Syst Rev.* 2011;2011(11):CD003553. doi:10.1002/14651858. CD003553.pub3

55. American College of Obstetricians and Gynecologists' Committee on Clinical Consensus–Gynecology. General approaches to medical management of menstrual suppression: ACOG clinical consensus no. 3. *Obstet Gynecol.* 2022;140(3):528-541. doi:10.1097/AOG.0000000000004899

56. Hubacher D, Lopez L, Steiner MJ, Dorflinger L. Menstrual pattern changes from levonorgestrel subdermal implants and DMPA: systematic review and evidence-based comparisons. *Contraception.* 2009;80(2):113-118.

57. Zieman M, Guillebaud J, Weisberg E, Shangold GA, Fisher AC, Creasy GW. Contraceptive efficacy and cycle control with the Ortho Evra/Evra transdermal system: the analysis of pooled data. *Fertil Steril.* 2002;77(2 suppl 2):S13-S18.

58. Kaneshiro B, Edelman A. Contraceptive considerations in overweight teens. *Curr Opin Obstet Gynecol.* 2011;23(5):344-349. doi:10.1097/GCO.0b013e328348ec82

59. Bonny AE, Ziegler J, Harvey R, Debanne SM, Secic M, Cromer BA. Weight gain in obese and nonobese adolescent girls initiating depot medroxyprogesterone, oral contraceptive pills, or no hormonal contraceptive method. *Arch Pediatr Adolesc Med.* 2006;160(1):40-45. doi:10.1001/archpedi.160.1.40

60. Le YL, Rahman M, Berenson AB. Early weight gain predicting later weight gain among depot medroxyprogesterone acetate users. *Obstet Gynecol.* 2009;114(2 Pt 1):279-284. doi:10.1097/AOG.0b013e3181af68b2

61. Cheung TS, Goldstuck ND, Gebhardt GS. The intrauterine device versus oral hormonal methods as emergency contraceptives: a systematic review of recent comparative studies. *Sex Reprod Healthc.* 2021;28:100615.

62. Salcedo J, Cleland K, Bartz D, Thompson I. Society of Family Planning Clinical Recommendation: emergency contraception. *Contraception.* 2023;121:109958. doi:10.1016/j.contraception.2023.109958

63. Ramanadhan et al The Levonorgestrel-Releasing Intrauterine Device as Emergenc… : Obstetrics & Gynecology (lww.com)

64. FSRH 2021 FSRH CEU Statement: Response to Recent Publication Turok et al. (2021) - February 2021 - Faculty of Sexual and Reproductive Healthcare

65. Jatlaoui TC, Curtis KM. Safety and effectiveness data for emergency contraceptive pills among women with obesity: a systematic review. *Contraception.* 2016;94(6):605-611.

66. Glasier A, Cameron ST, Blithe D, et al. Can we identify women at risk of pregnancy despite using emergency contraception? Data from randomized trials of ulipristal acetate and levonorgestrel. *Contraception.* 2011;84(4):363-367.

67. Moreau C, Trussell J. Results from pooled Phase III studies of ulipristal acetate for emergency contraception. *Contraception.* 2012;86(6):673-680.

68. ACOG committee opinion no. 740: gynecologic care for adolescents and young women with eating disorders. *Obstet Gynecol.* 2018;131(6):e205-e213. doi:10.1097/AOG.0000000000002652

69. ACOC committee opinion no. 740: gynecologic care for adolescents and young women with eating disorders. *Obstet Gynecol.* 2018;131(6):e205-e213. doi:10.1097/AOG.0000000000002652

70. Lantzouni E, Grady R. Eating disorders in children and adolescents: a practical review and update for pediatric gynecologists. *J Pediatr Adolesc Gynecol.* 2021;34(3):281-287. doi:10.1016/j.jpag.2021.01.010

71. American College of Obstetricians and Gynecologists' Committee on Adolescent Health Care. Options for Prevention and Management of Menstrual Bleeding in Adolescent Patients Undergoing Cancer Treatment: ACOG Committee Opinion, Number 817. *Obstet Gynecol.* 2021;137(1):e7-e15. doi:10.1097/AOG.0000000000004209. Erratum in: Obstet Gynecol. 2022;140(2):344.

72. American College of Obstetricians and Gynecologists' Committee on Adolescent Health Care. Options for prevention and management of menstrual bleeding in adolescent patients undergoing cancer treatment: ACOG committee opinion, number 817. *Obstet Gynecol.* 2021;137(1):e7-e15. doi:10.1097/AOG.0000000000004209. Erratum in: *Obstet Gynecol.* 2022;140(2):344.

73. Huguelet PS, Sheehan C, Spitzer RF, Scott S. Use of the levonorgestrel 52-mg intrauterine system in adolescent and young adult solid organ transplant recipients: a case series. *Contraception.* 2017;95(4):378-381.

74. Paulen ME, Folger SG, Curtis KM, Jamieson DJ. Contraceptive use among solid organ transplant patients: a systematic review. *Contraception.* 2010;82(1):102-112.

75. Pietrzak B, Kaminski P, Wielgos M, Bobrowska K, Durlik M. Combined oral contraception in women after renal transplantation. *Neuro Endocrinol Lett.* 2006;27(5):679-682.

76. Pietrzak B, Bobrowska K, Jabiry-Zieniewicz Z, et al. Oral and transdermal hormonal contraception in women after kidney transplantation. *Transplant Proc.* 2007;39(9):2759-2762.

77. Curtis KM, Martins SL. Progestogen-only contraception and bone mineral density: a systematic review. *Contraception.* 2006;73(5):470-487. doi:10.1016/j.contraception.2005.12.010

78. Lessan-Pezeshki M, Ghazizadeh S, Khatami MR, et al. Fertility and contraceptive issues after kidney transplantation in women. *Transplant Proc.* 2004;36(5):1405-1406.

79. Zerner J, Doil KL, Drewry J, Leeber DA. Intrauterine contraceptive device failures in renal transplant patients. *J Reprod Med.* 1981;26(2):99-102.

80. Carmine L. Contraception for adolescents with medically complex conditions. *Curr Probl Pediatr Adolesc Health Care*. 2018;48(12):345-357.

81. Zapata LB, Paulen ME, Cansino C, Marchbanks PA, Curtis KM. Contraceptive use among women with inflammatory bowel disease: a systematic review. *Contraception*. 2010;82(1):72-85.

82. Curtis KM, Mohllajee AP, Martins SL, Peterson HB. Combined oral contraceptive use among women with hypertension: a systematic review. *Contraception*. 2006;73(2):179-188.

83. Hatcher RA. *Contraceptive Technology*. 21st rev. ed. Ardent Media; 2018.

84. National High Blood Pressure Education Program Working Group on High Blood Pressure in Children and Adolescents. The fourth report on the diagnosis, evaluation, and treatment of high blood pressure in children and adolescents. *Pediatrics*. 2004;114(suppl 2):555-576.

85. Whelton PK, Carey RM, Aronow WS, et al. 2017 ACC/AHA/AAPA/ABC/ACPM/AGS/APhA/ASH/ASPC/NMA/PCNA guideline for the prevention, detection, evaluation, and management of high blood pressure in adults: executive summary: a report of the American College of Cardiology/American Heart Association Task Force on Clinical Practice Guidelines. *Circulation*. 2018;138(17):e426-e483.

86. Gordon CM, Zemel BS, Wren TAL, et al. The determinants of peak bone mass. *J Pediatr*. 2017;180:261-269.

87. Clark MK, Sowers M, Levy BT, Tenhundfeld P. Magnitude and variability of sequential estradiol and progesterone concentrations in women using depot medroxyprogesterone acetate for contraception. *Fertil Steril*. 2001;75(5):871-877.

88. Cromer BA, Stager M, Bonny A, et al. Depot medroxyprogesterone acetate, oral contraceptives and bone mineral density in a cohort of adolescent girls. *J Adolesc Health*. 2004;35(6):434-441.

89. Scholes D, LaCroix AZ, Ichikawa LE, Barlow WE, Ott SM. Change in bone mineral density among adolescent women using and discontinuing depot medroxyprogesterone acetate contraception. *Arch Pediatr Adolesc Med*. 2005;159(2):139-144.

80. Kaunitz AM, Arias R, McClung M. Bone density recovery after depot medroxyprogesterone acetate injectable contraception use. *Contraception*. 2008;77(2):67-76.

Ovarian Fertility Preservation for Children and Adolescents

Olga Kciuk and Stephanie Marie Cizek

INTRODUCTION

When a pediatric or adolescent patient is planning to undergo a therapy that may affect their fertility in the future, medical organizations including the American Society of Clinical Oncology,[1] the American Society for Reproductive Medicine,[2,3] the American College of Obstetricians and Gynecologists,[4] and the American Academy of Pediatrics[5] agree that offering a full range of fertility preservation treatments is the standard of care. The field of fertility preservation is still often referred to as *oncofertility* because many patients undergoing cancer treatment are at risk of infertility and subfertility, but fertility preservation is not just for patients with cancer. Many patients with nononcology diagnoses undergo gonadotoxic therapies, such as patients with lupus receiving multiple rounds of cyclophosphamide or those with congenital anemias undergoing hematopoietic stem cell transplants. Some patients have conditions that may predispose them to primary ovarian insufficiency (POI), such as Turner syndrome. Any patient with Turner syndrome who has achieved menarche should be considered for fertility preservation.[6] Although the magnitude of the fertility risk is unclear, transgender male patients undergoing gender-affirming testosterone therapy are also candidates for fertility preservation.[7] See Table 23.1 for examples of conditions that may necessitate gonadotoxic therapies. Fertility preservation options exist also for patients with testes; however, this chapter will focus on options for young patients with ovaries.

Patients should be fully informed about the effects that their conditions and/or recommended treatments could have on future hormonal and fertility-related outcomes. In qualitative studies, some patients describe the risk of infertility as more devastating than the cancer diagnosis

itself.[8,9] Adolescent patients and their families value early, frequent, and matter-of-fact conversations about fertility preservation, even when options are limited.[10]

TREATMENTS THAT AFFECT FERTILITY

Different therapies have differing effects on the organs and processes required for fertility. Fig. 23.1 summarizes the ways that the hypothalamic-pituitary-gonadal axis and the reproductive tract can be affected.

Chemotherapy

Chemotherapy can result in ovarian insufficiency in a class- and dose-dependent manner. According to the longitudinal Childhood Cancer Survivor Study, 6% of cancer survivors experience acute ovarian insufficiency (defined as primary amenorrhea or permanent amenorrhea within 5 years of diagnosis or treatment).[12] Over the longer term, 9% of cancer survivors experience POI or premature menopause.[13] Chemotherapeutic agents, especially alkylating agents, promote follicular apoptosis, cortical fibrosis, and depletion of the follicle pool by recruitment and burnout.[11] The resulting estrogen depletion can cause vaginal dryness and dyspareunia, affect sexual function, and decrease bone density.

Radiation

Radiation effects on fertility vary based on the location (cranial, pelvic, or total body irradiation [TBI]) and dose of treatment. Radiation to the hypothalamus or pituitary gland is associated with decreased fertility in a dose-dependent fashion, by altering release of follicle-stimulating hormone (FSH), luteinizing hormone (LH), and thyroid-stimulating hormone (TSH). Radiation-related deficiencies

TABLE 23.1 Conditions That May Necessitate Gonadotoxic Therapies

Oncologic Conditions	Anemia	Autoimmune	Other
Lymphoma (e.g., HL, NHL)	Aplastic anemia	Multiple sclerosis	SCID
Sarcoma	Fanconi anemia	SLE	HLH
• Ewing	Diamond-Blackfan anemia	Nephrotic syndrome	Wiskott-Aldrich
• Soft tissue	Sickle cell anemia	Rheumatoid arthritis	Metabolic storage defects
• Bone	Thalassemia	Early/evolving POI	Mucopolysaccharidosis
Leukemia (e.g., AML, ALL)			Amyloidosis
Embryonal tumor			Gaucher disease
• Retinoblastoma			Turner syndrome
• Neuroblastoma			DSD conditions
• Nephroblastoma (Wilms tumor)			Transgender patients
Ovarian tumors			

Predicted gonadotoxicity is dependent on the type of treatment planned.
ALL, Acute lymphoblastic leukemia; *AML*, acute myelocytic leukemia; *DSD*, differences of sex development; *HL*, Hodgkin lymphoma; *HLH*, hemophagocytic lymphohistiocytosis; *NHL*, non-Hodgkin lymphoma; *POI*, primary ovarian insufficiency; *SCID*, severe combined immunodeficiency; *SLE*, systemic lupus erythematosus.
(Adapted from Appiah LC. Fertility Preservation for Adolescents Receiving Cancer Therapies. Clin Obstet Gynecol. 2020;63(3): 574-587. doi:10.1097/GRF.0000000000000547.)[11]

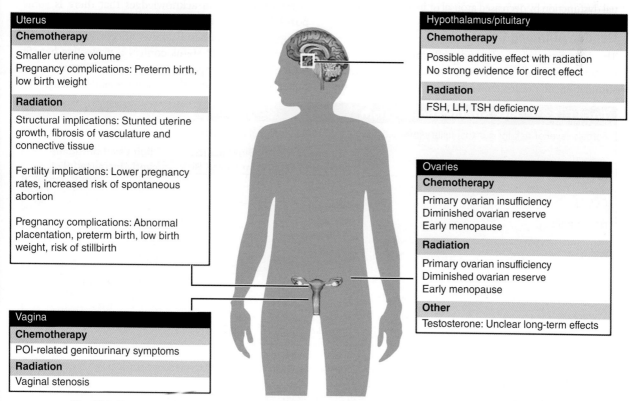

Fig. 23.1 Summary of gonadotoxic and fertility-impairing effects of chemotherapy, radiation, and hormonal treatment.

in FSH and LH can lead to hypogonadotropic hypogonadism and have effects on ovarian and sexual function.[14] At the level of the ovaries, pelvic radiation and TBI promote follicular apoptosis and depletion of the follicle pool.[15] Radiation to the pelvis and TBI can also result in endometrial, myometrial, and vascular damage to the uterus. This can lead to increased risk of spontaneous abortion, abnormal placentation and placental function, fetal growth restriction, fetal malposition, and premature labor.[15] Prepubertal patients who undergo pelvic and abdominal radiation therapy can have stunted uterine growth.[16] Finally, pelvic radiation and TBI can have deleterious effects on vaginal tissues, including fibrosis and atrophy, resulting in pain and loss of function.

Surgery

In the setting of planned pelvic surgery, the long-term fertility and endocrine effects of removal of reproductive organs should be considered and discussed with the patient. In addition to direct effects of resection of the ovaries, tubes, and/or uterus, pelvic adhesions can result in tubal factor infertility, and postoperative nerve damage can lead to sexual dysfunction by decreased arousal or inability to orgasm.

Gender-Affirming Care

The long-term effect of gender-affirming testosterone therapy on ovarian function remains uncertain. Ovarian stimulation after testosterone exposure is often medically feasible, but the process of stimulation and retrieval is not always desired by patients. Before testosterone treatment, discussion of fertility preservation options is beneficial, both to understand fertility preservation offerings and to consider optimal timing for an individual patient.[7]

CLINICAL CARE PATHWAY FOR FERTILITY PRESERVATION

Assess Pubertal Status

The patient's baseline pubertal status should be assessed by clinical history and physical examination (as described in Chapter 11).

Assess Gonadotoxicity Risk

Risk of gonadotoxicity is highest with certain forms of chemotherapy and with pelvic or total body radiation therapy. The risk stratification tool in Table 23.2 takes into account pubertal status, recommended therapy, and expected total dose to stratify the risk of any planned therapy into minimally increased, significantly increased, and high level of increased risk of POI. This classification system acknowledges that there is some possibility of harm with even low-risk therapies. It also recognizes that pubertal status affects POI risk. Although prepubertal status confers a protective benefit for a given dose range, it is important to note that prepubertal patients are still at risk for gonadotoxicity.

TABLE 23.2   Risk Stratification System

Female level of risk for gonadal failure/infertility above that for the general population

		Minimally Increased Risk	Significantly Increased Risk	High Level or Significantly Increased Risk
Alkylators CED g/m²[a]	Prepubertal	CED <8	8–12	>12
	Pubertal	CED <4	4–8	>8
Heavy metal		Cisplatin Carboplatin		
HSCT				Alkylator ± TBI Myeloablative and reduced intensity
Radiation exposure	Ovary Prepubertal		<15 Gy	≥15 Gy
	Pubertal		<10 Gy	≥10 Gy
	Hypothalamus	22–29.9 Gy	>30–39.9 Gy	>40 Gy

[a]CED, Cyclophosphamide equivalent dose. Calculators are available online to aid in calculating an individual patient's CED based on the planned or prior chemotherapy regimen. For example, one may be found at: https://fertilitypreservationpittsburgh.org/fertility-resources/fertility-risk-calculator/.

(Adapted from Meacham LR, Burns K, Orwig KE, Levine J. Standardizing risk assessment for treatment-related gonadal insufficiency and infertility in childhood adolescent and young adult cancer: the Pediatric Initiative Network Risk Stratification System. *J Adolesc Young Adult Oncol.* 2020;9(6):662-666. doi:10.1089/jayao.2020.0012.) The original reference also presents a similar risk stratification tool for male patients, not included in this chapter.

Assess Medical and Surgical Candidacy for Fertility Preservation

Baseline fertility status: Postmenarchal patients should have baseline fertility laboratory testing, which typically includes serum FSH, LH, estradiol, and anti-müllerian hormone (AMH). These tests identify people who at baseline may already be experiencing POI from prior treatments or related to their underlying disease. AMH can predict successful oocyte cryopreservation, although it is unknown if it is able to predict future in vitro or in vivo successful use of tissue after ovarian tissue cryopreservation (OTC). Antral follicle counts (AFCs) to predict oocyte cryopreservation procedural success are typically obtained via transvaginal ultrasound, which is not recommended for prepubertal patients or for postpubertal patients who are never sexually active and/or nonconsenting.

Medical candidacy: A patient's medical status must be considered before any fertility preservation procedure. Patients with airway limitations such as a mediastinal mass may not be safe candidates for surgical procedures. Severely cytopenic and/or immunocompromised patients may also incur higher surgical risks, which should be considered. The time frame in which the gonadotoxic

therapy needs to be started also dictates the ability to do fertility preservation.

During fertility preservation treatment: If OTC is considered, minimally invasive approaches may allow chemotherapy to start the same day as the procedure;[18] if for some reason an open surgical technique is required, this may require a longer recovery time before starting treatment. Oocyte cryopreservation results in supraphysiologic levels of estrogen, which for some patients (for example, those with sickle cell anemia) may incur additional venous thromboembolism (VTE) risks. If feasible, collaborative procedures such as combining OTC with central line placement may minimize anesthesia events for the patient and reduce costs.

After fertility preservation treatment: Significant procedural complication rates are extremely low. For OTC, complication rates are reported to be <1%.[19] Typical pain management medications may be restricted (for example, avoiding nonsteroidal antiinflammatory drugs in a patient with thrombocytopenia), so appropriate alternative pain management modalities should be considered. Table 23.3 summarizes fertility preservation options for young patients with ovaries.

TABLE 23.3 Summary of Fertility Preservation Options for Young Patients With Ovaries

Technique	Typical Candidates	Time Frame Required	Considerations for Pediatric/Adolescent Patients
Oocyte cryopreservation[a]	Postmenarchal	2–3 weeks	Young patients may not be able to tolerate hormone self-injections, multiple (usually transvaginal) ultrasounds
Ovarian tissue cryopreservation	Premenarchal patients or patients of any age who either wish to avoid the process of oocyte cryopreservation or do not have the required time before gonadotoxic treatment	1–2 days	Partial oophorectomy may be possible; because of small size of ovaries, prepubertal patients typically require whole oophorectomy
Ovarian shielding	Candidates planning abdominal or pelvic radiation therapy	Used during treatment	
Oophoropexy	Candidates planning pelvic radiation therapy	1–2 days	More compact anatomy, may not always be feasible to move ovary out of radiation field
GnRH analogue therapy			Although menstrual suppression can be beneficial to reduce bleeding in the setting of chemotherapy-induced myelosuppression, GnRH analogues are NOT a proven fertility preservation method

GnRH, Gonadotropin-releasing hormone.
[a]Embryo cryopreservation requires a sperm partner/donor and is usually not a feasible option in young patients.

Oocyte Cryopreservation

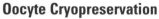

In the adolescent population, oocyte cryopreservation (OC), or egg freezing, is the fertility preservation procedure with the strongest evidence base for resulting pregnancy and live birth. In OC, injectable medications (e.g., gonadotropins) are used to hyperstimulate ovarian follicle development over about 10 to 14 days. Follicle maturation is monitored using ultrasound. This is followed by a procedure, most commonly performed under sedation, in which mature oocytes are retrieved by ultrasound-guided aspiration. The retrieved oocytes are cryopreserved using vitrification. To use the cryopreserved oocytes to achieve pregnancy in the future, the oocytes are fertilized with sperm, and embryo transfer is performed. Embryo cryopreservation, in which sperm is used to perform in vitro fertilization (IVF) immediately after oocyte retrieval to create an embryo, is not common in the adolescent population and is legally restricted in some jurisdictions. During the OC process, ultrasound monitoring and oocyte retrieval are usually performed transvaginally, although for some people a transabdominal approach may be possible. OC is available primarily to postmenarchal teens, as ovaries that have not been exposed to endogenous gonadotropin stimulation may be less likely to respond to stimulation medications. The OC process takes about 2 weeks and requires psychological readiness to undergo ovarian stimulation and the retrieval procedure; this can be difficult for very young postmenarchal patients or people with dysphoria related to gynecologic procedures or hormones. The cost of frozen oocyte storage may not be covered by insurance providers and can be a major barrier.[20]

Ovarian Tissue Cryopreservation

OTC is the fertility preservation option available for premenarchal children or postmenarchal patients who do not have the time required to complete OC or cannot tolerate the procedure of OC. As of 2019, the American Society for Reproductive Medicine considers OTC to be an established medical procedure, no longer an experimental one.[2] For OTC, a laparoscopic unilateral oophorectomy is performed under general anesthesia. The ovarian cortex, which contains primordial follicles, is isolated, divided into small fragments, and cryopreserved.[21] Cryopreserved ovarian tissue can then be transplanted surgically in the future, both to achieve hormonal function and to achieve pregnancy. Ovarian tissue transplantation can be orthotopic, with fragments

of ovarian cortex surgically tunneled into an existing ovary or placed in a peritoneal pocket in the ovarian fossa, or heterotopically, for example, subcutaneously in an arm. In the latter case, IVF must be performed to achieve pregnancy; however, in orthotopic transplantation (OTT), spontaneous pregnancies have been described. The live birth rate after OTC and OTT is up to 40%.[22,23] The risks of this method include the surgical risks of the oophorectomy procedure and the shorter history of this procedure. As of 2020, there have been more than 200 live births using cryopreserved ovarian tissue.[22] The cost of tissue storage can similarly be a barrier to pursuing OTC.[20] Although cost of the surgery itself can be prohibitive, coordination with other planned procedures (e.g., port-a-cath placement) can help to lower fees.

Ovarian Transposition

Ovarian transposition (OT) is the gold standard for fertility preservation in the setting of planned pelvic radiation, for example, for cervical or rectal cancer. Using a laparoscopic approach, the ovaries are mobilized from their usual location in the pelvis and attached to the abdominal wall outside of the field of radiation. Blood supply is maintained through the infundibulopelvic ligament. Hormonal function is maintained, although depending on the transposed location of the ovaries, IVF is likely necessary for pregnancy in the future. The drawbacks of this method include the surgical risks of the transposition procedure and the risk of scattered radiation reaching the ovaries despite their transposed location.[11]

Ovarian/Pelvic Shielding

During TBI, for example, in the setting of stem cell transplant, a lead shield external to the body is placed over the pelvis with a goal of protecting ovarian and uterine tissue. There is a lack of data on whether the decreased dose of TBI resulting from ovarian shielding is associated with increased relapse rate.[11]

Pharmacologic Ovarian Suppression

It has been theorized that gonadotropin-releasing hormone analogues (GnRHas) administered during gonadotoxic therapies may have a protective effect on fertility by suppressing ovarian tissue at a time of high risk for rapid follicle activation and burnout. Systematic reviews of adult women undergoing chemotherapy for breast cancer showed that GnRHa co-administration increased the likelihood of having preserved ovarian function in this population, although pregnancy rates were unchanged.[24] In other populations, data have been conflicting, and no protective fertility effect has been demonstrated.[25] The 2018 American Society of Clinical Oncology (ASCO) recommendations[1] do not support using GnRHa in place of proven fertility preservation methods. However, the menstrual suppression achieved with GnRHa can be beneficial to reduce bleeding in the setting of chemotherapy-induced myelosuppression. If other methods of fertility preservation are not feasible, administration of GnRHa can be discussed as an unproven alternative.[1]

Family Building Alternatives

Fertility preservation counseling should always include a discussion of alternative methods for family building, including using donor oocytes, gestational surrogacy, partnering with someone who has children, or adoption. It should also not be assumed that every person desires to raise children.

SHARED DECISION MAKING

Everyone who receives therapy known to be gonadotoxic should have a documented discussion about their risks of fertility before the gonadotoxic treatment is administered, using the risk stratification protocols as discussed previously, and should be referred for fertility preservation if desired.[2,4] All available fertility preservation options should be offered. Providers who do not feel comfortable or knowledgeable enough to have these discussions should refer to a fertility-trained specialist.

Fertility conversations should be a shared decision-making discussion. Having the discussion itself, regardless of whether a patient ultimately pursues fertility preservation, has been consistently shown to be an important factor in reducing posttreatment regret.[26] Pre-triaging patients into those who should or should not have a fertility discussion, based on factors such as perceived financial status or even prognostic considerations, is ethically fraught and risks paternalism; in general, all patients who are undergoing gonadotoxic therapies should have a pretreatment fertility discussion. All options should be discussed in the framework of risks, benefits, alternatives, and indications in language that the patient and family can understand. Concerns for

overwhelming the patient and family at the time of diagnosis and care planning should also be considered; it may be helpful to provide more than one counseling session, allowing for patient processing and follow-up opportunities for questions.

MONITORING AFTER GONADOTOXIC TREATMENT

Monitoring for posttreatment gonadal insufficiency is recommended in childhood cancer survivors, regardless of whether fertility preservation procedures have been performed.[27,28] Although no clear guidelines are established, a potential standardized protocol for POI surveillance has been proposed (Table 23.4).[29] Throughout monitoring, it is important to counsel patients that spontaneous pregnancy can occur. In the setting of POI in adolescence, there is a 5% to 10% chance of pregnancy related to spontaneous ovulation.[30] For patients who are not planning a pregnancy, use of effective contraception is recommended.

During treatment, temporary ovarian suppression may occur because of the effects of the treatment itself or adjunctive medications used for menstrual suppression (such as GnRHa). Therefore it is *not* recommended to

---

TABLE 23.4 Suggested Protocol for Posttreatment Monitoring for POI Starting 12 Months After Treatment

Prepubertal	Clinical: • Linear growth spurt • Tanner staging • Menstrual calendar • Hypoestrogenic symptoms Laboratory: • Consider FSH, LH, estradiol, AMH q2–3 years until age of typical puberty
Postpubertal	Clinical: • Menstrual calendar • Hypoestrogenic symptoms Laboratory: • Annual FSH, LH, estradiol, AMH *Note that hormonal medications such as birth control may mask clinical symptoms and can affect laboratory values.*

AMH, Anti-müllerian hormone; *FSH,* follicle-stimulating hormone; *LH,* luteinizing hormone.

perform ovarian function testing (FSH, LH, estradiol, AMH) within the first year after treatment completion.[29,31]

Prepubertal and peripubertal patients receiving treatment that may result in ovarian insufficiency (POI or hypothalamic causes) should be asked about hypoestrogenic symptoms and monitored clinically using sexual maturity rating and menstrual calendars in order to ensure that the patient undergoes a normal puberty.[27]

Prepubertal patients would typically have low FSH, LH, and estradiol values, and blood work may be done either intermittently or deferred completely until a patient is nearing the typical age of puberty. AMH, which can be predictive of the number of oocytes able to be obtained with OC, is otherwise less reliable for prediction of fertility. However, there are some data that a downtrending AMH may be a harbinger of impending POI, even in prepubertal patients.[32]

Postpubertal patients who have previously undergone treatments that are intermediate- or high-risk for POI should consider annual FSH, LH, estradiol, and AMH monitoring. This allows (1) early initiation of hormone therapy if POI is identified and (2) if a patient previously declined or was unable to pursue fertility preservation, normal values may indicate an opportune and unique window in which fertility preservation may be undertaken before POI occurs. In addition, a downtrending AMH or intermittently elevated FSH value may represent evolving POI and indicate a more urgent window of time in which fertility preservation may still be pursued, if desired.[33] Patients who are using hormone contraception may still be followed with AMH (not FSH, LH, or estradiol). Although AMH can be decreased by hormonal contraception, nonhormonal contraception such as copper intrauterine devices (IUDs) should not affect AMH, and progesterone IUDs have less of an effect compared with other hormone contraception.[34,35]

BARRIERS TO FERTILITY PRESERVATION CARE

Patients face significant barriers to accessing fertility preservation counseling and treatments. Table 23.5 provides a nonexhaustive summary of barriers to fertility preservation care.

Provider Barriers

In the United States, referral rates for fertility preservation are low; 56% of adolescent and young adult females report having never had a discussion of fertility preservation options before starting cancer treatment.[36] Referral rates improve after implementation of fertility preservation programs.[37,38] As gonadotoxic treatments are usually being administered by providers who are not fertility specialists, the burden falls on referring providers to (1) understand the fertility risks of treatments they are administering and (2) identify and systematically refer patients at risk of gonadotoxicity to an appropriate fertility-trained specialist. Lack of provider

TABLE 23.5 Summary of Barriers to Fertility Preservation

Barriers to Fertility Preservation Care	Strategies to Reduce Barriers
Provider barriers • Referring providers: lack of awareness of treatment risks or fertility preservation options, incorrect knowledge about fertility preservation process, avoiding or deprioritizing fertility discussions • Lack of local fertility-trained specialists	• Provider education • Standardized referral protocols • Identify local fertility-trained specialists, use telehealth if none locally
Systems barriers • Lack of local tissue cryopreservation facility • Nonstandardized referral processes	• Safe shipping of tissue to outside cryopreservation facilities • Electronic medical record tools such as opt-out referrals and alerts • Periodic quality control queries to assess if candidate patients were missed

Cost barriers
• Lack of insurance coverage for fertility preservation
• Insurance mandates for infertility often do not include fertility preservation
• High cost of procedures or related medications
• Annual storage fees for frozen tissue
	• Avoid assumptions
	  • Do not assume a patient cannot afford
	  • Do not assume insurance will not cover—coverage is constantly increasing
	• Insurance mandates to cover fertility preservation
	• Hospital measures to reduce costs of care

awareness of gonadotoxicity of treatments or awareness of options for fertility preservation may be an important barrier. Misinformation about fertility preservation treatments may also be a barrier; for example, in one study in which an institution reported a 24- to 48-hour turnaround to provide a fertility consultation, three quarters of referring providers thought the process would take longer.[39]

Systems Barriers

When the referring physician desires to make a referral, there may be a lack of local fertility-trained specialists, or patients may not have all fertility preservation options available. OTC was labeled experimental until 2019,[2] and until that time a hospital had to have a research protocol in place to offer this procedure. However, with the experimental label removed, many hospitals still do not have the program support or the logistical requirements to offer OTC, and patients may need to travel to access OTC. Adult-trained fertility specialists may also have practice barriers precluding young patients from being seen or may not feel comfortable discussing fertility options with young patients and their families. Pediatric and adolescent gynecology (PAG) represents a growing field in medicine, but there are still some large geographic areas without PAG providers. The growing use of telemedicine may help increase options for patient access in this area.

Nonstandardized referral processes place additional burdens on referring providers to individually identify and refer patients who may be candidates for fertility preservation. To avoid this, it is recommended that opt-out referral processes be implemented; this essentially creates a "pause" point for referring providers to assess the fertility risks of a planned treatment.[40]

Cost

Infertility is traditionally defined as the inability to conceive within 1 year of regular, unprotected intercourse, and infertility treatments have historically been very poorly covered by insurance in the United States.[41] Fertility preservation is treatment for people who *are not yet infertile,* often very young people; insurance coverage and laws mandating insurance coverage therefore often exclude fertility preservation. As of this writing, in the United States, 12 states[42] have laws mandating insurance coverage for fertility preservation, although even among those 12 the mandates are variably wide (for example, some mandate private but not public insurances) and variably enforced.[41]

The cost of fertility treatments is substantial. OC and subsequent IVF can be in the tens of thousands, and surgery for OTC and subsequent OTT can be in the hundreds of thousands of dollars. Annual costs of storage for the frozen tissue can be in the hundreds of dollars per year.[20] The cost of care and the poor insurance coverage contribute dramatically to disparities in care.

Some proposed remedies include broadening insurance mandates to include all types of insurers. As infertility is a known possible, or even likely, outcome for people undergoing gonadotoxic treatments, fertility preservation should be considered part of the cost of those treatments. Institutional-wide and health care systems–wide cost reduction measures also could feasibly make fertility preservation more accessible for all people.

RESEARCH AND KNOWLEDGE GAPS

The field of fertility preservation has exploded in the last several decades, but there is still much that remains unknown:

- Improved understanding of gonadotoxic effects of drugs and therapies
- Development of in vitro oocyte maturation techniques, especially for prepubertal ovarian tissue
- Techniques to avoid reintroduction of malignancy for patients at risk of hematologic spread or who have malignancy within the ovarian tissue
- Pharmacologic ovarian suppression and potential beneficial impact on fertility risk

In addition, continuing to examine and improve the ethical framework around which fertility preservation exists remains an important aspect of care. For example, as laparoscopic techniques become safer, should patients at low risk of gonadotoxicity be offered OTC? Are we striking the optimal balance of provider recommendations, patient autonomy, and parental decision making for our young patients? What systems-based or individual biases contribute to disparities in care for fertility preservation? As this technology is quickly growing and changing, examination of ourselves and the systems we work in remains a constant and important aspect of this work.

KEY POINTS

- Fertility preservation should be discussed with any patient undergoing a potentially gonadotoxic therapy.
- Risk stratification tools can help guide the patient and provider on possible future fertility effects of planned therapy.
- Evaluating a patient for FP requires an assessment of pubertal status, gonadotoxicity risk of the planned treatment, and medical candidacy for OC and surgical treatments (OTC, OT).
- Baseline FSH, LH, estradiol, and AMH levels should be drawn to identify patients already experiencing POI from prior treatments or related to their underlying disease.
- Although pharmacologic ovarian suppression with GnRHas can be beneficial for menstrual suppression in the setting of myelosuppression, data are lacking about its effectiveness for fertility preservation for adolescents.
- Significant barriers to fertility preservation include lack of fertility-trained providers, nonstandardized referral processes, and cost of fertility preservation treatments.
- After undergoing therapies that may pose a risk to fertility, patients should be monitored clinically with annual pubertal/menstrual assessments. For prepubertal patients, there is growing evidence that downtrending annual AMH measurements may be a sign of impending POI. For postpubertal patients, annual FSH, LH, estradiol and AMH allow for early identification of POI.

REVIEW QUESTIONS

1. Which of the following patients would benefit from a referral to discuss fertility preservation?
   a. Prepubertal 9-year-old female status post unilateral salpingo-oophorectomy for germ cell tumor of the ovary planning to undergo chemotherapy with a cyclophosphamide equivalent dose of 7 g/m^2
   b. A 16-year-old transgender adolescent assigned female at birth and planning to start gender-affirming testosterone therapy
   c. A postpubertal 13-year-old female with planned radiation therapy for malignant brain tumor near the hypothalamus
   d. All of the above
2. A 14-year-old cisgender female plans to undergo cyclophosphamide therapy for sarcoma, to be started the next day. The primary team consults you, the gynecologist, to discuss starting gonadotropin-releasing hormone agonist therapy for fertility preservation. The patient describes regular, monthly menses lasting 4 to 5 days and requiring five to six pads per day. What is true about GnRHa administration in this context?
   a. GnRHa has been demonstrated to preserve ovarian function in children receiving chemotherapy.
   b. GnRHa should be used to decrease the risk of primary ovarian insufficiency.
   c. GnRHa may be considered for menstrual suppression in the setting of predicted myelosuppression, but evidence is lacking for decreasing the risk of primary ovarian insufficiency after cyclophosphamide.
   d. GnRHa should be considered both to provide menstrual suppression during therapy, and to decrease the risk of primary ovarian insufficiency from chemotherapy for patients with cancer.
3. A 3-year-old female with familial hemophagocytic lymphohistiocytosis (HLH) plans to undergo hematopoietic stem cell transplantation using a reduced-intensity chemotherapy regimen. What form of fertility preservation should be offered?
   a. Oocyte cryopreservation
   b. Ovarian tissue cryopreservation
   c. No fertility preservation is needed given the patient's prepubertal status
   d. Ovarian transposition

REFERENCES

1. Oktay K, Harvey BE, Partridge AH, et al. Fertility preservation in patients with cancer: ASCO clinical practice guideline update. *JCO*. 2018;36(19):1994-2001. doi:10.1200/JCO.2018.78.1914
2. Practice Committee of the American Society for Reproductive Medicine. Fertility preservation in patients undergoing gonadotoxic therapy or gonadectomy: a committee opinion. *Fertil Steril*. 2019;112(6):1022-1033. doi:10.1016/j.fertnstert.2019.09.013
3. Ethics Committee of the American Society for Reproductive Medicine. Access to fertility services by transgender and nonbinary persons: an ethics committee opinion. *Fertil Steril*. 2021;115(4):874-878. doi:10.1016/j.fertnstert.2021.01.049

4. ACOG committee opinion no. 747 summary: gynecologic issues in children and adolescent cancer patients and survivors. *Obstet Gynecol.* 2018;132(2):535-536. doi:10.1097/AOG.0000000000002764

5. Klipstein S, Fallat ME, Savelli S, et al. Fertility preservation for pediatric and adolescent patients with cancer: medical and ethical considerations. *Pediatrics.* 2020;145(3):e20193994. doi:10.1542/peds.2019-3994

6. Oktay K, Bedoschi G, Berkowitz K, et al. Fertility preservation in women with Turner syndrome: a comprehensive review and practical guidelines. *J Pediatr Adolesc Gynecol.* 2016;29(5):409-416. doi:10.1016/j.jpag.2015.10.011

7. Douglas CR, Phillips D, Sokalska A, Aghajanova L. Fertility preservation for transgender males: counseling and timing of treatment. *Obstet Gynecol.* 2022;139(6):1012-1017. doi:10.1097/AOG.0000000000004751

8. Armuand GM, Wettergren L, Rodriguez-Wallberg KA, Lampic C. Women more vulnerable than men when facing risk for treatment-induced infertility: a qualitative study of young adults newly diagnosed with cancer. *Acta Oncol.* 2015;54(2):243-252. doi:10.3109/0284186X.2014.948573

9. Logan S, Perz J, Ussher JM, Peate M, Anazodo A. Systematic review of fertility-related psychological distress in cancer patients: informing on an improved model of care. *Psycho-Oncology.* 2019;28(1):22-30. doi:10.1002/pon.4927

10. Taylor JF, Ott MA. Fertility preservation after a cancer diagnosis: a systematic review of adolescents', parents', and providers' perspectives, experiences, and preferences. *J Pediatr Adolesc Gynecol.* 2016;29(6):585-598. doi:10.1016/j.jpag.2016.04.005

11. Appiah LC. Fertility preservation for adolescents receiving cancer therapies. *Clin Obstet Gynecol.* 2020;63(3):574-587. doi:10.1097/GRF.0000000000000547

12. Chemaitilly W, Mertens AC, Mitby P, et al. Acute ovarian failure in the childhood cancer survivor study. *J Clin Endocrinol Metab.* 2006;91(5):1723-1728. doi:10.1210/jc.2006-0020

13. Sklar CA, Mertens AC, Mitby P, et al. Premature menopause in survivors of childhood cancer: a report from the childhood cancer survivor study. *J Natl Cancer Inst.* 2006;98(13):890-896. doi:10.1093/jnci/djj243

14. Crowne E, Gleeson H, Benghiat H, Sanghera P, Toogood A. Effect of cancer treatment on hypothalamic-pituitary function. *Lancet Diabetes Endocrinol.* 2015;3(7):568-576. doi:10.1016/S2213-8587(15)00008-X

15. Oktem O, Kim SS, Selek U, Schatmann G, Urman B. Ovarian and uterine functions in female survivors of childhood cancers. *Oncologist.* 2018;23(2):214-224. doi:10.1634/theoncologist.2017-0201

16. Griffiths MJ, Winship AL, Hutt KJ. Do cancer therapies damage the uterus and compromise fertility? *Hum Reprod Update.* 2020;26(2):161-173. doi:10.1093/humupd/dmz041

17. Meacham LR, Burns K, Orwig KE, Levine J. Standardizing risk assessment for treatment-related gonadal insufficiency and infertility in childhood adolescent and young adult cancer: the Pediatric Initiative Network Risk Stratification System. *J Adolesc Young Adult Oncol.* 2020;9(6):662-666. doi:10.1089/jayao.2020.0012

18. Jadoul P, Dolmans MM, Donnez J. Fertility preservation in girls during childhood: is it feasible, efficient and safe and to whom should it be proposed? *Hum Reprod Update.* 2010;16(6):617-630. doi:10.1093/humupd/dmq010

19. Beckmann MW, Dittrich R, Lotz L, et al. Fertility protection: complications of surgery and results of removal and transplantation of ovarian tissue. *Reprod Biomed Online.* 2018;36(2):188-196. doi:10.1016/j.rbmo.2017.10.109

20. Coker Appiah L, Fei YF, Olsen M, Lindheim SR, Puccetti DM. Disparities in female pediatric, adolescent and young adult oncofertility: a needs assessment. *Cancers (Basel).* 2021;13(21):5419. doi:10.3390/cancers13215419

21. Hinkle K, Orwig KE, Valli-Pulaski H, et al. Cryopreservation of ovarian tissue for pediatric fertility. *Biopreserv Biobank.* 2021;19(2):130-135. doi:10.1089/bio.2020.0124

22. Dolmans MM, von Wolff M, Poirot C, et al. Transplantation of cryopreserved ovarian tissue in a series of 285 women: a review of five leading European centers. *Fertil Steril.* 2021;115(5):1102-1115. doi:10.1016/j.fertnstert.2021.03.008

23. Shapira M, Dolmans MM, Silber S, Meirow D. Evaluation of ovarian tissue transplantation: results from three clinical centers. *Fertil Steril.* 2020;114(2):388-397. doi:10.1016/j.fertnstert.2020.03.037

24. Lambertini M, Moore HCF, Leonard RCF, et al. Gonadotropin-releasing hormone agonists during chemotherapy for preservation of ovarian function and fertility in premenopausal patients with early breast cancer: a systematic review and meta-analysis of individual patient–level data. *JCO.* 2018;36(19):1981-1990. doi:10.1200/JCO.2018.78.0858

25. Smith KL, Gracia C, Sokalska A, Moore H. Advances in fertility preservation for young women with cancer. *Am Soc Clin Oncol Educ Book.* 2018;38:27-37. doi:10.1200/EDBK_208301

26. Deshpande NA, Braun IM, Meyer FL. Impact of fertility preservation counseling and treatment on psychological outcomes among women with cancer: a systematic review. *Cancer.* 2015;121(22):3938-3947. doi:10.1002/cncr.29637

27. van Iersel L, Mulder RL, Denzer C, et al. Hypothalamic-pituitary and other endocrine surveillance among childhood cancer survivors. *Endocr Rev.* 2022;43(5):794-823. doi:10.1210/endrev/bnab040

28. Long-Term Follow-Up Guidelines for Survivors of Child-hood, Adolescent and Young Adult Cancers, Version 5.0. Published Online October 2018. www.survivorshipguide-lines.org

29. Molinari S, Parissone F, Evasi V, et al. Serum anti-Müllerian hormone as a marker of ovarian reserve after cancer treatment and/or hematopoietic stem cell transplantation in childhood: proposal for a systematic approach to gonadal assessment. *Eur J Endocrinol.* 2021;185(5):717-728. doi:10.1530/eje-21-0351

30. American College of Obstetricians and Gynecologists. ACOG committee opinion no. 605. Primary ovarian insufficiency in adolescents and young women. *Obstet Gynecol.* 2014;123(605):193-197.

31. Gupta AA, Lee Chong A, Deveault C, et al. Anti-müllerian hormone in female adolescent cancer patients before, during, and after completion of therapy: a pilot feasibility study. *J Pediatr Adolesc Gynecol.* 2016;29(6):599-603. doi:10.1016/j.jpag.2016.04.009

32. Brougham MFH, Crofton PM, Johnson EJ, Evans N, Anderson RA, Wallace WHB. Anti-Müllerian hormone is a marker of gonadotoxicity in pre- and postpubertal girls treated for cancer: a prospective study. *J Clin Endocrinol Metab.* 2012;97(6):2059-2067. doi:10.1210/jc.2011-3180

33. Kanakatti Shankar R, Dowlut-McElroy T, Dauber A, Gomez-Lobo V. Clinical utility of anti-mullerian hormone in pediatrics. *J Clin Endocrinol Metab.* 2022; 107(2):309-323. doi:10.1210/clinem/dgab687

34. Hariton E, Shirazi TN, Douglas NC, Hershlag A, Briggs SF. Anti-Müllerian hormone levels among contraceptive users: evidence from a cross-sectional cohort of 27,125 individuals. *Am J Obstet Gynecol.* 2021;225(5):515.e1-515.e10. doi:10.1016/j.ajog.2021.06.052

35. Nelson SM, Ewing BJ, Gromski PS, Briggs SF. Contraceptive specific anti-Müllerian hormone values in reproductive age women: a population study of 42,684 women. *Fertil Steril.* 2023;119(6):1069-1070. doi:10.1016/j.fertnstert.2023.02.019

36. Shnorhavorian M, Harlan LC, Smith AW, et al. Fertility preservation knowledge, counseling, and actions among adolescent and young adult patients with cancer: a population-based study. *Cancer.* 2015;121(19):3499-3506. doi:10.1002/cncr.29328

37. Korkidakis A, Lajkosz K, Green M, Strobino D, Velez MP. Patterns of referral for fertility preservation among female adolescents and young adults with breast cancer: a population-based study. *J Adolesc Young Adult Oncol.* 2019;8(2):197-204. doi:10.1089/jayao.2018.0102

38. Vu JV, Llarena NC, Estevez SL, Moravek MB, Jeruss JS. Oncofertility program implementation increases access to fertility preservation options and assisted reproductive procedures for breast cancer patients. *J Surg Oncol.* 2017;115(2):116-121. doi:10.1002/jso.24418

39. Boone AN, Arbuckle JL, Ye Y, Wolfson JA. How accurate is oncologist knowledge of fertility preservation options, cost, and time in female adolescents and young adults? *J Adolesc Young Adult Oncol.* 2023;12(1):110-117. doi:10.1089/jayao.2021.0212

40. Moravek MB, Appiah LC, Anazodo A, et al. Development of a pediatric fertility preservation program: a report from the Pediatric Initiative Network of the Oncofertility Consortium. *J Adolesc Health.* 2019;64(5):563-573. doi:10.1016/j.jadohealth.2018.10.297

41. Peipert BJ, Montoya MN, Bedrick BS, Seifer DB, Jain T. Impact of in vitro fertilization state mandates for third party insurance coverage in the United States: a review and critical assessment. *Reprod Biol Endocrinol.* 2022;20(1):111. doi:10.1186/s12958-022-00984-5

42. RESOLVE: The National Infertility Association. Insurance Coverage by State. Published August 27, 2021. https://resolve.org/learn/financial-resources-for-family-building/insurance-coverage/insurance-coverage-by-state/. Accessed January 30, 2023.

Differences of Sex Development: Overview and Clinical Guide

Gylynthia E. Trotman and Alla Vash-Margita

INTRODUCTION

Differences of sex development (DSDs; also known as *disorders of sex development*) is a group of congenital conditions of the urogenital and reproductive tracts that affects human sex determination and/or differentiation.[1] Sex differentiation and development involve a series of events and stages whereby the indifferent gonads, internal reproductive organs, and external genitalia progressively acquire male or female characteristics. In patients with DSDs, the typical development of chromosomal, gonadal, or anatomic sex is altered; karyotype, gonads, and phenotype do not correlate. The evaluation of an individual with DSD includes careful consideration of the medical, surgical, and psychosocial needs of the patient and family. Care is optimally provided in a patient-centered, multidisciplinary approach. Here we discuss the core clinical concepts and highlight discussion on a subset of specific DSD diagnoses.

BACKGROUND AND EMBRYOLOGY

Biologic sex is determined by the sex chromosomes complement that provide direction for an undifferentiated embryo to form along a male or female path.[2] Sex determination and differentiation is comprised of (1) chromosomal sex which refers to the sex chromosome complement (eg. XX, XY) and is established at fertilization. This guides the differentiation of (2) gonadal sex, which is the presence of testis or ovaries. The hormones produced from the gonad then determine the (3) phenotypic or anatomic sex, which refers to the appearance of internal and external genitalia. Multiple genes are involved in differentiation of the bipotential gonad, and

a mutation or error encoding these genes can lead to resulting altered development (Fig. 24.1).[3]

The gonads and reproductive tract are derived from the urogenital ridges. The paired urogenital ridges appear in the fourth week postfertilization and are composed of intermediate mesoderm covered by coelomic epithelium.[2] In addition to the reproductive tract, the urogenital ridge also develops into the kidneys and adrenal cortices.[4] Initially gonads are considered bipotential, as they are undifferentiated and may develop into testes or ovaries.[5]

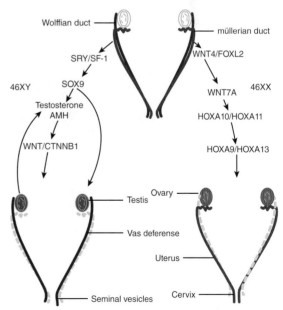

Fig. 24.1 Molecular mechanism of sex differentiation. (From Kyei-Barffour I, Margetts M, Vash-Margita A, Pelosi E. The embryological landscape of Mayer-Rokitansky-Kuster-Hauser syndrome: genetics and environmental factors. *Yale J Biol Med.* 2021;94[4]:657-672.)

Although numerous genes are involved in the process, *NR5A1* and Wilms tumor 1 have been identified as two genes instrumental to the development of the urogenital ridge into an undifferentiated or bipotential gonad, which will then subsequently form into testes or ovaries.[5]

At the sixth week of embryonic life, the initial stages of sexual differentiation are noted where under the presence of the *SRY* gene on the short arm of the Y chromosome (this is also known as the *testis-determining factor on the Y chromosome*), upregulation of SOX-9 occurs, and the undifferentiated gonad develops into testes, with the appearance of first Sertoli and then Leydig germ cells by week 8. The Sertoli cells begin producing anti-müllerian hormone (AMH) and Leydig cells produce testosterone.[4-6] The testes start to descend from the abdominal cavity around week 10, and the descent of the testes to the scrotum by the twenty-fifth to thirty-fifth weeks of development.[2] In the absence of *SRY*, there is a lack of Sertoli and Leydig cells, resulting in an upregulation of ovary-specific transcription factors by week 9. Germ cells then differentiate into oogonia, and under this influence by week 11 to 12, ovarian development subsequently

occurs.[4] The paramount importance of testicular differentiation for fetal sex development has prompted the use of the expression "sex determination" to refer to the differentiation of the bipotential or primitive gonads into testes.[5]

Initially, both of the paired Wolffian or mesonephric (male) and müllerian or paramesonephric (female) ducts are present. Under the influence of testosterone, the Wolffian ducts differentiate into male reproductive structures, whereas AMH secretion causes regression of the müllerian ducts, which are completely absent by week 10. In the absence of high concentrations of AMH and testosterone produced by testicular tissue, there is müllerian duct differentiation and Wolffian duct regression. The paired müllerian ducts develop into the fallopian tubes, uterus, cervix, and upper two-thirds of the vagina. The müllerian duct then meets with the urogenital sinus, which forms the lower vagina.[2,7,8] The Wolffian ducts form the epididymis, vas deferens, seminal vesicles, and common ejaculatory duct.[2,9]

The external genitalia, initially undifferentiated and composed of the genital tubercle, the labioscrotal folds, and the urogenital sinus, similarly undergo hormonally dependent differentiation around weeks 8 to 12[10] (Fig. 24.2).

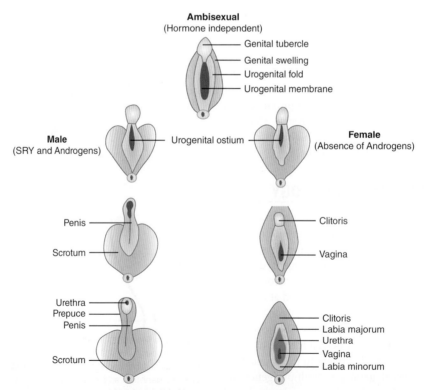

Fig. 24.2 Differentiation of external genitalia. (From Blaschko SD, Cunha GR, Baskin LS. Molecular mechanisms of external genitalia development. *Differentiation.* Oct;84[3]:261-268.)

Male external genital development requires (1) high levels of circulating testosterone, (2) 5-alpha reductase type 2 enzyme for the conversion of testosterone to dihydrotestosterone (DHT) in target organs, and (3) functional androgen receptors. DHT is a potent androgen that results in enlargement of the genital tubercle to a penis and fusion of the labioscrotal folds to form the scrotum. In the absence of elevated androgens, female external genitalia are formed.[10]

EPIDEMIOLOGY

DSD occur in about 1:4500 to 5000 live births and can be caused by atypical chromosomal, gonadal, or phenotypic sex caused by a variation from the typical sequence of sex development. There are generally three categories of DSD: (1) sex chromosome DSD, (2) 46,XY DSD, and (3) 46,XX DSD. Fig. 24.3 describes the three main groups of DSDs and differential diagnosis for each disorder.[1]

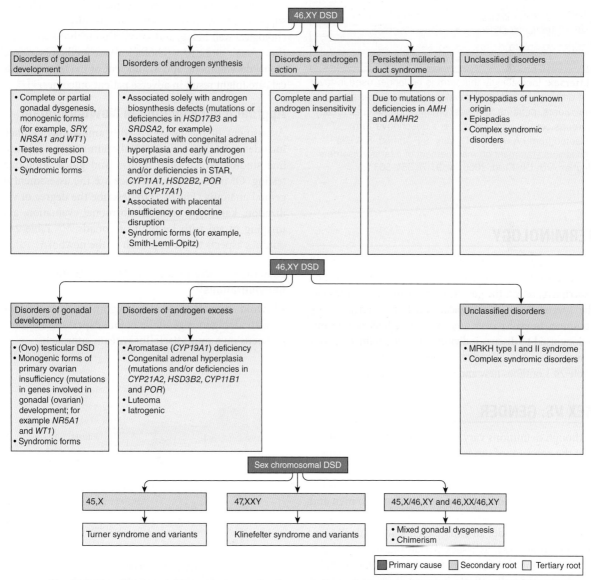

Fig. 24.3 Classification of differences in sex development. (From Cools M, Nordenström A, Robeva R, et al. Caring for individuals with a difference of sex development (DSD): a Consensus Statement. Nat Rev Endocrinol. Jul 2018;14(7):415-429. doi:10.1038/s41574-018-0010-8.)

TABLE 24.1 Evolution of Terminology in Patients with Differences of Sex Development

Updated Terminology	Historical Terminology
Differences in Sexual Development	• Disorder of Sexual Development • Intersex*
46,XX DSD	• Female pseudohermaphrodite
46,XY DSD	• Male pseudohermaphrodite
Ovotesticular DSD	• True hermaphrodite
46,XX testicular DSD	• XX sex reversal
46,XY complete gonadal dysgenesis	• XY sex reversal • Swyer syndrome

*__Intersex:__ Increasingly this term is no longer used in favor of differences in sexual development, however some providers, patients, families, organizations and advocacy groups continue to use this as a descriptive term.
(Adapted from I A Hughes, C Houk, S F Ahmed, P A Lee: Consensus statement on management of intersex disorders. Hughes Arch Dis Child. 2006 Jul; 91(7): 554–563.)

TERMINOLOGY

Terminology used to describe individuals with DSD should be sensitive to the concerns of the patient and family, be descriptive, reflect the genetic etiology, and accommodate the spectrum of phenotypical variation.[11] Terminology continues to evolve over time, and some historical terminology used to discuss individuals may be outdated, controversial, and/or offensive to some patients and families Table 24.1 outlines new and revised terminology.[11]

SEX VS. GENDER

Although definitions vary, it is important to understand that the concepts of sex and gender are not interchangeable. Gender is not to be thought of in a "male" or "female" context but is a social construct that refers to the roles, behaviors, and expectations attributed to men and women in a given society.[12,13] Concepts surrounding sexuality and gender in DSD patients are critically important to address, as issues pertaining to sex assignment and gonadal function may be complex. Gender dysphoria generally affects between 8.5% and 20% of individuals with DSDs.[14] Moreover, studies have shown

that sexuality and sexual function may be negatively affected.[15] Fortunately, the literature has supported overall good sexual well-being among patients who have had optimal medical care.[16]

EVALUATION

Most individuals with DSD will be diagnosed at birth or in the prenatal setting, whereas others will be diagnosed later, such as in the cases of delayed puberty, amenorrhea, or virilization in a girl.[11] For people with DSD, adequate support, quality of life, sexual aspects, physical and psychological well-being, and satisfaction with the treatment (hormonal, surgical, psychological) are predictors of good global development, and insufficient or inadequate medical care might result in adverse patient outcomes.[1,17,18]

Approach to Evaluation in Newborn/Infant

Assessment of the newborn with ambiguous genitalia includes careful history, physical examination, and baseline studies, which then inform and guide additional testing. Of particular importance are the assessment of genital anatomy (Fig 24.4) to describe the degree of virilization, karyotype analysis, hormonal evaluation, and imaging to aid with location of gonads.[18,19] Table 24.2 outlines aspects to the approach of the newborn.

Essentials of Diagnosis and Key Treatment Considerations[11]

• Avoid immediate gender assignment in individuals with ambiguous genitalia before expert evaluation.
• Focus on a multidisciplinary team approach.

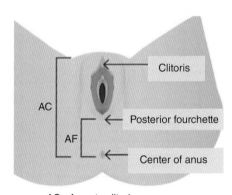

AC= Anus to clitoris
AF= Anus to posterior fourchette
Fig. 24.4 Measurement for anogenital ratio.

TABLE 24.2 Evaluation of the Newborn/Infant for Differences in Sex Development

Approach to Newborn/Infant

History	• Prenatal History • Exposures: danazol, testosterone, phenytoin, spironolactone • Maternal virilization: placental aromatase deficiency, luteoma, theca lutein cyst, androgen-producing adrenal/ovarian tumors • Family history: women in the family (both sides) primary amenorrhea, infertility (no children), unexplained infant deaths Construct Pedigree via consultation with genetics. • Parental consanguinity? • Ethnicity
Physical exam	• Careful examination for other anomalies • Symmetry of external genitalia • Presence of palpable gonads • Genital pigmentation • Extent of labioscrotal fusion • Measure length and diameter of phallus • Location of urethral meatus • Number of perineal openings • Presence of posterior labial fusion • Estimation of anogenital ratio (AF/AC) **(Fig. 24.4)** • For phenotypical girls: distance from the base of the phallus (clitoris) to the posterior fourchette should be approximately 2/3 of the distance from the base of the phallus (clitoris) to the anus
Laboratory evaluation	• Electrolytes • 17-hydroxyprogesterone • Testosterone, DHEAS, androstenedione • LH, FSH, AMH • Plasma renin activity • Dihydrotestosterone • Urinary steroids • Stimulation tests (ACTH, GnRH)
Genetic evaluation	• Karyotype & FISH • Microarray • Sequencing: DSD Gene Panel or Whole exome sequencing
Imaging	• Pelvic ultrasound and MRI: ultrasound is first-line imaging modality • Renal ultrasound will document presence and structure of kidneys • Genitogram (A test in which pelvic ultrasound is used in concert with injection of contrast dye in the urogenital sinus): in complex types of DSD this modality will help delineate urogenital sinus, vagina and cervix thus helping with the diagnosis and possible surgical planning

ACTH, Adrenocorticotropic hormone; *AMH,* anti-müllerian hormone; *DHEAS,* dehydroepiandrosterone sulfate; *FISH,* fluorescence in situ hybridization; *FSH,* follicle-stimulating hormone; *GnRH,* gonadotropin-releasing hormone; *LH,* luteinizing hormone; *AC,* anus to clitoris; *AF,* anus to posterior fourchette.

- Ensure open communication with patients and families with respect and autonomy for patient and family concerns.
- Support the individual in expressing their gender identity as they grow.
- Address any critical associated medical concerns and treatment as needed.
- Discuss endogenous sex steroid adequacy and indications for hormone replacement therapy.
- Consider indications and counseling for surgical management, including gonadectomy and genital surgery, in a patient-centered approach with a focus on patient well-being.
- Discuss impact on fertility and options for fertility preservation where available.

A patient-centered and multidisciplinary care approach with psychosocial support and education is critical to the care (Fig. 24.5). For example, if a newborn is diagnosed with ambiguous genitalia, an algorithm is followed (Fig. 24.6).[20]

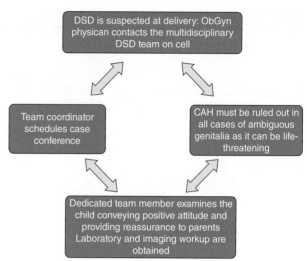

Fig. 24.6 Algorithm if ambiguous genitalia is noted. *CAH,* Congenital adrenal hyperplasia; *DSD,* difference of sex development.

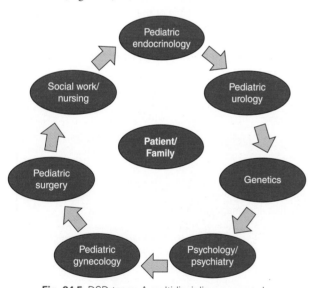

Fig. 24.5 DSD team: A multidisciplinary approach.

Assessment of Genital Anatomy and Gender Assignment

For the newborn with ambiguous genitalia, a variety of methods are used to describe the extent of virilization of the external genitalia, with an aim to communicate the phenotype of an individual. The Quigley scale is a grading system that defines seven classes between "fully masculinized" and "fully feminized" genitalia.[21] The Prader staging is useful to communicate the extent of virilization in 46,XX patients and comprises five stages: 0 (female phenotype, normal clitoris) to V (male phenotype with clitoris appearing as male phallus)[22] (Figs. 24.7[23] and 24.8). The external masculinization score (EMS) is a scoring system ranging from 0 to 12 used to classify the degree of undervirilization of a 46,XY patient. Modified, nonbinary tools, aimed to be more objective and inclusive are in the process of development and validation.

Gender assignment of a child with ambiguous genitalia can be difficult for families and clinicians.[24] The approach

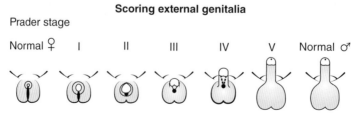

Fig. 24.7 Prader staging tool for evaluation of genital virilization. (From Sperling M, editor. Pediatric endocrinology, ed 2 (p 406). Philadelphia: Saunders.)

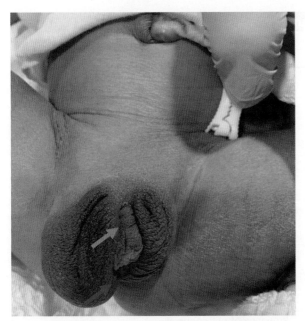

Fig. 24.8 Severely virilized patient with mosaic DSD karyotype 46,XY/45,XO: Rugated labia majora, fusion of labia majora *(red arrow)*, clitoromegaly *(green arrow)*, Prader stage 4 (urogenital sinus with single opening at the base of the clitoris (not seen in this photo). (Courtesy Alla Vash-Margita, MD.)

to sex of rearing decisions in DSD patients has changed fundamentally over time and involves many factors. Influencing factors for sex assignment include specific DSD diagnosis, genital appearance or extent of virilization or feminization (i.e., Prader stage and phallus length), fertility potential, therapeutic and surgical options, and familial views or circumstances including cultural factors.[25,26] Regardless of the gender assigned, providers should understand that as a child grows, they will express their gender identity and should be provided support and resources to allow for gender expression.[27]

Approach to Evaluation in the Adolescent

For the adolescent patient, in addition to a detailed history, evaluation for the presence and sequence of secondary sex characteristics, including androgen or estrogen effect, growth patterns, primary amenorrhea, or virilization, is completed. As the adolescent is gaining autonomy in their care, they should be included in discussions surrounding their diagnosis and care, including medical, surgical options, gender identity, sexuality and sexual function, and fertility potential as age and maturity appropriate.

Treatment Considerations

Management for individuals with DSD is complex and should focus on fostering the well-being of the child and the future adult.[28]

Hormone replacement. Some patients with DSD may have impaired sex steroid production because of gonadal failure/variable function or their gonads removed before, during, or after adolescence, thus requiring hormone replacement therapy (HRT). The goals of HRT are to induce puberty and/or maintain secondary sexual characteristics with adequate circulating sex steroids (estradiol or testosterone), optimize bone health, and promote physical and social well-being.[29]

In biologic females with DSD and absence of endogenous estrogen, HRT with exogenous estrogen is offered for those who identify as females. For pubertal induction, formulations of estrogen are typically introduced at a low dose, gradually increasing to an adult replacement dose over 1 to 2 years. In the presence of a uterus, progesterone is added when the adult dose of estrogen is attained, or earlier if menarche occurs. Pubertal induction using the natural estrogen 17-beta-estradiol is preferable to synthetic or equine estrogens, and this can be administered via oral or transdermal routes.[30,31]

In males who require HRT, exogenous treatment with intramuscular testosterone esters is usually used. Alternatively, testosterone gels and patches may also be used.[31] Optimal hormone replacement throughout the age spectrums is still evolving.[32]

Surgical management. Considerations for surgical management vary and include feminizing genitoplasty with clitoral reduction (clitoroplasty), external genitalia reconstruction, and gonadectomy.[11,33] The medical management in early childhood has been criticized from an ethical point of view, and some advocate for a moratorium on any feminizing or masculinizing operations except for medical emergencies.[11,28] Given the vast heterogeneity of DSD, there is no clear consensus on optimal timing for surgical management. However, our knowledge of the various conditions, outcomes, and quality-of-life measures have improved. DSD care today involves a more patient-centered approach, which has led to a shift from early to later genital surgery, with postponing of surgical management all together in many cases.[1,18,34]

Genital surgery. Table 24.3 highlights arguments for early for delayed genitoplasty.

TABLE 24.3   **Vaginoplasty: Early Versus Late Surgery**

EARLY SURGERY		LATE SURGERY	
Advantages	Disadvantages	Advantages	Disadvantages
Reinforcement of sex of rearing	Scarring at the introitus, necessitating repeated surgeries; potential impact on sexual function	Allows individual to participate in informed consent process	Blood loss and infections are more common in adult patients
Relieve of parental tension regarding the ambiguity of the genitalia	Necessity of revisions of the clitoris in adolescence because of regrowth of tissue in puberty	Potentially reduces need for further surgery in adulthood	Fewer surgeons have experience with late (delayed?) vaginoplasty
Belief that procedure performed early enough in life would be forgotten by the patient	Inability of patient to participate in shared decision making	Allows for vaginal dilation by patient	No consensus regarding the technique used for late vaginoplasties
	Procedure completed prior to gender self-identification	Larger caliber of the proximal vagina leads to a better end result at the level of anastomosis	
		Presence of estrogens allows for easier tissue plane identification and postoperative healing	

Any surgical intervention in neonates and infants that leads to irreversible changes should be done with the utmost caution.[18,34]

Goals of early genital surgery should focus on functionality such as to address issues of urinary tract obstruction or infections and not cosmesis. It is now recommended that surgery be considered only in cases of severe virilization (Prader III, IV, and V).[11] There is limited evidence on patient viewpoints; however, a study composed of 459 individuals with 46,XX and 46,XY DSD found that individuals who had early genital surgery were more likely to approve of it. Participant perspectives varied by diagnosis, gender, history of surgery, and contact with support groups.[35] At this time a few medical centers in the United States have stopped offering vaginoplasty and clitoroplasty for patients too young to participate in the decision making (outside of medical necessity) even in complex cases.[1,36]

Gonadectomy. Gonadectomy is indicated to reduce the risk of developing a malignant germ cell tumor in patients with Y chromatin present. However, the risk of malignancy is based on the underlying etiology. The highest risk is noted in patients with gonadal dysgenesis and partial androgen insensitivity syndrome (PAIS)

with intraabdominal gonads. Other conditions confer much lower risk.[37,38] Table 24.4 provides a key tool outlining malignancy risk assessment, which can inform surgical timing decisions. As gonadectomy necessitates lifelong HRT and removes fertility potential, risk stratification is important in the discussion of optimal timing of gonadectomy. Whereas early removal is typically recommended for diagnoses carrying a high risk of tumor, delayed removal after pubertal development is complete, and patient consent can be obtained if recommended.[18] An increasing number of adults with a DSD have retained gonads. However, to date there are no clear guidelines for monitoring or screening for malignancy in addition, and often surveillance imaging and gonadal biopsies are considered.[1]

Fertility preservation. Individuals with DSD often have inherent subfertility. Their infertility risks are the result of (1) abnormal gonadal development, (2) progressive gonadal failure over the first two decades of life, (3) gonadectomy for malignancy risk, (4) abnormal hormone production, resulting in impaired gamete production, (5) discordance between gonadal type and gender identity, leading to an assumption of infertility, and (6) anatomic barriers.[39,40] The emerging and

TABLE 24.4 Key Tool Outlining Malignancy Risk Assessment

DSD	Malignancy Risk (%)	Risk	Management of the Gonads
Gonadal dysgenesis with Y chromosome, gonad located intraabdominally	15-35	High	Gonadectomy[a]
PAIS, nonscrotal gonad	50		Gonadectomy[a]
Turner with Y chromosome	12	Intermediate	Gonadectomy[a]
17-β-HSD	28		Surveillance is acceptable
PAIS, scrotal gonad	Unknown		Biopsy[b] and radiation(?)
CAIS	2	Low	Biopsy and ?
Ovotestes DSD	3		Testicular tissue removal(?)
Turner (absent Y chromosome)	1		No action
5α-reductase	0	No risk (?)	Unresolved

(From Morin J, Peard L, Saltzman AF. Gonadal malignancy in patients with differences of sex development. Transl Androl Urol. 2020 Oct;9(5):2408-2415 Looijenga LH, Hersmus R, Oosterhuis JW, Cools M, Drop SL, Wolffenbuttel KP. Tumor risk in disorders of sex development (DSD). Best Pract Res Clin Endocrinol Metab. 2007 Sep;21(3):480-95.)

CAIS, Complete androgen insensitivity syndrome; *17-β-HSD,* 17-β-hydroxysteroid dehydrogenase deficiency; *PAIS,* partial androgen insensitivity syndrome.
[a]– At time of diagnosis
[b]– At puberty
?– Consensus, but further studies are needed

expanding field of oncofertility has made fertility preservation options viable for some individuals with DSD, and novel studies on germ cell quantity in a variety of DSD conditions typically thought to have no or very limited fertility prospective suggests that fertility potential may be greater than previously thought.[41] Although fertility potential is known to be an important predictor of quality of life, clinicians should make no assumptions as to an individual's desires for biologic parenthood. Moreover, alternative options for family building, including adoption, fostering, use of donor oocytes or sperm, and gestational surrogacy, should be discussed with patients and families.

SEX CHROMOSOME DSD

Klinefelter Syndrome

Klinefelter syndrome (KS), Online Mendelian Inheritance in Man (OMIM; https://www.omim.org) #400045, is the most common form of sex chromosome (X-linked) aneuploidy, with an incidence of 1 in 500 to 1000 births.[42] The most common karyotype is 47,XXY, with other less frequent variants also reported. The nondisjunction of the sex chromosomes during the first or second meiotic division leads to this type of DSD. The müllerian ducts regress because the testes produce AMH. The male internal ducts (Wolffian) are normal

because of adequate production of testosterone. Puberty is typically delayed or absent; thus diagnosis is commonly made during adolescence. Classically, the individual shows signs of hypogonadism and has elevated levels of gonadotropins (e.g., hypergonadotropic hypogonadism). On physical examination gynecomastia and small firm testes are the cardinal stigmata of KS.[43] See Table 24.5.

Historically, infertility was universal. Currently, fertility can be achieved in up to 64% of patients with KS via testicular sperm extraction and intracytoplasmic sperm injection (TESE/ICSI).[44]

Turner Syndrome

Turner syndrome (TS), OMIM #300082, is the most common sex chromosome abnormality in females and is the most common etiology for primary amenorrhea and delayed puberty.[45,46] TS occurs in approximately 1/2500 live-born girls and is a common genetic cause of spontaneous abortion, accounting for 1/15.[47,48] Diagnosis requires characteristic physical features and complete or partial absence of a sex chromosome. 45,XO accounts for 50% of cases, with the remaining cases comprising mosaic karyotypes such as 45,X/46,XX.[46,49]

The diagnosis of TS can occur at a wide range of ages, from prenatal diagnosis to diagnosis in adulthood, given the variable genetic and phenotypic presentations.[32]

TABLE 24.5 Phenotypical and Endocrine Features of the Klinefelter Syndrome

Feature	Findings
Growth (height)	Tall stature
External Genitalia	
Male	• Normal penis • Ambiguous genitalia • Hypospadias
Female	• Enlarged clitoris • Urogenital sinus
Internal Genitalia	
Male	• Low libido • Small, soft testes • Azoospermia • Ovotestis, unilateral • Fibrous ovarian stroma • Primordial ovarian follicles • Seminiferous tubules without germ cells, rete testis, or Leydig cells
Endocrine features	• Low testosterone • Elevated follicle-stimulating hormone (FSH) • Elevated luteinizing hormone (LH)

Classic TS is associated with reduced adult height and gonadal dysgenesis presenting as streak gonads. In individuals with classic TS, the germ cells develop normally; however, accelerated loss of oocytes results in rapid depletion and primary ovarian insufficiency.[50] This leads to insufficient circulating levels of female sex steroids resulting in absent pubertal development and infertility.[51] Other findings include but are not limited to webbed neck, broad chest and wide-spaced nipples, cardiac and renal abnormalities, sensorineural hearing loss, ophthalmologic problems, thyroid abnormalities, metabolic syndrome, inflammatory bowel disease, and neurocognitive issues. There are fewer related health conditions in patients with certain mosaic karyotypes.[32]

Spontaneous puberty has been reported in 14% of TS patients with 45,X and up to a third of patients with mosaicism.[32] The majority of the girls with TS, however, require induction of puberty and estrogen/progestin replacement therapy to achieve adequate breast development, uterine maturation, and peak bone mass.

Growth hormone (GH) therapy is used to improve adult height.[52] Patients with TS typically do not present with ambiguity in terms of sex assignment, and gender dysphoria is comparable to that of the general population. Turner mosaic patients with Y chromosome material have an increased risk of malignancy, even in infancy and childhood, and timely gonadectomy is warranted at the time of diagnosis of the Y material.[53] See Table 24.4.

There are reported rates of spontaneous pregnancy in 2% to 5% of patients with TS; however, the majority of patients will have eventual infertility. As such, early counseling on fertility preservation options is integral. Fertility preservation can be accomplished through ovarian tissue cryopreservation (OTC) or oocyte cryopreservation in patients with evidence of fertility potential based on ovarian reserve testing.[54] However, many patients with TS will employ donor oocytes as a path to parenthood. Whether conception is spontaneous or assisted reproductive technology is employed, pregnancy in patients with TS is associated with increased maternal morbidity and mortality, mainly owning to cardiovascular risks, as well as increased fetal/neonatal risks. As such, preconception screening and counseling are critical for affected individuals seeking pregnancy.[55,56]

46,XY DSD

Androgen Insensitivity Syndrome

Complete androgen insensitivity syndrome (CAIS), OMIM #300068, is defined as an X-linked recessive DSD in which androgen resistance is caused by mutations in the androgen receptor (AR) gene located on Xq12. The prevalence of CAIS is approximately 1:20,000 to 1:64,000 male births. Aromatization of endogenous testosterone production during puberty will lead to the development of secondary female sex characteristics. Impairment of androgen receptor function leads to an unvirilized or typically female phenotype with scant pubic hair. Typically, a child with CAIS will be assigned female gender and will be raised as female. On physical examination and imaging, CAIS is characterized by female external genitalia; absence of the uterus and fallopian tubes; no Wolffian duct development; testes located in the abdomen, inguinal canal, or labioscrotal region; and a blind-ending vagina. Genetic testing reveals a 46,XY karyotype.

Two diagnostic clinical scenarios of CAIS presentation are as follows:

1. Female child with inguinal hernia → suspect CAIS → workup shows testes in inguinal canal (as content of hernia) → perform vaginoscopy to see if cervix is visualized. If no cervix is seen → karyotype should be performed[57]
2. Primary amenorrhea in an adolescent with female secondary sex characteristics → evaluation shows elevated testosterone levels and ultrasound reveals no uterus

Once a diagnosis of CAIS is made, clinical care should address the following major concerns:

1. Management of the gonads: Historically, gonads were removed at the time of diagnosis because of concern for malignancy (i.e., gonadoblastoma, seminoma, or germ cell neoplasia in situ [GCNIS]). Subsequently, growing evidence indicated that because of the low rate of malignancy early in life, prophylactic gonadectomy may be deferred until at least after puberty. In a recent systematic review of 15 studies including 456 patients, malignancy was detected in only 1.3% and after 12 years of age in patients with CAIS (see Table 24.4).[58] In general, the accepted practice is to maintain gonads in situ until after puberty, allowing for optimal pubertal development and participation of a more mature patient in health care decisions.
2. Gender assignment: The majority of individuals with 46,XY CAIS choose female gender identity. According to a recent systematic review and meta-analysis, all patients with CAIS were raised as females, and the prevalence of gender identity query or gender identity disorder (GID) was low, at 1.7% (4/238).[59]
3. Creation of the vagina: In individuals who desire to lengthen the vagina and facilitate sexual intercourse, nonsurgical self-dilation of the vaginal pouch is the first line of treatment because of its less invasive character and high success rate. Various surgical techniques are available to lengthen the vagina in case self-dilation is not desired or could not be accomplished, but the best treatment remains controversial.[60-66] Timing of vaginoplasty remains unclear as well. Arguably, the most appropriate time to undergo surgical creation of the vagina is in adolescence. Most studies (including studies dedicated to vaginal aplasia in müllerian anomalies) recommend that such intervention is to be undertaken when the

patient is emotionally mature and expresses a desire to engage in sexual activity.[67-70]

4. Hormonal replacement therapy: HRT is an integral part of care for these patients. If an adolescent underwent surgery before puberty, HRT should be offered at the average age of pubertal development after a shared decision is achieved between the patient, caregivers, and providers. If a patient chooses female gender identity, estrogen hormone replacement is traditionally used. The optimal regimen of hormone replacement remains unknown. Progestin addition is not required, as individuals with CAIS do not have a uterus; therefore protection of the endometrium is not required.
5. Fertility counseling: Spontaneous pregnancy is not possible. Germ cells have been detected in the intraabdominal gonads; therefore there is a possibility of future fertility, although this approach is strictly experimental at this time.[41]

Partial Androgen Insensitivity Syndrome

PAIS is an X-linked recessive type of 46,XY DSD, OMIM# 312300, that results in the partial inability of the cell to respond to androgens. Individuals produce age-appropriate androgen levels but have undermasculinized external genitalia because of defects in androgen action. The phenotype in PAIS is highly variable, ranging from a penis with penoscrotal or perineoscrotal hypospadias and cryptorchidism to labioscrotal swellings burying a micropenis, looking feminized.[71] Infants with PAIS are assigned to either male or female sex, depending on the degree of masculinization.

Because of this heterogeneity in the phenotype, it is difficult to estimate the prevalence of this condition. Many individuals with PAIS are raised as males, although a clear recommendation on sex of rearing remains elusive in PAIS, and gender identity is much more fluid among persons born with PAIS.[27]

The risk of germ cell tumor is higher compared with CAIS, at approximately 15%.[37,72]

For individuals who choose female gender and wish to engage in penetrative vaginal intercourse, vaginoplasty may be offered. Self-dilation and surgical techniques would be employed similarly as described for individuals with CAIS.

For the individuals who choose male gender and demonstrate readiness for pubertal development, pubertal induction should be offered around age 12 years by administering low-dose testosterone esters (testosterone enanthate, cypionate, and propionate) and slowly increasing to mimic typical pubertal development.[73]

The options for fertility preservation for individuals with PAIS are limited. However, studies are evaluating any potential viable gonadal tissue cryopreserved for future use.[63,74]

Ovotesticular DSD

Ovotesticular DSD, OMIM# 400045, is associated with different karyotypes, including 46,XX (60% of the cases), mosaic 46,XX/XY (30% of the cases), and 46,XY (10% of the cases). In this condition, a combination of the bilateral ovotestes or a healthy ovary or testis with a contralateral ovotestis can be detected. Ovotesticular DSD is characterized by the presence of both ovarian and testicular tissues. The overall incidence has been reported as 1 out of 100,000 live births. Genital appearance is dependent on the type and function of the gonadal tissue present. In cases where gonads contain ovarian tissue, such gonads are usually functional.[75-77]

A small number of pregnancies have been reported in ovotesticular DSD females. In a cohort of 22 patients, 3 patients had normal uteri and 2 of them had pregnancy and childbirth.[78] Another study that followed patients since 1974 describes 26 pregnancies in 14 patients with ovotesticular DSD, with 20 healthy babies born.[76] The risk for malignant germ cell tumors in ovotesticular DSD is exceedingly low, with only nine cases reported to date (see Table 24.4).[79]

The decision on sex of rearing in ovotesticular DSD is often considered based on the potential for fertility as a female.[78] At present, there are no clear reports on GID prevalence in this condition. Individuals with ovotesticular DSD who choose male gender identity may proceed with the removal of müllerian structures and unilateral gonad (ovary) and subsequent intramuscular testosterone injections, with resultant male phenotype and normal sperm concentration even after cessation of the injections.[80]

Complete Gonadal Dysgenesis

This type of DSD is a 46,XY DSD, OMIM# 233420, with a prevalence of 1:80,000 individuals. It is characterized by normal external female genitalia, uterus and fallopian tubes, and bilateral streak gonads (Fig. 24.9). This condition will usually present in the adolescent period as primary amenorrhea and absent pubertal development.

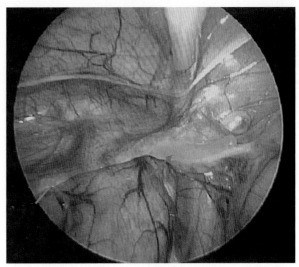

Fig. 24.9 Panoramic view of the pelvis in a 10-month-old patient with 46,XY DSD complete gonadal dysgenesis who underwent bilateral gonadectomy: Right streak gonad *(blue arrow)*; fundus of the hypoestrogenic uterus *(green arrow)*. (Courtesy Alla Vash-Margita, MD.)

Diagnosis is often delayed, as individuals typically appear female without any signs of virilization.

Dysgenetic streak gonads have a high potential for malignancy.[81] Germ cell tumor prevalence is around 15% to 35% in conditions associated with gonadal dysgenesis, with the most common cancers being gonadoblastoma, carcinoma in situ (CIS) with potential development into dysgerminoma, and seminoma (see Table 24.4). The widely accepted recommendation is that patients with XY,CGD have bilateral gonadectomy at the time of diagnosis in order to prevent the development of malignancy[82] (Fig. 24.10).

There is a low prevalence of gender dysphoria in complete gonadal dysgenesis (CGD) patients raised as females.[59,83] Typically, a female gender is chosen as sex of rearing, which is congruent with female external genitalia.[59,83]

In a study by Finlayson and colleagues, none of the patients with complete or partial gonadal dysgenesis had germ cells.[41] Infertility was considered universal in the past. These individuals have a normal uterus, so current advancements in reproductive fertility led to the ability of individuals with CGD to become pregnant via egg donation and embryo transfer. To date, however,

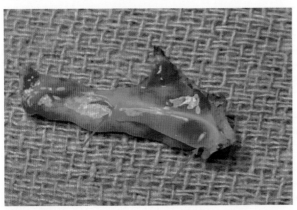

Fig. 24.10 A 10-month-old patient with 46,XY DSD complete gonadal dysgenesis: streak gonad removed; pathology consistent with gonadoblastoma. Two poles of the gonad *(blue arrows)*. (Courtesy Alla Vash-Margita, MD.)

there is limited evidence of pregnancies in individuals with CGD of that achieved after in vitro fertilization (IVF).[84-86]

46,XX DSD

Congenital Adrenal Hyperplasia

Congenital adrenal hyperplasia (CAH) comprises a family of autosomal recessive disorders that disrupt adrenal steroidogenesis. The most common form is caused by 21-hydroxylase deficiency (21-OHD) associated with mutations in the *CYP21A2* gene, which is located at chromosome 6p21 and occurs in ~95%.[87] Other less common virilizing forms include but are not limited to 3-β-hydroxysteroid dehydrogenase and 11-β-hydroxylase deficiencies.[86] CAH is the most common cause of the masculinized female and ambiguous genitalia at birth.[88] The incidence is about ~1:14,000 to 1:18,000 births; however, the condition is more prevalent in small geographic regions such as the Alaskan Yupiit.[89]

21-Hydroxylase deficiency (21-OHD) leads to an underproduction of cortisol and aldosterone, which results in increased adrenocorticotropic hormone (ACTH) production. Clinical presentation varies based on the severity of 21-OHD and ranges from salt-losing and simple virilizing seen in the early-onset or classic form to the milder late-onset or nonclassic form of congenital adrenal hyperplasia (NCCAH)[87,90] (Fig. 24.11).

Classic 21-OHD CAH is subdivided into two forms: (1) salt wasting, which is most common occurring in 75% to 80% of affected individuals, and (2) simple virilizing.[91] Classic 21-OHD CAH is a life-threatening condition owing to deficiencies of cortisol, aldosterone, and adrenaline. This is potentially fatal because of the resulting hyponatremia, hypoglycemia, hyperkalemia, and hypotension if not recognized within the first 2 to 3 weeks of life; hence neonatal screening programs exist worldwide.[87,91,92] Simple virilization occurs in the remaining 2% to 25% of patients and is not associated with severe electrolyte abnormalities.[91]

Because of elevated testosterone, affected females are virilized at birth, with phenotype ranging from slight clitoromegaly to complete masculinization of the external genitalia, which is most often described by Prader stage. Despite excessive prenatal androgen exposure, the uterus and ovaries are present and the Wolffian ducts regress. In severe forms, the urogenital sinus persists.[87,89]

Adolescents and Adults

The nonclassic (mild) form is associated with *CYP21A2* mutations that retain 20% to 50% of enzyme activity.[92] It has a reported frequency of 1:200 in the US population.[89]

Evaluation for NCCAH is made by testing for elevated 17OHP (Table 24.6).[89] Patients diagnosed with NCCAH may present with similar clinical features of polycystic ovary syndrome (PCOS) and include hirsutism, abnormal or absent menses, and infertility, with hirsutism being the most common presenting feature.[87,93]

Treatment

Treatment of CAH varies based on severity and includes administration of steroids, cortisol, and mineralocorticoid to prevent life-threatening electrolyte abnormalities and progressive virilization. These patients also require evaluation and ongoing management for typical linear growth and pubertal development. Regularization of menses, prevention of progression of hirsutism with the use of antiandrogen and estrogen-/progestin-containing preparations, and preservation of fertility in adolescents and adults are paramount.[87,89]

Gender Assignment

Most individuals with CAH and modest virilization (Prader scale 0–3) are designated female at birth.[94] The overall prevalence of gender dysphoria in CAH is 5% according to a recent systematic literature review and

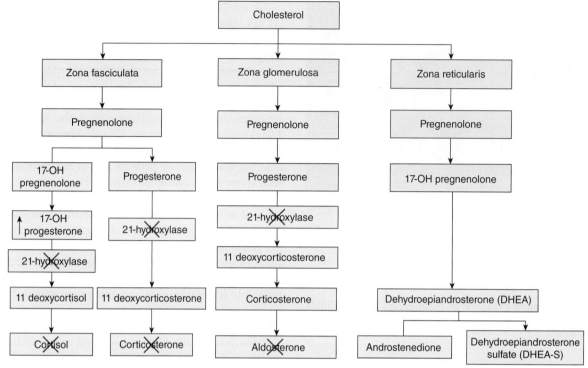

Fig. 24.11 21-Hydroxylase deficiency in CAH: Affected steroidogenesis. (From Prentice P. Guideline review: congenital adrenal hyperplasia clinical practice guideline 2018. *Arch Dis Child Educ Pract Ed.* 2021;106[6]: 354-357. doi:10.1136/archdischild-2019-317573)

TABLE 24.6 **Diagnosis of Nonclassical Congenital Adrenal Hyperplasia**	
17OHP Level (should be obtained in the early morning (before 8 AM)	**Interpretation**
<200 ng/dL	NCCAH is ruled out
200 and 1,000 ng/dL	Need for additional testing with cosyntrin stimulation test
>1,000 ng/dL	NCCAH is confirmed

meta-analysis.[59] In the same study patients with CAH reared as females had 4% gender dysphoria, whereas patients reared as males had significantly higher dysphoria at 15%.[59]

Surgery

Controversy exists regarding the necessity and timing of genitoplasty in girls with CAH.[35,95,96] Consensus guidelines recommend feminizing genitoplasty only in cases of severe virilization, undertaken via a multidisciplinary approach, involving extensive discussion and shared decision making.[11,97] For patients in which the decision is made to proceed with surgical management, feminizing genitoplasty typically includes vaginoplasty, clitoroplasty, or a combination of both and is undertaken in infancy or later in adolescence.[87,95]

Fertility

Fertility rates in females with CAH depend on phenotype and are inversely proportional to the severity of the disease. Subfertility rates are higher in those patients with suboptimal control, partially because of suboptimal ovulation, and patients wishing for fertility should be counseled regarding this.[88]

Consultation with a reproductive specialist is recommended to increase ovulation and discuss options for oocyte cryopreservation when appropriate. NCCAH is associated with higher pregnancy rates, particularly among those treated with glucocorticoids, and live birth rates comparable to the general population.[98]

KEY POINTS

- DSD is a group of complex conditions with variations in presentation, diagnosis, and ongoing care.
- Multidisciplinary teams are the preferred models of health care for this patient population (see Fig. 24.5).
- A patient-centered care approach with psychosocial support and education is critical to the care, with emphasis placed on fostering the well-being of the child and the future adult.
- All aspects of care such as fertility potential, surgical considerations, and hormone replacement should be conducted in a patient-/family-centered approach.

REVIEW QUESTIONS

1. The development of male external genitalia requires:
   a. 5-alpha reductase type 2 enzyme
   b. Low circulating testosterone
   c. Secretion of anti-müllerian hormone (AMH) from the Leydig germ cells
2. The indication for gonadectomy in a patient with DSD is:
   a. Decrease the risks of malignant transformation of a gonadoblastoma
   b. Ensure the sex of rearing aligns with gender identity
   c. Required in a patient with Turner syndrome 45,XO
3. Congenital adrenal hyperplasia is a group of autosomal recessive disorders caused by:
   a. Mutations in the androgen receptor (AR) gene
   b. Disruption of adrenal steroidogenesis
   c. Rapid depletion of oogonia

ACKNOWLEDGMENTS

The authors would like to acknowledge the support of Alyssa Grimshaw, MBA, MSLIS, Harvey Cushing/John Hay Whitney Medical Library, Yale University, United States, for organization of the bibliography and Isaac Kyei-Barffour, MPhil, molecular and cellular biologist, University of Cape Coast, Department of Biomedical Sciences, Ghana, for graphic design.

REFERENCES

1. Cools M, Nordenström A, Robeva R, et al. Caring for individuals with a difference of sex development (DSD): a consensus statement. *Nat Rev Endocrinol.* 2018;14(7):415-429. doi:10.1038/s41574-018-0010-8.
2. Aatsha P, Krishan K. Embryology, sexual development. In: *StatPearls [Internet].* Treasure Island, FL: StatPearls Publishing; 2023 Jan.
3. Kyei-Barffour I, Margetts M, Vash-Margita A, Pelosi E. The embryological landscape of Mayer-Rokitansky-Kuster-Hauser syndrome: genetics and environmental factors. *Yale J Biol Med.* 2021;94(4):657-672.
4. Witchel SF. Disorders of sex development. *Best Pract Res Clin Obstet Gynaecol.* 2018;48:90-102. doi:10.1016/j.bpobgyn.2017.11.005.
5. Rey R, Josso N, Racine C. Sexual differentiation. In: *Endotext [Internet].* South Dartmouth, MA: MDText.com, Inc.; 2000.
6. Lucas-Herald AK, Bashamboo A. Gonadal development. *Endocr Dev.* 2014;27:1-16. doi:10.1159/000363608.
7. Cunha GR, Robboy SJ, Kurita T, et al. Development of the human female reproductive tract. *Differentiation.* 2018;103:46-65. doi:10.1016/j.diff.2018.09.001.
8. Roly ZY, Backhouse B, Cutting A, et al. The cell biology and molecular genetics of Müllerian duct development. *Wiley Interdiscip Rev Dev Biol.* 2018;7(3):e310. doi:10.1002/wdev.310.
9. Shaw G, Renfree MB. Wolffian duct development. *Sex Dev.* 2014;8(5):273-280. doi:10.1159/000363432.
10. Blaschko SD, Cunha GR, Baskin LS. Molecular mechanisms of external genitalia development. *Differentiation.* 2012;84(3):261-268. doi:10.1016/j.diff.2012.06.003.
11. Hughes IA, Houk C, Ahmed SF, Lee PA. Consensus statement on management of intersex disorders. *Arch Dis Child.* 2006;91(7):554-563. doi:10.1136/adc.2006.098319.
12. Phillips SP. Defining and measuring gender: a social determinant of health whose time has come. *Int J Equity Health.* 2005;4:11. doi:10.1186/1475-9276-4-11.
13. Wagner J, Sackett-Taylor AC, Hodax JK, Forcier M, Rafferty J. Psychosocial overview of gender-affirmative care. *J Pediatr Adolesc Gynecol.* 2019;32(6):567-573. doi:10.1016/j.jpag.2019.05.004.
14. Furtado PS, Moraes F, Lago R, Barros LO, Toralles MB, Barroso Jr U. Gender dysphoria associated with disorders of sex development. *Nat Rev Urol.* 2012;9(11):620-627. doi:10.1038/nrurol.2012.182.
15. Kreukels BPC, Cohen-Kettenis PT, Roehle R, et al. Sexuality in adults with differences/disorders of sex development (DSD): findings from the DSD-LIFE Study. *J Sex Marital Ther.* 2019;45(8):688-705. doi:10.1080/0092623x.2019.1610123.
16. Engberg H, Strandqvist A, Berg E, et al. Sexual function in women with differences of sex development or premature loss of gonadal function. *J Sex Med.* 2022;19(2):249-256. doi:10.1016/j.jsxm.2021.11.003.
17. Ernst MM, Chen D, Kennedy K, et al. Disorders of sex development (DSD) web-based information: quality

survey of DSD team websites. *Int J Pediatr Endocrinol.* 2019;2019:1. doi:10.1186/s13633-019-0065-x.

18. Hiort O, Birnbaum W, Marshall L, et al. Management of disorders of sex development. *Nat Rev Endocrinol.* 2014;10(9):520-529. doi:10.1038/nrendo.2014.108.

19. Sathyanarayana S, Grady R, Redmon JB, et al. Anogenital distance and penile width measurements in The Infant Development and the Environment Study (TIDES): methods and predictors. *J Pediatr Urol.* 2015;11(2): 76.e1-e6. doi:10.1016/j.jpurol.2014.11.018.

20. Consortium on the Management of Disorders of Sex Development. *Clinical Guidelines for the Management of Disorders of Sex Development in Childhood.* Intersex Society of North America; 2006. https://dsdguidelines.org/htdocs/clinical/.

21. Quigley CA, De Bellis A, Marschke KB, el-Awady MK, Wilson EM, French FS. Androgen receptor defects: historical, clinical, and molecular perspectives. *Endocr Rev.* 1995;16(3):271-321. doi:10.1210/edrv-16-3-271.

22. Makiyan Z. Systematization of ambiguous genitalia. *Organogenesis.* 2016;12(4):169-182. doi:10.1080/15476278.2 016.1210749.

23. Stokowski L. Congenital adrenal hyperplasia: an endocrine disorder with neonatal onset. *Crit Care Nurs Clin N Am.* 2009;21(2):195-212. https://doi.org/10.1016/j.ccell. 2009.01.008.

24. Gürbüz F, Alkan M, Çelik G, et al. Gender identity and assignment recommendations in disorders of sex development patients: 20 years' experience and challenges. *J Clin Res Pediatr Endocrinol.* 2020;12(4):347-357. doi:10.4274/jcrpe.galenos.2020.2020.0009.

25. Markosyan R, Ahmed SF. Sex assignment in conditions affecting sex development. *J Clin Res Pediatr Endocrinol.* 2017;9(suppl 2):106-112. doi:10.4274/jcrpe.2017. S009.

26. Finlayson C, Rosoklija I, Aston CE, et al. Baseline characteristics of infants with atypical genital development: phenotypes, diagnoses, and sex of rearing. *J Endocr Soc.* 2019;3(1):264-272. doi:10.1210/js.2018-00316.

27. Fisher AD, Ristori J, Fanni E, Castellini G, Forti G, Maggi M. Gender identity, gender assignment and reassignment in individuals with disorders of sex development: a major of dilemma. *J Endocrinol Invest.* 2016;39(11):1207-1224. doi:10.1007/s40618-016-0482-0.

28. Wiesemann C, Ude-Koeller S, Sinnecker GH, Thyen U. Ethical principles and recommendations for the medical management of differences of sex development (DSD)/intersex in children and adolescents. *Eur J Pediatr.* 2010;169(6):671-679. doi:10.1007/s00431-009-1086-x.

29. Birnbaum W, Bertelloni S. Sex hormone replacement in disorders of sex development. *Endocr Dev.* 2014;27: 149-159. doi:10.1159/000363640.

30. Hewitt J, Zacharin M. Hormone replacement in disorders of sex development: current thinking. *Best Pract Res Clin Endocrinol Metab.* 2015;29(3):437-447. https://doi.org/10.1016/j.beem.2015.03.002.

31. Palmert MR, Dunkel L. Clinical practice. Delayed puberty. *N Engl J Med.* 2012;366(5):443-453. doi:10.1056/NEJMcp1109290.

32. Shankar RK, Backeljauw PF. Current best practice in the management of Turner syndrome. *Ther Adv Endocrinol Metab.* 2018;9(1):33-40. doi:10.1177/2042018817746291.

33. Hemesath TP, de Paula LCP, Carvalho CG, Leite JCL, Guaragna-Filho G, Costa EC. Controversies on timing of sex assignment and surgery in individuals with disorders of sex development: a perspective. *Front Pediatr.* 2018;6:419. doi:10.3389/fped.2018.00419.

34. Diamond M, Garland J. Evidence regarding cosmetic and medically unnecessary surgery on infants. *J Pediatr Urol.* 2014;10(1):2-6. doi:10.1016/j.jpurol.2013.10.021.

35. Bennecke E, Bernstein S, Lee P, et al. Early genital surgery in disorders/differences of sex development: patients' perspectives. *Arch Sex Behav.* 2021;50(3):913-923. doi:10.1007/s10508-021-01953-6.

36. DiSandro M, Merke DP, Rink RC. Review of current surgical techniques and medical management considerations in the treatment of pediatric patients with disorders of sex development. *Horm Metab Res.* 2015;47(5):321-328. doi:10.1055/s-0035-1547292.

37. Cools M, Drop SL, Wolffenbuttel KP, Oosterhuis JW, Looijenga LH. Germ cell tumors in the intersex gonad: old paths, new directions, moving frontiers. *Endocr Rev.* 2006;27(5):468-484. doi:10.1210/er.2006-0005.

38. Morin J, Peard L, Saltzman AF. Gonadal malignancy in patients with differences of sex development. *Transl Androl Urol.* 2020;9(5):2408-2415. doi:10.21037/tau-19-726.

39. Finlayson C, Johnson EK, Chen D, et al. Proceedings of the Working Group Session on Fertility Preservation for Individuals with Gender and Sex Diversity. *Transgend Health.* 2016;1(1):99-107. doi:10.1089/trgh.2016.0008.

40. Johnson EK, Finlayson C, Rowell EE, et al. Fertility preservation for pediatric patients: current state and future possibilities. *J Urol.* 2017;198(1):186-194. doi:10.1016/j.juro.2016.09.159.

41. Finlayson C, Fritsch MK, Johnson EK, et al. Presence of germ cells in disorders of sex development: implications for fertility potential and preservation. *J Urol.* 2017;197(3 Pt 2):937-943. doi:10.1016/j.juro.2016.08.108.

42. Johns Hopkins University. OMIM: An Online Catalog of Human Genes and Genetic Disorders. https://www.omim.org/.

43. Zitzmann M, Aksglaede L, Corona G, et al. European Academy of Andrology guidelines on Klinefelter Syndrome Endorsing Organization: European Society of Endocrinology. *Andrology.* 2021;9(1):145-167. doi:10.1111/andr.12909.

44. Barros P, Cunha M, Barros A, Sousa M, Dória S. Clinical outcomes of 77 TESE treatment cycles in non-mosaic Klinefelter syndrome patients. *JBRA Assist Reprod.* 2022;26(3):412-421. doi:10.5935/1518-0557.20210081.

45. Reindollar RH, Byrd JR, McDonough PG. Delayed sexual development: a study of 252 patients. *Am J Obstet Gynecol.* 1981;140(4):371-380. doi:10.1016/0002-9378(81)90029-6.

46. Saenger P. Turner's syndrome. *N Engl J Med.* 1996;335(23):1749-1754. doi:10.1056/nejm199612053352307.

47. Sybert VP, McCauley E. Turner's syndrome. *N Engl J Med.* 2004;351(12):1227-1238. doi:10.1056/NEJMra030360.

48. Gravholt CH, Andersen NH, Conway GS, et al. Clinical practice guidelines for the care of girls and women with Turner syndrome: proceedings from the 2016 Cincinnati International Turner Syndrome Meeting. *Eur J Endocrinol.* 2017;177(3):G1-G70. doi:10.1530/eje-17-0430.

49. Hjerrild BE, Mortensen KH, Gravholt CH. Turner syndrome and clinical treatment. *Br Med Bull.* 2008;86:77-93. doi:10.1093/bmb/ldn015.

50. De Vos M, Devroey P, Fauser BC. Primary ovarian insufficiency. *Lancet.* 2010;376(9744):911-921. doi:10.1016/s0140-6736(10)60355-8.

51. Gravholt CH. Clinical practice in Turner syndrome. *Nat Clin Pract Endocrinol Metab.* 2005;1(1):41-52. doi:10.1038/ncpendmet0024.

52. van Pareren YK, de Muinck Keizer-Schrama SM, Stijnen T, et al. Final height in girls with Turner syndrome after long-term growth hormone treatment in three dosages and low dose estrogens. *J Clin Endocrinol Metab.* 2003;88(3):1119-1125. doi:10.1210/jc.2002-021171.

53. Coyle D, Kutasy B, Han Suyin K, et al. Gonadoblastoma in patients with 45,X/46,XY mosaicism: a 16-year experience. *J Pediatr Urol.* 2016;12(5):283.e1-283.e7. doi:10.1016/j.jpurol.2016.02.009.

54. Oktay K, Bedoschi G. Fertility preservation in girls with Turner syndrome: limitations, current success and future prospects. *Fertil Steril.* 2019;111(6):1124-1126. doi:10.1016/j.fertnstert.2019.03.018.

55. Karnis MF. Fertility, pregnancy, and medical management of Turner syndrome in the reproductive years. *Fertil Steril.* 2012;98(4):787-791. doi:10.1016/j.fertnstert.2012.08.022.

56. Calanchini M, Aye CYL, Orchard E, et al. Fertility issues and pregnancy outcomes in Turner syndrome. *Fertil Steril.* 2020;114(1):144-154. doi:10.1016/j.fertnstert.2020.03.002.

57. Deeb A, Hughes IA. Inguinal hernia in female infants: a cue to check the sex chromosomes? *BJU Int.* 2005;96(3):401-403. doi:10.1111/j.1464-410X.2005.05639.x.

58. Barros BA, Oliveira LR, Surur CRC, Barros-Filho AA, Maciel-Guerra AT, Guerra-Junior G. Complete androgen insensitivity syndrome and risk of gonadal malignancy: systematic review. *Ann Pediatr Endocrinol Metab.* 2021;26(1):19-23. doi:10.6065/apem.2040170.085.

59. Babu R, Shah U. Gender identity disorder (GID) in adolescents and adults with differences of sex development (DSD): a systematic review and meta-analysis. *J Pediatr Urol.* 2021;17(1):39-47. doi:10.1016/j.jpurol.2020.11.017.

60. Ismail IS, Cutner AS, Creighton SM. Laparoscopic vaginoplasty: alternative techniques in vaginal reconstruction. *BJOG.* 2006;113(3):340-343. doi:10.1111/j.1471-0528.2005.00845.x.

61. Michala L, Cutner A, Creighton SM. Surgical approaches to treating vaginal agenesis. *BJOG.* 2007;114(12):1455-1459. doi:10.1111/j.1471-0528.2007.01547.x.

62. Thomas JC, Brock JW III. Vaginal substitution: attempts to create the ideal replacement. *J Urol.* 2007;178(5):1855-1859. doi:10.1016/j.juro.2007.07.007.

63. Gargollo PC, Cannon Jr GM, Diamond DA, Thomas P, Burke V, Laufer MR. Should progressive perineal dilation be considered first line therapy for vaginal agenesis? *J Urol.* 2009;182(suppl 4):1882-1889. doi:10.1016/j.juro.2009.03.071.

64. Ozkan O, Erman Akar M, Ozkan O, Doğan NU. Reconstruction of vaginal agenesis. *Ann Plast Surg.* 2011;66(6):673-678. doi:10.1097/SAP.0b013e3181edd50c.

65. Routh JC, Laufer MR, Cannon Jr GM, Diamond DA, Gargollo PC. Management strategies for Mayer-Rokitansky-Kuster-Hauser related vaginal agenesis: a cost-effectiveness analysis. *J Urol.* 2010;184(5):2116-2121. doi:10.1016/j.juro.2010.06.133.

66. ACOG committee opinion no. 728: Müllerian agenesis: diagnosis, management, and treatment. *Obstet Gynecol.* 2018;131(1):e35-e42. doi:10.1097/aog.0000000000002458.

67. Alessandrescu D, Peltecu GC, Buhimschi CS, Buhimschi IA. Neocolpopoiesis with split-thickness skin graft as a surgical treatment of vaginal agenesis: retrospective review of 201 cases. *Am J Obstet Gynecol.* 1996;175(1):131-138. doi:10.1016/s0002-9378(96)70262-4.

68. Schätz T, Huber J, Wenzl R. Creation of a neovagina according to Wharton-Sheares-George in patients with Mayer-Rokitansky-Küster-Hauser syndrome. *Fertil Steril.* 2005;83(2):437-441. doi:10.1016/j.fertnstert.2004.06.079.

69. Brucker SY, Gegusch M, Zubke W, Rall K, Gauwerky JF, Wallwiener D. Neovagina creation in vaginal agenesis: development of a new laparoscopic Vecchietti-based procedure and optimized instruments in a prospective comparative interventional study in 101 patients. *Fertil Steril.* 2008;90(5):1940-1952. doi:10.1016/j.fertnstert.2007.08.070.

70. Fotopoulou C, Sehouli J, Gehrmann N, Schoenborn I, Lichtenegger W. Functional and anatomic results of amnion vaginoplasty in young women with Mayer-Rokitansky-Küster-Hauser syndrome. *Fertil Steril.* 2010;94(1):317-323. doi:10.1016/j.fertnstert.2009.01.154.

71. Hughes IA, Davies JD, Bunch TI, Pasterski V, Mastroyan-nopoulou K, MacDougall J. Androgen insensitivity syndrome. *Lancet.* 2012;380(9851):1419-1428. doi:10.1016/s0140-6736(12)60071-3.

72. Looijenga LH, Hersmus R, Oosterhuis JW, Cools M, Drop SL, Wolffenbuttel KP. Tumor risk in disorders of sex development (DSD). *Best Pract Res Clin Endocrinol Metab.* 2007;21(3):480-495. doi:10.1016/j.beem.2007.05.001.

73. Dunkel L, Quinton R. Transition in endocrinology: induction of puberty. *Eur J Endocrinol.* 2014;170(6):R229-R239. doi:10.1530/eje-13-0894.

74. Finney EL, Johnson EK, Chen D, et al. Gonadal tissue cryopreservation for a girl with partial androgen insensitivity syndrome. *J Endocr Soc.* 2019;3(5):887-891. doi:10.1210/js.2019-00023.

75. El-Sherbiny M. Disorders of sexual differentiation: I. Genetics and pathology. *Arab J Urol.* 2013;11(1):19-26. doi:10.1016/j.aju.2012.11.005.

76. Bayraktar Z. Potential autofertility in true hermaphrodites. *J Matern Fetal Neonatal Med.* 2018;31(4):542-547. doi:10.1080/14767058.2017.1291619.

77. Nihoul-Fékété C, Thibaud E, Lortat-Jacob S, Josso N. Long-term surgical results and patient satisfaction with male pseudohermaphroditism or true hermaphroditism: a cohort of 63 patients. *J Urol.* 2006;175(5):1878-1884. doi:10.1016/s0022-5347(05)00934-1.

78. Deng S, Sun A, Chen R, Yu Q, Tian Q. Gonadal dominance and internal genitalia phenotypes of patients with ovotesticular disorders of sex development: report of 22 cases and literature review. *Sex Dev.* 2019;13(4):187-194. doi:10.1159/000507036.

79. Li Z, Liu J, Peng Y, Chen R, Ge P, Wang J. 46,XX Ovotesticular disorder of sex development (true hermaphroditism) with seminoma: a case report. *Medicine (Baltimore).* 2020;99(40):e22530. doi:10.1097/md.0000000000022530.

80. Abd Wahab AV, Lim LM, Mohamed Tarmizi MH. Ovotesticular disorders of sex development: improvement in spermatogonia after removal of ovary and müllerian structures. *J Pediatr Adolesc Gynecol.* 2019;32(1):74-77. doi:10.1016/j.jpag.2018.09.006.

81. Dieckmann KP, Pichlmeier U. Clinical epidemiology of testicular germ cell tumors. *World J Urol.* 2004;22(1):2-14. doi:10.1007/s00345-004-0398-8.

82. McCann-Crosby B, Mansouri R, Dietrich JE, et al. State of the art review in gonadal dysgenesis: challenges in diagnosis and management. *Int J Pediatr Endocrinol.* 2014;2014(1):4. doi:10.1186/1687-9856-2014-4.

83. Kreukels BPC, Köhler B, Nordenström A, et al. Gender dysphoria and gender change in disorders of sex development/intersex conditions: results from the DSD-LIFE Study. *J Sex Med.* 2018;15(5):777-785. doi:10.1016/j.jsxm.2018.02.021.

84. Chen MJ, Yang JH, Mao TL, Ho HN, Yang YS. Successful pregnancy in a gonadectomized woman with 46,XY gonadal dysgenesis and gonadoblastoma. *Fertil Steril.* 2005;84(1):217. doi:10.1016/j.fertnstert.2004.11.087.

85. Plante BJ, Fritz MA. A case report of successful pregnancy in a patient with pure 46,XY gonadal dysgenesis. *Fertil Steril.* 2008;90(5):2015.e1-e2. doi:10.1016/j.fertnstert.2008.04.043.

86. Creatsas G, Deligeoroglou E, Tsimaris P, Pantos K, Kreatsa M. Successful pregnancy in a Swyer syndrome patient with preexisting hypertension. *Fertil Steril.* 2011;96(2):e83-e85. doi:10.1016/j.fertnstert.2011.05.061.

87. Witchel SF. Congenital adrenal hyperplasia. *J Pediatr Adolesc Gynecol.* 2017;30(5):520-534. doi:10.1016/j.jpag.2017.04.001.

88. Kalra R, Cameron M, Stern C. Female fertility preservation in DSD. *Best Pract Res Clin Endocrinol Metab.* 2019;33(3):101289.

89. Speiser PW, Arlt W, Auchus RJ, et al. Congenital adrenal hyperplasia due to steroid 21-hydroxylase deficiency: an Endocrine Society Clinical Practice Guideline. *J Clin Endocrinol Metab.* 2018;103(11):4043-4088. doi:10.1210/jc.2018-01865.

90. Prentice P. Guideline review: congenital adrenal hyperplasia clinical practice guideline 2018. *Arch Dis Child Educ Pract Ed.* 2021;106(6):354-357. doi:10.1136/archdischild-2019-317573.

91. Ginalska-Malinowska M. Classic congenital adrenal hyperplasia due to 21-hydroxylase deficiency – the next disease included in the neonatal screening program in Poland. *Dev Period Med.* 2018;22(2):197-200. doi:10.34763/devperiodmed.20182202.197200.

92. Mallappa A, Merke DP. Management challenges and therapeutic advances in congenital adrenal hyperplasia. *Nat Rev Endocrinol.* 2022;18(6):337-352. doi:10.1038/s41574-022-00655-w.

93. Pall M, Azziz R, Beires J, Pignatelli D. The phenotype of hirsute women: a comparison of polycystic ovary syndrome and 21-hydroxylase-deficient nonclassic adrenal hyperplasia. *Fertil Steril.* 2010;94(2):684-689. doi:10.1016/j.fertnstert.2009.06.025.

94. Ozbey H, Darendeliler F, Kayserili H, Korkmazlar U, Salman T. Gender assignment in female congenital adrenal hyperplasia: a difficult experience. *BJU Int.* 2004;94(3):388-391. doi:10.1111/j.1464-410X.2004.04967.x.

95. Sturm RM, Durbin-Johnson B, Kurzrock EA. Congenital adrenal hyperplasia: current surgical management at academic medical centers in the United States. *J Urol.* 2015;193(suppl 5):1796-1801. doi:10.1016/j.juro.2014.11.008.

96. Wang LC, Poppas DP. Surgical outcomes and complications of reconstructive surgery in the female congenital adrenal hyperplasia patient: what every endocrinologist should know. *J Steroid Biochem Mol Biol.* 2017;165 (Pt A):137-144. doi:10.1016/j.jsbmb.2016.03.021.

97. Lee PA, Nordenström A, Houk CP, et al. Global disorders of sex development update since 2006: perceptions,

approach and care. *Horm Res Paediatr.* 2016;85(3): 158-180. doi:10.1159/000442975.

98. Eyal O, Ayalon-Dangur I, Segev-Becker A, Schachter-Davidov A, Israel S, Weintrob N. Pregnancy in women with nonclassic congenital adrenal hyperplasia: time to conceive and outcome. *Clin Endocrinol (Oxf).* 2017;87(5):552-556. doi:10.1111/cen.13429.

Complex Genitourinary Anomalies

Kate McCracken and Shruthi Srinivas

INTRODUCTION

Caring for patients with complex genitourinary anomalies can be challenging. These patients are anatomically complicated with nuanced disease processes. Here, we will focus on three common genitourinary anomalies: anorectal malformations, cloacal malformations, and genitourinary sinuses (Box 25.1). These patients are closely followed in clinic; undergo multiple operative interventions; and face unique challenges when it comes to quality of life, bowel habits, urination, and sexual function and reproduction.

ANORECTAL MALFORMATIONS AND CLOACAL MALFORMATIONS

Overview and Definition

Anorectal malformations (ARMs) occur along a wide spectrum in both boys and girls.[1] Severity ranges from easily treated with good functional outcomes to severe, with other involved organ systems, a need for complex reconstruction, and poorer functional outcomes. Overall, a diagnosis of "anorectal malformation" is a buzzword. Understanding the anatomy underlying a patient's individual diagnosis is key to understanding their

---

> **BOX 25.1** **Complex Genitourinary Anomalies in Pediatric and Adolescent Gynecology**
>
> - Anorectal malformations
> - Cloacal malformations: single outflow or common channel
> - Urogenital sinus

---

functional status, future outcomes, and individual challenges and needs.

ARMs can be loosely divided into the following categories (Figs. 25.1 and 25.2)[2]:

- Imperforate anus without fistula (see Fig. 25.1A): Absence of normal anal opening.
- Perineal fistula (see Fig. 25.1B and Fig. 25.2A): Abnormal anal opening outside of the sphincter muscle complex but within the perineum.
- Vestibular fistula (see Fig. 25.1C and Fig. 25.2B): Abnormal anal opening outside of the sphincter muscle complex within the vulvar vestibule of the female genitalia. Vestibular fistula is the most common female ARM.
- Vaginal fistula (see Fig. 25.1C and Fig. 25.2C): Abnormal anal opening outside of the sphincter muscle complex within the vagina.
- Cloacal malformation (see Fig. 25.1D): Rectum, vagina, and urinary tract form a single outflow system (common channel) rather than three separate tracts; generally divided into long common channel (>3 cm) or short common channel (<3 cm).
- Rectal atresia: Normal anal canal with a stricture proximal to the dentate line.

ARMs occur in approximately 1 in 5000 live births.[3] Historically, imperforate anus was the first described ARM. Classified in the early 18th century, surgeons were encouraged to divide the membrane theorized to be overlying the anal opening.[4] Patients with low imperforate anus did well with this operation; patients with high imperforate anus did not. The operation for a high imperforate anus evolved over time. The modern approach, known as the *posterior sagittal anorectoplasty* (PSARP), was defined in 1980.[5] This involves complete exposure of the anorectal region by incising all muscle

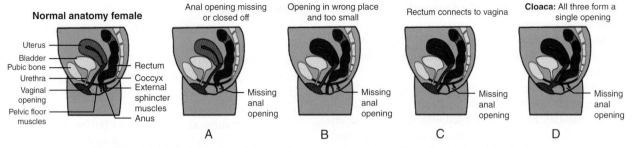

Fig. 25.1 Anatomic illustration of the most common anorectal malformations in female patients.

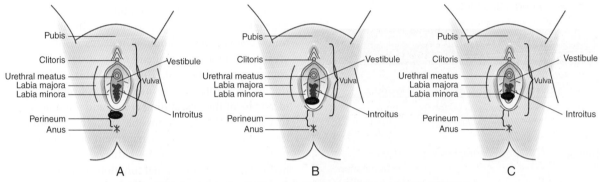

Fig. 25.2 Anatomic illustration of perineal, vestibular, and vaginal fistulas.

structures behind the rectum. Colloquially referred to as a *pull-through,* the PSARP allows for the opportunity to restore continence in children with ARMs.

Etiology and Pathophysiology

There are several theories regarding the etiology of ARM, but no one pinpointed cause.[6] There are many associated congenital abnormalities, including trisomy 21, Currarino syndrome, and VACTERL associations (vertebral defects, anal atresia, cardiac defects, tracheo-esophageal fistula, renal anomalies, and limb abnormalities). These represent only about 11% of the population with ARM.[7] Pathologically, an ARM is defined by an ectopic anus.[8] One theory involves the development of the cloaca, a common channel that contains the urinary tract, female reproductive tract, and gastrointestinal tract.[9] Around the seventh week of gestation, these structures separate. Abnormal development of the anorectal septum to separate these structures may lead to the formation of ARMs.

History and Physical: Initial Evaluation

Most patients with ARMs are diagnosed as newborns. A thorough physical examination is extremely critical,

including a perineal examination and a complete examination to identify associated anomalies. Specifically, the anus should be identified as in the center of the sphincter complex. It must also be of appropriate size. If patients have concerning physical examination findings, surgeon evaluation is warranted, and an examination under anesthesia may be performed.

In females with concern for ARM, a close examination of the vulvar vestibule and vagina should also be performed, as this can help identify the presence of a rectovestibular fistula, rectovaginal fistula, or other vaginal malformation (i.e., distal vaginal atresia). This examination can be performed using a labial traction to fully visualize the vestibule (see chapter 4, Figure 4.1 and 2.2) and, in some cases, vaginoscopy to examine the vagina. Often an examination under anesthesia is combined with cysto-vaginoscopy. This affords the opportunity to understand the type of ARM and the patient's unique anatomy—including the relationship between the urethra, vagina, and rectum; the length of the common channel (in cloaca malformations); and the number of cervices present (zero, one, or two). This information helps preoperative surgical planning.

A minority of ARMs can be diagnosed prenatally, often because of the presence of other associated anomalies.[10-12] This may facilitate delivery in a specialized center and more appropriate predelivery counseling for patients and families.

Because of the high coincidence of chromosomal abnormalities and syndromes, especially with VACTERL abnormalities, patients diagnosed with ARM should undergo a thorough workup for these associated symptoms[10] (Table 25.1). Additionally, the sacral ratio should be calculated via sacral radiograph images, as this may provide prognostic information for future continence.[11]

Management

Management of ARMs depends on the health of the child and the type of ARM. In unstable patients, urgent operation may be warranted regardless of the child's associated comorbidities; in stable patients, full assessment may help optimize for surgical intervention.

The major surgical decision is to pursue a primary operation, with an early pull-through, or delayed operation, with an early colostomy and delayed pull-through. Indications for a colostomy and delayed primary repair include a flat perineum, meconium in the urine, distal gas high above the pelvis, and cloaca.[5] The initial colostomy decompresses stool; a mucous fistula is also created with the proximal end of the distal colon to decompress the distal end. The goal in this initial operation is to create two stomas—the colostomy should ideally be of the descending colon, and the mucous fistula small and as far as possible from the colostomy. A key component of early management of cloaca malformations is protection of the kidneys. The presence of hydrocolpos can affect renal function, and a renal ultrasound is used to evaluate for hydronephrosis and/or hydroureter. Decompression of the hydrocolpos and subsequent improvement of hydronephrosis can be performed via clean intermittent catheterization via the common channel or vaginostomy.

Definitive surgical management with a "pull-through" procedure varies based on the type of ARM. Most operations begin with an examination under anesthesia, which allows the provider opportunity to identify anatomy. Operative choice then depends on the malformation type (Table 25.2). Pull-through may or

TABLE 25.1 Workup for VACTERL Abnormalities

Involved Organ System	Examples	Workup
Vertebral	Butterfly vertebrae Hemi-vertebrae	Spinal ultrasound Spinal x-rays
Anus	Imperforate anus	Physical examination
Cardiac	Ventricular septal defect Atrial septal defect Patent ductus arteriosus	Cardiac echo-cardiography
TE (trachea/esophagus)	Tracheo-esophageal fistula Esophageal atresia	Physical examination Nasogastric tube placement
Renal	Horseshoe kidney	Renal ultrasound
Limb	Radial hypoplasia	Limb x-rays

TABLE 25.2 Operative Interventions for ARM ("Pull-Throughs")

Intervention	Population	Description
Posterior sagittal ano-rectoplasty (PSARP)[14]	Rectoperineal fistula	Posterior sagittal incision, mobilization of rectum, and transposition/placement within the sphincter complex
Posterior sagittal ano-rectoplasty (PSARP)	Rectovestibular fistula and imperforate anus without fistula	Generation of two walls between the rectum and the urethra via separation of the common septum in addition to traditional PSARP
Posterior sagittal ano-rectal-vaginal-urethral-plasty (PSARVUP)[15]	Cloacal malformation <3 cm	Posterior sagittal approach as in the PSARP followed by mobilization of the vagina and urethra together with eventual separation
PSARVUP with laparotomy or laparoscopy	Cloacal malformation >3 cm	PSARVUP with additional maneuvers to ensure adequate length of the urethra and the vagina to the perineum if anatomically feasible; may include creation of a neovagina (using a bowel graft)

may not be done with an ostomy for protection at the same time. If not previously performed, a thorough assessment of the female reproductive tract is necessary to accurately determine anatomy.[12] Vaginoscopy provides information on the presence or absence of a longitudinal vaginal septum and number of cervices, which helps understand the müllerian anatomy. Additionally, an inspection of müllerian structures via laparoscopy or at the time of other abdominal procedures allows accurate assessment of the upper reproductive tract.[13] The likelihood of an associated gynecologic anomaly increases with the complexity of the ARM (rectoperineal fistula 5%, rectovestibular fistula 18%, cloacal malformation 68%). Understanding the upper reproductive tract anatomy, lower reproductive tract anatomy, and the relationship to the urinary and colorectal tracts optimizes preoperative reconstructive planning and aids in anticipatory guidance and counseling for patients and families.

Given the complexity of the primary operation, it is not uncommon for these patients to require reoperations. Early reoperations are often technical or anatomic for reasons such as anal stricture, acquired atresia, anal mislocation, and rectal prolapse. Simple reoperations include examinations under anesthesia with dilation of the anal opening or injection of Botox. More complicated reoperative interventions involve laparoscopic drainage of abscesses, laparotomy for bowel obstruction, and more. For patients with ARM who have trouble remaining continent of stool after pull-through, an operative antegrade continence enema (ACE) may be offered.[16] This involves using the appendix as a channel to catheterize and perform antegrade enemas through the colon to improve emptying and decrease fecal incontinence episodes. Additional urologic procedures may be necessary for urinary continence.

Prognosis

The goal with all children is effective anatomic reconstruction that allows for postoperative bowel and bladder continence and optimization of future reproductive function. Children who are continent have improved quality of life.[17] Continence is affected by the type of ARM, the sacral ratio, and the presence or absence of a tethered cord. The higher the ARM, the lower the chance of postoperative continence; low sacral ratio and presence of tethered cord also negatively affect continence. However, fecal incontinence is rarely predictable and requires close follow-up.[18]

Several strategies have been developed over the past decades to address incontinence in this population. In the early years, regular toilet training is encouraged, and laxatives can be used for regular and easy bowel movements. If constipation develops, patients can undergo bowel management programs, an intensive 1-week therapy where providers develop a tailored enema recipe that allows patients to remain clean for at least a 24-hour period.[19-21] This multidisciplinary program improves continence overall. In cases of abnormal anatomy after initial operation, redo PSARP can successfully restore continence and improve quality of life.[22]

Gynecologic Considerations

Children with ARM require lifelong follow-up. Puberty is a critical time for females with ARM and brings unique challenges.[23] Assuming normal growth, the timing and tempo of puberty should be similar to their peers without ARM. Thelarche typically occurs at age 10 and menarche at age 12. Understanding which reconstructive procedures the patient has undergone, the upper reproductive tract anatomy, and lower reproductive tract anatomy is imperative. A patient's unique müllerian and vaginal anatomy may increase their risk of a menstrual outflow tract obstruction. Outflow tract obstructions can occur at various anatomic levels—the vaginal introitus, vagina, anastomosis of native to neovagina, cervix, or uterus.

Key components of pubertal assessment for females with ARM includes (1) menstrual history (assessment of menarche, menstrual pattern, dysmenorrhea, and pelvic pain); (2) pelvic imaging (ultrasound and, in some cases, pelvic magnetic resonance imaging [MRI]) to confirm the müllerian anatomy and screen for an outflow tract obstruction; and (3) pelvic examination in the office or under anesthesia. Should a menstrual outflow tract obstruction be identified, thoughtful consideration to management options (medical, surgical, or both) and shared medical decision making is necessary. It may be necessary to perform additional surgical procedures to relieve the obstruction, and discussion on the impact of future sexual-reproductive function and fertility is essential. Additionally, a thorough examination should be performed before tampon use or vaginal intercourse to ensure the vaginal introitus is of adequate size.

Although gynecologic anatomy should be determined early, further anatomic abnormalities after reconstruction can occur.[24] In cloacal abnormalities, there is a high rate of associated gynecologic abnormalities.[25] Complications described include acquired rectovaginal fistula, posterior mislocated introitus, introital stenosis, and retained vaginal septum.

Research is still ongoing in understanding the full impact of ARM repair on fertility; however, most studies demonstrate a normal ability for women with ARM to become pregnant.[26-28] Although females with ARM have unique challenges, they should receive comprehensive sexual-reproductive health education and care similar to their peers without ARM.[29]

UROGENITAL SINUS

Overview and Definition

A urogenital sinus anomaly is a congenital condition in which the urethra and the vagina open into a common channel, without the associated ARM.[30] Similar embryologically to cloacal malformations, children with urogenital sinus reflect an interesting and unique group, as it is often a feature of disordered sexual differentiation.

Prevalence, Epidemiology, and History

Similar to ARMs and cloacal malformations, the embryology of urogenital sinuses is most important between the sixth and twelfth weeks of gestation, at which point the urogenital plate and folds form into the vaginal introitus and the labial folds. Urogenital sinuses are uncommon but are most often associated with congenital adrenal hyperplasia (CAH) and ambiguous genitalia. CAH is autosomally recessive and can be screened for on typical newborn screening.[31-33]

Etiology and Pathophysiology

CAH is most often an autosomal recessive disorder of the 21-hydroxylase enzyme, resulting traditionally in salt wasting and virilization.[31] Females typically experience clitoral enlargement and formation of the urogenital sinus as an effect of excess androgen. Depending on the severity, it may present in the newborn period and may also present at the onset of puberty. Although CAH is associated with external virilization, androgens have no effect on internal genitalia development; women with clitoromegaly resulting from androgen exposure will still have a normally developed uterus and ovaries. The urogenital sinus anomaly forms when the urethral groove, which normally remains open, begins to close in response to androgen stimulation to create the

normal male urethra. This disruption leads to the urogenital sinus.

History and Physical Examination

Children with CAH should be identified as part of traditional newborn screening. Generally, the more severe the virilization, the longer the common urogenital sinus; these abnormalities can be identified on initial physical examination, which may also include an examination under anesthesia with cysto-vaginoscopy. Prader's classification uses the PVE terms, in which genital ambiguity and urogenital sinus are classified by phallic length and width (P), location of vagina with respect to the bladder neck and perineal meatus (V), and the external genitalia appearance (E).[34] The PVE classification can aid in surgical planning and prognosis (Table 25.3).[35] Urogenital sinuses can be diagnosed on prenatal ultrasound, but this is uncommon.

Management

Definitive management of urogenital sinuses is surgical. The common channel must be separated to create a separate genital tract and urinary tract. In some situations, partial urogenital mobilization is adequate.[36] In low urogenital sinuses, a perineal approach, or "flap vaginoplasty," is effective, with or without a skin flap.[37] In patients with a high vaginal implantation into the urogenital sinus, a more significant operation is needed. Recent success has been described with the anterior sagittal transrectal approach, which allows for adequate exposure and facilitates separation of the structures.[38]

TABLE 25.3 **Prader Classification of Urogenital Sinus Abnormalities**	
Classification	**Characteristics**
Type 1 (P-1)	Clitoral hypertrophy
Type 2 (P-2)	Clitoral hypertrophy, urethral and vaginal orifices present and close to one another
Type 3 (P-3)	Clitoral hypertrophy with single urogenital orifice
Type 4 (P-4)	Penile clitoris, complete fusion of the labia majora
Type 5 (P-5)	Complete masculinization without testes

This approach has had good success with accurate division of the two structures and low rates of postoperative complications. In extremely virilized females, a total urogenital sinus mobilization may be required.[39]

Prognosis

As with ARMs, the main concerns after surgical correction of urogenital sinus malformations are in bladder continence and in future sexual-reproductive health and fertility. In patients who undergo total urogenital sinus mobilization, reduction clitoroplasty can be concurrently performed to decrease masculinization of external genitalia.[40] Not all patients and families choose to have the concurrent clitoroplasty. As always, shared medical decision making with comprehensive discussions about risks and benefits of surgical interventions is crucial. Fortunately, surgical management has demonstrated high rates of postoperative continence regardless of approach and good quality of life.[41,42] These children retain orgasmic potential and sexual attraction, and some experience cross-gender identity development.[43] Psychosocially, patients should be closely followed by individuals with experience working with this population and knowledge of the unique challenges, such as in an experienced center for colorectal and pelvic reconstruction.

Gynecologic Considerations

Similar to patients with ARMs, patients with urogenital sinuses require early gynecologic care. Patients with urogenital sinus undergo similar vaginal reconstruction, which should be closely monitored. The association with ovarian or uterine pathology is lower in patients with urogenital sinus; however, patients should still be followed. As with other complex urogenital malformations, there may be a need for additional surgical procedures during puberty. In the case of a patient with CAH and prior genitoplasty, assessment of the vaginal introitus is important before tampon use or vaginal intercourse. If introital or vaginal stenosis is present, management options include vaginal dilation, introitoplasty, or redo vaginoplasty. The use of buccal mucosa grafts for introitoplasty and vaginoplasty has been promising.

Additionally, children with urogenital sinus and associated CAH face unique challenges at the time of adolescence. Children with CAH have a roughly 50% incidence of precocious puberty, with an increased incidence of primary amenorrhea, oligomenorrhea, and hirsutism.[44] Menstrual irregularities are common in this population

and should be managed medically. In children who desire it, early treatment can help in developing a phenotypically female appearance and normalization of the hypothalamic-pituitary-adrenal axis.

> **KEY POINTS**
>
> - Thorough physical examinations, including perineal, vaginal, urologic, and anal, are essential in the newborn to identify ARMs, cloacal malformations, and urogenital sinuses.
> - Individuals with these malformations experience unique challenges regarding continence (urinary and fecal) and sexual-reproductive health and should be managed by specialized providers with experience in these areas.
> - Surgical management is often complex and is a tailored approach with shared medical decision making focusing on the individual characteristics of a patient's anatomic malformation.

REVIEW QUESTIONS

1. Which of the following abnormalities is traditionally associated with congenital adrenal hyperplasia and involves virilization of the female patient?
   a. Rectal atresia
   b. Rectovestibular fistula
   c. Urogenital sinus
   d. Cloacal malformation
   e. Imperforate anus

2. What is the most common anorectal malformation in the female population?
   a. Imperforate anus
   b. Rectal atresia
   c. Rectovestibular fistula
   d. Perineal fistula
   e. Cloacal malformation
   f. Urogenital sinus

3. A newborn female in the nursery has failed to pass meconium. On physical examination, there is a smooth perineum without an anal dimple. The vaginal and urethral openings are both appropriately sized and located. There is no family history of any genetic abnormalities, and the patient had no concerning prenatal screening. Which of the following should be performed?
   a. Computed tomography (CT) abdomen/pelvis
   b. Echocardiogram

c. Meta-iodobenzylguanidine (MIBG) scan

d. MRI brain

e. Barium enema

REFERENCES

1. Levitt MA, Peña A. Anorectal malformations. *Orphanet J Rare Dis.* 2007;2(1):33. doi:10.1186/1750-1172-2-33

2. Anorectal Malformations. https://reference.medscape.com/medline/abstract/7728507. Accessed October 25, 2022.

3. Smith ED. Incidence, frequency of types, and etiology of anorectal malformations. *Birth Defects Orig Artic Ser.* 1988;24(4):231-246.

4. Yesildag E, Muñiz RM, Buyukunal SNC. How did the surgeons treat neonates with imperforate anus in the eighteenth century? *Pediatr Surg Int.* 2010;26(12):1149-1158. doi:10.1007/s00383-010-2672-8

5. Peña A, Devries PA. Posterior sagittal anorectoplasty: important technical considerations and new applications. *J Pediatr Surg.* 1982;17(6):796-811. doi:10.1016/S0022-3468(82)80448-X

6. Wang C, Li L, Cheng W. Anorectal malformation: the etiological factors. *Pediatr Surg Int.* 2015;31(9):795-804. doi:10.1007/s00383-015-3685-0

7. American Journal of Medical Genetics Part A – Wiley Online Library. Chromosomal Anomalies in the Etiology of Anorectal Malformations: A Review. 2011. https://onlinelibrary.wiley.com/doi/full/10.1002/ajmg.a.34253. Accessed October 25, 2022.

8. Rintala RJ. Anorectal malformations—management and outcome. *Semin Neonatol.* 1996;1(3):219-230. doi:10.1016/S1084-2756(96)80040-6

9. Smith CA, Avansino J. Anorectal malformations. In: *StatPearls.* StatPearls Publishing; 2022. http://www.ncbi.nlm.nih.gov/books/NBK542275/. Accessed October 25, 2022.

10. PMC. VACTERL/VATER Association. https://www.ncbi.nlm.nih.gov/pmc/articles/PMC3169446/. Accessed October 25, 2022.

11. Macedo M, Martins JL, Freitas Filho LG. Sacral ratio and fecal continence in children with anorectal malformations. *BJU Int.* 2004;94(6):893-894. doi:10.1111/j.1464-410X.2004.05053.x

12. Levitt MA, Bischoff A, Breech L, Peña A. Rectovestibular fistula—rarely recognized associated gynecologic anomalies. *J Pediatr Surg.* 2009;44(6):1261-1267. doi:10.1016/j.jpedsurg.2009.02.046

13. Pradhan S, Vilanova-Sanchez A, McCracken KA, et al. The Mullerian Black Box: Predicting and defining Mullerian anatomy in patients with cloacal abnormalities and the need for longitudinal assessment. *J Pediatr Surg.* 2018;53(11):2164-2169. doi:10.1016/j.jpedsurg.2018.05.009

14. Bischoff A, Peña A, Levitt MA. Laparoscopic-assisted PSARP — the advantages of combining both techniques for the treatment of anorectal malformations with recto-bladderneck or high prostatic fistulas. *J Pediatr Surg.* 2013;48(2):367-371. doi:10.1016/j.jpedsurg.2012.11.019

15. Peña A. Total urogenital mobilization—an easier way to repair cloacas. *J Pediatr Surg.* 1997;32(2):263-268. doi:10.1016/S0022-3468(97)90191-3

16. Rangel SJ, Lawal TA, Bischoff A, et al. The appendix as a conduit for antegrade continence enemas in patients with anorectal malformations: lessons learned from 163 cases treated over 18 years. *J Pediatr Surg.* 2011;46(6):1236-1242. doi:10.1016/j.jpedsurg.2011.03.060

17. Bai Y, Yuan Z, Wang W, Zhao Y, Wang H, Wang W. Quality of life for children with fecal incontinence after surgically corrected anorectal malformation. *J Pediatr Surg.* 2000;35(3):462-464. doi:10.1016/S0022-3468(00)90215-X

18. Minneci PC, Kabre RS, Mak GZ, et al. Can fecal continence be predicted in patients born with anorectal malformations? *J Pediatr Surg.* 2019;54(6):1159-1163. doi:10.1016/j.jpedsurg.2019.02.035

19. Bischoff A, Levitt MA, Peña A. Bowel management for the treatment of pediatric fecal incontinence. *Pediatr Surg Int.* 2009;25(12):1027-1042. doi:10.1007/s00383-009-2502-z

20. Bischoff A, Levitt MA, Bauer C, Jackson L, Holder M, Peña A. Treatment of fecal incontinence with a comprehensive bowel management program. *J Pediatr Surg.* 2009;44(6):1278-1284. doi:10.1016/j.jpedsurg.2009.02.047

21. Wood RJ, Vilanova-Sanchez A, El-Gohary Y, et al. One-year impact of a bowel management program in treating fecal incontinence in patients with anorectal malformations. *J Pediatr Surg.* 2021;56(10):1689-1693. doi:10.1016/j.jpedsurg.2021.04.029

22. Wood RJ, Halleran DR, Ahmad H, et al. Assessing the benefit of reoperations in patients who suffer from fecal incontinence after repair of their anorectal malformation. *J Pediatr Surg.* 2020;55(10):2159-2165. doi:10.1016/j.jpedsurg.2020.06.011

23. Levitt MA, Stein DM, Peña A. Gynecologic concerns in the treatment of teenagers with cloaca. *J Pediatr Surg.* 1998;33(2):188-193. doi:10.1016/S0022-3468(98)90429-8

24. Vilanova-Sanchez A, Reck CA, McCracken KA, et al. Gynecologic anatomic abnormalities following anorectal malformations repair. *J Pediatr Surg.* 2018;53(4):698-703. doi:10.1016/j.jpedsurg.2017.07.012

25. Peña A, Levitt MA, Hong A, Midulla P. Surgical management of cloacal malformations: a review of 339 patients. *J Pediatr Surg.* 2004;39(3):470-479. doi:10.1016/j.jpedsurg.2003.11.033

26. Breech L. Gynecologic concerns in patients with anorectal malformations. *Semin Pediatr Surg.* 2010;19(2):139-145. doi:10.1053/j.sempedsurg.2009.11.019

27. Huibregtse ECP, Draaisma JMTH, Hofmeester MJ, Kluivers K, van Rooij IALM, de Blaauw I. The influence of anorectal malformations on fertility: a systematic review. *Pediatr Surg Int.* 2014;30(8):773-781. doi:10.1007/s00383-014-3535-5

28. Ahmad H, Knaus ME, Gasior AC, et al. Sexual and reproductive health outcomes in females with cloacal malformations and other anorectal malformations. *J Pediatr Adolesc Gynecol.* 2023;36(2):148-154. doi:10.1016/j.jpag.2022.10.008

29. Svetanoff WJ, Lawson A, Lopez JJ, et al. Unique evaluation and management considerations for adolescents with late gynecologic and colorectal issues in the setting of anorectal malformations. *J Pediatr Adolesc Gynecol.* 2023;36(3):315-320. doi:10.1016/j.jpag.2022.12.002

30. Thomas DM. The embryology of persistent cloaca and urogenital sinus malformations. *Asian J Androl.* 2020;22(2):124. doi:10.4103/aja.aja_72_19

31. Pignatelli D, Carvalho BL, Palmeiro A, Barros A, Guerreiro SG, Macut D. The complexities in genotyping of congenital adrenal hyperplasia: 21-hydroxylase deficiency. *Front Endocrinol.* 2019;10:432. doi:10.3389/fendo.2019.00432

32. Merke DP, Auchus RJ. Congenital adrenal hyperplasia due to 21-hydroxylase deficiency. *N Engl J Med.* 2020;383(13):1248-1261. doi:10.1056/NEJMra1909786

33. Speiser PW, Arlt W, Auchus RJ, et al. Congenital adrenal hyperplasia due to steroid 21-hydroxylase deficiency: an Endocrine Society Clinical Practice Guideline. *J Clin Endocrinol Metab.* 2018;103(11):4043-4088. doi:10.1210/jc.2018-01865

34. Rink RC, Adams MC, Misseri R. A new classification for genital ambiguity and urogenital sinus anomalies. *BJU Int.* 2005;95(4):638-642. doi:10.1111/j.1464-410X.2005.05354.x

35. Ogilvy-Stuart AL, Brain CE. Early assessment of ambiguous genitalia. *Arch Dis Child.* 2004;89(5):401-407. doi:10.1136/adc.2002.011312

36. Marei MM, Fares AE, Abdelsattar AH, et al. Anatomical measurements of the urogenital sinus in virilized female children due to congenital adrenal hyperplasia. *J Pediatr Urol.* 2016;12(5):282.e1-282.e8. doi:10.1016/j.jpurol.2016.02.008

37. Peña A, Filmer B, Bonilla E, Mendez M, Stolar C. Transanorectal approach for the treatment of urogenital sinus: preliminary report. *J Pediatr Surg.* 1992;27(6):681-685. doi:10.1016/S0022-3468(05)80090-9

38. Salle JLP, Lorenzo AJ, Jesus LE, et al. Surgical treatment of high urogenital sinuses using the anterior sagittal transrectal approach: a useful strategy to optimize exposure and outcomes. *J Urol.* 2012;187(3):1024-1031. doi:10.1016/j.juro.2011.10.162

39. Ludwikowski BM, González R. The surgical correction of urogenital sinus in patients with DSD: 15 years after description of total urogenital mobilization in children. *Front Pediatr.* 2013;1:41. doi:10.3389/fped.2013.00041

40. Jenak R, Ludwikowski B, Gonz ÁR. Total urogenital sinus mobilization: a modified perineal approach for feminizing genitoplasty and urogenital sinus repair. *J Urol.* 2001;165(6 Part 2):2347-2349. doi:10.1016/S0022-5347(05)66200-3

41. Palmer BW, Trojan B, Griffin K, et al. Total and partial urogenital mobilization: focus on urinary continence. *J Urol.* 2012;187(4):1422-1426. doi:10.1016/j.juro.2011.12.012

42. Braga LHP, Lorenzo AJ, Tatsuo ES, Silva IN, Pippi Salle JL. Prospective evaluation of feminizing genitoplasty using partial urogenital sinus mobilization for congenital adrenal hyperplasia. *J Urol.* 2006;176(5):2199-2204. doi:10.1016/j.juro.2006.07.063

43. Meyer-Bahlburg HFL, Gruen RS, New MI, et al. Gender change from female to male in classical congenital adrenal hyperplasia. *Horm Behav.* 1996;30(4):319-332. doi:10.1006/hbeh.1996.0039

44. Oliveira JC, Sousa FC, Campos ST, et al. Congenital adrenal hyperplasia in adolescence — a gynecological perspective. *Ginekol Pol.* 2022. doi:10.5603/GP.a2021.0248

Nonobstructive Reproductive Tract Anomalies*

Krista Childress and Katherine G. Hayes

INTRODUCTION, PREVALENCE, AND EPIDEMIOLOGY

Approximately 7% of those born with female anatomy will have differences in the formation of the reproductive tract, resulting in varying degrees of vaginal, uterine, or cervical development. These variations can either lead to an obstructive outflow tract, which causes pain, or a nonobstructive outflow tract, which is not usually associated with pain. Nonobstructive reproductive tract anomalies can present with variations at the level of the hymen, vagina, cervix, or uterus. The exact cause of these anomalies is unknown but is likely multifactorial, including both genetic and environmental factors. Nonobstructive anomalies can present at various times throughout life, including during childhood, after menarche, during an infertility workup, during prenatal or antepartum care, or during evaluation of another anatomic system or syndrome.[1,2]

PATHOPHYSIOLOGY OF DISEASE AND EMBRYOLOGY

At 4 weeks' gestational age, intermediate mesoderm is present and the mesonephros and paramesonephros begin their differentiation into müllerian and Wolffian ducts based on the presence or absence of the *SRY* gene and exposure to androgens. In the absence of the *SRY* gene, female anatomy develops. During gestational weeks 5 to 6, the mesonephros, metanephric ducts, and genital ridge form. Gestational weeks 7 to 8 are focused on cloacal division, further development of the paramesonephric ducts, and gonadal differentiation (ovary versus testis). The müllerian ducts fuse starting around 6 to 7 weeks and continue through the 14th week. The fused müllerian ducts interact with the urogenital sinus to form the sinovaginal bulb. Remnants of the Wolffian system may persist and result in broad ligament cysts, hydatids of Morgagni, paratubal cysts, and Gartner duct cysts. The genetic mechanism for differences in the development of müllerian ducts is not well understood in humans. Any defects in migration or fusion of these structures can lead to reproductive tract anomalies along with anomalies of other associated organ systems such as the renal system (Fig. 26.1).[1-4]

Classification Systems

There are multiple classification systems of müllerian anomalies, including the American Fertility Society (AFS) from 1979, which focused mostly on uterine anomalies; VCUAM classification (Vagina, Cervix, Uterus, Adnexa, associated Malformations), which was developed to be more precise and describe associated anomalies; and the European Society of Human Reproduction (ESHRE) and Embryology-European Society for Gynaecological Endoscopy (ESGE), which classified uterine anomalies separately from cervical and vaginal anomalies. More recently, the American Society for Reproductive Medicine (ASRM) Task Force for Müllerian Anomaly Classification recognized the need for a more thorough classification system to improve how we describe müllerian anomalies. This new system allows for standard communication between providers and results in improved clinical care. It has been

*Parts of this chapter are presented in concise and easy-to-grasp bullets.

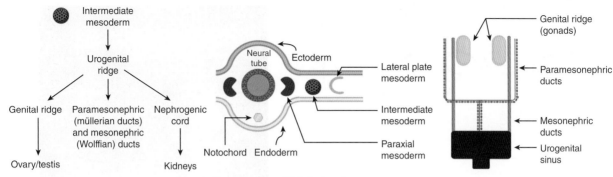

Fig. 26.1 Embryology.

published as the Müllerian Anomalies Classification 2021 (MAC2021), the main classification system used in the United States today.[2] An interactive tutorial can be found at https://connect.asrm.org/education/asrm-mac-2021/asrm-mac-2021?ssopc=1.

GENERAL CLINICAL PRESENTATION/EVALUATION

Nonobstructive anomalies of the reproductive tract are usually asymptomatic and are incidentally discovered on imaging for a gynecologic complaint, evaluation of another organ system, or during an infertility evaluation. They are not usually diagnosed on routine physical examination, as the external genitalia appear typical. Nonobstructive anomalies may present with a range of symptoms, including difficulty with tampon placement or pain with intercourse in the setting of a vaginal septum, recurrent pregnancy loss or other pregnancy complications, or even primary amenorrhea in the setting of müllerian agenesis.[1,4] Box 26.1 demonstrates the non-obstructive reproductive tract anomalies.

BOX 26.1   Nonobstructive Anomalies of the Müllerian Duct

Müllerian agenesis/MRKH
Unicornuate uterus
Uterine didelphys
Bicornuate uterus
Septate uterus
Arcuate/normal uterus
Longitudinal vaginal septum

MRKH, Mayer-Rokitansky-Küster-Hauser.

RELEVANT TESTING FOR NONOBSTRUCTIVE REPRODUCTIVE TRACT ANOMALIES

- Pelvic ultrasound (US)
- 3D US
- Pelvic magnetic resonance imaging (MRI)
- Hysterosalpingogram (HSG)
- Hysteroscopy
- Laparoscopy

DEFINITIONS AND CLINICAL PRESENTATION

Müllerian Agenesis

This congenital anomaly presents with the absence of a uterus and cervix along with most or all of the upper vagina. The ovaries are typically normal because they have a different embryologic origin. Variations of müllerian agenesis can include absence of a functional uterus but presence of unilateral or bilateral underdeveloped uterine remnants with no functional endometrium and thus no pain symptoms. There can also be functional endometrium in these structures (7%–10% of uterine remnants)[5] leading to symptoms, most notably cyclic pain (see Chapter 27).[2] Müllerian agenesis is sometimes more commonly known as *Mayer-Rokitansky-Küster-Hauser (MRKH) syndrome* (Fig. 26.2).[2]

Prevalence and epidemiology[5]:
- General population: 0.1%
- Müllerian anomalies: 5% to 10%

Manifestations of the disease:
- Normal pubertal breast development
- Primary amenorrhea and no pelvic pain

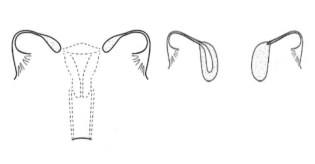
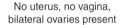
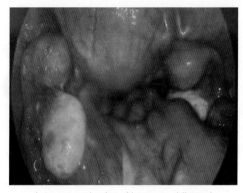

No uterus, no vagina, bilateral ovaries present

Diagram of uterine remnants on pelvic side wall

Laparoscopic view: No uterus, bilateral uterine remnants, bilateral ovaries.

Fig. 26.2 Müllerian agenesis variants.

Clinical presentation and examination: Patients are likely to present during evaluation for primary amenorrhea. Physical examination will be notable for a shortened vaginal canal (dimple to several centimeters long) and no palpable cervix or uterus on vaginal or rectal examination. Rudimentary uterine horns may be seen on imaging.

Differential diagnosis:
- Androgen insensitivity syndrome
- Distal vaginal agenesis
- Transverse vaginal septum
- Imperforate hymen
- Cervical agenesis

Testing/imaging relevant to condition:
- Chromosome analysis to confirm 46,XX
- Pelvic US and MRI to confirm no functional uterus

Management/treatment options: Patients born with agenesis of the uterus and vagina have important reproductive considerations:
- **No uterus:** These patients will be unable to carry a pregnancy. They do have ovaries and therefore can undergo oocyte retrieval and then have a surrogate carry the pregnancy. Though successful uterine transplantation followed by pregnancy and delivery have been reported, this is still experimental, very high risk, and currently not standard of care.
- **Vaginal creation**[2-4]: Multiple techniques are available for vaginal creation to allow for receptive intercourse:
  - **Vaginal dilation:** Sequential dilation to lengthen the native vaginal tissue to a satisfactory length.
    - Recommended first option
    - 99% effective

- Patient-facing resource addressing vaginal dilation in teens: https://www.dsdteens.org/taking-the-wheel/dilation-a-step-by-step-guide/.

Surgical:
- Simple reconstruction with insertion of a graft (i.e., McIndoe vaginoplasty with skin graft, buccal mucosa, peritoneum or Davydov procedure, artificial grafts, amnion)
- Surgical traction (i.e., Vecchietti procedure)
- Balloon
- Vulvovaginoplasty (i.e., Williams procedure)
- Bowel vaginoplasty

Other key clinical considerations:
- Screening for spinal stenosis (spine series)
- Screen for auditory deficits
- Always screen for renal anomalies/absence
- Consider peer support groups: https://www.beautifulyoumrkh.org/
- Offer referral for psychological support for patient and family

Essentials of diagnosis and key treatment considerations:
- Clinical presentation with primary amenorrhea and no pain.
- Examination reveals dimple or shortened blind-ending vagina and pubic hair, which differentiates müllerian agenesis from androgen insensitivity syndrome.
- Atrophic uterine remnants without functional endometrium that are not causing symptoms do not need to be removed.
- Pelvic MRI and chromosome analysis can confirm the diagnosis.

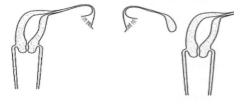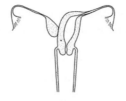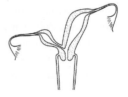

Unicornuate uterus

Unicornuate uterus with distal atrophic uterine remnant

Unicornuate uterus with associated atrophic uterine remnant

Unicornuate uterus with uterine body communicating at level of cervix

Fig. 26.3 Unicornate uterus variants.

Unicornuate Uterus

Müllerian anomaly that manifests in a single hemiuterus, cervix, and vagina on either the right or left side of the pelvis. The other müllerian duct does not develop or presents as rudimentary (uterine remnant) with no functional endometrium (no pain) or functional endometrium (see Chapter 27).[2] The uterine remnant can be located near or far from the well-developed unicornuate system. Contralateral uterine remnants (both functional and nonfunctional) are associated with unicornuate uterus approximately 70% of the time. This müllerian variant is also the most common one associated with renal anomalies (40%) (Fig. 26.3).[2]

Variants:
- **Unicornuate uterus with distal atrophic uterine remnant:** Unilateral hemiuterus and contralateral uterine remnant without functional endometrium, separate and distinct from the patent unicornuate uterus.
- **Unicornuate uterus with associated atrophic uterine remnant:** Unilateral hemiuterus and contralateral uterine remnant without functional endometrium separate but adjacent and touching the patent unicornuate uterus.
- **Unicornuate uterus with uterine horn communicating at the level of the uterus or cervix:** Unilateral hemiuterus with contralateral uterine remnant with functional endometrium and communicating with the unilateral hemiuterus via a tract allowing menstrual egress.

Prevalence and epidemiology[5]:
- General population: 0.03% to 0.1%
- Müllerian anomalies: 5% to 20%

Manifestations of the disease:
- Normal pubertal breast development
- Normal menstruation from patent unicornuate uterus
- Pregnancy risks: preterm labor, malpresentation, pregnancy loss

Testing relevant to condition: Pelvic US, 3D US, pelvic MRI, HSG

Clinical presentation and examination: Patients with a variant of a unicornuate uterus without obstructed uterine remnants are not likely to present with symptoms during their adolescent years. Physical examination will show a normal vagina and cervix and a relatively smaller uterine body deviated toward one side. The contralateral uterine remnant may be diagnosed as an ovarian or other adnexal mass on US; therefore pelvic MRI can be valuable to clarify the anatomy. Unicornuate variants can also be diagnosed during pregnancy and lead to preterm labor, malpresentation (i.e., breech presentation), and recurrent pregnancy loss.

Differential diagnosis:
- Uterus didelphys with obstructing longitudinal vaginal septum (obstructed hemivagina and ipsilateral renal anomaly [OHVIRA])
- Bicornuate uterus with two cervices (bicollis) with obstructing longitudinal vaginal septum
- Complete septate uterus with obstructing longitudinal vaginal septum

Management/treatment options:
- Renal US (40% association of renal anomalies with unicornuate uterus)[2]
- Surgical resection of the noncommunicating uterine remnant without functional endometrium is not necessary in asymptomatic patients
- Surgical resection of small functional communicating uterine remnant may be necessary to prevent pregnancy complications in the rudimentary structure
- Surgical resection or menstrual suppression in the setting of a symptomatic functional uterine remnant (see Chapter 27)[2]

Essentials of diagnosis and key treatment considerations:
- Asymptomatic clinical presentation in adolescents and young adults with regular menses given no obstructive symptoms.
- Can lead to pregnancy complications, including preterm labor, malpresentation, and recurrent pregnancy loss.
- Associated contralateral uterine remnants do not need to be surgically removed unless symptomatic or concern for pregnancy complications.
- Pelvic MRI or 3D US is important to determine the exact anatomy notable for solitary hemiuterus, cervix, and vagina.

Uterus Didelphys

This anomaly occurs when the two müllerian ducts fail to fuse. It presents as two widely separate uterine bodies connected at the level of the lower uterine segment or two separate cervices. This müllerian variant is often associated with a longitudinal vaginal septum dividing the vaginal canal into two cavities of variable sizes.[2] Patients may present with pain if one of the uteri is obstructed because of an anomaly at the level of the cervix or vagina (see Chapter 27) (Fig. 26.4)[2].

Variants:
- **Uterus didelphys and longitudinal vaginal septum:** Fibrous septum typically extends from between the two cervices to the introitus, creating two separate vaginal cavities. Vaginal opening and canal may be symmetric or asymmetric.
- **Uterus didelphys and longitudinal vaginal septum of variable length:** Short fibrous septum extending from the level of the cervix to variable lengths in the vagina. Septum may not be visible at the introitus.

Prevalence and epidemiology[5]:
- General population: 0.03% to 0.01%
- Müllerian anomalies: 5%

Manifestations of the disease:
- Normal pubertal breast development
- Normal menstruation from both patent uteri
- Tampon issues: difficulty with placement or bleeding around tampon
- Pregnancy risks: preterm labor, malpresentation, pregnancy loss

Testing relevant to condition: Pelvic US, 3D US, pelvic MRI, HSG, hysteroscopy

Clinical presentation and examination: Patients with uterus didelphys without obstructive variations are unlikely to present with symptoms during their adolescent years. Physical examination in the absence of a longitudinal vaginal septum will show a normal single vagina and two separate cervices. A longitudinal vaginal septum that extends the complete length of the vagina may be visible with simple labial traction at the introitus and can often be confused with a septate hymen. Vaginal examination will reveal two separate vaginal cavities with a separate cervix palpable at the top of each vaginal cavity. The vaginal openings may be asymmetric or symmetric. Patients can present with difficulty with tampon placement because of the vaginal septum or note that they often bleed around the tampon, given a tampon is only being placed in one of the vaginal cavities, allowing uncontrolled menstrual egress from the other vaginal cavity. Patients can also present with painful intercourse or avulsion of the vaginal septum during intercourse. These uterine variants can also be diagnosed during pregnancy and lead to preterm labor, malpresentation, and recurrent pregnancy loss. It is also possible for the longitudinal vaginal septum to first be diagnosed during labor.

Differential diagnosis:
- Bicornuate uterus
- Normal uterus with duplicated cervix

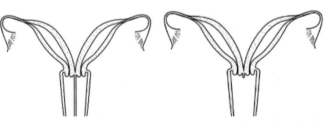

Uterus didelphys with and longitudinal vaginal septum

Uterus didelphys with and longitudinal vaginal septum of variable length

Fig. 26.4 Uterus didelphys variants.

- Unicornuate uterus with functional or nonfunctional uterine remnant
- Bicornuate bicollis ± longitudinal vaginal septum
- Complete septate uterus ± longitudinal vaginal septum

Management and treatment:

- Renal US given association with renal anomalies
- No surgical resection of either uterus is required if there are no obstructive symptoms.
- Associated longitudinal vaginal septum can be resected if symptomatic

Essentials of diagnosis and key treatment considerations:

- Usually asymptomatic unless associated with a longitudinal vaginal septum leading to issues with tampons or intercourse.
- Examination reveals two separate cervices ± two vaginal canals created by variable-length longitudinal vaginal septum.
- Surgical resection of one uterine body or the longitudinal vaginal septum is not required unless there are associated symptoms.
- Confirmation of uterine didelphys with pelvic MRI is important given the wide differential diagnosis associated with uterine duplication.

Bicornuate Uterus

Müllerian anomaly that occurs when the upper portion of the müllerian ducts fail to fuse while the distal portion fuses normally into the lower uterine segment, cervix, and upper vagina. Imaging shows two partially separate uterine bodies with an external fundal (serosal) indentation >1.0 cm with unification of the distal uterine body into one lower uterine segment.

Typical presentation: Usually presents with a single cervix (unicollis) and single vagina (Fig. 26.5).

Variants:

- **Bicornuate bicollis:** Two separate uterine bodies, external fundal cleft >1 cm, separate lower uterine segment cavities, two separate cervices.
  - ± Variable-length longitudinal vaginal septum: as described in uterus didelphys
  - ± Obstructive longitudinal vaginal septum: OH-VIRA (described in Chapter 27)

Prevalence and epidemiology[5]:

- General population: 0.3%
- Müllerian anomalies: 10%

Manifestations of disease:

- Normal pubertal breast development
- Normal menstruation from both patent uterine cavities
- Tampon issues: difficulty with placement or bleeding around tampon when vaginal septum present
- Painful intercourse: when vaginal septum present
- Pregnancy risks: preterm labor, malpresentation, pregnancy loss

Testing relevant to condition: 3D US, pelvic MRI, hysteroscopy

Clinical presentation and examination: Patients with bicornuate uterine variations have similar presentations to those with uterine didelphys.

Physical examination in the absence of a longitudinal vaginal septum will show a normal vagina and one cervix unless bicornuate bicollis is present. In this case two cervices will be palpable. A longitudinal vaginal septum of variable length may be present and is usually associated with two cervices.

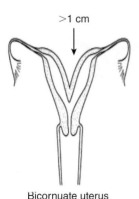
Bicornuate uterus

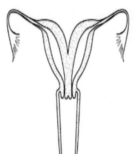
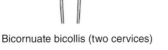
Bicornuate bicollis (two cervices)

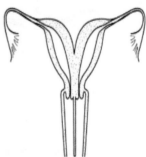
Bicornuate uterus bicollis and longitudinal vaginal septum

Fig. 26.5 Bicornuate uterus variants.

A combination of MRI, hysteroscopy, and/or laparoscopy can be used differentiate between bicornuate uterus and uterine didelphys. Bicornuate uterus differs from uterine didelphys because the bicornuate uterus has two uterine horns that communicate in the lower uterine segment. Uterine didelphys has two separate uteri and two cervices.

Bicornuate uterus differs from septate uterus in that the bicornuate uterus will have a fundal indentation or cleft measuring greater than 1 cm with two separate endometrial canals. The septate uterus has a smooth fundal contour, but the endometrium will have a >1 cm indent (see Fig. 26.6).

These uterine variants can also be diagnosed during pregnancy and lead to preterm labor, malpresentation, and recurrent pregnancy loss.

Differential diagnosis:
- Uterus didelphys ± longitudinal vaginal septum
- Normal or arcuate uterus
- Septate uterus

Management and treatment:
- Renal US to evaluate for associated renal anomaly
- Surgical reunification of the two uterine fundus is not recommended but has been described

Essentials of diagnosis and key treatment considerations:
- Usually asymptomatic unless associated with a longitudinal vaginal septum leading to issues with tampons or intercourse.
- Examination reveals one or two cervices ± two vaginal canals created by variable-length longitudinal vaginal septum.

- Differentiate from uterus didelphys and septate uterus by showing uterine horns and endometrial cavities symmetric in size with fundal indentation >1 cm and communication of the uterine horns near the lower uterine segment.
- Surgical reunification is not recommended.

Septate Uterus

Müllerian anomaly caused by failure of resorption during development. The classic presentation is a single uterine body externally, single cervix, and single vagina. The cavity of the uterus is separated by a fibrous muscular septum arising from the fundus and extending variable lengths into the lower uterine segment, cervical os, or even the vaginal canal. A septum is defined as having a depth of >1 cm and angle of the leading edge of the septum of <90 degrees into the uterine cavity[2] (Fig. 26.7).

Variants:
- **Partial septate uterus:** Serosal fundal indentation <1 cm, variable-length endometrial cavity septum extending from the fundus to the top of the cervix.
- **Complete septate uterus with duplicated cervices and longitudinal vaginal septum:** Single uterine body with septum that extends from the fundus through duplicated cervices, dividing the uterine cavity into two, and the septum extends variable lengths into the vagina as a longitudinal vaginal septum.
- **Complete septate uterus with septate cervix and longitudinal vaginal septum:** Single uterine body with a septum that extends from the fundus through

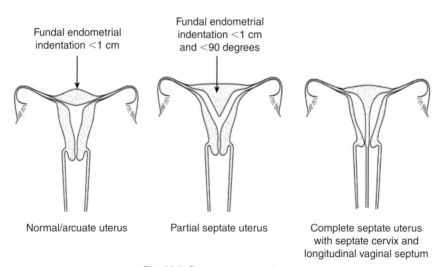

Fundal endometrial indentation <1 cm

Fundal endometrial indentation <1 cm and <90 degrees

Normal/arcuate uterus

Partial septate uterus

Complete septate uterus with septate cervix and longitudinal vaginal septum

Fig. 26.6 Septate uterus variants.

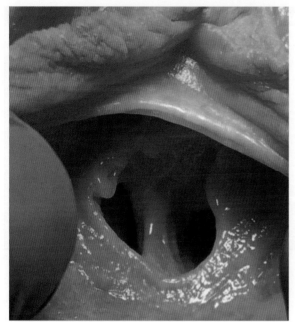

External genitalia and longitudinal vaginal septum with labial retraction

Fig. 26.7 Longitudinal vaginal septum.

a single cervix, dividing the uterine cavity into two, and the septum extends variable lengths into the vagina as a longitudinal vaginal septum.

Prevalence and epidemiology[5]:

- General population: 0.9% to 2%
- Müllerian anomalies: 55% (most common type)

Manifestations of the disease:

- Normal pubertal breast development
- Normal menstruation from patent uterine cavity
- Tampon issues: difficulty with placement or bleeding around tampon when vaginal septum present
- Painful intercourse: when vaginal septum present
- Pregnancy risks: preterm labor, malpresentation, pregnancy loss

Testing relevant to condition: pelvic US, 3D US, MRI, hysteroscopy, HSG

Clinical presentation and examination: Patients with septate uterine variations have similar presentations to those with uterine didelphys and bicornuate uterus.

Physical examination in the absence of a longitudinal vaginal septum will show a normal vagina and one cervix unless there is a complete uterine and vaginal septum, which can separate the vagina into two variable-length cavities.

A combination of MRI, hysteroscopy, and/or laparoscopy can be used to differentiate a septate uterus from bicornuate uterus, uterine didelphys, and arcuate uterus by showing a fundal serosal indentation of <1 cm and a septum separating the uterine cavity of variable lengths. As previously described, patients can present with difficulty with tampon placement because of a vaginal septum. Patients can also present with painful intercourse or avulsion of the vaginal septum during intercourse. These uterine variants can also be diagnosed during pregnancy and lead to preterm labor, malpresentation, and recurrent pregnancy loss.

Differential diagnosis:

- Uterus didelphys
- Bicornuate uterus
- Normal or arcuate uterus

Management and treatment:

- Renal US to evaluate for associated renal anomalies
- Hysteroscopic resection of the uterine septum to improve pregnancy outcomes
- ± Resection of the longitudinal septum if symptomatic

Essentials of diagnosis and key treatment considerations:

- Usually asymptomatic unless associated with a longitudinal vaginal septum leading to issues with tampons and intercourse or recurrent pregnancy loss because of uterine septum.
- Examination reveals one cervix ± two vaginal canals created by a variable-length longitudinal vaginal septum.
- Differentiate from uterus didelphys and bicornuate uterus by showing fundal serosal indentation of <1 cm, endometrial fundal indentation of >1 cm, and angle of leading edge <90 degrees.
- Arcuate uterus is considered a variant of normal.
- Surgical resection of a uterine septum can be done to prevent recurrent pregnancy loss.

Arcuate (Variant of Normal)

Endometrial fundal indentation of <1 cm and angle of leading edge >90 degrees (Fig. 26.7). A normal uterus has no endometrial fundal indentation. Table 26.1 provides a comparison between the different uterine configurations.

Longitudinal Vaginal Septum

Anomaly formed by incomplete fusion and resorption of the lower parts of the müllerian ducts. It presents as thin fibrous tissue extending along the long axis of the vagina creating two separate asymmetric or symmetric vaginal canals. The septum can be partial and of variable lengths

TABLE 26.1	Comparison of Similar Müllerian Anomaly Variants		
Condition	**Uterus/Fundus**	**Vaginal Septum**	**Cervix**
Uterine didelphys	Two widely spaced divergent uterine horns attached at the lower uterine segment or cervices	Common association: longitudinal vaginal septum OHVIRA: obstructed hemivagina	Two cervices
Bicornuate uterus	Deep fundal/serosal indentation >1 cm, separate endometrial canals that communicate	Common association when two cervices: longitudinal vaginal septum or OHVIRA	Can have one or two cervices (bicornuate bicollis)
Septate uterus	Fundal/serosal indentation <1 cm Endometrial fundal indentation >1 cm Angle of leading edge <90 degrees	Common association: longitudinal vaginal septum associated with septate cervix	Can have one or two cervices ± septum
Arcuate uterus (normal variant)	Endometrial fundal indentation of <1 cm and angle of leading edge >90 degrees	None	One cervix

OHVIRA, Obstructed hemivagina and ipsilateral renal anomaly.

along the vagina or extend the full length of the vagina from the cervix (or two cervices) to the introitus. Commonly associated with uterine duplication such as uterine didelphys and bicornuate bicollis and complete septate uterus, but can be associated with a solitary uterus. See variant discussion under uterus didelphys, bicornuate uterus, and septate uterus. Can also be associated with obstructive anomalies such as OHVIRA (see Chapter 27).[2]

Manifestations of disease:
- Normal pubertal breast development
- Normal menstruation from patent uterine cavity or cavities
- Difficulty with tampon placement or bleeding around tampon
- Painful intercourse

Testing relevant to condition: MRI, physical examination

Clinical presentation and examination: Patients with variants of longitudinal vaginal septum are often asymptomatic or can present with difficulty with tampon use, pain with intercourse, or avulsion of the septum during intercourse leading to heavy bleeding. Physical examination with simple labial retraction can often identify a longitudinal vaginal septum (see Fig. 26.7). It is important to differential a longitudinal vaginal septum from a hymenal variant, which only involves the tissue at the introitus. On vaginal examination, a longitudinal vaginal septum can be palpated more proximally in the vagina, extending variable lengths from the cervix or between

two cervices down the long axis of the vagina. Longitudinal vaginal septum is commonly associated with uterine duplication and cervical duplication (uterine didelphys/bicornuate bicollis) and can also lead to variable obstructive symptoms (see Chapter 27).[2]

Differential diagnosis:
- Hymen anomaly (septate or microperforate)
- Vaginal adhesions
- Incomplete transverse vaginal septum

Management and treatment:
- ± Resection of longitudinal septum if symptoms present

Essentials of diagnosis and key treatment considerations:
- Usually asymptomatic unless presenting with issues with tampon placement or intercourse.
- Examination reveals fibrous septum of variable lengths and one or two cervices depending on the associated uterine anomaly.
- Resection of the longitudinal vaginal septum is not required unless symptomatic.

SPECIAL CONSIDERATIONS FOR WOMEN AND GIRLS WITH NONOBSTRUCTIVE REPRODUCTIVE TRACT ANOMALIES

Approximately 30% to 40% of women with reproductive tract anomalies will have a concurrent urologic anomaly.[1-4] Müllerian anomalies may be seen in conjunction with differences of sex differentiation and in girls with anorectal malformations such as imperforate anus (25%) and cloacal anomalies (75%).[6,7]

Reproductive Considerations

Uterine anomalies that result because of a failure of unification/fusion of the two müllerian ducts, including uterus didelphys, bicornuate uterus, and unicornuate uterus, or failed canalization/resorption, including septate uterus, can be associated with reproductive complications. The smaller uterine capacity associated with these anomalies can lead to malpresentation (breech), preterm labor, low birth weight, and recurrent pregnancy loss. They can also be associated with infertility or inability to conceive. Uterine malformations have been reported in up to 18% of those with recurrent pregnancy loss and 7% of those diagnosed with infertility. Although a vaginal septum may not cause difficulty getting pregnant or preterm delivery, it may lead to labor dystocia, vaginal laceration, or bleeding complications during vaginal delivery. Therefore one should consider removal of the vaginal septum before vaginal delivery to reduce complications.[1]

SUPPLEMENTAL MATERIAL FOR CHAPTER

NASPAG Patient Handouts: https://www.naspag.org/patient-handouts

NASPAG Clinical Recommendations JPAG Collection: https://www.jpagonline.org/content/clinical_recommendations_collection

ASRM Müllerian Anomalies Classification 2021 Update: https://connect.asrm.org/education/asrm-mac-2021?ssopc=1

REVIEW QUESTIONS

1. A 15-year-old patient presents with difficulty placing a tampon. She feels like there is extra tissue in her vagina, and when she places the tampon completely, she often bleeds around it. What is the most common müllerian anomaly associated with this diagnosis?
   a. Unicornuate uterus
   b. Uterus didelphys
   c. Uterine agenesis
   d. Normal uterus

2. A 16-year-old patient is found to have a uterine didelphys on pelvic ultrasound during a workup for abdominal pain. She has no associated obstructive symptoms, and physical examination is notable for two palpable cervices. What other imaging study is recommended?
   a. Renal US
   b. X-ray
   c. Spine US
   d. None

3. A 17-year-old patient is diagnosed with a bicornuate uterus incidentally on pelvic US during a workup for abdominal pain. She and her mother ask many questions about her menstrual and reproductive future. Which statement is correct?
   a. Given the two uterine cavities, you will likely have heavier periods.
   b. Given the two uterine cavities, you will likely have more painful periods.
   c. Bicornuate uterus can be associated with preterm delivery and malpresentation.
   d. Because of your Müllerian anomaly, you will not be able to carry a pregnancy to term.

REFERENCES

1. Dietrich JE, Millar DM, Quint EH. Non-obstructive mullerian anomalies. *J Pediatr Adolesc Gynecol.* 2014;27(6):386-395.
2. Pfeifer SM, Attaran M, Goldstein J, et al. ASRM Mullerian anomalies classification 2021. *Fertil Steril.* 2021;116(5):1238-1252.
3. Grimbizis GF, Gordts S, Di Spiezio Sardo A, et al. The ESHRE-ESGE consensus on the classification of the female genital tract congenital anomalies. *Gynecol Surg.* 2013;10(3):199-212.
4. Dietrich JE, Millar DM, Quint EH. Obstructive reproductive tract anomalies. *J Pediatr Adolesc Gynecol.* 2014;27(6):396-402.
5. Bhagavath B, Greiner E, Griffiths K, et al. Uterine malformations: an update of diagnosis, management and outcomes. *Obstet Gynecol Surv.* 2017;72(6):377-392.
6. Wu CQ, Childress KJ, Traore EJ, Smith EA. A review of Mullerian anomalies and their urologic associations. *Urology.* 2021;151:98-106.
7. Moore SW. Association of anorectal malformations and related syndromes. *Pediatr Surg Int.* 2013;29(7):665-676.

Obstructive Reproductive Tract Anomalies*

Jennifer E. Dietrich and Katherine G. Hayes

INTRODUCTION, PREVALENCE, AND EPIDEMIOLOGY

Similar to nonobstructive reproductive tract anomalies, approximately 7% of those born with female reproductive anatomy will have differences in the formation of the reproductive tract, resulting in varying degrees of vaginal, uterine, or cervical development. Unfortunately, no distinct numbers exist regarding the percentage presenting with an obstructive versus nonobstructive reproductive tract anomaly. These anomalies occur based on their derivation from the müllerian ducts or from the urogenital sinus. Most women will present at the time of puberty, during delivery, or during an infertility workup. Earlier diagnosis may occur because of incidental findings of these conditions during the course of a workup for a urologic or spinal condition or during the course of evaluation for a syndrome. Referral to a specialist familiar with diagnosing and managing these conditions is important for the best outcomes.[1-3]

PATHOPHYSIOLOGY OF DISEASE AND EMBRYOLOGY

Please see this section in Chapter 26.

RELEVANT TESTING FOR OBSTRUCTIVE REPRODUCTIVE TRACT ANOMALIES

The most important testing for these anomalies relies on physical examination, followed by pelvic

*Parts of this chapter are presented in concise and easy-to-grasp bullets.

ultrasound and pelvic magnetic resonance imaging (MRI).[1]

DEFINITION AND CLINICAL PRESENTATION

Cervicovaginal Atresia and Cervical Dysgenesis

Patients born with cervicovaginal atresia typically have a small or normal-sized uterine body with the complete or partial absence of the cervix and vagina, which occurs by vacuolization of the paramesonephric tissue and may occur because of defects in canalization or defects in vertical development (Fig. 27.1).[1-5]

Prevalence and epidemiology: 1/80,000 to 100,000

Testing relevant to condition: Pelvic ultrasound and pelvic MRI

Manifestations of disease: Normal pubertal development and primary amenorrhea in the setting of pelvic pain that progressively worsens.

Clinical presentation and examination: Patients are likely to present early after the onset of (cryptic) menarche because the uterus quickly becomes distended leading to pain. Upon initial presentation, a blind-ending vaginal dimple will be noted with no mass (hematocolpos) appreciated on digital rectal examination. In rare cases, a vagina may have developed without development of the cervix in between. No bulge will be seen or palpable at the level of the vagina (see Fig. 27.2).

Imaging: An ultrasound should be obtained followed by an MRI to help confirm the diagnosis. It is important to confirm the absence of cervical stroma on imaging, as the current counseling on management is

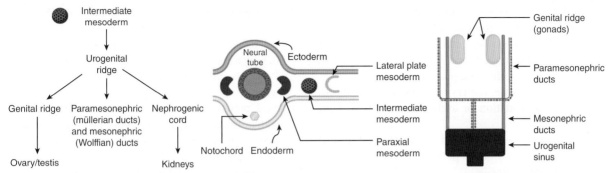

Fig. 27.1 Intermediate mesoderm is present at 4 weeks gestational age. The mesonephros and paramesonephros differentiate into müllerian and Wolffian at weeks 5-6, and the mesonephros, metanephric ducts and genital ridge form in response to androgen presence or absence. Any defects in the migration and fusion of the mesoderm (specifically intermediate mesoderm), which is responsible for the formation of many organ systems, may result in reproductive tract anomalies.

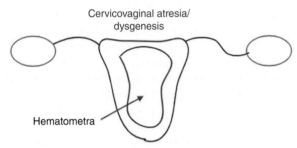

Fig. 27.2 Depiction of cervicovaginal agenesis with hematometra. (Figure developed with Biorender and permission granted by JE Dietrich.)

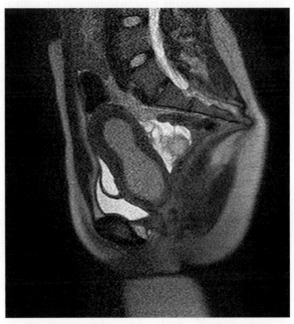

Fig. 27.3 MRI demonstrating hematometra and sagittal view of cervical agenesis. Note that the obstruction in above the level of the pubis. (Permission granted by JE. Dietrich.)

quite different in the presence or absence of a cervix (Fig. 27.3).[4]

Differential diagnosis: Includes complete müllerian aplasia, complete androgen insensitivity, lower vaginal atresia, and transverse vaginal septum and is often misdiagnosed as imperforate hymen.

Management/treatment options: Historically, patients with cervicovaginal atresia have been counseled on the recommendation for removal of the uterine body. Menstrual suppression can be used until the patient is ready to have definitive surgery, so there is no urgency to remove this remnant right away. This is related to reports of high rates of complications with attempts to create a cervix and vagina, including death. More recently, techniques have been described with successful creation of a neocervix and neovagina. The best review of varieties of cervical types is from John Rock and colleagues.[5] This paper echoed

the many different types that clinicians may encounter but attempts at unification have not improved obstetric outcomes. Therefore removal of the uterine remnant is recommended if patients fail menstrual suppression. This can be done laparoscopically or through an open laparotomy approach. Patients who undergo removal of the uterine body may be candidates for uterine transplant in the future. At this time, uterine transplant has also been well described for women with uterine factor infertility, but outcomes are limited, and in some countries, this remains an experimental procedure.[1,4-9]

Essentials of diagnosis and key treatment considerations:

- Clinical presentation of cyclic pelvic pain without menses.
- Examination reveals a blind-ending vaginal dimple in the setting of normal pubertal characteristics for cervicovaginal atresia.
- There may be variable vaginal and cervical development in cases of cervical dysgenesis.
- MRI of the pelvis confirms hematometra without hematocolpos or vaginal distension.
- See Chapter 26 on nonobstructive reproductive tract anomalies addressing treatment options for vaginal creation.

Obstructed Hemivagina With Ipsilateral Renal Anomaly

Patients born with obstructed hemivagina with ipsilateral renal anomaly (OHVIRA) have a müllerian anomaly resulting in uterine and cervical duplication and a partially formed longitudinal vaginal septum that has obstructed the outflow of one cervix (Fig. 27.4).[1-3,8,9]

Prevalence and epidemiology: Not known, but estimated to be between 0.16% and 10%

Relevant testing: Pelvic ultrasound, pelvic MRI, and examination

Manifestations of disease: A patient with OHVIRA will present with the onset of menarche at a typical age but will note progressively worsening dysmenorrhea. They may also complain of urinary and/or bowel symptoms. Patients with a perforation in the obstructing septum will often present in a delayed fashion.

Clinical presentation and examination: Patients present with normal puberty, having regular periods, but usually dysmenorrhea gets progressively worse, as one side is obstructed as it fills with menses (depending on the thickness of the septum and whether located in the lower, middle, or upper third of the vagina). Occasionally, these patients may experience constipation or urinary hesitancy. Some may present with a microperforation of the obstructed longitudinal vaginal septum, in which case they may not experience pelvic pain, but rather vaginal discharge, prolonged periods, spotting, or watery discharge. On physical examination a normal introitus and vaginal opening are noted. One may be able to appreciate a vaginal bulge from one side if the level of obstruction is distal within the vagina. One will not appreciate a one-sided bulge if the obstruction is in the middle or upper vagina. A bulge will be palpable on one side and a single cervix palpated on the unobstructed side. For the patient unable to undergo a vaginal examination, a rectal examination may be performed to assess the level of obstruction instead. In addition, a vaginoscopy under anesthesia may be performed to determine the location just before surgical repair. This can be very useful in the situation where a microperforation is suspected, given the vaginoscopy can help magnify any small perforated areas (Fig. 27.5).[10,11]

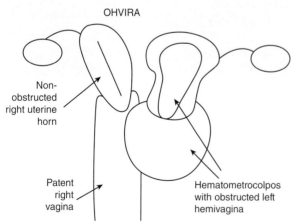

OHVIRA

Non-obstructed right uterine horn

Patent right vagina

Hematometrocolpos with obstructed left hemivagina

Fig. 27.4 Illustration of uterine didelphys with obstructed left hemivagina and hematocolpos. Image developed with Biorender. (Permission granted by JE Dietrich.)

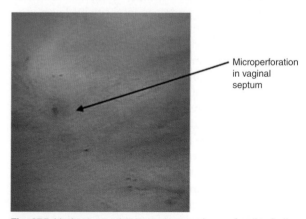

Microperforation in vaginal septum

Fig. 27.5 Vaginoscopy demonstrating a microperforation in the obstructed vaginal septum. (Permission granted by JE Dietrich.)

Imaging: An ultrasound should be obtained followed by an MRI to help confirm the diagnosis, the thickness of the vaginal septum, and the level of obstruction on the affected side (Fig. 27.6). In addition, MRI can help determine if there is an ipsilateral ectopic ureter draining to the obstructed hemivagina. Ultrasound gel or surgical lubricating jelly can be placed into the patent vagina to better delineate the obstructed septum.

Differential diagnosis: May be misdiagnosed as imperforate hymen or transverse vaginal septum. Uterine anatomy may be misdiagnosed with bicornuate or septate uterus.

Management/treatment options: In rare circumstances, these patients may have been diagnosed at an early age during a workup for a solitary kidney. Affected patients can see a pediatric and adolescent gynecologist earlier for anticipatory guidance on puberty and menarche. Interventions are typically not performed until menarche to optimize systemic estrogen levels, which promote vaginal healing and prevent stenosis. More commonly, patients are diagnosed secondary to progressively worsening abdominal pain with menses. Treatment involves excision of the obstructed longitudinal vaginal septum on the affected side, the same side on which the kidney is dysgenetic, malpositioned, or absent. Once the septum is excised, vaginoplasty, much like longitudinal vaginal septum excision, is performed by anastomosing the right and left sides of the vagina in the area where the two hemivaginas branch off separately.[1,2,7,8,9,11]

Essentials of diagnosis and key treatment considerations:

- Progressively worsening pelvic pain with menses.
- History of prolonged spotting after menses without pelvic pain symptoms, which brings about concern for an obstructed longitudinal vaginal septum with microperforation.
- History of vaginal discharge without pelvic pain symptoms, which brings about concern for an obstructed longitudinal vaginal septum with microperforation.
- History of solitary kidney, dysgenetic kidney, or renal anomaly.
- On vaginal examination a single cervix may be visualized or palpated with bulging of the left or right hemivagina, depending on the side obstructed. The side obstructed will be ipsilateral to the renal anomaly.
- MRI of the pelvis confirms uterine didelphys with hematometrocolpos caused by an obstructed hemivagina on the left or right.
- In the situation of microperforation, MRI will demonstrate a uterine didelphys, but may not show hematometrocolpos. In this circumstance an examination under anesthesia with vaginoscopy may help pinpoint the site of microperforation.

Lower (Distal) Vaginal Atresia/Agenesis

Patients born with lower vaginal atresia fail to develop the lower portion of the vagina. Typically, patients will have cyclic pain that may eventually become more constant. They may also experience urinary retention and difficulty with defecation. On examination a typical vaginal introitus is not seen. Rectal examination reveals a palpable mass in the vagina consistent with hematocolpos. An ultrasound can confirm the presence of the hematocolpos, but an MRI is recommended to better understand the distance from the leading edge of the vagina to the perineum (Figs. 27.7 and 27.8).[1-3,7-9]

Prevalence/epidemiology: Not known

Relevant testing: Pelvic ultrasound, pelvic MRI, and examination

Manifestations of disease: Normal pubertal development, cyclic pelvic pain over time with progressive worsening depending on the distance the atretic vagina is from the perineum.

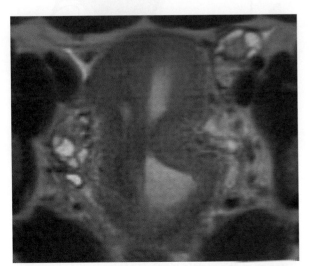

Fig. 27.6 MRI demonstrating coronal view of uterine didelphys with obstructed left hemivagina. (Permission granted by JE. Dietrich.)

Lower vaginal atresia

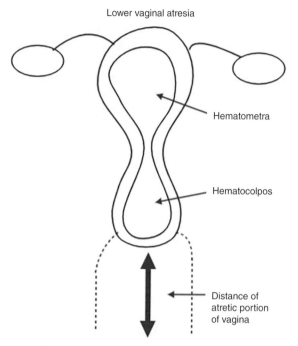

Fig. 27.7 Illustration of lower vaginal atresia or distal vaginal atresia. Developed with Biorender. (Permission granted by JE. Dietrich.)

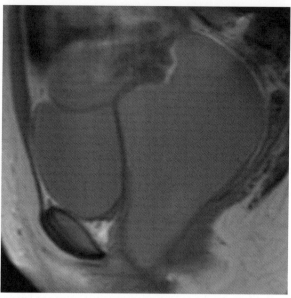

Fig. 27.8 MRI showing sagittal view of obstructed lower vagina, indicating lower vaginal atresia. Note how the vagina cones down rather than appearing flat, as this differentiate the condition from transverse vaginal septum. (Permission granted by JE Dietrich.)

Clinical presentation and examination: A vaginal dimple is seen with a less prominent vaginal bulge in cases where the obstruction is high or proximal and a more prominent bulge when the level of obstruction is low or distal. The tissue will appear pale pink and will not have a blue hue. For patients unable to tolerate a vaginal examination, a rectal examination may be performed to assess the level of obstruction instead.

Imaging: Pelvic ultrasound and pelvic MRI will demonstrate a hematometrocolpos that ends blindly with a curvature in the pelvis a variable distance from the perineum (Fig. 27.8).

Differential diagnosis: Includes complete müllerian aplasia, complete androgen insensitivity, transverse vaginal septum, and cervicovaginal atresia and is often misdiagnosed as imperforate hymen

Management/treatment options: Historically patients with lower vaginal atresia will undergo a vaginal pull-through procedure (see Fig. 27.9). When the distance from the perineum is 3 cm or less, a simple pull-through may be accomplished, whereby the

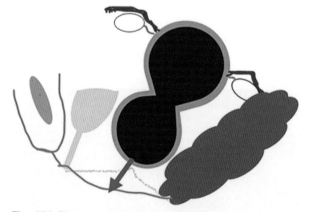

Fig. 27.9 Blue arrow on this sagittal illustration of the obstructed atretic vagina between the bladder and rectum, indicates the direction of the pull through operation to pull the vagina to the correct location on the perineum. (Permission granted by JE. Dietrich.)

surgeon pulls the vagina to the correct, more distal location and normal outlet position. When the distance of the atretic portion of the vagina is greater than 3 cm from the hidden hematocolpos to the perineum, two possible solutions exist. The first is to suppress the patient with hormones until the patient has reached maturity to undergo self-vaginal dilation. This allows for the patient to dilate the vaginal dimple to then meet the upper, obstructed vagina. Then the two vaginal portions can be anastomosed proximally to distally. Alternatively, another tissue graft may be used to bridge this distance. In either circumstance, when this distance spans >3 cm, there is a risk for subsequent vaginal stenosis, requiring dilation, modification, or reoperation.[1,3,7,12]

Essentials of diagnosis and key treatment considerations:
- Cyclic pelvic pain with absent menses in the setting of normal pubertal development.
- Vaginal dimple present without vaginal bulge or with bulge that is not blue hued.
- MRI of the pelvis demonstrates hematometrocolpos and a single uterus that is a variable distance from the perineum.

Functional Noncommunicating Uterine Horn

As discussed earlier, the uterus forms from two separate müllerian ducts that should come together in the midline and fuse. When there is incomplete development and decreased or no fusion, a noncommunicating uterine horn is formed (Fig. 27.10).[1-3]

Prevalence/epidemiology: Unknown

Relevant testing: Pelvic ultrasound and pelvic MRI

Manifestations of disease: Normal pubertal development. Pelvic pain that is usually cyclic and worse during menses but may improve between cycles sometimes. May be seen with Mayer-Rokitansky-Küster-Hauser (MRKH), duplication anomalies, and unicornuate uteri with obstructed horn on one side.

Clinical presentation and examination: Most patients will have a normal external genital examination, unless the diagnosis is MRKH. In MRKH, a blind-ending vaginal dimple may be present. No bulging is palpable or visualized from the introitus or within the vagina. This can only be elucidated with imaging.

Imaging: Pelvic ultrasound and pelvic MRI reveal a circular structure with a hematometra that is separate and has a cortex similar to uterine wall muscle (Fig. 27.11).

Differential diagnosis: May be misdiagnosed as a uterine fibroid, hemorrhagic ovarian cyst, or endometrioma.

Management/treatment options: These may present in a variety of circumstances, but in most instances, these uterine remnants are easily accessible laparoscopically

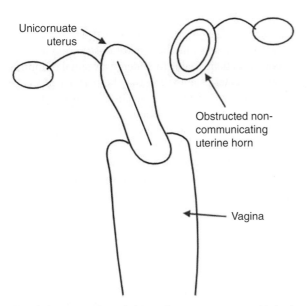

Fig. 27.10 Illustration of right unicornuate uterus and left obstructed noncommunicating horn. Figure developed with Biorender. (Permission granted by JE Dietrich.)

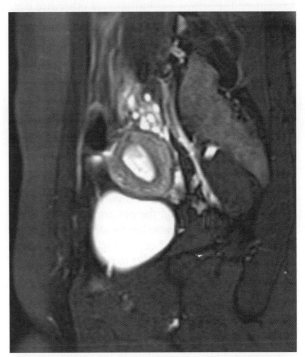

Fig. 27.11 MRI demonstrating hematometra within a noncommunicating obstructed uterine remnant horn (sagittal view). (Permission granted by JE Dietrich.)

and may be excised completely with a laparoscopic vessel sealing device or with a combination of cautery and cutting. Until a patient is ready to have surgery, menstrual suppression with hormonal treatment can be initiated.[1-3,7,13]

Essentials of diagnosis and key treatment considerations:

- Progressively worsening pelvic pain with menses.
- May be associated with unicornuate uterus, OHVIRA, or uterovaginal agenesis.
- On examination a single normal cervix may be visualized within the vagina.
- MRI of the pelvis demonstrates the anatomy distinctly with evidence of obstructed horns.

Transverse Vaginal Septum

Patients with a transverse vaginal septum are typically diagnosed around the time of puberty, when obstructed menstrual products cause pelvic pain. This is the result of failed canalization of the vagina and may occur in the upper, middle, or lower portion of the vagina. The most common presentation occurs in the upper vagina. The development of the uterus and cervix is unaffected. Patients with this condition can be diagnosed with an examination. The hymen and introitus are otherwise normal in these patients. A speculum can be placed into the vagina, but no cervix is visualized. Instead, a wall of tissue is seen initially. Occasionally these patients will develop a microperforation, in which case they may present with prolonged light menses or chronic vaginal discharge rather than pelvic pain (Fig. 27.12).[1-3,14]

Prevalence/epidemiology: 1/84,000

Relevant testing: Pelvic ultrasound, pelvic MRI, and examination

Manifestations of disease: Normal pubertal development, cyclic pelvic pain over time, with progressive worsening depending on the distance the transverse vaginal septum is from the perineum, the thickness of the septum, and whether located in the upper, middle, or lower third of the vagina. Pelvic ultrasound (US) followed by MRI of the pelvis. Microperforation is a special consideration, distinguished by distinct hymenal and vaginal layers that can be seen visually as separate on external examination. Low, middle, and upper septae may also be visualized with a speculum. In the situation of lower vaginal atresia, you cannot place a speculum in the vagina, whereas with transverse septae, you can place it until the level of obstruction is met.

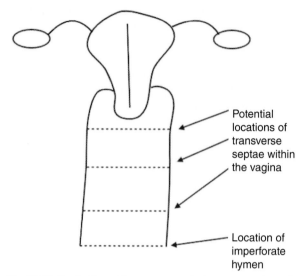

Fig. 27.12 Illustration of transverse vaginal septum and possible locations of the obstructed septa in the vaginal canal. Developed with Biorender. (Permission granted by JE Dietrich.)

Clinical presentation and examination: A normal introitus is seen along with a normal hymenal ring. When the transverse septum is low, it may be possible to place a small cotton-tipped applicator into the vagina to assess where the level of the obstruction is. The septum does not typically bulge outward but is flatter in appearance. A speculum can be placed into the vagina to determine the level of obstruction as well. For the patient unable to undergo a vaginal examination, a rectal examination may be performed to assess the level of obstruction instead. In addition, a vaginoscopy under anesthesia may be performed to determine the location just before surgical repair. This can be useful in the situation where a microperforation is suspected, given the vaginoscopy can help magnify any very small perforated areas.

Imaging: Pelvic US, pelvic MRI, and examination

Differential diagnosis: May be confused with lower vaginal atresia, vaginal aplasia, cervicovaginal atresia, or imperforate hymen.

Management/treatment options: A transverse vaginal septum should be fully excised regardless of the location within the vagina. A thin septum may be excised with cautery after needle mapping and subsequently the proximal and distal vaginas anastomosed together. In the case of a thicker septum, a Z-plasty technique may be required in order to aid with both lengthening of the vagina and increasing the vaginal caliber. These are complex surgeries, and therefore referral to a specialist is important.[1-3,14]

Essentials of diagnosis and key treatment considerations:

- Cyclic pelvic pain that gets progressively worse.
- Normal pubertal development.
- External genital examination is normal.
- Septum noted best by MRI of the pelvis and may be located in the lower, middle, or upper vagina.
- For those who can tolerate a speculum examination, a speculum may be placed, but a flat wall is seen rather than a cervix.
- Can present with microperforation.

Imperforate Hymen

This is a condition where the hymen fails to canalize and is the most distal level of obstruction occurring at the hymenal ring (Fig. 27.13).[1,2,15]

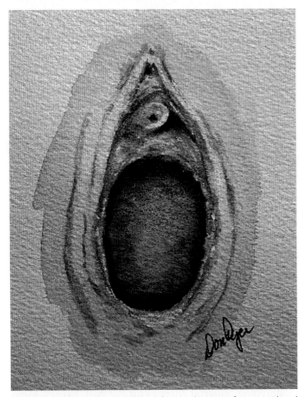

Fig. 27.13 Illustration of imperforate hymen from perineal view. Note the classic blue bulge of the hymen. (Permission granted by Dr. Donald Dyer.)

BOX 27.1 **Obstructive Anomalies of the Müllerian Ducts**

Cervicovaginal atresia and cervical dysgenesis
OHVIRA
Lower distal vaginal atresia/agenesis
Functional noncommunicating horn

OHVIRA, Obstructed hemivagina and ipsilateral renal anomaly.

BOX 27.2 **Anomalies of the Urogenital Sinus**

Transverse vaginal septum
Imperforate hymen

Prevalence/epidemiology: 1/2000 females

Relevant testing: Pelvic US and examination

Manifestations of disease: This results in cyclic pelvic pain and the progressive development of a blue-hued bulge at the perineum.

Clinical presentation and examination: The hymenal tissue is thin, and once the vagina and hymen become fully distended with menstrual products over months' or years' time, the pressure from the volume of menstrual fluid on the hymen results in a bulging effect and the bulged tissue appears bluish in color—a diagnostic hallmark. Patients may present with urinary retention or constipation as well.

Imaging: Pelvic US alone demonstrates a hematocolpos.

Differential diagnosis: When not presenting at puberty with hematometrocolpos, this may be confused with cervicovaginal atresia, müllerian aplasia, complete androgen insensitivity, transverse vaginal septum, or labial adhesions.

Management/treatment options: An imperforate hymen is addressed by removing the obstructed hymenal mucosa. In most cases, this is a thin membrane and can be easily accomplished with the use of cautery devices. Interrupted stitches are usually necessary for hemostasis and to minimize scarring later. There are several ways in which the tissue may be removed. Either an initial cruciate incision may be made or needle mapping to open initially in a horizontal plane or via an ellipse and then subsequently excising all remaining tissue in order to create a space large enough for a small speculum or two finger-breadths width. It is most important to know the location of the urethral meatus, because this can be distorted from stretched hymenal tissue as a result of the hematocolpos as well.[1,2,15]

Essentials of diagnosis and key treatment considerations:

- Pelvic pain that may be cyclic over many months.
- Normal pubertal development.
- External genital examination reveals a vaginal bulge with blue hue.
- May present with urinary retention and constipation.

SPECIAL CONSIDERATIONS FOR WOMEN AND GIRLS WITH OBSTRUCTIVE REPRODUCTIVE TRACT ANOMALIES

Approximately 30% to 40% of women with a müllerian anomaly will have a concurrent urologic anomaly.[1] Approximately 15% to 20% of women with this condition will have a concurrent spinal anomaly.[1] There is a higher risk of endometriosis among women with müllerian anomalies, especially those with outflow tract obstruction.[16-18] These anomalies may be seen in conjunction with disorders of sexual differentiation, depending on the underlying diagnosis.[1,16] Finally, approximately 25% of girls with imperforate anus will have a concurrent reproductive tract anomaly, and nearly 75% will have a concurrent reproductive tract anomaly with a cloacal anomaly.[16,19]

OBSTRUCTIVE REPRODUCTIVE TRACT ANOMALY RESEARCH GAPS

For surgical reconstruction, specifically for patients with vaginal agenesis and those who have undergone vaginal surgery for a vaginal pull-through excision of a longitudinal or transverse vaginal septum and have developed a stricture, more research studies are needed to understand the best options for vaginal replacement and vaginal lengthening. Several surgical techniques have been described and are appropriate options for patients failing vaginal dilation. Regardless, no single technique is superior, and surgery includes the potential for complications. Tissue engineering has come a long way, although to date there is a paucity of information regarding tissue scaffolding methods both in vivo and in vitro for neovagina creation.[18,19]

Imaging continues to improve over time, and ultrasonography is more widely available in most countries.

With the ability for modern ultrasonography to include three-dimensional tools, this becomes useful for evaluating müllerian anomalies as well, with similar sensitivity rates to MRI of the pelvis.[20,21]

The underlying pathophysiology leading to müllerian and vaginal anomalies remains elusive. Although more genetic studies are being conducted, no single genetic mutation or rearrangement explains all anomaly variants to date.[22]

Information is also lacking for obstetric outcomes. This population is diverse, and therefore it is more difficult to study each individual anomaly with respect to specific risks and outcomes. More studies are being conducted as more precise diagnoses are pinpointed and as specific populations are studied. One example of this is a recent study looking at intrauterine growth restriction (IUGR) among those with a müllerian anomaly. This meta-analysis demonstrated an increased risk with a pooled odds ratio (OR) of 1.9.[23] Other situations that would benefit from a more detailed look include the risks for breech presentation, cesarean delivery rates, and preterm labor.[24,25]

▮ REVIEW QUESTIONS

1. A 16-year-old patient is referred to you for absent menses. She started breast development around age 12 years and developed underarm hair and pubic hair around age 11 years. She denies any cyclic pelvic pain. On examination you note Tanner 5 breasts and pubic hair but no vaginal opening. She is noted to have a vaginal dimple that is not bulging. Laboratory testing shows normal gonadotropins and a 46,XX karyotype. Which of the following is the most likely diagnosis to consider ahead of imaging studies?
   a. Imperforate hymen
   b. Labial adhesions
   c. Uterovaginal agenesis
   d. Cervicovaginal atresia
2. A 12-year-old cisgender female presents to the emergency room with urinary retention and constipation that has worsened over 3 months' time. She has been seen by her pediatrician and treated for constipation but continues to struggle with this. She has been undergoing pubertal changes for the past 2 years. Mom notes that she has been complaining of pain for the past 6 months that has worsened. On examination she

has Tanner 5 breasts and Tanner 5 genitourinary development. She has a bulging hymen that looks blue or purplish. A pelvic ultrasound demonstrates a large hematocolpos. What is the most likely diagnosis?

a. Imperforate hymen
b. Labial adhesions
c. Urogenital sinus
d. Hematoma

3. Müllerian anomalies range in complexity. Which of the following imaging studies is the best to accurately describe and assess these anomalies?

a. KUB
b. CT scan
c. Gynecogram
d. MRI of the pelvis

SUPPLEMENTAL MATERIAL FOR CHAPTER

NASPAG Patient Handouts (https://www.naspag.org/naspag-patient-handouts).

Beautiful You MRKH – Support (https://www.beautifulyoumrkh.org).

NASPAG Clinical Recommendations JPAG Collection. Journal of Pediatric & Adolescent Gynecology (https://www.naspag.org/assets/docs/amenorrhea_2020.pdf and https://www.naspag.org/assets/docs/ohvira_2020.pdf).

ASRM Müllerian Anomalies Classification 2021 Update (https://www.fertstert.org/article/S0015-0282(21)02071-9/fulltext)

REFERENCES

1. Dietrich JE, Millar DM, Quint EH. Obstructive reproductive tract anomalies. *J Pediatr Adolesc Gynecol.* 2014;27(6):396-402. doi:10.1016/j.jpag.2014.09.001.
2. Grimbizis GF, Gordts S, Di Spiezio Sardo A, et al. The ESHRE–ESGE consensus on the classification of female genital tract congenital anomalies. *Gynecol Surg.* 2013;10(3):199-212.
3. Pfeifer SM, Attaran M, Goldstein J, et al. ASRM Müllerian anomalies classification 2021. *Fertil Steril.* 2021;116(5):1238-1252.
4. Mikos T, Lantzanaki M, Anthoulakis C, Grimbizis GF. Functional and reproductive outcomes following surgical management of congenital anomalies of the cervix: a systematic review. *J Minim Invasive Gynecol.* 2021;28(8):1452-1461.e16.
5. Rock JA, Roberts CP, Jones HW. Congenital anomalies of the uterine cervix: lessons learned from 30 cases managed clinically by a common protocol. *Fertil Steril.* 2010;94(5):1858-1863.
6. ACOG committee opinion no. 728: müllerian agenesis: diagnosis, management, and treatment. *Obstet Gynecol.* 2018;131(1):e35-e42.
7. Handa VL, Van Le L, eds. Chapter 40: congenital anomalies of the reproductive tract. In: *Telinde's Operative Gynecology.* 12th ed. 2019.
8. Atkinson E, Bennett MJ, Dudley J, et al. Consensus statement: the management of congenital genital tract anomalies in women. *Aust N Z J Obstet Gynaecol.* 2003;43(2):107-108.
9. Akhtar MA, Saravelos SH, Li TC, Jayaprakasan K, Royal College of Obstetricians and Gynaecologists. Reproductive implications and management of congenital uterine anomalies: scientific impact paper no. 62 November 2019. *BJOG.* 2020;127(5):e1-e13.
10. O'Flynn O'Brien KL, Bhatia V, et al. The prevalence of müllerian anomalies in women with a diagnosed renal anomaly. *J Pediatr Adolesc Gynecol.* 2021;34(2):154-160.
11. Santos XM, Dietrich JE. Obstructed hemivagina with ipsilateral renal anomaly. *J Pediatr Adolesc Gynecol.* 2016;29(1):7-10.
12. Mansouri R, Dietrich JE. Postoperative course and complications after pull-through vaginoplasty for distal vaginal atresia. *J Pediatr Adolesc Gynecol.* 2015;28(6):433-436.
13. Tian W, Chen N, Liang Z, et al. Clinical features and management of endometriosis among patients with MRKH and functional uterine remnants. *Gynecol Obstet Invest.* 2021;86(6):518-524.
14. Brander EPA, Vincent S, Mc Quillan SK. Transverse vaginal septum resection: technique, timing and the utility of dilation. A scoping review of the literature. *J Pediatr Adolesc Gynecol.* 2022;35(1):65-72.
15. Hamouie A, Dietrich JE. Imperforate hymen: clinical pearls and implications of management. *Clin Obstet Gynecol.* 2022;65(4):699-707.
16. Wu, CQ, Childress KJ, Traore EJ, Smith EA. A review of Müllerian anomalies and their urologic associations. *Urology.* 2021;151:98-106.
17. Freytag D, Mettler L, Maass N, Gunther V, Alkatout I. Uterine anomalies and endometriosis. *Minerva Med.* 2020;111(1):33-49.
18. Pitot MA, Bookwalter CA, Dudiak KM. Müllerian duct anomalies coincident with endometriosis: a review. *Abdom Radiol N Y.* 2020;45(6):1723-1740.
19. Moore SW. Association of anorectal malformations and related syndromes. *Pediatr Surg Int.* 2013;29(7):665-676.

20. Jakubowska W, Chabaud S, Saba I, Galbraith T, Berthod F, Bolduc S. Prevascularized tissue-engineered human vaginal mucosa: in vitro optimization and in vivo validation. *Tissue Eng Part A*. 2020;26(13-14):811-822.
21. Foster C, Daigle R, Rowe CK. Tissue engineering opportunities for vaginal replacement in a pediatric population. *Tissue Eng Part B Rev*. 2022;28(2):476-487.
22. Ergenoglu AM, Sahin Ç, Şimşek D, et al. Comparison of three-dimensional ultrasound and magnetic resonance imaging diagnosis in surgically proven Müllerian duct anomaly cases. *Eur J Obstet Gynecol Reprod Biol*. 2016;197:22-26.
23. Cekdemir YE, Mutlu U, Acar D, Altay C, Secil M, Dogan OE. The accuracy of three-dimensional ultrasonography in the diagnosis of Müllerian duct anomalies and its concordance with magnetic resonance imaging. *J Obstet Gynaecol*. 2022;42(1):67-73.
24. Chan N, Zhao S, Jolly A, et al. Perturbations of genes essential for Müllerian duct and wolffian duct development in Mayer Rokitansky Kuster Hauser syndrome. *Am J Hum Genet*. 2021;108(2):337-345.
25. Karami M, Jenabi E. The association between Müllerian anomalies and IUGR: a meta-analysis. *J Matern Fetal Neonatal Med*. 2019;32(14):2408-2411.
26. Belfort MA. Chapter 2.1: Operative techniques in obstetrics surgery. In: Adeyemi OA, Dietrich JE, eds. *Operative Concerns in Patients with Congenital Anomalies of the Reproductive Tract and External Genitalia*. Lippincott Williams and Wilkins; 2022.
27. Cahen-Peretz A, Sheiner E, Friger M, Walfisch A. The association between Müllerian anomalies and perinatal outcome. *J Maternal Fetal Neonatal Med*. 2019;32(1):51-57.

Neonatal Ovarian Cysts

Ashli Lawson

INTRODUCTION

Neonatal ovarian cysts are rare, but they are the most common cystic abdominal finding in neonatal imaging.[1] Cysts are usually discovered in the third trimester at 28 weeks gestation or later.[2] The cyst may be simple (fluid filled) or complex (heterogenous appearing) and is usually a result of maternal and placental hormone exposure. Regardless of appearance, almost all cysts in this period are benign and spontaneously resolve.[2] Of those that do not resolve or that are large, there is variation in management practices. Antenatal cyst aspiration has scant outcome data and therefore should not be routinely done. If a cyst persists with certain characteristics past the neonatal period, surgery should be considered. Of those operated on as infants, the most common pathology is remote torsion. Other pathology includes functional cysts, cystadenomas, and mature teratomas/dermoid cysts.

DISEASE DEFINITION

Neonatal ovarian cysts are masses on the ovary that are found during the antenatal period through the first 28 days of life. They can be simple or complex. Because of the nature of ultrasound, they can be confused with cysts of gastrointestinal or genitourinary origin.

PREVALENCE AND EPIDEMIOLOGY

About 30% of female neonates have notable ovarian follicles.[3,4] However, antenatal diagnosis of prominent ovarian cysts (>4 cm) is rare, occurring in about 1/2500 female fetuses.[4] Because of the advances in imaging

capabilities, this incidence is increasing. Risk factors for neonatal ovarian cysts include maternal preeclampsia, maternal diabetes, polyhydramnios, and rhesus isoimmunization.[2] It is not clear if these risk factors are directly related to ovarian cyst development or instead are incidentally found because of increased third-trimester antenatal fetal surveillance.

ETIOLOGY AND PATHOPHYSIOLOGY

Although the etiology is not completely understood, neonatal ovarian cysts are likely driven by maternal and placental hormones.[2] These circulating hormones stimulate the fetal ovaries, which subsequently develop functional cysts. Most functional cysts will spontaneously resolve (slowly involuting) usually by month 12 of life.[5,6] However, some will develop a hemorrhagic component and/or may undergo torsion, both of which are more likely with cysts greater than 4 cm, have complex components, and are persistent.

TESTING

Neonatal ovarian cysts are typically identified during routine antenatal ultrasounds. Cysts <2 cm are presumed follicles and do not need follow-up testing. Most experts suggest surveillance ultrasounds for masses >4 cm. The interval for this surveillance is variable, but most agree that a postnatal ultrasound and a follow-up ultrasound no more than 6 months later are reasonable.[1,4,7] If a mass is >6 cm and appears complex, it is more likely to be surgically managed.[7,8] Because of the extreme rarity of malignancy in this age group and maternal-placental transfer of traditional ovarian tumor markers, there are no recommended serum markers for neonatal ovarian masses.

MANIFESTATIONS OF DISEASE

The majority of neonatal ovarian cysts are asymptomatic. Of those that have symptoms, they include mass effect with compression of surrounding viscera (including inferior vena cava compression or urinary obstruction), rupture or hemorrhage of the cyst (with or without secondary effects on surrounding anatomy), or symptoms of torsion.

CLINICAL PRESENTATION AND EVALUATION

Most neonatal ovarian cysts are found during routine antenatal ultrasounds. Depending on the size and characteristics of the mass, follow-up ultrasounds may be appropriate.

There is no classic clinical picture of the neonate or infant with an ovarian cyst, but when referring or evaluating this child, the provider should inquire about the baby's demeanor (are they consolable when fussy), their urine output, and review their growth curve. Similarly, there is no standardization of surveillance. Experts recommend follow-up imaging based on the baby's clinical picture, cyst size, and cyst characteristics.

IMAGING TECHNIQUE AND FINDINGS

When identified on neonatal ultrasound, cysts are typically simple, anechoic, and <3 cm. Of the neonatal cysts that are larger, the majority are between 3 and 6 cm.[2] When performing serial ultrasounds, it is important to compare the progression of the cyst characteristics, including size, contour, echogenicity, and location, to help elucidate the pathophysiology and need for repeat imaging or surgical management. Cysts that are persistent in size and changing from simple to heterogenous are more likely to undergo surgical evaluation. A pediatric radiologist should note any signs pointing to nonovarian origin (such as the "gut signature"). The "gut signature" is five alternating echogenic layers of the bowel wall. When seen around a cyst that abuts more bowel, as in Fig. 28.1, this suggests an enteric duplication cyst.[9] Enteric duplication cysts are congenital cysts that have a gastrointestinal tract epithelium with a smooth muscle

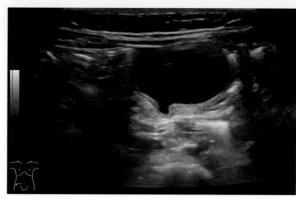

Fig. 28.1 Gut signature on an enteric duplication cyst.

envelope and abut the alimentary tract. They are often symptomatic within the first 2 years of life, but can pose life-threatening complications; therefore an expedited pediatric surgery consult is recommended.

PHYSICAL EXAMINATION

On physical examination of a neonate or infant, start by assessing their growth curve to confirm appropriate weight gain. On abdominal examination, the mass may or may not be appreciated. If there is adnexal torsion, it is likely remote (in utero); therefore peritoneal signs should prompt evaluation for nonovarian pathology.

DIFFERENTIAL DIAGNOSIS

- Ovarian mass: follicle, hemorrhagic component with or without torsion, cystadenoma, dermoid
- Genital anomalies: hydrometrocolpos, cloacal anomaly
- Urologic anomalies: urinary outflow tract obstruction (with enlarged bladder and/or hydroureter), renal cyst, urachal cyst
- Gastrointestinal anomalies: mesenteric cyst, enteric duplication cyst, duodenal atresia, volvulus
- Neoplasms: presacral teratoma, neuroblastoma, lymphangioma

MANAGEMENT AND TREATMENT OPTIONS

There is no clear guidance on management of neonatal cysts. Management is either expectant with serial imaging or surgical with aspiration of the cyst contents or removal of the mass. Removal of the mass may be with a cystectomy or an oophorectomy if autoamputation from remote torsion has already occurred. However, given that most cysts will resolve by 12 months with expectant management, this should be the first line of treatment. In addition, because neonatal ovarian masses are usually asymptomatic and the risk of malignancy is exceedingly rare, surgical intervention should be timed to balance the need for intervention, risks of general anesthesia, and the risks of the need for postoperative analgesics. Intrauterine aspiration of fetal ovarian cysts has been studied and "did not lead to a significant reduction of neonatal interventions."[10] By 6 months of age, if a mass is persistently >4 cm or complex, surgery should be considered; however, clinical context is needed. In general, when surgery is performed, torsion is found about 20% of the time.[2] The risk of torsion was also increased if the cyst was >4 cm (odds ratio [OR] 30.8, 95% confidence interval [CI] 8.6–110.0) or complex appearing (OR 59.1, 95% CI 24.7–141.0). At the time of surgery, ovarian-sparing surgery should be performed if possible. Historically, though, there are higher rates of oophorectomy if undergoing surgery (25.1%, 95% CI 17.2%–34.0%) and if the mass is >4 cm (OR 58.9, 95% CI 19.2–181.0) or complex (OR 35.1, 95% CI 17.0–72.7), likely because of autoamputation.[2] Autoamputation will appear as a strictured infundibulopelvic ligament with separate adnexa in varying stages of necrosis. The higher rates of autoamputation likely reflect the remote or antenatal torsion event.

Expectant management of some infants with complex masses has shown complete resolution of autoamputation by 12 months.[11] A case of premenarchal ovarian torsion also had signs of what was likely unrecognized neonatal torsion.[12]

SPECIAL CONSIDERATIONS FOR THIS POPULATION

Intrauterine cyst aspiration has not been shown to reduce further neonatal interventions.[10]

Although general anesthesia is relatively safe, it is not without risks. The Pediatric Perioperative Cardiac Arrest (POCA) Registry was formed to characterize the patients associated with perioperative cardiac arrest. The registry found that cardiac arrest was rare (1.4/10,000), but more common in children less than 1 year old and those with severe underlying disease.[13,14] Other anesthetic and surgical risks include respiratory and cardiovascular depression

from intraoperative and postoperative medications.[13,14] Because of these findings, postanesthesia management is individualized and based on postconception age of the infant, their gestation at delivery, other comorbidities, and type of surgery. Postanesthesia management may require admission for monitoring, including of analgesics.

A laparoscopic approach is preferred in the neonate for an adnexal mass. During umbilical entry, there should be extra attention to increased risk of umbilical vein complications. Stab incisions with direct placement of instruments are often used instead of trocars for the assisting ports. If an open approach is needed, a mini laparotomy around the umbilicus should be done rather than a Pfannenstiel incision.

RESEARCH GAPS

There is no data-driven consensus on management for neonatal adnexal masses. Textbook guidance is based on expert opinion from prior retrospective case series and cohort studies.

> ### KEY POINTS
>
> - Neonatal ovarian cysts <3 cm are likely follicles, they are common, and they will spontaneously regress.
> - Neonatal ovarian cysts >4 cm are rare, but most resolve on their own.
> - Almost all neonatal ovarian cysts have benign pathology.
> - Serial ultrasounds for ovarian cysts <4 cm after birth should be the first line of care unless other concerns are present.
> - Neonatal ovarian cysts that are >4 to 6 cm, complex, and persistent at 6 to 12 months old are more likely to undergo surgical evaluation.
> - Torsion is usually a fetal event.
> - In utero cyst aspiration does not change outcomes.

▮ REVIEW QUESTIONS

1. A 20-week anatomy scan of an XX fetus reveals multiple bilateral adnexal simple cysts ~2 to 3 cm each. What is the likely pathology and course of these cysts by 12 months?
   - **a.** Cystadenomas, spontaneous resolution
   - **b.** Functional cysts, spontaneous resolution
   - **c.** Cystadenomas, persistent
   - **d.** Functional cysts, persistent

2. You are seeing a 6-month-old for evaluation of a persistent adnexal cyst. It was first seen at 20 weeks' gestation as a 4-cm simple cyst. At a 32-week gestation ultrasound it was 6 cm with a reticular hyperechoic pattern. At 6 months old the cyst was still present, measuring about 5 cm and complex in nature. The infant is growing well with no change in GI or GU habits and a soft abdomen. What is your recommendation?
   a. Referral to a pediatric gynecologist or pediatric surgeon to discuss surgical options
   b. Proceed to nearest ER to rule out ovarian torsion
   c. Prescribe antibiotics for pelvic inflammatory disease
   d. Perform computed tomography scan to elucidate origin of mass

3. At 4 hours of life, a newborn has their initial newborn examination, which demonstrates a single perineal opening with no anus and shortened labia. The pregnancy was uncomplicated with a term vaginal delivery; however, a "midline pelvic simple cystic structure" was noted at a 32-week ultrasound. What is the most likely malformation and cystic structure in this infant?
   a. Difference in sexual development, hydroureter
   b. Congenital adrenal hyperplasia, urogenital sinus
   c. Cloacal anomaly, hydrocolpos
   d. Imperforate hymen, mucocolpos

REFERENCES

1. Trinh TW, Kennedy AM. Fetal ovarian cysts: review of imaging spectrum, differential diagnosis, management, and outcome. *Radiographics.* 2015;35(2):621-635. doi:10.1148/rg.352140073
2. Bascietto F, Liberati M, Marrone L, et al. Outcome of fetal ovarian cysts diagnosed on prenatal ultrasound examination: systematic review and meta-analysis. *Ultrasound Obstet Gynecol.* 2017;50(1):20-31. doi:10.1002/uog.16002
3. Bryant AE, Laufer MR. Fetal ovarian cysts: incidence, diagnosis and management. *J Reprod Med.* 2004;49(5):329-337.
4. Cesca E, Midrio P, Boscolo-Berto R, et al. Conservative treatment for complex neonatal ovarian cysts: a long-term follow-up analysis. *J Pediatr Surg.* 2013;48(3):510-515. doi:10.1016/j.jpedsurg.2012.07.067
5. Rialon KL, Akinkuotu A, Fahy AS, Shelmerdine S, Traubici J, Chiu P. Management of ovarian lesions diagnosed during infancy. *J Pediatr Surg.* 2019;54(5):955-958. doi:10.1016/j.jpedsurg.2019.01.027
6. Papic JC, Billmire DF, Rescorla FJ, Finnell SM, Leys CM. Management of neonatal ovarian cysts and its effect on ovarian preservation. *J Pediatr Surg.* 2014;49(6):990-994. doi:10.1016/j.jpedsurg.2014.01.040
7. Silva CT, Engel C, Cross SN, et al. Postnatal sonographic spectrum of prenatally detected abdominal and pelvic cysts. *AJR Am J Roentgenol.* 2014;203(6):W684-W696. doi:10.2214/AJR.13.12371
8. Cho MJ, Kim DY, Kim SC. Ovarian cyst aspiration in the neonate: minimally invasive surgery. *J Pediatr Adolesc Gynecol.* 2015;28(5):348-353. doi:10.1016/j.jpag.2014.10.003
9. Cheng G, Soboleski D, Daneman A, Poenaru D, Hurlbut D. Sonographic pitfalls in the diagnosis of enteric duplication cysts. *AJR Am J Roentgenol.* 2005;184(2):521-525. doi:10.2214/ajr.184.2.01840521
10. Diguisto C, Winer N, Benoist G, et al. In-utero aspiration vs expectant management of anechoic fetal ovarian cysts: open randomized controlled trial. *Ultrasound Obstet Gynecol.* 2018;52(2):159-164. doi:10.1002/uog.18973
11. Trotman GE, Zamora M, Gomez-Lobo V. Non-surgical management of the auto-amputated adnexa in the neonate: a report on two cases. *J Pediatr Adolesc Gynecol.* 2014;27(2):107-110. doi:10.1016/j.jpag.2013.06.019
12. Gupta N, Nigam A, Tripathi R, De A. Unilateral tubo-ovarian agenesis with contralateral adnexal torsion in a premenarchal girl. *BMJ Case Rep.* 2018;2018:bcr 2017224157. doi:10.1136/bcr-2017-224157
13. Morray JP, Geiduschek JM, Ramamoorthy C, et al. Anesthesia-related cardiac arrest in children: initial findings of the Pediatric Perioperative Cardiac Arrest (POCA) Registry. *Anesthesiology.* 2000;93(1):6-14. doi:10.1097/00000542-200007000-00007
14. Bhananker SM, Ramamoorthy C, Geiduschek JM, et al. Anesthesia-related cardiac arrest in children: update from the Pediatric Perioperative Cardiac Arrest Registry. *Anesth Analg.* 2007;105(2):344-350. doi:10.1213/01.ane.0000268712.00756.dd

Adnexal Masses in Infants, Children, and Adolescents

Sari Kives and Valerie Bloomfield

INTRODUCTION

Adnexal lesions occur in infants, children, and adolescents with varying frequency and may represent ovarian or tubal pathology. Consideration of a patient's age, pubertal status, clinical presentation, and physical examination serves to inform appropriate investigations and management. Through this chapter, we will outline an approach to adnexal masses in neonatal, pediatric, and adolescent patients and describe key diagnostic and management principles.

THE FETUS AND NEONATE

Fetal ovarian cysts are often diagnosed incidentally during antenatal imaging. The vast majority of fetal cysts are functional and likely form secondary to stimulation from fetal follicle-stimulating hormone, maternal estrogen, and placental human chorionic gonadotropin (HCG).[1-3] Diagnosis of an ovarian neoplasm in utero, such as a teratoma, cystadenoma, or malignancy, is uncommon.[4] Approximately 30% to 70% of female fetuses will have a functional cyst identified on imaging.[3,5,6] Incidence increases with increasing gestational age and some maternal complications of pregnancy, including hypertensive disorders of pregnancy, diabetes mellitus, and alloimmunization. Among live-born female neonates, the incidence of ovarian cysts is estimated to be 1 in 2500.[7]

Diagnostic criteria for a fetal ovarian cyst include (1) female fetus, (2) nonmidline cystic structure, (3) normal-appearing urinary tract, and (4) normal-appearing gastrointestinal tract.[1] The differential diagnosis for cystic lesions in the fetal abdomen is broad, with gastrointestinal and urinary anomalies considered (Table 29.1).

TABLE 29.1 Differential Diagnosis of Fetal Abdominal Cystic Lesions
Gynecologic Origin
• Ovarian cyst
• Hydrometrocolpos
Gastrointestinal Origin
• Intestinal duplication cyst
• Mesenteric cyst
• Choledochal cyst
• Omental cyst
Urinary Origin
• Ureteric cyst
• Bladder diverticulum
Other
• Lymphangioma
• Anterior myelomeningocele

Most ovarian lesions are diagnosed at 28 weeks of gestational age or beyond.[8,9] Many antenatal cysts persist during the pregnancy with minimal change; some cases of complete resolution have been documented in utero.[1,4,6] The most common complication of fetal ovarian cysts is antenatal adnexal torsion, which complicates 20% to 40% of cases.[4]

After delivery, there is rapid withdrawal of maternal estrogen and progesterone. As such, neonatal follicle-stimulating hormone levels rapidly increase, peak at 3 to 4 months of age, then fall to prepubertal levels by the second year of life.[10,11] After withdrawal of ovarian stimulation, the majority of functional cysts will resolve spontaneously. Predictors for cyst resolution include diameter less than 40 mm and simple characteristics on ultrasound imaging. In contrast, complex cysts measuring more than 40 mm in diameter are less likely to resolve spontaneously.[4] Complex cystic characteristics on antenatal and postnatal imaging may predict loss of ipsilateral ovarian function secondary to antenatal torsion and autoamputation of the ovary.[4-6]

Antenatal Management

Management of fetal ovarian cysts remains an area of study. Serial ultrasounds are recommended to follow cyst size and characteristics. Evolution of a simple and anechoic cyst to a complex mass suggests intrauterine torsion with or without adnexal autoamputation. Risk factors for antenatal torsion include cyst diameter greater than 40 mm and complex appearance on ultrasound.[4] Case reports have described rare antenatal complications secondary to large fetal ovarian cysts, including polyhydramnios likely secondary to cord compression, bowel obstruction, pulmonary hypoplasia, and hemorrhage.[12-16]

Prenatal aspiration has been considered in an effort to reduce the risk of torsion and need for postnatal surgery. To date, studies have suggested prenatal aspiration increases rates of intrauterine resolution and reduces rates of postnatal oophorectomy; however, studies are limited by small sample sizes and low quality.[17] Further study is required to inform evidence-based practice. The mode of delivery is based on obstetric indications.

Neonatal and Infant Management

Neonates with suspected ovarian cysts should undergo postnatal imaging to confirm the diagnosis. To date, there is significant variation in the management of neonatal cysts. Early surgical intervention was previously considered as a strategy to prevent loss of ovarian tissue secondary to ovarian torsion or hemorrhage.[4] However, despite the goal of ovarian-sparing surgery, most surgical interventions resulted in oophorectomy.[4] Older literature cited a concern about underlying malignancy as a rationale for early surgical management.[18] However, epidemiologic studies have consistently demonstrated neonatal ovarian cysts to be functional with an exceedingly low rate of neoplasms; as such, concerns for malignancy should not inform management decisions.[3,4,18,19] Most neonates can be managed expectantly given high rates of resolution within the first year of life.

Bascietto and colleagues describe spontaneous resolution of 70% of all simple cysts and 80% resolution of all cysts less than 40 mm in diameter.[4] Even complex cysts suspicious for antenatal torsion will often resolve spontaneously within 6 to 18 months.[6,20] In the event of antenatal torsion with adnexal autoamputation, a wandering cystic lesion may be seen throughout the pelvis and abdomen; again, expectant management is considered, as several studies have documented resolution of these lesions over time.[20,21] Caregivers should be counseled about signs and symptoms of adnexal torsion, including pain or inconsolable crying, feeding intolerance, abdominal distention, and fevers.

Intervention with postnatal aspiration or surgical management is considered in the event of symptomatic or persistent, nonresolving lesions. Bryant and Laufer suggest the use of percutaneous aspiration for simple ovarian cysts greater than 60 mm to reduce the risk of ovarian torsion. Cyst recurrence was documented in up to 30% of patients.[1] Predictors for nonresolution requiring surgical management include greater than 60 mm diameter at the time of diagnosis and complex characteristics.[1,20,22] Whenever possible, ovarian cystectomy is preferred to salpingo-oophorectomy to preserve functional ovarian tissue.

ADNEXAL LESIONS IN CHILDREN AND ADOLESCENTS

Adnexal lesions can represent ovarian (neoplastic and nonneoplastic) and nonovarian lesions in children and adolescents. The incidence of each pathology varies based on age and pubertal status. As demonstrated by Hermans and colleagues, most ovarian lesions are benign in childhood and adolescence.[23] A bimodal distribution is noted with a nadir in incidence in early childhood (Fig. 29.1).

Next, we will review nonneoplastic ovarian lesions, neoplastic ovarian lesions, and nonovarian adnexal masses.

Nonneoplastic Ovarian Lesions
Functional Ovarian Cysts

Functional ovarian cysts typically develop secondary to stimulation from pituitary gonadotropins. Follicular cysts form when a dominant follicle fails to ovulate and involute, resulting in a thin-walled cystic structure. Similarly, fluid accumulation in a physiologic corpus luteum can result in a thicker-walled cystic structure

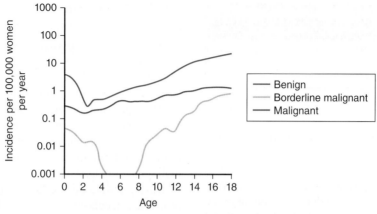

Fig. 29.1 Incidence of adnexal masses stratified by benign, borderline, and malignant pathology on a logarithmic scale among children and adolescents. (Hermans AJ, Kluivers KB, Janssen LM, et al. Adnexal masses in children, adolescents and women of reproductive age in the Netherlands: A nationwide population-based cohort study. Gynecol Oncol. Oct 2016;143(1):93-97. doi:10.1016/j.ygyno.2016.07.096.)

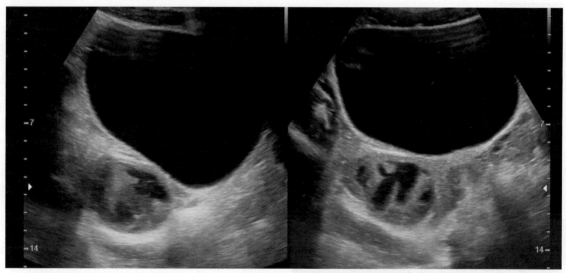

Fig. 29.2 Ultrasound imaging of the pelvis. The right ovary contains a hemorrhagic cyst characterized by a heterogeneous cyst. A reticular "cobweb" pattern is noted with a retracting clot. (Published with patient permission.)

within the ovary reaching up to 8 cm.[24] Cyst walls become vascularized before regression; cysts can undergo hemorrhagic transformation with intracystic and/or intraabdominal hemorrhage.[25]

Hemorrhagic cysts have been described as great imitators, as their clinical presentation with acute-onset pain may be confused for ovarian torsion.[26] Imaging can also be difficult to interpret, with a broad differential diagnosis including ovarian torsion, neoplasm, or tubo-ovarian

abscess. Careful review with radiology colleagues with consideration of the clinical context is important before planning intervention. In the event of cyst rupture, hemoperitoneum can develop with associated anemia and potential hemodynamic instability. Characteristic ultrasound findings of hemorrhagic cysts are highlighted in Fig. 29.2.

As noted earlier, functional cysts account for nearly all antenatal and neonatal cysts secondary to stimulation

TABLE 29.2   **Triad of McCune-Albright Syndrome**
Peripheral precocious puberty
Café-au-lait skin lesions
Fibrous dysplasia bone lesions

from fetal/neonatal gonadotropins and maternal and placenta hormones. Functional cysts account for nearly 30% to 50% of ovarian lesions in adolescents with stimulation from pituitary gonadotropins.[27-29] In contrast, functional ovarian lesions in childhood are uncommon, given low prepubertal gonadotropin levels. Functional cysts within childhood should prompt consideration of endocrinopathies such as precocious puberty, including McCune-Albright syndrome (Table 29.2).[2]

Endometrioma

Endometriomas are benign ovarian masses of ectopic endometrium. Incidence within adolescents is not well defined but may occur in up to one-third of patients with surgically documented endometriosis.[28,30] In addition to an adnexal lesion on ultrasound characterized by a unilocular cyst with homogenous ground-glass echoes, patients will typically describe cyclic and acyclic pelvic pain (Fig. 29.3). Moreover, patients often describe associated bladder and bowel symptoms such as dyschezia and dysuria and dyspareunia.[27,29-32]

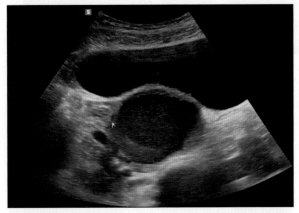

Fig. 29.3 Transabdominal ultrasound image of an ovarian endometrioma characterized by a unilocular cyst, low-level echoes, and homogenous hemorrhagic debris that appears like "ground glass." (Published with patient permission.)

Ovarian Neoplasms

Ovarian neoplasms—benign, borderline, and malignant—account for approximately 2% of all tumors in children and adolescents.[33] Incidence is approximately 2.6 per 100,000 girls per year.[34] Lesions can be classified based on cell line of origin, including germ cell tumor (GCT), epithelial tumor, or sex cord stromal tumor (SCST). Each tumor type is characterized by clinical presentations and imaging findings (Table 29.3). Classic ultrasound findings for mature cystic teratomas are highlighted in Fig. 29.4.

During childhood, GCTs account for more than 70% of ovarian neoplasms (Fig. 29.5). In adolescents, germ cell and epithelial lesions occur at similar rates. Sex cord stromal lesions are most common in early childhood, accounting for approximately 20% of cases, and are rare in later childhood and adolescence.

Of all ovarian malignancies in children and adolescents, the majority are diagnosed in adolescents aged 15 to 19 years.[35] Age-adjusted rates of ovarian malignancy in children ≤9 years old is 0.102 per 100,000 per year compared with 1.072 per 100,000 per year in children aged 10 to 19.[35] Although the incidence of malignancy is 10-fold higher in adolescents, the proportion of malignant lesions is highest in childhood (Fig. 29.6).[23] This reflects low rates of functional, benign ovarian lesions in childhood, as the hypothalamic-pituitary-ovarian axis remains quiescent.

Borderline ovarian neoplasms are uncommon in children and account for 2% to 4% of ovarian lesions in adolescents.[23]

Nonovarian Pathologies

Paratubal and paraovarian cysts represent congenital remnants of the paramesonephric and mesonephric ducts. Ultrasound identifies paratubal cysts as simple, anechoic cystic lesions, which may be mistaken as ovarian in origin. Paratubal cysts are benign in nature but can be associated with acute pathology such as adnexal torsion.

Additional tubal pathologies should be considered within the sexually active adolescent population, including ectopic pregnancy and tubo-ovarian abscess.

CLINICAL PRESENTATION

Ovarian lesions in children and adolescents have a wide range of clinical presentations based on mass size and underlying pathology. Knowledge of gynecologic

TABLE 29.3   Common Clinical Presentations and Imaging Characteristics of Ovarian Neoplasms by Cell Line

Cell Line Origin	Clinical Features	Examples	Classic Imaging Characteristics
Germ Cell Origin			
Develop from primordial ovarian germ cells	• GCTs are the most common ovarian neoplasms of childhood and adolescence • Can present with rapid growth and onset of symptoms • Malignant GCT commonly limited to a single ovary (stage 1A disease); bilateral ovarian involvement occurs in 10%–20% of cases	Benign neoplasms account for 90% of GCTs 1. Mature cystic teratoma 2. Gonadoblastoma Malignant neoplasms 1. Immature teratoma 2. Dysgerminoma 3. Endodermal sinus tumors 4. Mixed germ cell tumors 5. Choriocarcinoma	• Mature cystic teratomas present as a unilocular cystic mass with a hyperechoic nodule, with distal acoustic shadowing, presence of fat and calcifications, and dot-dash pattern • Commonly present as heterogenous lesions given the mix of germ cell origins • Dysgerminoma typically presents as a solid, heterogeneous mass • Highly vascularized
Epithelial Origin			
Develop from epithelial cells of the ovary	• Second most common neoplasm in adolescent patients; uncommon in childhood • Typically slow growing and can attain large sizes	Benign: 70% of epithelial lesions 1. Serous cystadenoma 2. Mucinous cystadenoma Borderline: 20% of epithelial lesions 1. Borderline serous cystadenoma 2. Borderline mucinous cystadenoma Malignant: <10% of epithelial lesions 1. Serous adenocarcinoma 2. Mucinous adenocarcinoma	• Unilocular or multilocular thin-walled cysts • Absence of enhancing septations or solid components • Mucinous tumors may have fluid levels because of mucin layering • May contain vascular septations or solid components
Sex Cord Stromal Tumors			
Develop from the sex cord cells (Sertoli or granulosa cells) or stromal cells (fibroma, thecoma)	• Account for <10% of ovarian neoplasms in children and adolescents • May produce hormones (estrogen or androgens) • Hormone-related symptoms include precocious puberty abnormal uterine bleeding, acne, hirsutism, clitoromegaly, or voice deepening	Benign 1. Thecoma 2. Fibroma Malignant 1. Juvenile granulosa cell tumor 2. Sertoli-Leydig tumor	• Typically unilateral and solid • Finding of solid ovarian mass, ascites, and pleural effusion suggestive of Meigs syndrome, most often associated with fibroma • Commonly unilateral, with nonspecific appearance • Can be solid-cystic in appearance • Can be large; average diameter 16 cm

GCT, Germ cell tumor; *NMDA*, N-methyl-D-aspartate receptor.

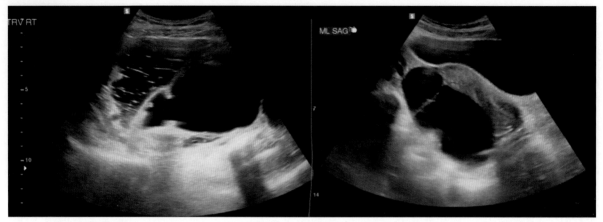

Fig. 29.4 Classic ultrasound findings of a mature cystic teratoma include anechoic cystic contents, dot-dash pattern, and solid Rokitansky nodule. (Published with patient permission.)

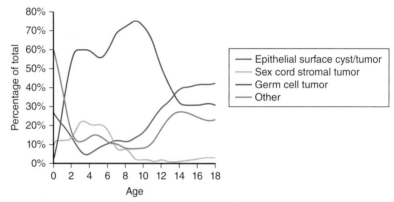

Fig. 29.5 Proportion of ovarian neoplasm by cell line among children and adolescents. (Hermans AJ, Kluivers KB, Janssen LM, et al. Adnexal masses in children, adolescents and women of reproductive age in the Netherlands: A nationwide population-based cohort study. Gynecol Oncol. Oct 2016;143(1):93-97. doi:10.1016/j.ygyno.2016.07.096.)

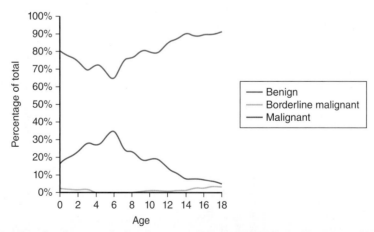

Fig. 29.6 Proportion of malignancy of adnexal masses. (Hermans AJ, Kluivers KB, Janssen LM, et al. Adnexal masses in children, adolescents and women of reproductive age in the Netherlands: A nationwide population-based cohort study. Gynecol Oncol. Oct 2016;143(1):93-97. doi:10.1016/j.ygyno.2016.07.096.)

anatomy, typical pubertal progression, and common ovarian pathologies within a given age group are important when considering a patient's presentation.

Pelvic pain is the most common complaint in children and adolescents presenting with an adnexal mass, accounting for up to 70% of presentations.[23,29,31,36-39] Patients may describe a history of abdominopelvic discomfort or aching. Given that pain symptoms often correlate with lesion size, there may be associated symptoms of fullness or bloating. Severe, acute-onset pain may suggest an ovarian mass has been complicated by adnexal torsion or hemorrhage.[23,29,31,36-39]

Alternatively, patients may present with a palpable abdominal or pelvic mass. In childhood, the ovary migrates from the lower thoracic vertebrae, ultimately reaching the pelvis by puberty. Given this anatomy, ovarian etiology should be considered for any palpable abdominal mass in childhood. In fact, ovarian masses account for approximately 20% of abdominal masses in children.[18,39,40] In contrast, in adolescent patients, the adnexa sit within the bony pelvis, and lesions only become palpable abdominally with increasing size.

Patients presenting with hormonally active tumors, such as sex cord-stromal tumors (SCSTs), may present with symptoms of endocrinopathy. In prepubertal children, clinicians should inquire about symptoms of isosexual precocious puberty, including breast development, increased growth velocity, and vaginal bleeding. A detailed history about the sequence and rapidity of symptoms will help to distinguish between normal pubertal development and potential underlying pathology. In the case of an estrogen-secreting tumor (granulosa cell tumor), pubertal patients may describe abnormal uterine bleeding. Prepubertal and pubertal patients with androgen-secreting tumors (Sertoli-Leydig tumor) may describe symptoms of virilization, including hirsutism, voice changes, and clitoromegaly (see Table 29.3).[41]

Sexually active adolescents are at risk of pathologies such as pelvic inflammatory disease with tubo-ovarian abscess or ectopic pregnancy. A confidential psychosocial history should be conducted to identify risk factors. Please refer to Chapter 2 on approaches to the confidential history.

Physical Examination

Vital signs, including height and weight, should be measured and compared with age-appropriate normal values. Height and weight trajectories should be plotted on growth curves. Sexual maturity staging of breasts and pubic hair allows for assessment of pubertal status when appropriate. Chapter 5 for more information on sexual maturity ratings.

A thorough abdominal examination should be completed. In addition to palpating for lesion size and mobility, clinicians can assess for tenderness or acute findings such as peritonitis. Masses that are fixed or nodular on palpation associated with ascites and lymphadenopathy are rare but suspicious of malignancy.

In pediatric and younger adolescent patients, the pelvic examination is commonly deferred. Older sexually active patients may be able to tolerate a single-digit bimanual examination to assess lesion laterality, size, and mobility. Alternatively, a single-digit rectal examination can be considered in nonsexually active patients. If concerns for pelvic inflammatory disease or tubo-ovarian abscess exist, a pelvic examination can identify cervical motion tenderness and tenderness of the uterus and adnexa. Similarly, a speculum examination may be tolerated in some adolescents to collect cervical swabs and assess for purulent cervical discharge.

Investigations

Investigations should follow a comprehensive history and physical examination.

Transabdominal ultrasonography is first line for infants, children, and adolescents presenting with a clinical history or physical examination suggestive of an adnexal mass. Ultrasonography should be performed and interpreted by radiologists with expertise in gynecologic imaging whenever possible. In addition to assessing lesion etiology and size, ultrasound characteristics can aid in identifying underlying pathology (see Table 29.1).

Magnetic resonance imaging (MRI) or computed tomography may be considered when ultrasound is inconclusive. Cross-sectional imaging can be helpful in patients at risk of malignancy to assess lesion characteristics, ascites, lymphadenopathy, and metastatic spread.

Blood work and further laboratory investigations should be tailored to a patient's presentation:
- Complete blood count
  - Anemia may reflect acute bleeding in the event of a hemorrhagic cyst or ruptured ectopic pregnancy
  - Elevated white blood cell count with left shift may suggest an infectious process such as pelvic inflammatory disease
  - Thrombocytosis may be seen as an acute-phase reactant in acute infection or a metastatic process

- Beta-HCG
  - In nonsexually active patients, can suggest ovarian germ cell neoplasm
  - In sexually active patients with an adnexal mass, can suggest germ cell neoplasm, ectopic pregnancy, or pregnancy-associated ovarian lesions such as corpus luteal cyst
- Vaginal or cervical swabs for sexually transmitted infection
  - Presence of chlamydia or gonorrhea infection in a sexually active adolescent may suggest tubo-ovarian abscess

INVESTIGATION OF A SUSPICIOUS ADNEXAL MASS

Clinicians are challenged to identify patients at risk of malignancy through history, physical examination, and investigations. As described, most children and adolescents with adnexal masses have benign lesions which can be managed with conservative, ovarian-sparing therapies. Accurate preoperative risk assessment aims to predict which patients are at risk of malignancy and will benefit from an oncologic approach with surgical staging.

Review of clinical history can highlight risk factors for malignancy. Oltmann and colleagues report that patients presenting with a chief complaint of abdominal mass or precocious puberty were more likely to have a malignant rather than benign lesion (odds ratio 4.84 and 5.67, respectively). In contrast, pain is not a distinguishing factor for benign or malignant disease.[39] As described earlier, patients presenting between the ages of 1 and 8 years have a threefold increase in the risk of malignant diagnosis compared with infants and adolescents.[39]

Although tumor markers are not validated among pediatric and adolescent patients, they may be considered as part of a comprehensive workup for suspected malignancy (Table 29.4).[42] Clinicians should be aware that values must be interpreted within age-specific normal values. Within pediatric and adolescent patients, abnormal tumor markers differentiate a malignant mass with a high negative predictive value of 94.4% but poor positive predictive value (17.1%).[42] The performance of individual tumor markers to predict malignancy is poor. For example, although associated with dysgerminoma, lactate dehydrogenase (LDH) is a nonspecific marker that does not independently distinguish between benign and malignant processes.[43] Similarly, alpha fetal protein (AFP) can be elevated in malignant lesions, such as yolk sac tumors and immature teratomas, as well as benign lesions such as dermoid cysts.[42]

For patients with malignant diagnoses on final pathology, tumor markers that were elevated preoperatively can be useful to monitor for disease response to systemic therapy (such as chemotherapy) and in surveillance for recurrence after treatment completion.

Ultrasound characteristics associated with malignant ovarian lesions have been described (Table 29.5). Size thresholds of 5 to 8 cm have been proposed within the literature as increased risk of malignancy; Oltmann and colleagues found that lesions greater than 8 cm in diameter predicted malignancy with an odds ratio of 19.0. Solid or solid-cystic masses also have an increased odds ratio for malignancy (10.13 and 3.62, respectively).[39]

TABLE 29.4   Tumor Markers Associated With Ovarian Neoplasms

	Ca-125	CEA	AFP	b-HCG	LDH	Estradiol	Inhibin	Testosterone
Germ cell tumors								
Teratoma			X		X			
Dysgerminoma					X			
Choriocarcinoma				X				
Mixed germ cell tumor			X	X	X			
Epithelial tumor	X	X						
Sex cord stromal tumors								
Granulosa cell tumor						X	X	
Sertoli-Leydig tumor							X	X

AFP, Alpha fetal protein; *b-HCG,* beta human chorionic gonadotropin; *Ca-125,* cancer antigen 125; *CEA,* carcinoembryonic antigen; *LDH,* lactate dehydrogenase.

TABLE 29.5 **Imaging Characteristics Associated With Ovarian Malignancy**
• Diameter ≥5–8 cm
• Solid lesion
• Solid-cystic lesion
• Papillary projections
• Thick septations with vascularity
• Abdominal or pelvic ascites
• Metastatic lesions

Additional findings on imaging including the ovarian crescent sign, lesion complexity (thick septations, solid nodules, or papillary components), hypervascularity, and ascites are associated with malignancy. Metastatic disease is suspected in the event of bilateral ovarian lesions.[42]

Several ultrasound and MRI risk stratification tools have been developed and validated in adult populations https://www.acr.org/Clinical-Resources/Reporting-and-Data-Systems/O-RADS; https://www.acr.org/-/media/ACR/Files/RADS/O-RADS/ACR-Guidance-App.pdf. The Ovarian-Adnexal Reporting and Data System promotes the use of consistent terminology and interpretation of imaging, improves the accuracy of assignment of malignant risk, and provides recommendations for management dependent on risk.[44] An alternative reporting system includes the International Ovarian Tumor Analysis (IOTA).[45] To date, these protocols have not been validated in pediatric and adolescent populations.

Several authors have proposed a combination of laboratory investigations with imaging to better risk-stratify patients. Rogers and colleagues report that combining lesion size (≥8 cm) with the presence of complex features on ultrasound predicts malignancy with a positive predictive value of 37%.[42] Similarly, Madenci and colleagues reviewed 502 patients who underwent surgical management of adnexal masses, including 44 patients with malignancy on final pathology. They identified patients with heterogenous lesions with positive tumor markers and patients with solid tumors ≥9 cm to be at the highest risk for malignancy. In contrast, cystic lesions <9 cm were at low risk for malignancy.[46]

Efforts to develop improved predictive tools are ongoing. The Decision Tree System was proposed by Stanković; this algorithm incorporates clinical presentation and ultrasound findings to risk-stratify ovarian lesions. Study authors suggest the algorithm predicted malignancy with a positive predictive value of 86% and negative predictive value of 96%.[47] However, retrospective application of this algorithm to a Canadian population did not reproduce such robust results.[48]

Similarly, Lawrence and colleagues retrospectively reviewed children and adolescents who underwent surgery for ovarian neoplasms and found the rate of oophorectomy for benign lesions was independently associated with provider specialty, premenarchal status, preoperative suspicion for malignancy, larger lesion size, and presence of a solid component. The authors proposed a clinical approach to the management of adnexal masses aimed at reducing rates of oophorectomy for functional and benign neoplasms.[49] Efforts to prospectively validate this decision tool are ongoing.

Minneci and colleagues describe a multicenter collaboration to develop a consensus-based preoperative algorithm to reduce unnecessary oophorectomies, defined as oophorectomy for benign neoplasm on final pathology. The rate of unnecessary oophorectomy decreased from 16% before implementation of the algorithm to 8.4% after implementation. The algorithm demonstrated high sensitivity and specificity in detection of benign neoplasms (91.6% and 90.0%, respectively). Further studies are required to understand the use of this algorithm in clinical practice.[50]

MANAGEMENT

The approach to the management of adnexal lesions is guided by clinical presentation and suspected underlying pathology. With all adnexal lesions in pediatric and adolescent patients, an emphasis on careful preoperative collaboration with radiology, pediatric and adolescent gynecology, and pediatric surgery is important, with a goal of optimizing ovarian-sparing approaches.

Expectant Management

Expectant management of functional cysts in adolescents is the mainstay of therapy. Most functional cysts will resolve within 2 to 3 months; an ultrasound should be arranged to document normal-appearing adnexa at that time.[27,29,37] Even in the event of a hemorrhagic cyst with hemoperitoneum, most patients can be managed with supportive care including adequate analgesia. Although investigations documenting anemia and hemoperitoneum necessitate cautious surveillance, neither are absolute indications for surgical management. Similar to functional cysts, ultrasound should be repeated in approximately 3 months to document resolution. While expectantly managing ovarian lesions, patients should be counseled about the risk of ovarian torsion and need to present if sudden-onset, ipsilateral pain with associated nausea, vomiting, and fever appear.

Use of combined hormonal contraceptives can be considered to prevent future functional and hemorrhagic cysts in the adolescent population. This is achieved by suppression of pituitary follicle-stimulating hormone and luteinizing hormone, thereby suppressing ovarian stimulation.[51] As such, hormonal suppression will not change the natural history of an existing cyst. Adolescents should be prescribed combined hormonal contraceptives containing at least 30 mcg of ethinyl estradiol for bone health and adequate suppression of the hypothalamic-pituitary-ovarian axis.[52]

Surgical Management

Surgical management is recommended for nonresolving functional cysts, acute pathology such as ovarian torsion, and suspected ovarian neoplasms. Surgical intervention aims to resolve symptoms and achieve accurate tissue diagnosis. Whenever possible, surgical approaches that spare the ovarian cortex, such as cystectomy, are preferred. Cystectomy is preferred to cyst aspiration, as it is associated with lower rates of recurrence and allows for a pathologic diagnosis.[37] Laparoscopic techniques have been demonstrated safe within pediatric and adolescent populations and are associated with improved postoperative recoveries.[53,54]

Additional minimally invasive techniques have been described in the management of suspected benign ovarian neoplasms. A mini-laparotomy can allow for controlled drainage of the cystic contents, followed by exteriorization of the ovary to facilitate cystectomy (Fig. 29.7). This technique is helpful when large cystic size precludes safe laparoscopic entry. Some recommend this technique when managing suspected teratomas. Spillage of teratoma contents can result in chemical peritonitis with postoperative pain, fevers, and granulomatous deposits; cyst drainage through a mini-laparotomy and subsequent open cystectomy was proposed as a strategy to reduce spill risk and subsequent sequela.[55] Interestingly, although laparoscopy is associated with a higher rate of intraabdominal teratoma rupture, the literature reports very low rates of complications overall, supporting a laparoscopic approach when possible.[56,57] With any operative technique, preservation of the

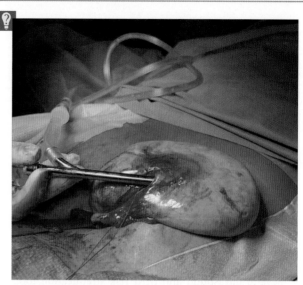

Fig. 29.7 Minimally invasive approach to ovarian cystectomy. A suprapubic mini-laparotomy (3–4 cm) is developed. The ovarian cortex is purse-stringed with suture, and the cyst is aspirated with a sharp gallbladder trocar. Constant traction on the purse-string suture minimizes spill. Once sufficiently drained, the entire adnexa can be delivered through the abdominal wall to perform a cystectomy. (Picture published with patient permission.)

functional ovarian tissue is paramount, with efforts to reduce trauma and the use of electrocautery to the ovarian cortex.

Patients should be counseled that the final pathology will be reviewed after cystectomy. In the event of unexpected malignancy, patients may require additional surgical interventions such as salpingo-oophorectomy or surgical staging.

Suspected malignancies are often managed by multidisciplinary teams, including pediatric gynecologists, general surgeons, urologists, and oncologists. Surgical staging typically involves unilateral salpingo-oophorectomy, lymphadenectomy of abnormal nodes (firm or enlarged), sampling of ascites or pelvic washings, and biopsies of the omentum and peritoneum. The contralateral ovary should be inspected and biopsied if abnormal.[58] Appropriate preoperative investigations and multidisciplinary collaboration inform the surgical approach and recommendation for adjuvant or neoadjuvant therapies. Recommendations for postoperative surveillance are guided by final pathology.

Postoperative Surveillance

To date, there are no validated algorithms for postoperative surveillance after ovarian cystectomy. For any functional cyst requiring operative management, such as hemorrhagic cyst, a follow-up ultrasound can be considered 1 to 2 months postoperatively as part of routine care. Beyond this, ultrasound surveillance for recurrence is discouraged, as functional cysts are common and do not require intervention unless symptomatic.

Patients who have undergone surgical management of a mature cystic teratoma may benefit from surveillance to monitor for recurrence. Studies report rates of recurrence in the ipsilateral or contralateral ovary ranging from 3% to 20%.[59-63] Limited data regarding timing are available, with one study suggesting a mean time to recurrence of 3 years.[62] Given the paucity of data, surveillance protocols vary, with clinicians often considering ultrasound surveillance for 1 to 3 years postoperatively.

FUTURE DIRECTIONS

Adnexal lesions occur in infants, children, and adolescents with varying frequency and represent functional ovarian lesions, ovarian neoplasms, and nonovarian pathology. Although the majority of lesions are benign, malignancies do occur within the patient population and require careful diagnostic consideration. Ongoing efforts to improve algorithms that predict malignancy will serve to better identify patients who can be safely managed with ovarian-sparing therapies.

KEY POINTS

- Fetal and neonatal ovarian cysts are most often functional in nature and can be managed expectantly with serial imaging until lesion resolution.
- Ultrasonography is considered first line for imaging adnexal lesions in infants, children, and adolescents.
- In childhood, most ovarian lesions are benign neoplasms (most often germ cell neoplasms) with low rates of functional lesions given the quiescent hypothalamic-pituitary-ovarian axis.
- Within adolescents, up to half of adnexal lesions are functional in nature, which can be managed expectantly with serial imaging to assess for resolution.
- Surgical management is considered for nonresolving lesions, acute pathology (such as ovarian torsion), and suspected neoplasms; whenever appropriate, ovarian-sparing therapy is preferred to oophorectomy to preserve endocrine function and fertility.

REVIEW QUESTIONS

1. Which of the following imaging characteristics is not suggestive of the most common benign ovarian neoplasm in childhood?
   a. Cystic lesion
   b. Dot-dash pattern
   c. Presence of solid nodule
   d. Increased vascularity
2. Which tumor markers would be most helpful in a prepubertal child presenting with a solid-cystic mass, rapid breast development and vaginal bleeding?
   a. Human chorionic gonadotropin (HCG)
   b. Ca-125
   c. Inhibin B
   d. Lactate dehydrogenase (LDH)
3. Which of the following characteristics do not help risk-stratify a lesion as benign or malignant?
   a. Vascularity
   b. Patient age/pubertal status
   c. Presentation with abdominal or pelvic pain
   d. Lesion size

REFERENCES

1. Bryant AE, Laufer MR. Fetal ovarian cysts: incidence, diagnosis and management. *J Reprod Med.* 2004;49(5): 329-337.
2. Strickland JL. Ovarian cysts in neonates, children and adolescents. *Curr Opin Obstet Gynecol.* 2002;14(5):459-465. doi:10.1097/00001703-200210000-00004
3. Brandt ML, Helmrath MA. Ovarian cysts in infants and children. *Semin Pediatr Surg.* 2005;14(2):78-85. doi:10.1053/j.sempedsurg.2005.01.002
4. Bascietto F, Liberati M, Marrone L, et al. Outcome of fetal ovarian cysts diagnosed on prenatal ultrasound examination: systematic review and meta-analysis. *Ultrasound Obstet Gynecol.* 2017;50(1):20-31. doi:10.1002/uog.16002
5. Chen L, Hu Y, Hu C, Wen H. Prenatal evaluation and postnatal outcomes of fetal ovarian cysts. *Prenat Diagn.* 2020;40(10):1258-1264. doi:10.1002/pd.5754
6. Tyraskis A, Bakalis S, Scala C, et al. A retrospective multicenter study of the natural history of fetal ovarian cysts. *J Pediatr Surg.* 2018;53(10):2019-2022. doi:10.1016/j.jpedsurg.2018.02.049
7. Sakala EP, Leon ZA, Rouse GA. Management of antenatally diagnosed fetal ovarian cysts. *Obstet Gynecol Surv.* 1991; 46(7):407-414. doi:10.1097/00006254-199107000-00001

8. Trinh TW, Kennedy AM. Fetal ovarian cysts: review of imaging spectrum, differential diagnosis, management, and outcome. *Radiographics.* 2015;35(2):621-635. doi:10.1148/rg.352140073

9. Silva CT, Engel C, Cross SN, et al. Postnatal sonographic spectrum of prenatally detected abdominal and pelvic cysts. *AJR Am J Roentgenol.* 2014;203(6):W684-W696. doi:10.2214/AJR.13.12371

10. Lucaccioni L, Trevisani V, Boncompagni A, Marrozzini L, Berardi A, Lughetti L. Minipuberty: looking back to understand moving forward. *Front Pediatr.* 2020;8:612235. doi:10.3389/fped.2020.612235

11. Kuiri-Hänninen T, Sankilampi U, Dunkel L. Activation of the hypothalamic-pituitary-gonadal axis in infancy: minipuberty. *Horm Res Paediatr.* 2014;82(2):73-80. doi:10.1159/000362414

12. Bornstein E, Barnhard Y, Ferber A, Segarra P, Divon MY. Acute progression of a unilateral fetal ovarian cyst to complex bilateral cysts causing acute polyhydramnios. *J Ultrasound Med.* 2006;25(4):523-526. doi:10.7863/jum.2006.25.4.523

13. Wang L, Shimizu E, Ikeda T, et al. Huge fetal ovarian cyst. *Clin Case Rep.* 2020;8(4):774-775. doi:10.1002/ccr3.2734

14. Landrum B, Ogburn PL, Feinberg S, et al. Intrauterine aspiration of a large fetal ovarian cyst. *Obstet Gynecol.* 1986;68(suppl 3):11S-14S.

15. Abolmakarem H, Tharmaratnum S, Thilaganathan B. Fetal anemia as a consequence of hemorrhage into an ovarian cyst. *Ultrasound Obstet Gynecol.* 2001;17(6):527-528. doi:10.1046/j.1469-0705.2001.00443.x

16. Hassan R, Chong YC, Khairun Nisa M, Yew CG, Tan PG, Mazlin J. Hemorrhage in a fetal ovarian cyst. *J Neonatal Surg.* 2017;6(2):49. doi:10.21699/jns.v6i2.505

17. Tyraskis A, Bakalis S, David AL, Eaton S, De Coppi P. A systematic review and meta-analysis on fetal ovarian cysts: impact of size, appearance and prenatal aspiration. *Prenat Diagn.* 2017;37(10):951-958. doi:10.1002/pd.5143

18. Cass DL, Hawkins E, Brandt ML, et al. Surgery for ovarian masses in infants, children, and adolescents: 102 consecutive patients treated in a 15-year period. *J Pediatr Surg.* 2001;36(5):693-699. doi:10.1053/jpsu.2001.22939

19. Brandt ML, Luks FI, Filiatrault D, Garel L, Desjardins JG, Youssef S. Surgical indications in antenatally diagnosed ovarian cysts. *J Pediatr Surg.* 1991;26(3):276-281; discussion 281-282. doi:10.1016/0022-3468(91)90502-k

20. Safa N, Yanchar N, Puligandla P, et al. Treatment and outcomes of congenital ovarian cysts: a study by the Canadian Consortium for Research in Pediatric Surgery (CanCORPS). *Ann Surg.* 2022;277(5):e1130-e1137. doi:10.1097/SLA.0000000000005409

21. Trotman GE, Zamora M, Gomez-Lobo V. Non-surgical management of the auto-amputated adnexa in the neonate: a report on two cases. *J Pediatr Adolesc Gynecol.* 2014;27(2):107-110. doi:10.1016/j.jpag.2013.06.019

22. Diguisto C, Winer N, Benoist G, et al. In-utero aspiration vs expectant management of anechoic fetal ovarian cysts: open randomized controlled trial. *Ultrasound Obstet Gynecol.* 2018;52(2):159-164. doi:10.1002/uog.18973

23. Hermans AJ, Kluivers KB, Janssen LM, et al. Adnexal masses in children, adolescents and women of reproductive age in the Netherlands: a nationwide population-based cohort study. *Gynecol Oncol.* 2016;143(1):93-97. doi:10.1016/j.ygyno.2016.07.096

24. Jain KA. Sonographic spectrum of hemorrhagic ovarian cysts. *J Ultrasound Med.* 2002;21(8):879-886. doi:10.7863/jum.2002.21.8.879

25. Levine D, Patel MD, Suh-Burgmann EJ, et al. Simple adnexal cysts: SRU Consensus Conference update on follow-up and reporting. *Radiology.* 2019;293(2):359-371. doi:10.1148/radiol.2019191354

26. Allen L, Fleming N, Strickland J, Millar H. Adnexal masses in the neonate, child and adolescent. In: Sanfilippo J, Lara-Torre E, Gomez-Lobo V, eds. *Sanfilippo's Textbook of Pediatric and Adolescent Gynecology.* 2nd ed. CRC Press; 2019:137-150.

27. Kirkham YA, Kives S. Ovarian cysts in adolescents: medical and surgical management. *Adolesc Med State Art Rev.* 2012;23(1):178-191, xii.

28. Deligeoroglou E, Eleftheriades M, Shiadoes V, et al. Ovarian masses during adolescence: clinical, ultrasonographic and pathologic findings, serum tumor markers and endocrinological profile. *Gynecol Endocrinol.* 2004;19(1):1-8. doi:10.1080/09513590410001712895

29. Kirkham YA, Lacy JA, Kives S, Allen L. Characteristics and management of adnexal masses in a Canadian pediatric and adolescent population. *J Obstet Gynaecol Can.* 2011;33(9):935-943. doi:10.1016/s1701-2163(16)35019-8

30. Shim JY, Laufer MR. Adolescent endometriosis: an update. *J Pediatr Adolesc Gynecol.* 2020;33(2):112-119. doi:10.1016/j.jpag.2019.11.011

31. Kelleher CM, Goldstein AM. Adnexal masses in children and adolescents. *Clin Obstet Gynecol.* 2015;58(1):76-92. doi:10.1097/GRF.0000000000000084

32. Jermy K, Luise C, Bourne T. The characterization of common ovarian cysts in premenopausal women. *Ultrasound Obstet Gynecol.* 2001;17(2):140-144. doi:10.1046/j.1469-0705.2001.00330.x

33. Renaud EJ, Sømme S, Islam S, et al. Ovarian masses in the child and adolescent: an American Pediatric Surgical Association Outcomes and Evidence-Based Practice

Committee systematic review. *J Pediatr Surg.* 2019;54(3): 369-377. doi:10.1016/j.jpedsurg.2018.08.058

34. Taskinen S, Fagerholm R, Lohi J, Taskinen M. Pediatric ovarian neoplastic tumors: incidence, age at presentation, tumor markers and outcome. *Acta Obstet Gynecol Scand.* 2015;94(4):425-429. doi:10.1111/aogs.12598

35. Brookfield KF, Cheung MC, Koniaris LG, Sola JE, Fischer AC. A population-based analysis of 1037 malignant ovarian tumors in the pediatric population. *J Surg Res.* 2009;156(1):45-49. doi:10.1016/j.jss.2009.03.069

36. Salvador S, Scott S, Glanc P, et al. Guideline no. 403: initial investigation and management of adnexal masses. *J Obstet Gynaecol Can.* 2020;42(8):1021-1029.e3. doi:10.1016/j.jogc.2019.08.044

37. Northridge JL. Adnexal masses in adolescents. *Pediatr Ann.* 2020;49(4):e183-e187. doi:10.3928/19382359-20200227-01

38. Hermans AJ, Kluivers KB, Wijnen MH, Bulten J, Massuger LF, Coppus SF. Diagnosis and treatment of adnexal masses in children and adolescents. *Obstet Gynecol.* 2015;125(3):611-615. doi:10.1097/AOG.0000000000000665

39. Oltmann SC, Garcia N, Barber R, Huang R, Hicks B, Fischer A. Can we preoperatively risk stratify ovarian masses for malignancy? *J Pediatr Surg.* 2010;45(1): 130-134. doi:10.1016/j.jpedsurg.2009.10.022

40. Templeman C, Fallat ME, Blinchevsky A, Hertweck SP. Noninflammatory ovarian masses in girls and young women. *Obstet Gynecol.* 2000;96(2):229-233. doi:10.1016/s0029-7844(00)00929-7

41. Schneider DT, Orbach D, Ben-Ami T, et al. Consensus recommendations from the EXPeRT/PARTNER groups for the diagnosis and therapy of sex cord stromal tumors in children and adolescents. *Pediatr Blood Cancer.* 2021;68(suppl 4):e29017. doi:10.1002/pbc.29017

42. Rogers EM, Casadiego Cubides G, Lacy J, Gerstle JT, Kives S, Allen L. Preoperative risk stratification of adnexal masses: can we predict the optimal surgical management? *J Pediatr Adolesc Gynecol.* 2014;27(3):125-128. doi:10.1016/j.jpag.2013.09.003

43. von Allmen D. Malignant lesions of the ovary in childhood. *Semin Pediatr Surg.* 2005;14(2):100-105. doi:10.1053/j.sempedsurg.2005.01.005

44. Andreotti RF, Timmerman D, Strachowski LM, et al. O-RADS US Risk Stratification and Management System: a consensus guideline from the ACR Ovarian-Adnexal Reporting and Data System Committee. *Radiology.* 2020;294(1):168-185. doi:10.1148/radiol.2019191150

45. Timmerman D, Valentin L, Bourne TH, et al. Terms, definitions and measurements to describe the sonographic features of adnexal tumors: a consensus opinion from the International Ovarian Tumor Analysis (IOTA) Group.

Ultrasound Obstet Gynecol. 2000;16(5):500-505. doi:10.1046/j.1469-0705.2000.00287.x

46. Madenci AL, Levine BS, Laufer MR, et al. Preoperative risk stratification of children with ovarian tumors. *J Pediatr Surg.* 2016;51(9):1507-1512. doi:10.1016/j.jpedsurg.2016.05.004

47. Stanković ZB, Sedlecky K, Savić D, Lukač BJ, Mažibrada I, Perovic S. Ovarian preservation from tumors and torsions in girls: prospective diagnostic study. *J Pediatr Adolesc Gynecol.* 2017;30(3):405-412. doi:10.1016/j.jpag.2017.01.008

48. Goldberg HR, Kives S, Allen L, Navarro OM, Lam CZ. Preoperative risk stratification of adnexal masses in the pediatric and adolescent population: evaluating the decision tree system. *J Pediatr Adolesc Gynecol.* 2019;32(6): 633-638. doi:10.1016/j.jpag.2019.07.005

49. Lawrence AE, Gonzalez DO, Fallat ME, et al. Factors associated with management of pediatric ovarian neoplasms. *Pediatrics.* 2019;144(1):e20182537. doi:10.1542/peds.2018-2537

50. Minneci PC, Bergus KC, Lutz C, et al. Reducing unnecessary oophorectomies for benign ovarian neoplasms in pediatric patients. *JAMA.* 2023;330(13):1247-1254. doi:10.1001/jama.2023.17183

51. ESHRE Capri Workshop Group. Ovarian and endometrial function during hormonal contraception. *Hum Reprod.* 2001;16(7):1527-1535. doi:10.1093/humrep/16.7.1527

52. Di Meglio G, Crowther C, Simms J. Contraceptive care for Canadian youth. *Paediatr Child Health.* 2018;23(4): 271-277. doi:10.1093/pch/pxx192

53. Winton C, Yamoah K. Ovarian torsion and laparoscopy in the paediatric and adolescent population. *BMJ Case Rep.* 2020;13(5):e232610. doi:10.1136/bcr-2019-232610

54. Toker Kurtmen B, Divarci E, Ergun O, Ozok G, Celik A. The role of surgery in antenatal ovarian torsion: retrospective evaluation of 28 cases and review of the literature. *J Pediatr Adolesc Gynecol.* 2022;35(1):18-22. doi:10.1016/j.jpag.2021.08.007

55. Agboola AA, Uddin K, Taj S, et al. Dermoid cyst spillage resulting in chemical peritonitis: a case report and literature review. *Cureus.* 2022;14(9):e29151. doi:10.7759/cureus.29151

56. Childress KJ, Santos XM, Perez-Milicua G, et al. Intraoperative rupture of ovarian dermoid cysts in the pediatric and adolescent population: should this change your surgical management? *J Pediatr Adolesc Gynecol.* 2017;30(6): 636-640. doi:10.1016/j.jpag.2017.03.139

57. Savasi I, Lacy JA, Gerstle JT, Stephens D, Kives S, Allen L. Management of ovarian dermoid cysts in the pediatric and adolescent population. *J Pediatr Adolesc Gynecol.* 2009;22(6):360-364. doi:10.1016/j.jpag.2008.12.008

58. Billmire D, Vinocur C, Rescorla F, et al. Outcome and staging evaluation in malignant germ cell tumors of the ovary in children and adolescents: an intergroup study. *J Pediatr Surg.* 2004;39(3):424-429; discussion 424-429. doi:10.1016/j.jpedsurg.2003.11.027

59. Rogers EM, Allen L, Kives S. The recurrence rate of ovarian dermoid cysts in pediatric and adolescent girls. *J Pediatr Adolesc Gynecol.* 2014;27(4):222-226. doi:10.1016/j.jpag.2013.11.006

60. Knaus ME, Onwuka AJ, Abouelseoud NM, et al. Recurrence rates for pediatric benign ovarian neoplasms. *J Pediatr Adolesc Gynecol.* 2023;36(2):16-166. doi:10.1016/j.jpag.2022.11.006

61. Chabaud-Williamson M, Netchine I, Fasola S, et al. Ovarian-sparing surgery for ovarian teratoma in children. *Pediatr Blood Cancer.* 2011;57(3):429-434. doi:10.1002/pbc.23070

62. Taskinen S, Urtane A, Fagerholm R, Lohi J, Taskinen M. Metachronous benign ovarian tumors are not uncommon in children. *J Pediatr Surg.* 2014;49(4):543-545. doi:10.1016/j.jpedsurg.2013.09.019

63. Templeman CL, Hertweck SP, Scheetz JP, Perlman SE, Fallat ME. The management of mature cystic teratomas in children and adolescents: a retrospective analysis. *Hum Reprod.* 2000;15(12):2669-2672. doi:10.1093/humrep/15.12.2669

Laparoscopic Considerations in the Pediatric and Teen Patient

Alexzandra Adler and Patricia S. Huguelet

Laparoscopic surgery is an important topic in pediatric and adolescent gynecology (PAG) and is becoming the mainstay of operative management for many conditions in this patient population. This chapter aims to outline preoperative, intraoperative, and postoperative considerations for pediatric and adolescent patients undergoing laparoscopic surgery for gynecologic concerns.

PREOPERATIVE CONSIDERATIONS

Informed Consent

Informed consent is imperative for any gynecologic procedure in pediatric and adolescent patients. Most states require a decision maker for those patients under the age of 18. Because most patients presenting to a pediatric and adolescent gynecologist will be under the age of 18, the patient's decision maker must be present. The decision maker should be the legal guardian of the patient, which can include a parent, appointed legal guardian, or court-appointed legal guardian. Cases of life-threatening surgical emergency, pregnancy, or an emancipated minor may not require a legal guardian for informed consent depending on state laws, so it is recommended that providers become familiar with the laws in the state in which they practice.[1-6]

Clinicians should also consider involving the patient in the informed consent process when of appropriate age and development in order to allow the patient to participate and provide assent. This allows the patient to demonstrate an understanding of the indications, risks, and benefits of the procedure and allow the patient to actively participate in their own health care decision making.[1-4] However, this may pose an ethical dilemma in the event the patient opposes the legal guardian and refuses the proposed treatment; thus it is important to understand the laws regarding refusal of lifesaving care in the state they practice.

When possible, and especially with elective gynecologic surgeries, it is recommended that providers schedule a preoperative visit to counsel patients and guardians on the details of the procedure, including the risk and benefits of surgery, alternatives to the procedure, and potential effects on fertility.[2,3,5] The preoperative visit allows the patient, family members, and/or legal guardians to ask relevant questions before obtaining informed consent.

Anatomic Differences in the Pediatric and Adolescent Patient

The subspecialty of PAG continues to grow and expand, resulting in providers who are uniquely trained to understand the anatomic and physiologic differences in the pediatric and adolescent population compared with adults. Pediatric and adolescent anatomy differs based on both the patient's age and pubertal development.

Newborn females will have effects from estrogen exposure in utero, which manifests as a pronounced clitoris and thickened labia majora and minora. Newborn females may also experience light vaginal discharge and/or spotting in the first several weeks to 18 months of life. Estrogen levels then reach a nadir around the age of 3 to 8 years old, resulting in increasingly atrophic external genitalia with a smaller clitoris and external urethral meatus and smaller and more translucent hymenal ring, compared with the adolescent and adult patient (Fig. 30.1). Additionally, the neonatal uterus is much smaller before pubertal onset, measuring approximately 3.5 cm in length and 1.5 cm in width on average.[1,7]

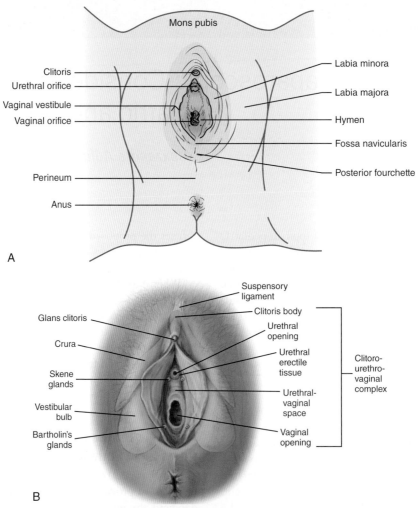

Fig. 30.1 (A) Prepubertal versus (B) postpubertal genital anatomy. (A, From Kristin S. Stukus, Noel S. Zuckerbraun, Review of the Prepubertal Gynecologic Examination: Techniques and Anatomic Variation, Clinical Pediatric Emergency Medicine, 2009;10(1):3-9; B, From Bradley and Daroff's Neurology in Clinical Practice, 7th ed. Elsevier Inc.)

Prepuberatal females have a distinctly erythematous posterior vestibule because of increased capillary density, which can lead to increased bleeding if disrupted (Fig. 30.2). The cervix in prepubertal females takes up approximately two-thirds of the cervico-uterine length, resulting in a spade-shaped uterus. The fundus grows throughout childhood and results in a tubular-shaped uterus as the fundus and cervix become equivalent in size. Additionally, the ovaries in prepubertal patients are abdominal structures and do not descend down into the pelvis until after pubertal onset. As a result of longer fallopian tubes, a smaller uterus, and higher position of the ovary in the pelvis, there is an increased risk of ovarian and tubal torsion in the pediatric and adolescent population.[1,7-10] The bladder is also higher in the abdomen and extended more cranially than in adults, which can affect positioning of laparoscopic ports.[6-9]

Pediatric and adolescent gynecologic surgeons should also be aware of differences in hymenal shape, as this may affect surgical planning in the event of the need for uterine manipulation or vaginal surgery. Differences include annular, crescent, redundant, teardrop, microperforated, septated, and imperforate hymenal shapes. Fig. 30.3 includes two specific variations: the septate hymen and annular hymen.

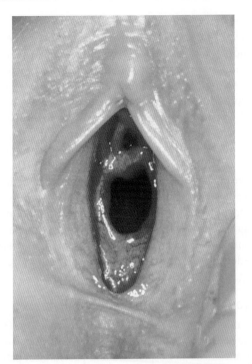

Finally, pediatric and adolescent patients have two unique characteristics that affect laparoscopic entry. The first characteristic is the integrity of the abdominal wall and how it varies with age. There are significant laxity and pliability in the abdominal wall in newborns and infants. The fascial wall tension and strength progressively increase throughout childhood and puberty; therefore the entry forces needed for a young child may be significantly lower than that needed for an adolescent. Moreover, the abdominal wall strength of an adolescent may be significantly greater than that of an adult. The second unique characteristic is the short distance from the abdominal wall to the major abdominal vessels, including the aorta, inferior vena cava (IVC), and the left common iliac vein. This distance is much shorter compared with the adult population and can result in inadvertent injury to the major pelvic vessels if laparoscopic port placement is not adjusted to account for this difference.[1-3,6-8,11,12]

Preoperative Imaging

Preoperative imaging is an important step in surgical planning for many pediatric and adolescent conditions that require laparoscopic surgery. The initial imaging

Fig. 30.2 Erythema at posterior vestibule in prepubertal patient. (Reproduced with permission from North American Society of Pediatric and Adolescent Gynecology Pedi-Gyn Slide Set.)

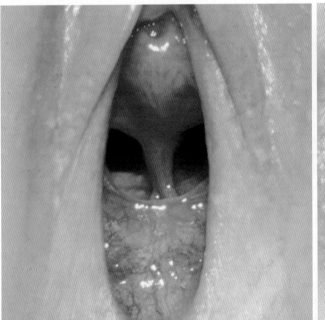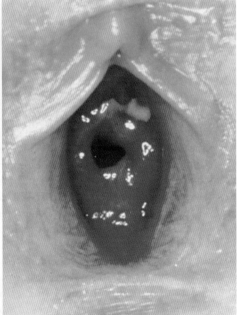

Fig. 30.3 Septate hymen and annular hymen. (Reproduced with permission from North American Society of Pediatric and Adolescent Gynecology Pedi-Gyn Slide Set.)

modality of choice for a pelvic mass is a transabdominal ultrasound of the pelvis. Transvaginal ultrasound is unnecessary and should not be performed in pediatric and adolescent patients, particularly if they have not been sexually active. In some settings where transabdominal imaging quality is poor, both transrectal and transperineal approaches have been described to obtain adequate imaging, especially in the setting of patients with distal vaginal agenesis or transverse vaginal septa, where knowledge of the distance between the perineum and thickness of the obstruction is critical to surgical planning.[1,2,9,13]

Magnetic resonance imaging (MRI) should be considered in the setting of suspected reproductive tract anomalies or if there is concern for malignancy. MRI in such circumstances allows for full evaluation of the gastrointestinal, genitourinary, and lymphatic systems in addition to the pelvic structures. MRI may also aid in surgical planning for patients with transverse septa or distal vaginal agenesis to help determine septal thickness and distance from introitus to the level of obstruction.[1,2,13] In these clinical scenarios, placement of a vitamin E or fish oil capsule at the perineum may help delineate the location of the introitus, as the capsule contains fat and appears hyperdense on imaging.[2,13]

Of note, diagnosis of uterine or vaginal anomalies by imaging alone before puberty can be challenging because of the small size of the prepubertal uterus and lack of endometrial stimulation, which would otherwise distend the uterus and vagina in the setting of a reproductive tract obstruction.[14]

Antibiotic Prophylaxis

Antibotic prophylaxis at the time of laparoscopic surgery is important in both the pediatric and adolescent and adult populations to reduce the risk of surgical site infections.[1,2,15] The Centers for Disease Control and Prevention (CDC) recommends preoperative antibiotic prophylaxis for clean-contaminated cases that involve entry into the genitourinary, gastrointestinal, and alimentary tracts. Surgeries involving the adnexal structures alone (fallopian tubes and ovaries) do not require antibiotic prophylaxis.

General guidelines for preoperative antibiotic prophylaxis are provided by the 2013 statement from the American Society of Health-Systems Pharmacists. Recommendations typically include a single dose of antibiotics administered within 60 minutes of surgical incision and redosage based on the half-life of the antibiotic. First- and second-generation cephalosporins

are generally recommended as first line for prophylaxis.[1,2,16] Table 30.1 summarizes specific guidelines, including dosages and redosing intervals, for pediatric and adolescent patients undergoing gynecologic surgery. Of note, it is recommended that surgeons avoid fluoroquinolones in pediatric patients because of concerns regarding the development of arthropathy.[16] However, the data are sparse on use of fluoroquinolones in pediatric patients, including a specific age range in which to avoid this class of drugs.

Dosing for the pediatric and adolescent patient is typically weight based. If the patient weighs more than 40 kg, antibiotic dosing calculations on a milligram-per-kilogram basis will generally result in doses that exceed recommended adult thresholds. It is therefore recommended that in pediatric patients weighing more than 40 kg, standard adult dosing should be used.

Venous Thromboembolism Prophylaxis

The most common cause of venous thrombolism (VTE) in the pediatric population is thrombosis of an indwelling central catheter in hospitalized and postsurgical patients. Other risk factors include sepsis, congenital thrombotic disorders, underlying malignancy, tobacco use, use of oral contraceptive pills (OCPs), pregnancy, and obesity.[1,2,17]

Data regarding use of VTE prophylaxis in pediatric and adolescent patients are limited, especially in those less than 13 years old, but it has been shown that the risk of surgery-related VTE is lower in patients under 13 years of age.[1,17] Morgan and colleagues found the risk of VTE is negligible in patients under 13 years of age, and routine chemoprophylaxis in this patient population is not recommended.[1,17] It has been proposed that the decreased risk of VTE in this patient population is caused by physiologic differences in the hemostatic system. Patients under 13 years old have approximately 50% less circulating vitamin K–dependent clotting factors, twice the amount of specific thrombin inhibitors, and 25% lower ability to produce thrombin.[17] As a result, it is generally recommended to avoid chemical VTE prophylaxis in patients less than 13 years old, as the risk of chemical prophylaxis outweighs the potential benefit.

Some hospital systems and institutions have developed guidelines and scoring systems to determine at-risk patients based on both patient risk factors—including obesity, use of OCPs, immobility, inherited factors, malignancy, or congenital heart disease—and surgical risk factors such as type and length of sugery. We recommend

TABLE 30.1 Recommended Dosing and Redosing of Commonly Prescribed Antimicrobials for Surgical Prophylaxis

Antimicrobial	Adult Dosing	Pediatric Dosing	Recommended Redosing Interval From Initial Dose (h)
Ampicillin-sulbactam	3 g (2 g ampicillin, 1 g sulbactam)	50 mg/kg of ampicillin component	2
Ampicillin	2 g	50 mg/kg	2
Aztreonam	2 g	30 mg/kg	2
Cefazolin[a]	2 g (3 g if ≥120 kg)	30 mg/kg	4
Cefuroxime	1.5 g	50 mg/kg	4
Cefotaxime	1 g	50 mg/kg	3
Cefoxitin	2 g	40 mg/kg	2
Cefotetan[a]	2 g	40 mg/kg	6
Ceftriaxone	2 g	50–75 mg/kg	n/a
Ciprofloxacin[c]	400 mg	10 mg/kg	n/a
Clindamycin[b]	900 mg	10 mg/kg	6
Ertapenem	1 g	15 mg/kg	n/a
Fluconazole	400 mg	6 mg/kg	n/a
Gentamicin[b]	5 mg/kg (based on dosing weight)	2.5 mg/kg (based on dosing weight)	n/a
Levofloxacin[c]	500 mg	10 mg/kg	n/a
Metronidazole	500 mg	15 mg/kg	n/a
Moxifloxacin[c]	400 mg	10 mg/kg	n/a
Piperacillin-tazobactam	3.375 g	Infants (2–9 mo): 80 mg/kg of piperacillin component Children (>9 mo and ≤40 kg): 100 mg/kg of piperacillin component	2
Vancomycin	15 mg/kg	15 mg/kg	n/a
Oral antibiotics for colorectal surgery (used for mechanical bowel preparation)			
Erythromycin base	1 g	20 mg/kg	n/a
Metronidazole	1 g	15 mg/kg	n/a
Neomycin	1 g	15 mg/kg	n/a

[a]Recommend as first-line agents.
[b]Recommend use of gentamicin and clindamycin for patients with β-lactam antibiotic allergies.
[c]Recommend avoiding use of fluoroquinolones in pediatric patients.
(From Dale W. Bratzler, E. Patchen Dellinger, Keith M. Olsen et.al: Clinical Practice Guidelines for Antimicrobial Prophylaxis in Surgery. Surgical Infections. Vol. 14, No. 1, 2013. https://doi.org/10.1089/sur.2013.9999)

that providers consult their institution-specific guidelines to determine those patients who meet criteria for chemical prophylaxis.

Low-molecular-weight heparins (LMWHs) are the mainstay of chemical prophylaxis in adults and children. LMWHs are preferred to unfractionated heparin (UFH) and warfarin, given the more predictable pharmocokinetics, minimal need for serum monitoring, less alteration in the case of underlying disease, less interaction with concurrent medications, and greater ease of administration, as they are administered subcutaneously instead of intravenously. LMWHs also have less incidence of heparin-induced thrombocytopenia and osteoporosis as compared with UFH. Clinicians should be aware of the patient's kidney function before administration of LMWHs, as these medications are renally cleared.

TABLE 30.2 Low-Molecular-Weight Heparin (Enoxaparin) Dosing in Children by Weight and/or Age			
Patient Age and Weight	Dose	Route	Timing
<5 kg or <2 mo	0.75 mg/kg	Subcutaneous	Twice daily
5–45 kg or >2 mo	0.5 mg/kg	Subcutaneous	Twice daily
>45 kg (regardless of age)	40 mg	Subcutaneous	Once daily

(Morgan J, Checketts M, Arana A, et al. Prevention of perioperative venous thromboembolism in pediatric patients: Guidelines from the Association of Paediatric Anaesthetists of Great Britain and Ireland (APAGBI). Paediatr Anaesth. 2018;28(5):382-391. doi:10.1111/pan.13355)

Table 30.2 provides dosage recommendations for the most commonly used LMWH, enoxaparin, which was adopted from Morgan and colleagues.[17]

Physiologic and Preoperative Anesthetic Considerations

Pediatric and adolescent patients respond differently than adults to the physiologic changes caused by laparoscopy and carbon dioxide insufflation; therefore it is important to operate with an anesthesia provider experienced in pediatric and adolescent physiology.[9,18]

Potential contraindications to laparoscopic surgery include history of significant cardiopulmonary disease and preexisting pulmonary disease. Pneumoperitoneum at the time of laparoscopy increases pressure on the patient's diaphragm, causes cephalic displacement of the diaphragm, and may compromise venous return. Patients with underlying cardiac and pulmonary disease should be medically optimized before any planned procedure, which ideally occurs in the preoperative ambulatory setting with a pediatric anesthesiologist.

INTRAOPERATIVE CONSIDERATIONS

Vaginal Examination and Uterine Manipulation

A thorough examination of the external genitalia is recommended before proceeding with surgery to assess for deviations from normal anatomy, including commonly occurring hymenal variants. This typically will occur in the operating room once the patient is anesthetized and will help to avoid inadvertent trauma if uterine manipulation is required. It is recommended to avoid speculum examinations in pediatric patients to prevent trauma to the hymen, instead using vaginoscopy to visualize the lower and upper vaginal tract. Vaginoscopy involves the use of a camera and distension fluid to visualize the vagina, as with hysteroscopy and cystoscopy. Indications for vaginoscopy include concern for vaginal foreign body, assessment of vaginal bleeding or suspected vaginal masses, and identification of anatomy.

- Video demonstration explaining the indications and set up required for vaginoscopy and hysteroscopy in PAG https://youtu.be/-YVifd5uVx8
  - Pediatric Vaginoscopy and Hysteroscopy Procedures - YouTube

Uterine manipulation is not necessary in most pediatric and adolescent laparoscopic cases. The utility of the uterine manipulator is limited because of the shorter uterine fundus and longer cervix in pediatric patients. When necessary, a sponge stick placed within the vaginal canal, a small Hulka dilator, or a small cervical dilator fixed to a tenaculum can be substituted to allow for a smaller manipulator if uterine manipulation is necessary.[1,6] The risk of uterine perforation in the pediatric population is proposed to be comparable to that of the postmenopausal woman given the hypoestrogenic nature of the prepubertal vagina, cervix, and uterus. This should be taken into consideration when determining the need for uterine manipulation.[1]

In older adolescents, typical uterine manipulators that are used in adults may be employed, including the Hulka dilator, HUMI/ZUMI and acorn dilators (which also allow for chromopertubation to assess tubal patency), and V-care dilators. Although hysterectomies are uncommon in the adolescent population, they are done, for example, for gender-affirming care, in acute lifesaving settings, and/or when all other measures to control bleeding have failed. V-care dilators are particularly useful when uterine manipulation is required for laparoscopic hysterectomy, to help delineate the cervico-uterine junction and push the ureter away from the vaginal cuff (Fig. 30.4).

- Video demonstration of V-care uterine manipulation for laparoscopic hysterectomy VCare® Plus and VCare® DX Plus - CONMED Product Video (youtube.com)
  - Inserting the V-Care Uterine Manipulator - YouTube

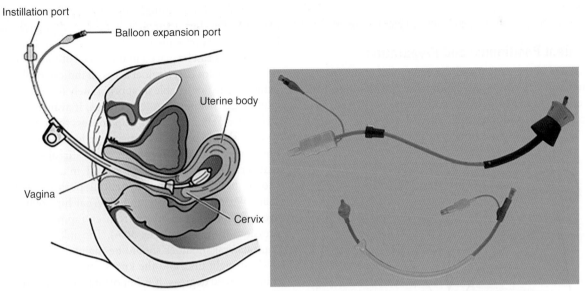

Fig. 30.4 Uterine manipulators. (Left Panel from Nancymarie Phillips, Anita Hornacky: Berry & Kohn's Operating Room Technique. 14th edition. Elsevier 2022.)

Surgical Scrub Preparation

Surgical preparation of the external genitalia and abdomen is often sufficient in pediatric and adolescent patients, as vaginal dissection and uterine manipulation are often not indicated. However, vaginal surgical preparation is indicated in the setting of vaginal surgery or when uterine manipulation will assist with planned laparoscopic surgery. Vaginal preparation can be achieved in the pediatric population with a Toomey syringe inserted just beyond the hymenal fenestration to allow for passive flow of fluid out the vagina and to help avoid any inadvertent trauma to the hymenal tissue.[1,2,6] If a Toomey syringe is unavailable, sponges can be cut to a smaller size or ring forceps can be used to carefully introduce a small unfolded sponge into the vagina, presoaked with surgical prep.

Surgical preparation solutions include sterile normal saline, chlorhexidine-alcohol, and povidone-iodine. The American College of Obstetricians and Gynecologists (ACOG) currently recommends surgical site skin preparations with an alcohol-based agent, usually chlorhexidine-alcohol with 2% chlorhexidine in 70% isopropyl alcohol, unless contraindicated. Povidone-iodine preparations are currently the only U.S. Food and Drug Administration–approved solutions for vaginal surgical site preparation; however, solutions of chlorhexidine

gluconate with low concentrations of alcohol are also safe and effective for off-label use as a vaginal surgical preparation, especially in the setting of iodine allergies.[19] The manufacturer packing labels can also provide specific instructions regarding appropriate length and technique of abdominal and vaginal preparation.

Urinary Foley Catheter Placement

Determination of whether a urinary Foley catheter is needed will depend on the type and length of surgery. It is often sufficient to have the patient void before the procedure or use a straight catheter to empty the bladder at the onset of the case; however, longer cases with more complex dissection may require an indwelling Foley catheter. The urinary catheter allows for bladder decompression to minimize inadvertent trauma to the bladder during surgical dissection and can allow for backfilling of the bladder in order to more easily identify the bladder intraoperatively if needed. Ultimately, determination of need for a urinary Foley catheter is at the discretion of the surgeon.

Standard adult-sized catheters are often too large for the pediatric and adolescent patient. For patients 5 to 12 years old, it is recommended surgeons use a 10-French Foley catheter. Many surgeons use the French-sized catheter to match the patient's age and adjust accordingly. For those patients greater than 12 years old, surgeons may need to increase to a size 12 French Foley catheter or larger.[1,2,6,20]

Patient Positioning and Preparation

The age of the patient and the equipment at the institution will determine the appropriate positioning of the patient. Younger patients will likely be placed in a frog-legged position when vaginal access is required (Fig. 30.5). If vaginal surgery or uterine manipulation is unnecessary, then younger pediatric patients can be placed in the dorsal supine position. With appropriate growth and development, older pediatric and adolescent patients can be placed in the dorsal lithotomy position to allow for easy vaginal access if indicated. Shorter patients may not be able to appropriately fit in standard adult-sized Yellofin or Allen stirrups. If available, pediatric-sized Yellofin stirrups help address this concern.

Care should be taken to ensure patients are correctly positioned in the appropriately sized stirrups to avoid inadvertent nerve compression and injury. The hips should be positioned in a neutral position without sharp flexion, abduction, and external hip rotation to avoid femoral nerve injury from entrapment or compression of the nerve (Fig. 30.6). The ankle, knee, and contralateral shoulder should be maintained in a relatively straight line, and the knees should not be flexed more than 90 degrees. It is important to ensure that the heels are properly seated in the heels of the boots and there are not pressure points on the calf. Care should also be taken not to lean on the patient's inner thigh during surgery, as this can also result in femoral nerve

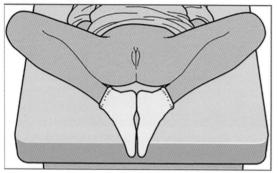

Fig. 30.5 Frog-legged position. (From Roberts, James R, et al. *Roberts and Hedges' Clinical Procedures in Emergency Medicine and Acute Care.* 7th ed., Philadelphia, Pa, Elsevier, 2019.)

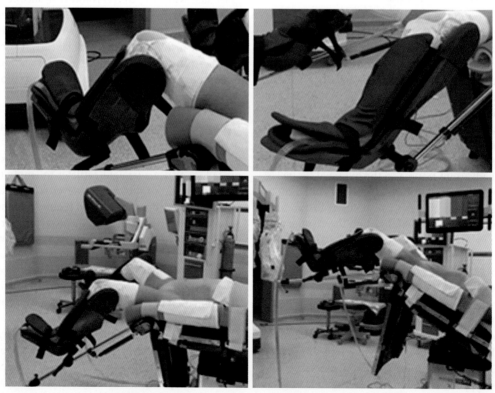

Fig. 30.6 Patient positioning of lower extremities at laparoscopy.

compression. Injury to the femoral nerve can present with paresthesia to the anteromedial aspect of the thigh and medial aspect of the calf. Additionally, if the motor fibers are involved, the patient may report difficulty with ambulation because of weakness with hip flexion, hip adduction, and knee extension, which classically presents as falling when trying to get out of bed or difficulty walking up stairs.[21,22]

The patient's legs should also be placed in the middle of the boot of the Yellofin stirrup, with extra padding applied if needed to the lateral portion of the knee to avoid compression of the common peroneal nerve where it passes on the lateral side of the popliteal fossa and around the fibular neck. Common peroneal nerve injury presents with paresthesias at the dorsum of the foot and lateral surface of the leg. Damage to the motor component of the nerve results in loss of foot dorsiflexion, loss of toe extension, and loss of lateral rotation of the ankle, commonly referred to as *foot drop.*[21,22]

Arms can be tucked at the side of the patient's body, similar to adult gynecologic laparoscopic surgery, thereby optimizing the surgeon's position when operating on the pelvic structures (Fig. 30.7A). The arms should be placed at the side in a pronated position with the thumb pointing superiorly and the fingertips facing the side of the body (see Fig. 30.7B). The arms will then be placed adjacent to the body with the use of a draw sheet. Care should be taken to place a foam pad or other protective material under the elbow to avoid ulnar nerve compression. The ulnar nerve is vulnerable to injury as it passes close to the medial epicondyle. If compressed against a hard surface for an extended period, injury to the ulnar nerve may occur, presenting as sensory loss or paresthesia in the medial 1.5 fingers; when motor nerves are affected, the patient may present with a claw hand.[21,22]

- Patient Positioning for Gynecologic Laparoscopic Surgery (preventing postoperative neuropathies)
  - Preventing postoperative neuropathies: Patient positioning for minimally invasive procedures (youtube.com)

Laparoscopic Entry and Port Placement

Veress, direct, and open laparoscopic entry have all been described in pediatric and adolescent laparoscopic surgery. A Cochrane review from 2015 suggested that the benefit for open technique over Veress needle or direct entry was a lower risk of failed entry,

but no statistically significant increased risk of injury was associated with any of the entry techniques in adult laparoscopic surgery.[1,11]

Pediatric and adolescent patients have two unique characteristics to take into consideration with laparoscopic entry. Abdominal integrity varies greatly, with significant laxity and pliability present in the abdominal wall in newborns and infants and fascial tension and strength progressively increasing as patients age. Additionally, the distance from the abdominal wall to large abdominal vessels, including the aorta, IVC, and left common iliac artery and vein, is significantly shorter in pediatric and adolescent patients.

- Video demonstration of patient positioning and Veress needle abdominal entry technique in gynecologic surgery:
  - Abdominal entry In laparoscopic gynecologic surgery (youtube.com)
- Video demonstration of Open Hassan abdominal entry technique:
  - Open/Hasson's Abdominal Entry for Laparoscopy - step by step (youtube.com)

The confluence of the abdominal wall layers at the base of the umbilicus provides the thinnest site of entry to the abdomen and therefore is the preferred site of entry for gynecologic laparoscopic surgery in pediatric, adolescent, and adult patients.

After entry, ancillary port placements are necessary to allow for tissue retraction, dissection, and resection. Several structures, including the umbilicus, the anterior superior iliac spine (ASIS), and the pubic symphysis, should be considered before placement of additional ports to avoid inadvertent neurovascular injuries. The inferior epigastric artery travels along the lateral third of the posterior surface of the rectus abdominis muscle and lateral to the medial umbilical ligaments. Notably, the inferior epigastric arteries lie deep to the rectus abdominis muscles and are unfortunately poorly transilluminated through the skin with the laparoscope but can be visualized in most cases intraabdominally using direct visualization with the laparoscope. Most neurovascular injuries can be avoided by placing the accessory ports superior to the ASIS and >6 cm from the abdomen's midline (Fig. 30.8). Accessory port placement in this location also allows for proper ergonomics and adequate access to pelvic organs, resulting in improved ease of surgery.[1,2,9,21]

Several case reports in the literature have described an increased risk of fascial herniation with smaller

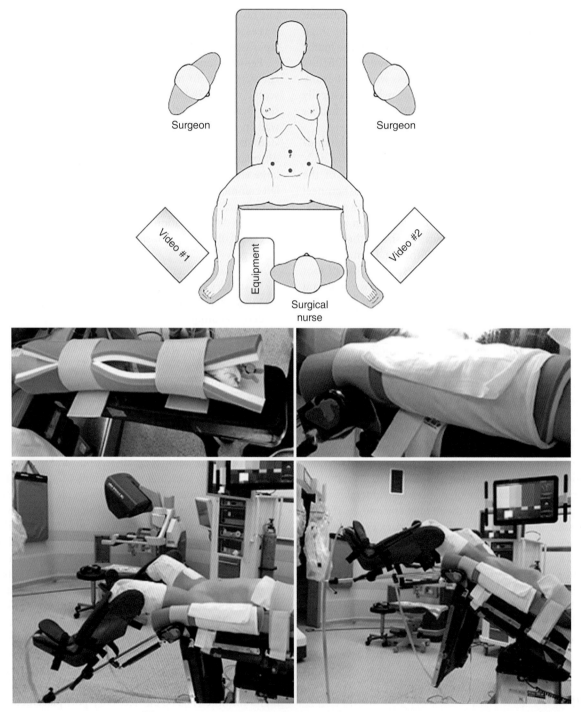

Fig. 30.7 Patient positioning of upper extremities at laparoscopy.

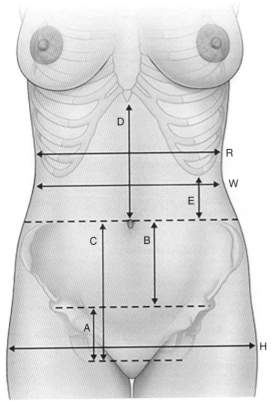

Fig. 30.8 Abdomen and laparoscopic port placement in child/teen.

pain before patients are able to verbally express what they are feeling.[23,24] Despite these limitations, adequate treatment of pain is imperative because undertreated pain can lead to maladaptive physiologic outcomes, including persistent postoperative pain and sensitization. Often, the responsibility to ensure adequate pain control is placed on the guardian. Pain control can be hindered by numerous factors, including guardians' misconceptions about analgesic side effects, fears of addiction, and tolerance.[24,25] Numerous studies have attempted to evaluate the most effective interventions to treat pediatric postoperative pain, including around-the-clock versus as-needed analgesic pain medications, training in pain assessment, nurse coaching, and education on distractions; however, no intervention has been identified as superior to another.[23-25]

Pain is subjective, and severity should be assessed individually for each patient. Numerous tools have been developed to assess pain intensity in pediatric and adolescent patients. The Children's Hospital of Eastern Ontario Pain Scale (CHEOPS) and Face, Legs, Activity, Cry and Consolability (FLACC) may be used to assess pain severity for infants and children less than 5 years old. These are visual charts to assess physical characteristics of pain and guide analgesic administration (Figs. 30.9 and 30.10).[24] Patients greater than 5 years old are typically able to begin to describe the severity of their pain and become increasingly expressive with age. Tools for pain assessment in this age group use a combination of observation and verbal description of their pain. The Wong-Baker FACES Pain Rating Scale, Oucher Scale, Revised Faces Pain Scale (Fig. 30.11), and Visual Analogue Scale (VAS; Fig. 30.12) are frequently used by nurses and other staff in the hospital to assess pain in this patient population.[24]

The 2012 practice guidelines for pain management in the perioperative setting recommend premedication in

diameter port sites in pediatric patients compared with adult patients. Herniations in even 3- to 5-mm incisions have been noted; thus routine closure of the fascia at these port sites should be considered. Despite this recommendation, there is no consensus on what age range of patients to recommend fascial closure for port sites ≤5 mm.[1,2,6,9] The fascia should be reapproximated in port sites that are greater than 10 mm regardless of age.[21]

When considering monopolar and bipolar cautery, adjustments are often made based on age. Similarly, maximum distension pressures are lower in pediatric patients (Box 30.1).

POSTOPERATIVE CONSIDERATIONS

Postoperative Pain Management

Pain in the pediatric patient population has been historically undertreated. This is likely multifactorial and in part the result of difficulty assessing the severity of

Children's Hospital of Eastern Ontario Pain Scale (CHEOPS)[a]

Item	Behavioral	Score	Definition
Cry	No cry	1	Child is not crying.
	Moaning	2	Child is moaning or quietly vocalizing silent cry.
	Crying	2	Child is crying, but the cry is gentle or whimpering.
	Scream	3	Child is in full-lunged cry; sobbing: May be scored with complaint or without complaint.
Facial	Composed	1	Child has neutral facial expression.
	Grimace	2	Score only if definite negative facial expression.
	Smiling	0	Score only if definite positive facial expression.
Child verbal	None	1	Child is not talking.
	Other complaints	1	Child complains, but not about pain, e.g., "I want to see mommy" or "I am thirsty."
	Pain complaints	2	Child complains about pain.
	Both complaints	2	Child complains about pain and about other things, e.g., "It hurts; I want my mommy."
	Positive	0	Child makes any positive statement or talks about others things without complaint.
Torso	Neutral	1	Body (not limbs) is at rest; torso is inactive.
	Shifting	2	Body is in motion in a shifting or serpentine fashion.
	Tense	2	Body is arched or rigid.
	Shivering	2	Body is shuddering or shaking involuntarily.
	Upright	2	Child is in a vertical or in upright position.
	Restrained	2	Body is restrained.
Touch	Not touching	1	Child is not touching or grabbing at wound.
	Reach	2	Child is reaching for but not touching wound.
	Touch	2	Child is gently touching wound or wound area.
	Grab	2	Child is grabbing vigorously at wound.
	Restrained	2	Child's arms are restrained.
Legs	Neutral	1	Legs may be in any position but are relaxed; includes gentle swimming or discrete movements.
	Squirming/ kicking	2	Definitive uneasy or restless movements in the legs and/or striking out with foot or feet.
	Drawn up/tensed	2	Legs tensed and/or pulled up tightly to body and kept there.
	Standing	2	Standing, crouching, or kneeling.
	Restrained	2	Child's legs are being held down.

View full size

[a] Recommended for children 1 to 7 years old; a score greater than 6 indicates pain.
  Face, Legs, Activity, Cry, Consolability Scale

Fig. 30.9 Children's Hospital of Eastern Ontario Pain Scale (CHEOPS).

Categories	Scoring		
	0	**1**	**2**
Face	No particular expression or smile	Occasional grimace or frown, withdrawn, disinterested	Frequent to constant frown, clenched jaw, quivering chin
Legs	Normal position or relaxed	Uneasy, restless, tense	Kicking, or legs drawn up
Activity	Lying quietly, normal position, moves easily	Squirming, shifting back and forth, tense	Arched, rigid, or jerking
Cry	No cry (awake or asleep)	Moans or whimpers, occasional complaint	Crying steadily, screams or sobs, frequent complaints
Consolability	Content, relaxed	Reassured by occasional touching, hugging, or being talked to, distractible	Difficult to console or comfort

Each of the five categories, (F) Face; (L) Legs; (A) Activity; (C) Cry; (C) Consolability, is scored from 0 to 2, which results in a total score between 0 and 10.

Fig. 30.10 Face, Legs, Activity, Cry, and Consolability (FLACC).

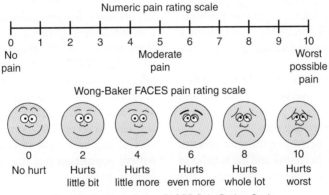

Fig. 30.11 Wong-Baker FACES Pain Rating Scale.

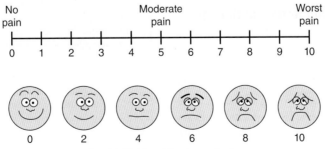

Fig. 30.12 Visual Analogue Scale.

the preoperative setting with two or more analgesics with multimodal mechanisms of action. This includes the use of a combination of acetaminophen, nonsteroidal antiinflammatory drugs (NSAIDs), narcotics, muscle relaxants, and/or neuraxial anesthesia when appropriate. Appropriate analgesic therapy depends on patient age, weight, and comorbidity and should be administered with guidance from the anesthesia provider.[25] Discussion with anesthesia providers regarding the usefulness of epidural anesthesia or transverse abdominus plane (TAP) block or quadratus lumborum (QL) block placement should be considered to aid in management of postoperative pain.

Over the past decade, surgeons have started implementing enhanced recovery after surgery (ERAS) protocols in adult gynecology, as well as in adult and pediatric colorectal surgery and urology. More recently, pediatric gynecologists have also implemented ERAS guidelines to enhance patient recovery after surgery, including a focus on non-narcotic pain management and earlier return to school and other activities.[26] Based on these guidelines, our institution has developed a specific ERAS protocol for pediatric and adolescent patients undergoing abdominal surgery at Children's Hospital Colorado, that includes the use of preoperative and postoperative neuromodulating medication (Fig. 30.13).

Most hospitals specializing in pediatric and adolescent care have dedicated pain services for patients and can be a useful adjunct for those patients with significant and unrelenting postoperative pain.

Ultimately, there is no consensus on the most effective regimen for postoperative pain control and the benefits of scheduled versus as-needed analgesic regimens. Thus pain control must be unique to the patient, and the aforementioned tools can help guide both the provider and guardians in managing the patient's postoperative pain.

Outpatient Recovery and Return to School Activities

Consideration should be given to when surgical procedures are scheduled to minimize disruption to school, home, and social activities for the patient. Worldwide, school absenteeism in girls and young women is commonly attributed to gynecologic issues, including heavy menstrual bleeding, which has been shown to significantly affect educational opportunities and social mobility, further highlighting the importance of minimizing disruption to normal daily activities.[3] Accommodations for school and after-school activities may be necessary, especially in the setting of an unplanned or emergent gynecologic procedure.

The postoperative visit is important for both the patient and guardian to review the procedure performed, confirm the definitive diagnosis and review pathology results, discuss the likelihood of recurrence, review any anticipated impact on fertility, and assess recovery of the patient.[1] This allows the patient and guardian to ask questions and allows the provider to assess for deviations from expected postoperative recovery.

Weight-based lifting restrictions for laparoscopic surgery are often dependent on size and number of port sites and are recommended to help reduce the risk of fascial herniation. Children and adolescents typically self-limit their own activity because of postoperative discomfort. Patients are often advised to use discomfort as a guide for when to start incorporating activities back into their daily lives. Typically, 6 weeks after the procedure, weight-lifting restrictions are stopped and patients can resume all normal activities.

CONCLUSIONS

Laparoscopy for gynecologic procedures in pediatric and adolescent patients allows for shorter hospital stays, faster recovery, less postoperative pain, less adhesion formation, better cosmetic results, potentially less effect on future fertility, and potentially improved visualization.[6-9,20,26-28] The steps to laparoscopic gynecologic surgery in pediatric and adolescent patients are similar; however, PAG surgeons should be aware of several anatomic and physiologic differences in this patient population that may require alterations in surgical technique.

KEY POINTS

- Laparoscopy allows for shorter hospital stays, faster recovery, less postoperative pain, less adhesion formation, better cosmetic results, potentially less effect on future fertility, and potentially improved visualization.
- Most states require a decision maker to facilitate informed consent for gynecologic procedures for pediatric and adolescent patients. Providers should be familiar with the laws surrounding informed consent in the state in which they practice.
- Two unique characteristics in pediatric and adolescent patients that affect laparoscopic entry include the variation in the integrity of the abdominal wall (wall tension and strength progressively increase throughout childhood and puberty) and the short distance from the abdominal wall to the major abdominal vessels including the aorta, IVC, and left common iliac vein.

	Process measure	Gynecology procedures
Preoperative	Counsel about ERAS	Patient instructions handouts + education video = phone = clinic = set expectations
	Carbohydrate load	16–20 oz Gatorade or Apple Juice between 3 and 2 hours prior to **start** time (note that ERAS cases at CHCO have special circumstance to gate NPO times to start time, not arrival time, please communicate accordingly with your patients)
	Avoid prolonged fasting	Regular diet night before, no prolonged clear-liquid diet
	No bowel prep	✓
	Pre-medications	Gabapentin 5 mg/kg TID PO started day prior to surgery, acetaminophen 15 mg/kg PO × 1 in preop
	Antibiotic prophylaxis	Case-appropriate within 60 min prior to incision
Intraoperative	Regional anesthesia	Pre-incision 1-shot blocks (ESP, QL, TAP) for larger incisions or local infiltration of laparoscopic port sites
	Avoiding excess drains	No intraperitoneal or subcutaneous drains
	Euvolemia	Target near zero fluid balance (prefer LR = albumin)
	Normothermia	36–38°C (during skin-to-skin time)
	Minimizing opioids	< 0.3 mg/kg IV morphine equivalents (< 0.3 mcg/kg IV fentanyl or < 0.045 mg/kg IV hydromorphone or < 0.3 mg/kg IV morphine)
	Lap- or robot-assisted	When technically feasible
	DVT prophylaxis	SCDs if any: age ≥ 14, family or personal prior DVT/PE, coag disorder, BMI ≥ 30, expected case duration > 90 min
Postoperative	No nasogastric tube	✓
	N/V prophylaxis	prn ondansetron, miralax 17 g PO daily
	Early feeding	Regular POD #0
	Early mobilization	Out of bed by POD #0
	Non-opioid pain meds (avoid NSAIDs if bilateral grade IV or V reflux, known CKD, solitary kidney, allergy)	Scheduled acetaminophen 10 mg/kg PO Q6hrs (max 650 mg), Ibuprofen 10 mg/kg PO Q6hrs (max 600 mg), gabapentin 5 mg/kg PO TID (max 300 mg)
	Early D/C IVF	✓
	Early D/C of excess drains	N/A
	Minimizing opioids	< 0.15 mg/kg IV morphine equivalents per day (< 0.3 mg/kg/day PO oxycodone [suggested 0.05 mg/kg PO Q4hrs prn breakthrough pain] or < 0.0225 mg/kg/day IV hydromorphone [suggested 0.005 mg/kg IV Q3hrs prn breakthrough pain] or < 0.1125 mg/kg/day [suggested 0.02 mg/kg/day PO Q3hrs prn breakthrough pain]

Fig. 30.13 ERAS protocol at Children's Hospital Colorado.

KEY POINTS—cont'd

- The umbilicus is the preferred site of laparoscopic entry in pediatric and adolescent patients. Accessory ports should be placed superior to the ASIS and >6 cm from the abdomen's midline to allow for proper ergonomics, adequate access to pelvic organs, and avoidance of most neurovascular injuries.
- Preoperative antibiotic recommendations are similar to recommendations for adult patients undergoing gynecologic procedures, the major difference being weight-based dosing for pediatric patients.
- VTE chemoprophylaxis is typically not indicated. LMWHs are preferred if chemoprophylaxis is indicated.
- Pain in pediatric and adolescent patients is often undertreated. Several pain assessment tools have been developed to assess pain more objectively. Ultimately, a multimodal approach (acetaminophen, NSAIDs, narcotics, muscle relaxants, and/or neuraxial anesthesia when appropriate) should be used to manage postoperative pain.

■ REVIEW QUESTIONS

1. Which laparoscopic entry techniques have been described in the pediatric and adolescent patient undergoing gynecologic surgery?
   a. Veress
   b. Direct
   c. Open
   d. All of the above
2. Postoperative venous thromboembolism (VTE) prophylaxis is not often indicated; however, a small subset of patients with risk factors may require chemoprophylaxis. What is the medication of choice for deep venous thromboembolism (DVT) chemoprophylaxis in pediatric and adolescent patients undergoing gynecologic surgery?
   a. Low-molecular-weight heparin
   b. Unfractionated heparin
   c. Warfarin
   d. Aspirin
3. Correct preoperative patient positioning is imperative to avoid nerve compression and injury. What physical examination findings would you expect with a femoral nerve injury?
   a. Loss of sensation to the upper anterior thigh, mons pubis, and labia majora
   b. Loss of sensation to the upper thigh and inner leg and difficulty with knee extension
   c. Loss of sensation to the medial and distal thigh and difficulty with adduction of the thigh
   d. Loss of sensation to the anterior and lateral thigh

REFERENCES

1. Casey J, Yunker A, Anderson T. Gynecologic surgery in the pediatric and adolescent populations: review of perioperative and operative considerations. *J Minim Invasive Gynecol.* 2016;23(7):1033-1039. doi:10.1016/j.jmig.2016.07.005
2. Chan SH, Lara-Torre E. Surgical considerations and challenges in the pediatric and adolescent gynecologic patient. *Best Pract Res Clin Obstet Gynaecol.* 2018;48:128-136. doi:10.1016/j.bpobgyn.2017.10.007
3. Crouch NS, Molyneux MK. Adolescent gynaecology: anaesthetic and peri-operative care implications. *Anaesthesia.* 2021;76(suppl 4):39-45. doi:10.1111/anae.15406
4. Katz AL, Webb SA. Informed consent in decision-making in pediatric practice. *Pediatrics.* 2016;138(2):e20161485. doi:10.1542/peds.2016-1484
5. Informed consent and shared decision making in obstetrics and gynecology. *Obstet Gynecol.* 2021;137(2):392-393. doi:10.1097/aog.0000000000004248
6. Mansuria SM, Sanfilippo JS. Pediatric and adolescent gynecologic laparoscopy. *Infertil Assist Reprod.* 2008;52(3):82-90. doi:10.1017/CBO9780511547287.012
7. Kim HB, Cho HY, Park SH, Park ST. Laparoscopic ovarian surgery in children and adolescents. *J Soc Laparoendosc Surg.* 2015;19(1):1-7. doi:10.4293/JSLS.2014.00253
8. Raźnikiewicz A, Korlacki W, Grabowski A. Evaluation of the usefulness of laparoscopy in the diagnosis and treatment of adnexal pathologies in the pediatric population. *Wideochir Inne Tech Maloinwazyjne.* 2020;15(2):366-376. doi:10.5114/wiitm.2020.93998
9. Raźnikiewicz A, Korlacki W, Grabowski A. The role of laparoscopy in paediatric and adolescent gynaecology. *Wideochir Inne Tech Maloinwazyjne.* 2020;15(3):424-436. doi:10.5114/wiitm.2020.97817
10. Shipps HP. Pediatric gynecology. *J Med Soc N J.* 1962;59:8-13. doi:10.5005/jp/books/11481_11
11. Ahmad G, Gent D, Henderson D, O'Flynn H, Phillips K, Watson A. Laparoscopic entry techniques. *Cochrane Database Syst Rev.* 2015;2015(8):CD006583. doi:10.1002/14651858.CD006583.pub4
12. Buisson P, Leclair MD, Podevin G, Laplace C, Lejus C, Heloury Y. Laparoscopic surgery in children. *Arch Pediatr.* 2005;12(9):1407-1410. doi:10.1016/j.arcped.2005.03.042

13. Amies Oelschlager AME, Berger-Chen SW. Management of acute obstructive uterovaginal anomalies. *Obstet Gynecol.* 2019;133(6):1290-1291. doi:10.1097/AOG.0000000000003282

14. Oelschlager AEA. Diagnosis and management of hymenal variants: ACOG committee opinion no. 780. *Obstet Gynecol.* 2019;133(6):e372-e376. doi:10.1097/AOG.0000000000003283

15. Committee of Practice Bulletins – Gynecology. ACOG practice bulletin: clinical management guidelines for obstetrician-gynecologists prevention of infection after gynecologic procedures. *Obstet Gynecol.* 2018;131(6):e172-e189.

16. Bratzler DW, Dellinger EP, Olsen KM, et al. Clinical practice guidelines for antimicrobial prophylaxis in surgery. *Surg Infect (Larchmt).* 2013;14(1):73-156. doi:10.1089/sur.2013.9999

17. Morgan J, Checketts M, Arana A, et al. Prevention of perioperative venous thromboembolism in pediatric patients: guidelines from the Association of Paediatric Anaesthetists of Great Britain and Ireland (APAGBI). *Paediatr Anaesth.* 2018;28(5):382-391. doi:10.1111/pan.13355

18. Misauno MA, Ojo EO, Uba AF. Laparoscopic paediatric surgery: a potential for paradigm shift in developing countries. *African J Paediatr Surg.* 2012;9(2):140-142. doi:10.4103/0189-6725.99401

19. Kallen AN. Perioperative pathways: enhanced recovery after surgery. *ACOG Comm Opin.* 2018;132(3):801-802.

20. Pelizzo G, Nakib G, Calcaterra V. Pediatric and adolescent gynecology: treatment perspectives in minimally invasive surgery. *Pediatr Rep.* 2019;11(4):64-71. doi:10.4081/pr.2019.8029

21. Hoffman BL, Schorge JO, Schaffer JI, Halvorson LM, Bradshaw KD, Cunningham FG. Minimally invasive surgery. In: *Williams Gynecology.* 2nd ed. McGraw-Hill; 2018:1094-1184. doi:10.1136/tsaco-2018-000290

22. Abdalmageed OS, Bedaiwy MA, Falcone T. Nerve injuries in gynecologic laparoscopy. *J Minim Invasive Gynecol.* 2017;24(1):16-27. doi:10.1016/j.jmig.2016.09.004

23. Chorney JML, Twycross A, Mifflin K, Archibald K. Can we improve parents' management of their children's postoperative pain at home? *Pain Res Manag.* 2014;19(4):115-124. doi:10.1155/2014/938352

24. Zieliński J, Morawska-Kochman M, Zatoński T. Pain assessment and management in children in the postoperative period: a review of the most commonly used postoperative pain assessment tools, new diagnostic methods and the latest guidelines for postoperative pain therapy in children. *Adv Clin Exp Med.* 2020;29(3):365-374. doi:10.17219/acem/112600

25. American Society of Anesthesiologists. Practice guidelines for acute pain management in the peri-operative setting. *Anesthesiology.* 2012;116(2):248-273.

26. Grabowski A, Korlacki W, Pasierbek M. Laparoscopy in elective and emergency management of ovarian pathology in children and adolescents. *Wideochir Inne Tech Maloinwazyjne.* 2014;9(2):164-169. doi:10.5114/wiitm.2014.41626

27. Velde EAT, Bax NMA, Tytgat SHAJ, et al. Minimally invasive pediatric surgery: increasing implementation in daily practice and resident's training. *Surg Endosc Other Interv Tech.* 2008;22(1):163-166. doi:10.1007/s00464-007-9395-5

28. Igwe AO, Talabi AO, Adumah CC, et al. Mitigating the challenges of laparoscopic paediatric surgery in Ile Ife: the trend so far and lessons learnt. *Afr J Paediatr Surg.* 2020;17(3-4):68-73. doi:10.4103/ajps.AJPS_32_20

ANSWERS

CHAPTER 1

1. Correct Answer: A. Current recommendations include screening all nonpregnant women every 5 to 10 years, starting in adolescence, with HgB and/or HCT. Employ selective screening if the patient has at least one risk factor for anemia (e.g., diet low in iron-rich foods, history of iron deficiency anemia, excessive menstrual bleeding, poverty, and/or food insecurities). Answers B to E are recommended components of universal health screening during annual health supervision visits for adolescents per the American Academy of Pediatrics.

2. Correct Answer: C. The first dose of HPV vaccine is routinely recommended at age 11 years old. The vaccination can be started at age 9 years. Only two doses of HPV vaccine are needed if the first dose was given before the 15th birthday. In a two-dose schedule of HPV vaccine, the minimum interval is 5 months between the first and second dose. Children aged 9 to 14 years who receive two doses less than 5 months apart will require a third dose of HPV vaccine. In a three-dose schedule of HPV vaccine, the minimum intervals are 4 weeks between the first and second dose, 12 weeks between the second and third dose, and 5 months between the first and third dose. If the HPV vaccination schedule is interrupted, earlier vaccine doses do not need to be repeated. There is no maximum interval of time between doses—only a minimum time between doses for vaccine efficacy. Patients do need to complete the two-dose or three-dose series depending on whether the first dose was received before age 15 years for maximum protection from HPV. The nonvalent HPV vaccine protects against nine HPV types (6, 11, 16, 18, 31, 33, 45, 52, and 58). HPV vaccination can prevent over 90% of cancers caused by HPV, including cervical, vaginal, vulvar, and anal cancers and precancers.

3. Correct Answer: E. Assessing screen time (including social media use) and physical activity is part of the "A," Activities category. The "H" in the HEADSS mnemonic is for Home, "E" is for Education/employment, and "SS" is for "Sexuality/relationships" and "Suicide/depression" categories.

CHAPTER 2

1. Correct Answer: D. This is the correct answer because health care providers are mandated reporters when abuse is suspected or has occurred. Answer A is incorrect. This disclosure does not warrant disclosure to a parent/guardian. Answer B is incorrect. Minors are entitled to confidential care in all states for treatment of sexually transmitted infections. Answer C is incorrect. More than half the states and the District of Columbia have laws explicitly allowing all individuals to consent to contraceptive care or those at a certain age (e.g., 12 or 14) and older to consent to this care. Nineteen states allow only specific categories of minors to consent to contraceptive services. Four states have no explicit case law or policy. (https://www.guttmacher.org/state-policy/explore/overview-minors-consent-law)

2. Correct Answer: C. To establish rapport, after introducing yourself, you can ask the patient to introduce themselves, and if they do not indicate, ask them their preferred pronouns. Answer A is incorrect. This would not be the first question asked. Generally, time should be made for teen and parent to be interviewed together, then teen alone. If the patient is 18 or older, explicit permission should be asked if a parent should be allowed in any part of the visit due to HIPAA privacy laws. Answer B is incorrect. This is important to obtain, but it would not be the first question asked to establish rapport with a patient. Answer D is incorrect. This would not be the first question asked of the teen.

3. Correct Answer: B. The verbal conversation the practitioner has with a patient can be kept confidential, unless there is disclosure by the patient of abuse or safety concerns (suicide, homicide). Answer A is incorrect. Unless a piece of the medical record is created that would not be visible to anyone who has access to the chart, this cannot be assured. Many systems have created this in the history section of the note (HEADSSS, SHADESS questions) but cannot ensure this in the assessment and plan. Answer C is

incorrect. This is dependent on the parameters set up for the patient portal and who is the primary "owner" of the portal and who is the proxy. It is always important to clarify this with the patient. Most adolescents may not be aware that their parents are the primary owners, even in systems that make parent the proxy, not the owner. Whoever's email is associated with the portal as a primary email would be the individual receiving the information. Answer D is incorrect. Explanation of benefits is generally sent to the owner of the insurance policy, who is the parent/guardian in most cases, even for patients who are over 18. Many young adults, until age 26 years, are insured under their parent/guardian's health insurance. Only 14 states have safeguards protecting confidentiality for insured individuals. (https://www.guttmacher.org/state-policy/explore/protecting-confidentiality-individuals-insured-dependents)

CHAPTER 3

1. Correct Answer: D. Clinicians caring for TGD patients should help patients find inclusive mental health providers especially if they are desiring medical or surgical therapy. Answer A is incorrect. More adolescents than adults identify as gender diverse. Answer B is incorrect. Providers should encourage the staff to use a patient's name and pronouns. Answer C is incorrect. Gynecologists can and should care for transfeminine individuals.

2. Correct Answer: B. Erythrocytosis is one of the most important risks of testosterone use and is an independent risk factor to venous thromboembolism in transmasculine individuals. Hypertension, elevated prolactin and a fasting LDL of 101 are not inherint risks of testosterone in typical range dosing.

3. Correct Answer: D. Currently there is no contraindication to any contraceptive option based on gender identity.

CHAPTER 4

1. Correct Answer: C. Restraining a patient to examine them should be avoided unless they are under 2 years of age if caregivers are agreeable.[7]

2. Correct Answer B. A speculum exam in a prepubertal child, in the office setting, is NEVER appropriate. If you suspect an infection, then vaginal swabs or lavage can be performed to obtain a culture. If you are worried about a foreign body or lesion, then vaginoscopy either at the bedside or in the operating room should be performed.[9]

3. Correct Answer: D. In North America, screening for cervical cancer is indicated only starting at age 21 to 25 years old depending on the province or state you live in. The reason being that the benefits of cervical cancer screening do not outweigh the harms in a younger age group. Also, in young women, most HPV (human papillomavirus) infections go away on their own. Screening people less than 21 years old often leads to unnecessary treatment, which can have side effects.[10,11]

CHAPTER 5

1. Correct Answer: B. This 11-year-old patient is in SMR III based on breast examination and is in their growth spurt, which occurs before menarche. They are already experiencing physiologic leukorrhea, indicating rising levels of estrogen, and for most this precedes menarche by ~6 to 12 months. Answer A is incorrect. This patient is not experiencing delayed puberty, and thelarche and skeletal growth seem appropriate in timeline and are occurring before menarche. Answer C is incorrect. Although maternal and sibling pubertal changes are a good estimate of pubertal timing, the patient in this case is showing other signs, indicating a possible earlier menarche than their mother. Answer D is incorrect. Height growth potential continues for 2 to 2.5 years after menarche.

2. Correct Answer: C. This 8-year-old has a completely normal prepubertal physical examination. There is no evidence of puberty. The light hairs on the mons may be categorized at SMR stage 2; however, pubarche significant of sexual development pubic hair is categorized more at SMR stage 3 with pigmentation and thickening of the hairs. Mons hair growth can occur before axillary hair, but there are cases when the axillary hair develops first and can be normal. Answers A, B, and D are incorrect. Neither laboratory workup, imaging, or medical intervention is needed in this case. Adrenarchal development at younger than 8 years of age would be concerning for premature adrenarche.

3. Correct Answer: A. Breasts at SMR stage 3 and 5 can appear similar in contour, and overall breast size is

not always helpful, as it is not a marker of pubertal change. Based on normal pubertal steps, menarche would be most likely to have occurred already at SMR 5 (typically in SMR 4 breast stage) and would be helpful in differentiating an SMR 3 from SMR 5 breast examination. Answer B is incorrect. Although the growth spurt should be complete by the time of menarche, it may still be occurring during SMR 3 development. Answer C is incorrect. A patient's report of pubic hair is wonderful but may lack the specificity on the distribution and texture that we rely on for pubic hair SMR staging. Answer D is incorrect. Breast tenderness is highly variable and not specific to any one SMR stage. It can occur at the time of breast budding (SMR 2), and may continue throughout later stages of puberty and adulthood, often in a cyclical nature related to menses.

CHAPTER 6

1. Correct Answer: C. A girl with features of Turner syndrome who has ovarian insufficiency will have an elevated FSH if bone age is at least 10 years. Answers A and D are incorrect. A pubertal child with functioning ovaries can have an FSH of 9 IU/L and estradiol of 96 pg/mL. Answer B is incorrect. A prepubertal child will have an LH below the limits of assay detection.
2. Correct Answer: D. The child has had normal pubertal timing and development without any evidence of a syndrome, and her cyclic pelvic pain suggests she may be having menstrual sloughing without evacuation of vaginal blood. This strongly suggests imperforate hymen. Answer A is incorrect. A webbed neck is often seen in Turner syndrome, which in 90% of girls will not result in menarche. Answer B is incorrect. Delta-shaped ears can be seen in CHARGE syndrome, which is often accompanied by delayed puberty with late or no development of secondary sex characteristics. Answer C is incorrect. Children with Russell-Silver syndrome have a small mandible and triangular facies; they can experience central precocious puberty.
3. Correct answer: B. A child with a hypothalamic hamartoma can have central precocious puberty, which can be suppressed until additional physical and emotional growth occur. Suppression is best accomplished using an growth hormone-releasing hormone (GHRH)

analogue that stops pulsatile LH and FSH release. Answer A is incorrect. Hormone replacement with transdermal estrogen and oral progesterone would continue menses and bone age advancement and compromise final adult height. Answer C is incorrect. An aromatase inhibitor is sometimes used for children with McCune-Albright syndrome, a cause of peripheral sexual precocity, to lower estrogen levels but does not have a mechanism of action to prevent LH and FSH stimulation of the ovaries. Answer D is incorrect. Intramuscular depot progesterone injections would not prevent bone age maturation, so final height would be compromised, and unpredictable menstrual bleeding might still occur.

CHAPTER 7

1. Correct Answer: C. Constipation is often associated with urethral prolapse. Answer A is incorrect. Urethral prolapse occurs in states of hypoestrogen and is not associated with precocious puberty. Answer B is incorrect. Chronic pulmonary conditions with sustained increased intra-abdominal pressure may be associated with urethral prolapse, not allergic rhinitis. Answer D is incorrect. Uterine prolapse is rare and not associated with urethral prolapse.
2. Correct Answer: D. Although usually sporadic, risk factors for infantile hemangiomas include prematurity, advanced maternal age, placental abnormalities, female gender, and low birth weight.
3. Correct Answer: A. The treatment of CPP includes long-acting GnRH analogue therapy until the normal age of pubertal onset. Answer B is incorrect. Cystectomy is reserved for an adrenal or ovarian tumor. Answers C and D are incorrect. Aromatase inhibitors and selective estrogen receptor modulators are considered in the treatment of McCune-Albright syndrome.

CHAPTER 8

1. Correct Answer: B. This is the correct answer because menstrual periods lasting longer than 7 days in duration may be an indicator of an underlying bleeding disorder or other concern, and therefore those patients require investigation. Answer A is incorrect. Individuals who have not started menses by 13 years of age do not require further investigation unless

there is a lack of breast development/pubertal development. Individuals with breast development who have not started their menses by age 15 may also require more investigation. Answer C is incorrect. This individual is 2 years post menarche, and the average cycle length intervals can vary between 21 and 45 days. Most menstrual cycles become more regular in time, and those who are older at age of menarche may have anovulatory cycles for longer than those with earlier menarche. Answer D is incorrect. It is a red flag if menstrual periods occur only every 3 months or less.

2. Correct Answer: C. This is the correct answer because the majority of dysmenorrhea in adolescents and young adults is primary and is associated with a normal ovulatory cycle and no pelvic pathology. Answer A is incorrect. Primary dysmenorrhea is mitigated by prostaglandin release and prostaglandin-mediated uterine contractions. Answer B is incorrect. Any individual with period complaints needs to be supported and appropriate treatment offered (even if menstrual symptoms reported are considered "normal" or nonpathologic). Periods need not interfere in someone's functioning. Answer D is incorrect. Dysmenorrhea is common in adolescents and tends to get less common as people age.

3. Correct Answer: D. This is correct because studies have shown that Black adolescents begin puberty and menstruation earlier than their White peers, whereas Latinx youth have menarche between the two. It is important to note that the effects of structural racism on pubertal onset have not been adequately researched. Answer A is incorrect. The age of menarche varies globally, with the onset of both puberty and menarche appearing to occur later in lower-income countries (LICs), likely secondary to suboptimal nutritional status. Answer B is incorrect. Many variables have been identified as potential contributors to timing of menarche; for example, higher weight/BMI, more robust nutritional status, and higher socioeconomic status have all been linked with earlier onset of menarche around the world. Physical activity, sleep quality, and emotional stressors may also be important contributors to pubertal timing. Answer C is incorrect. The median age of menarche across well-nourished individuals in HICs has been relatively stable for several decades, at 12.4 years of age.

CHAPTER 9

1. Correct Answer: B. An immature hypothalamic-pituitary-ovarian axis is the single most common cause of AUB in an adolescent. Answers A, C, and D are incorrect as they are not common in this age group

2. Correct Answer: B. Adolescents with HMB should undergo a workup for bleeding disorder. Eight days of bleeding is considered prolonged, and the patient has additional risk factors of frequent pad changes and nosebleeds. Answers A, C, and D are incorrect because they do not qualify as heavy menstrual bleeding

3. Correct Answer: D. All options may decrease bleeding over time, but norethindrone acetate is the only option used in the acute setting.

CHAPTER 10

1. Correct Answer: A. Functional impairment dysmenorrhea leads to a major impact on a person's work and/or school. It is a leading cause of recurrent short-term school absenteeism for adolescent girls in addition to having a negative impact on sleep, per the American College of Obstetricians and Gynecologists (ACOG). Practice Bulletin "Dysmenorrhea and Endometriosis in the Adolescent."[5] Answers B, C, and D are incorrect. Primary dysmenorrhea does not have an impact on fertility, nor does endometrial cancer. Endometriosis can negatively affect fertility rates; however, it does not affect endometrial cancer risk.

2. Correct Answer: E. Endometriosis has been found in all body parts listed. Most commonly found in the dependent portions of the abdominal cavity, lesions are also found along the surface of the bladder and ovary. Literature reviews include a compilation of pulmonary endometriosis, which can be diagnosed via biopsy and characterized by catamenial hemoptysis. Halban's theory of lymphatic/vascular spread supports remote locations of endometriosis.

3. Correct Answer: C. According to a recent Cochrane Database Systematic Review, NSAIDs appear to be a very effective treatment for dysmenorrhea. Answer A is incorrect. Laparoscopy has a role in the diagnostic process in cases of pelvic pain/dysmenorrhea resistant to NSAIDs and various regimens of hormonal methods. This approach may be also used in cases

where the patient and family want to have a definitive diagnosis with a histologic technique. Answer B is incorrect. GnRH antagonists are reserved for dysmenorrhea cases resistant to NSAIDs and hormonal regulation and, ideally, for cases with biopsy-proven endometriosis because of the significant side effect profile. Answer D is incorrect. Oral contraceptive pills may be prescribed as the next step if dysmenorrhea is not controlled with NSAIDs.

CHAPTER 11

1. Correct Answer: C. The patient's presentation, specifically her history of an eating disorder and low BMI, are most suggestive of functional hypothalamic amenorrhea, a common cause of secondary amenorrhea. Answers A, B, and D are incorrect. Her history is not consistent with the other listed etiologies.
2. Correct Answer: B. The most common cause of secondary amenorrhea is pregnancy, and this should be checked in every patient before considering other causes. Answers A, C, and D are incorrect. Although the other tests listed are indicated in further evaluation of secondary amenorrhea, the first step would be to rule out pregnancy, as it is the most common cause of secondary amenorrhea.
3. Correct Answer: D. This is the correct answer because it is important to perform a karyotype test in patients presenting with primary amenorrhea to determine whether a Y chromosome is present. This will further help determine the etiology of the patient's complaints and may have further implications for treatment. Answer A is incorrect. Although a serum FSH is indicated, a karyotype is more helpful in determining an etiology of the patient's presentation. Answers B and C are incorrect. Abnormal serum prolactin and TSH are less likely to cause a primary amenorrhea with absent müllerian structures.
4. Correct Answer: D. This is the correct answer because the patient described has polycystic ovary syndrome (PCOS). All of the choices have been implicated in the pathogenesis of PCOS. In this disease process, insulin resistance is hypothesized to alter normal hypothalamic hormonal feedback, causing an elevation in LH and FSH, increased androgens (e.g., testosterone) from theca interna cells, and a decreased rate of follicular maturation, resulting in unruptured follicles (cysts) and anovulation.

CHAPTER 12

1. Correct Answer: D. Menarche typically occurs 2 to 2.5 years after breast development begins. We do not start medications for suppression until after this occurs. Answers A to C are incorrect. In addition to not wanting to put patients on medications before they need it (potentially for years), it is possible that the patient may have very light periods that do not bother her. We always discuss waiting until menarche to assess whether medication is necessary.
2. Correct Answer: B. Recommend progestin-only pills. Answers A and D are incorrect. As this patient has a history of a deep venous thrombosis, she should not take the estrogen component of a combined hormonal option. This includes a combined pill and the vaginal ring. Answer C is incorrect. It is also important to remember that even with medical comorbidities, patients can still be sexually active.
3. Correct Answer: D. All answers are correct. It is important to remember that in addition to addressing a patient's chief concern, one should offer education as part of a reproductive health visit. In addition to addressing safety, healthy relationships, and sex and sexuality, this should include topics such as physiologic changes of puberty, safe online practices, consent, and sexual abuse.

CHAPTER 13

1. Correct Answer: C. Energy remaining for bodily functions and physiologic processes after energy for exercise has been used. Answers A, B, and D are incorrect. RED-S is based on a mismatch between energy taken in through diet and calories expended through exercise. Energy availability is what remains after subtracting exercise energy expenditure from energy intake, based on fat-free mass. This remaining energy is what is left to support daily physiologic bodily functioning. Low energy availability and relative deficiency can have negative effects on the human body in a variety of domains: menstrual disorders, impaired bone health, gastrointestinal conditions, hematologic findings, immune function, cardiovascular health, endocrinologic abnormalities, impaired athletic performance, injury, and psychological stress.

$$\text{Energy Availability} = \frac{\begin{array}{c}\text{Energy Intake (in kcal)}\\ -\text{Exercise Energy}\\ \text{Expenditure (in kcal)}\end{array}}{\text{Fat-Free Mass (in kg)}}$$

2. Correct Answer: D. An imbalance between energy intake and expenditure results in hormonal disruption. Answers A to C are incorrect. RED-S is a more comprehensive term for the condition previously known as the female athlete triad and describes the sequelae of the energy imbalance that can occur in athletes who do not meet their daily nutritional needs, resulting in low energy availability (EA). Low EA results in impairments in physiologic bodily functioning, particularly menstruation and bone health. The energy deficiency may be an unintentional mismatch between energy intake and energy spent through exercise or may be intentional because of the presence of disordered eating. Athletes with RED-S can be underweight, normal weight, or overweight. The presence of RED-S is dependent on a state of low EA. Low EA results in hormonal disruptions, which can affect menstrual patterns and cause menstrual dysfunction ranging from amenorrhea to infrequent/ irregular periods. It is not normal or appropriate for athletes to have changes to their menstrual pattern because of increased activity.

3. Correct Answer: C. Increasing energy intake is of critical importance for patients with identified energy deficits. Restoration of adequate daily energy availability is the preferred treatment for RED-S. Answer A is incorrect. If menstrual dysfunction is a concern, combined hormonal oral contraceptive pills will usually induce menstruation in athletes with amenorrhea, but will only mask the underlying problem. Combined oral contraceptives downregulate IGF-1 and increase sex hormone–binding globulin, which may further impair bone growth in oligomenorrheic athletes. Answer B is incorrect. Vitamin D supplementation should be advised if patients are deficient, but there is no available evidence that it protects bone health in amenorrheic athletes. Answer D is incorrect. First-line management for RED-S is restoration of energy availability and elimination of the energy-deficient state. If energy availability is not improved with increases in intake, then reductions in energy expenditure should be considered.

Cessation of all physical activity may be required for athletes who are unable to improve energy availability with increased intake, but only after attempts to augment energy intake.

CHAPTER 14

1. Correct Answer: D. These lesions are at risk for later breast cancer development and should be monitored closely in adulthood after excision in adolescence. Answer A is incorrect. Although it is a mass, it is benign with no increased risk of malignancy. Answer B is incorrect. Diffuse hard tissue may be palpated and is influenced by hormone imbalance; it does not predispose to malignancy. Answer C is incorrect. Although it can abscess and present with purulent discharge, this occurs with obstruction of the areolar tubercle and is not predisposing to malignancy.

2. Correct Answer: C. This patient displays signs of delayed or absent puberty. If no signs of breast development are present by age 13, further evaluation for an underlying cause is warranted. Answer A is incorrect. No secondary sexual characteristics by age 13 prompts concern for delayed puberty evaluation. Answer B is incorrect. Delay in initiating further evaluation could delay diagnosis of other underlying etiologies causing lack of breast development. Answer D is incorrect. After all pathology is excluded, surgical referral should not be considered until 18 years of age.

3. Correct Answer: D. Pregnancy can often cause breast discharge, even if not a typical milky substance, so it is prudent to exclude pregnancy before presuming the discharge is the result of other causes. Answer A is incorrect. Although this may decrease nipple discharge if due to mechanical nature, further evaluation to exclude pregnancy is warranted before these instructions only. Answer B is incorrect. A fasting prolactin is most accurate at excluding intracranial process; no need to repeat lab if in normal range. Answer C is incorrect. There are no data to support that vitamin E decreases milk production; although there are limited data on its effect with breast pain.

CHAPTER 15

1. Correct Answer: D. This is the correct answer because asymptomatic cases should be managed

conservatively, and most cases are expected to improve as child approaches puberty. Answer A is incorrect. Medical management with estrogen therapy is recommended in causes of mild to moderate symptoms with labial adhesions or concern for near obstruction of urethral meatus. This patient is asymptomatic. Answer B is incorrect. Antibiotics are not used as medical management for labial adhesions, especially those for patients who are asymptomatic and have no concerns for vulvovaginitis. Answer C is incorrect. Surgery is reserved for cases involving urinary retention, significant concern for obstruction of the urethral meatus, or recurrent dense labial adhesions that have already failed a trial of medical management.

2. Correct Answer: D. This is the correct answer because in a retrospective case series looking at causes of vulvar aphthous ulcers, viral syndromes were more frequently identified among patients with active ulcers. EBV and CMV have been most frequently identified in serologic testing. Answer A is incorrect. This is an apocrine disorder secondary to chronic follicular occlusion. This results in painful, deep, pustules and subcutaneous nodules that can form sinus tracts throughout the vulva and pelvis. It is not known to form ulcers. Answer B is incorrect. This is a rare disease association with systemic findings of ocular inflammation, genital ulcers, and mouth ulcers. It is important to consider this in the differential of recurrent ulcerations, especially in the setting of oral ulcers or other gastrointestinal ulcers. This is not the most likely cause. Answer C is incorrect. Bacterial vulvar infections can result in vulvovaginitis or, even in rare cases, labial abscesses in young children. They are not known to cause vulvar ulcers.

3. Correct Answer: D. This is the correct answer because given poor perineal hygiene, respiratory and enteric bacterial organisms are the most likely cause identified in cases of prepubertal vulvovaginitis. Answer A is incorrect. This usually causes anal itching patterns at nighttime because pinworms lay their eggs around the anus at night, causing itching and irritation. It can also cause vulvar itching as well but less often. Answer B is incorrect. Viral infections like EBV, CMV, influenza A, or even COVID-19 have been associated with vulvar aphthous ulcer formation, not vaginal discharge. Answer C is incorrect. The most common foreign object in the vagina is toilet paper and is usually associated with prepubertal vaginal bleeding or spotting in addition to malodorous vaginal discharge.

CHAPTER 16

1. Correct Answer: B. This is the correct answer because first-line management for concerns regarding labial hypertrophy or dissatisfaction involves counseling regarding anatomic variations and providing reassurance of normal anatomy. Answer A is incorrect. Labial asymmetry is not abnormal; in fact, it is quite common. Although asymmetry may resolve or persist with age, it is not inherently abnormal. Answer C is incorrect. Surgical correction—labiaplasty—should be reserved for individuals with persistent functional impairment documented on repeat assessments and with appropriate counseling and psychological assessment and ethical considerations. It is therefore not the best next step for this patient. Answer D is incorrect. There are no data to suggest that hormonal contraceptives contribute to labial enlargement or asymmetry.

2. Correct Answer: C. This is the correct answer because wedge resection labiaplasty uses removal of a wedge of tissue with anastomosis of the labia minora. This technique carries the risk of tissue necrosis of the anastomosed tissue. Answer A is incorrect. Vulvovaginal candidiasis is not caused by longer or asymmetric labia minora, and surgical alteration of the labia does not have any relationship to vaginitis caused by yeast. Answer B is incorrect. There are no objective data to show that labiaplasty improves sexual function or treats dyspareunia. There is a theoretical risk that removal of sensitive labia skin may result in alteration of sexual sensation, although this is not well studied. Answer D is incorrect. Edge resection labiaplasty removes the distal edge of the labia, which may alter the natural pigmentation and texture of the labia minora.

3. Correct Answer: D. This is the correct answer because the adolescent must be able to freely assent for labiaplasty, without influence from family members or caretakers. In addition to physical pubertal development, assessment of adolescent emotional maturity and readiness is necessary. Cosmetic labiaplasty for individuals under the age of 18 is illegal in many jurisdictions.

CHAPTER 17

1. Correct Answer: B. This is the correct answer because one study evaluating patients with a history of assault and a comparison group of patients with recent consensual sex found that the posterior fourchette was the genital area most likely injured in both groups. Answers A and C are incorrect. The vaginal side wall and labia are not the most common locations of genital injury. Answer D is incorrect. Although the hymen may show signs of trauma or injury after sexual assault, it is not the most common location when the two groups were compared.

2. Correct Answer: C. This is the correct answer because pediatric perineal lacerations should be repaired with a small-caliber, dissolvable suture, like 3-0 or 4-0 polyglactin. Answer A is incorrect. A PDS suture takes an extended period to dissolve and is not appropriate for vulvar tissues. Answer B is incorrect. A silk suture is a permanent suture. Answer D is incorrect. Monocryl is an appropriate suture type. However, the size of the suture is too large for pediatric perineal laceration repair.

3. Correct Answer: C. This is the correct answer because vulvar dermatosis, like lichen sclerosus, may be confused with trauma because both can present with subepithelial hemorrhages that can look similar to abrasions or contusions. They may also present with vaginal bleeding. Answer A is incorrect. Bite wounds are at increased risk of infection, and antibiotics should considered. Answer B is incorrect. Most straddle injuries (79%–87%) can be managed conservatively. Answer D is incorrect. Topical estrogen cream may help with healing by promoting granulation tissue and reducing inflammation.

CHAPTER 18

1. Correct Answer: D. This is the correct answer because the definition of POI is oligomenorrhea/amenorrhea ≥4 months and FSH >25 IU/L on two occasions >4 weeks apart. FSH needs to be repeated >4 weeks after the initial test. Answer A is incorrect. Pelvic ultrasound is not the most appropriate next step in evaluating POI. Although it may be helpful in identifying any structural abnormalities of the ovaries, it cannot definitively diagnose POI. Answer B is

incorrect. Consulting rheumatology is not necessary for evaluating POI. Given her family history of Hashimoto thyroiditis, there may be an autoimmune component to her POI; however, with a normal TSH, this is less likely. Answer C is incorrect. Starting OCPs is not the most appropriate next step in evaluating POI. OCPs can help regulate menstrual cycles but may mask the symptoms of POI and delay the diagnosis.

2. Correct Answer: C. This is the correct answer because this patient meets the criteria for POI. Given the short stature and POI, you should evaluate for Turner syndrome or mosaic Turner syndrome with a chromosome analysis. Answer A is incorrect. Consulting endocrinology would be appropriate if the patient's diagnosis remains unclear after chromosome analysis or if there are other endocrine concerns beyond POI. Answer B is incorrect. Starting OCPs would not be appropriate until the cause of the patient's amenorrhea is determined. OCPs may mask underlying hormonal imbalances or delay diagnosis. Answer D is incorrect. The patient already meets the criteria for POI since two sets of laboratory tests (FSH, LH, and estradiol) were already obtained. Repeating these tests is not necessary.

3. Correct Answer: B. This is the correct answer because this patient has a long-standing history of POI and is thus at risk of low bone density or osteoporosis. A DXA scan is recommended. Answer A is incorrect. Checking estradiol levels may not provide additional information in this case, as the patient is already on maintenance HRT. Answer C is incorrect. Checking FSH levels may also not provide much additional information, as the patient has a known history of POI. Answer D is incorrect. Starting her on vitamin D supplementation may be a good idea, but it does not address the concern of low bone density or osteoporosis, which is the main issue at hand.

CHAPTER 19

1. Correct Answer: B. The international PCOS guideline endorses the application of the NIH Criteria for diagnosing PCOS in adolescents. The criteria are menstrual dysregulation and clinical and/or biochemical hyperandrogenism. Oligomenorrhea is a common feature of menstrual dysregulation in adolescents with PCOS. Answer A is incorrect. An elevated LH is

commonly seen in PCOS; however, it is not a diagnostic criterion. Answer C is incorrect. The current adult sonographic diagnostic criteria may not sufficiently differentiate PCOS from normal adolescent ovarian morphology. Therefore polycystic ovaries on ultrasound is not recommended to be used as part of the diagnostic criteria in adolescents. Answer D is incorrect. Many adolescents diagnosed with PCOS have a history of premature adrenarche; however, this alone is not part of the diagnostic criteria.

2. Correct Answer: B. Adolescents with PCOS are at an increased risk of developing type 2 diabetes mellitus, not type 1 diabetes. However, type 1 diabetes may predispose to secondary PCOS. Answer A is incorrect. Adolescents with PCOS are at an increased risk of having anxiety and depression; therefore mental health screening is recommended. Answer C is incorrect. There is an increased risk of nonalcoholic fatty liver disease among all patients with PCOS regardless of BMI, so screening of ALT/AST is recommended. Answer D is incorrect. Metabolic syndrome is common in those with PCOS because of obesity and possibly hyperandrogenism as well.

3. Correct Answer: C. The first-line screening for non-classical CAH should be measuring a morning serum 17-hydroxyprogesterone level. Obtaining an afternoon 17-hydroxyprogesterone level may lead to false-negative results, as the hormone levels are typically highest in the morning. Answer A is incorrect. The Endocrine Society clinical practice guideline on CAH caused by 21-hydroxylase deficiency recommends an ACTH stimulation test be performed if basal 17-hydroxyprogesterone level is between 200 and 1000 ng/dL (6 and 30 nmol/L), but not as first-line screening because of the increased cost and burden of this testing for the patient. Answer B is incorrect. Genetic testing may be useful if ACTH stimulation testing results are indeterminate but are not recommended as first-line screening. Answer D is incorrect. A thorough clinical examination is necessary; however, diagnosing clitoromegaly on examination does not confirm CAH. Additionally, many patients with non-classical CAH will not have clitoromegaly.

CHAPTER 20

1. Correct Answer: A. Minors may consent to STI services (testing and treatment) in all states without parental notification. In some states, HIV testing is explicitly included in this, though specific state laws regarding HIV testing and treatment vary. A minor's ability to consent for contraceptive services varies from state to state as well.

2. Correct Answers: A and C. Routine STI screening in sexually active females includes gonorrhea and chlamydia, using a NAAT. Testing for *Trichomonas* may be considered as well. Answer B is incorrect. All adolescents should not be screened for HPV. Answer D is incorrect. Routine testing for HSV is not recommended in asymptomatic patients. Cervical cancer screening begins at 21 years of age, and a Pap smear is currently the recommended test.

3. Correct Answer: C. This patient meets the criteria for a diagnosis of PID, with adnexal tenderness on bimanual examination and other signs and symptoms of STI. Treatment of PID includes ceftriaxone, doxycycline, and metronidazole for 14 days to treat *N. gonorrhoeae*, *C. trachomatis*, and anaerobic organisms. This patient is well-appearing, is able to return for follow-up, and would be a candidate for outpatient treatment of PID. Answers A, B, and D are incorrect.

CHAPTER 21

1. Correct Answer: C. This is the correct answer because this is what the patient asked for, you reviewed all the options available, and this is what the patient ultimately chose for contraception. Answer A is incorrect. Shared decision making is an important part of counseling and choice of contraception options. Answer B is incorrect. An IUD is reasonable to offer, but again, shared decision making includes listening to the patient and avoiding bringing personal bias to the discussion. Answer D is incorrect. Although you can involve a parent depending on the patient's choice and state laws, ultimately the decision rests with the patient.

2. Correct Answer: C. This is the correct answer because there are no data to support that OC users gain more weight than non-OC users. Answers A, B and D are incorrect.

3. Correct Answer: C. This is the correct answer because laws vary state by state. Please consult the Guttmacher Institute state-by-state guidelines cited in the chapter for more information. Answer A is incorrect. For many states, an IUD is considered

contraception and can be placed without parental knowledge or consent, but there are more complex situations even in such states when things like anesthesia, or intellectual disability, or complications from IUD insertion occur and confidentiality cannot be guaranteed. Answer B is incorrect. There are many states where an IUD can be placed without parental knowledge or consent, but it is important to be cognizant of both the laws and the nuances of patient care with regard to consent for procedures, even for contraception, for minors.

CHAPTER 22

1. Correct Answer: E. We would want to avoid an estrogen containing method and shift to progesterone only. Not C because of the thrombophilia, want to avoid estrogen containing contraception methods.

2. Correct Answer: C. Topiramate is a weak inducer of cytochrome P-450, which may reduce the efficacy of estrogen-containing contraceptives when they are used in conjunction. Answer A is incorrect. Migraine with aura confers an increased risk for stroke that is deemed unacceptable, or category 4 by the CDC US MEC. Answer B is incorrect. There are many methods that are not induced by topiramate. Shared decision making should be employed to find the best method that allows the patient to continue using the topiramate, if she chooses. Answer D is incorrect. Topiramate is not induced by DMPA.

3. Correct Answer: E. Answer A is correct because the levonorgestrel emergency contraceptive pill may be less effective in those with BMI $\geq$ 30 kg/m2. Answer B is correct because the contraceptive patch may be less effective in patients weighing more than 91.1 kg. Answer C is incorrect because the risk of thromboembolism does increase with increasing BMI. Answer D is incorrect because contraceptive efficacy of progestin only pills is not affected by BMI.

CHAPTER 23

1. Correct Answer: D. Based on risk stratification, patient C has the highest risk of experiencing treatment-related gonadotoxicity as a result of hypothalamic radiation exposure. However, all of the patients described would benefit from assessment and counseling on fertility preservation before starting planned therapies.

Patients and family members alike find early fertility preservation counseling beneficial, and multiple societies including ACOG and AAP, consider this standard of care.

2. Correct Answer: C. For this postpubertal adolescent whose kidney function necessitates rapid initiation of cyclophosphamide therapy, GnRHa therapy offers menstrual suppression. GnRHa co-administration with chemotherapy for breast cancer increased the likelihood of having preserved ovarian function for adult women, but data have been conflicting in other populations. Because other methods of fertility preservation are not feasible based on time and medical comorbidity, administration of GnRHa can be discussed as an unproven alternative. Answers A, B, and D are incorrect because GnRHas have only been shown to increase the likelihood of preserving ovarian function (but not pregnancy rates) in adult women undergoing chemotherapy for breast cancer, but there is not conclusive data that this is true for pediatric populations or people with other cancers.

3. Correct Answer: B. Consideration of fertility preservation is important in the setting of hematopoietic stem cell transplantation (HSCT) for nononcologic diagnoses such as HLH. Answers A, C, and D are incorrect. HSCT confers a high level of increased risk for gonadotoxicity regardless of pubertal status. For other forms of chemotherapy, gonadotoxicity risk is still present for prepubertal patients, but more likely to happen at higher doses compared with a postpubertal patient. Even reduced-intensity regimens are thought to confer a high risk of POI, with only a few single-agent regimens potentially conferring less risk. For this 3-year-old patient, ovarian tissue cryopreservation is the option most likely to be successful for preservation of ovarian function and future fertility. Ovarian stimulation for oocyte cryopreservation would be unlikely to be successful for this prepubertal patient. Ovarian transposition is used only in the setting of planned pelvic radiation. Although higher doses of chemotherapy are generally needed to cause primary ovarian insufficiency in prepubertal patients compared to postpubertal patients, most conditioning chemotherapy regimens in the setting of stem cell transplants would be expected to pose a risk of primary ovary insufficiency, and fertility preservation should be offered to all patients.

CHAPTER 24

1. Correct Answer: A. Male external genital requires (1) high levels of circulating testosterone, (2) 5-alpha reductase type 2 enzyme for the conversion of testosterone to dihydrotestosterone (DHT) in target organs, and (3) functional androgen receptors. Answer B is incorrect. High circulating testosterone from Leydig cells is required. Answer C is incorrect. AMH is secreted from Sertoli cells and is responsible for müllerian duct regression.

2. Correct Answer: A. Gonadectomy is indicated to reduce the risk of developing a malignant germ cell tumor in patients with Y chromatin present. Answer B is incorrect. Gender identity is a person's innermost concept of self and is independent of biologic sex. Answer C is incorrect. Turner syndrome 45,XO does not confer an increased risk of malignancy, and gonadectomy is not indicated.

3. Correct Answer: B. CAH comprises a family of autosomal recessive disorders that disrupt adrenal steroidogenesis. The most common form is caused by 21-hydroxylase deficiency (21-OHD) associated with mutations in the *CYP21A2* gene. Answer A is incorrect. Complete androgen insensitivity syndrome (CAIS) is an X-linked recessive DSD in which androgen resistance is caused by mutations in the AR gene. Answer C is incorrect. Rapid depletion of oogonia leads to primary ovarian insufficiency.

CHAPTER 25

1. Correct Answer: C. Congenital adrenal hyperplasia is associated with a 21-hydroxylase deficiency, which presents with female virilization, consistent with a urogenital sinus. Answers A, B, D, and E are incorrect. Rectal atresia, rectovestibular fistula, cloacal malformations, and imperforate anus are not associated with congenital adrenal hyperplasia.

2. Correct Answer: C. The most common anorectal malformation in the female population is a rectovestibular fistula, in which the rectum connects to just outside the vagina. Answer A is incorrect. Although imperforate anus was the first described anorectal malformation, it is not the most common. Answers B, D, E, and F are incorrect. Rectal atresia, perineal fistulas, cloacal malformations, and urogenital sinuses are all less common.

3. Correct Answer: B. The patient has concern for imperforate anus, which raises concern for a possible VACTERL association. The patient should undergo an echocardiogram looking for potential congenital cardiac abnormalities before discussing surgical fixation. Answer A is incorrect. A CT abdomen/pelvis would not be indicated and would likely not demonstrate any actionable pathology. Answer C is incorrect. An MIBG scan is indicated for neuroendocrine tumors, which are not associated with imperforate anus. Answer D is incorrect. A brain MRI would be ordered if concern for intracranial neoplasm existed, which is not present in this patient. Answer E is incorrect. With an imperforate anus without a perineal opening, a barium enema would be logistically impossible.

CHAPTER 26

1. Correct Answer: B. Longitudinal vaginal septum is often associated with uterine duplication such as uterus didelphys and bicornuate bicollis. Answer A is incorrect. Longitudinal vaginal septum is not associated with unicornuate uterus. Answer C is incorrect. Uterine agenesis is usually associated with no uterus, uterine remnants, and shortened vagina. Answer D is incorrect. Although longitudinal vaginal septum can occur with normal uterus, it more commonly occurs in the setting of uterine duplication.

2. Correct Answer: A. Renal abnormalities are associated with müllerian anomalies up to 40% of the time; therefore it is important to evaluate the kidneys after diagnosis of a müllerian anomaly. Answer B is incorrect. An x-ray would not provide important anatomic information. Answer C is incorrect. Spinal abnormalities are not common enough with simple uterine didelphys to warrant screening. Answer D is incorrect. Renal US is indicated.

3. Correct Answer: C. As a result of the smaller-capacity uterus, bicornuate uterus is associated with preterm labor, malpresentation (i.e., breech), and pregnancy loss. Answers A and B are incorrect. There is no literature to support this. Answer D is incorrect.

CHAPTER 27

1. Correct Answer: C. These patients present with normal pubertal development, given they have normal ovaries and a 46,XX karyotype. Although some

patients may present with cyclic pain from uterine remnants, this is less common. These patients should be evaluated for renal and spinal concerns as well. Answer A is incorrect. This diagnosis would present with a vaginal bulge with blue hue and is associated with cyclic pain in addition to progressively worsening constipation and urinary dysfunction. Answer B is incorrect. This diagnosis commonly presents in prepubertal children and resolves the majority of the time as puberty ensues. Answer D is incorrect. These patients will present with normal pubertal development, but present early with pelvic pain, given the level of obstruction is located high within the reproductive tract.

2. Correct Answer: A. This is a classic presentation for this condition. Answer B is incorrect. Labial adhesions are most commonly seen in the prepubertal age group. This condition is not associated with hematocolpos. Answer C is incorrect. This type of condition is commonly associated with disorders of sexual development. In this situation, a urethral and vaginal opening are present but are first joined by a common channel that has the appearance of one genital opening aside from the anus. Answer D is incorrect. The bulging of the hymen looks blue and may give one that impression, but given the bulging is in the area of the hymen and there is no trauma history, this is not the diagnosis.

3. Correct Answer: D. This is the gold standard for imaging müllerian anomalies. Answer A is incorrect. Although this study may help elucidate if there is a mass effect or constipation, it will not accurately pick up the reproductive organs. Answer B is incorrect. CT scans can help differentiate bony structures from soft tissue organs, but the level of detail is limited. This can be a useful study to order in the setting of abscess or infection concerns, such as an appendicitis. Answer C is incorrect. This can be a good option to understand complex anomalies of the urogenital sinus or cloaca. This study involves use of contrast media during x-ray evaluation to map out hollow spaces. If a space is blocked, it would not be accurately mapped.

CHAPTER 28

1. Correct Answer: B. About 30% to 50% of female fetuses will have simple cysts <3 cm seen in their adnexa. These represent normal follicles likely being stimulated by maternal and placental hormones. After birth and transferred hormones wear off, these follicles will become atretic and spontaneously resolve. Answer A and C are incorrect. Cystadenomas are rare in the infant. They are benign neoplasms that are usually unilateral and larger than 4 cm. Also, a cystadenoma will persist. Answer D is incorrect because most functional cysts will spontaneously resolve once maternal hormones have worn off.

2. Correct Answer: A. This mass is likely a remote ovarian or adnexal torsion. It progressed from a 4-cm simple mass to a 6-cm complex mass and is persistent at 6 months old as a complex 5-cm cyst. This warrants a pediatric gynecologist or pediatric surgeon consult for possible surgical management. This likely represents a remote (in utero) torsion. Answer B is incorrect. Since the child is well appearing and this is likely a remote event, there is no need for emergent evaluation. Answers C and D are incorrect. This is not pelvic inflammatory disease and does not need a different imaging modality.

3. Correct Answer: C. This newborn has a single perineal orifice with no anal opening, which represents a cloaca (a confluence of the gastrointestinal and genitourinary systems). The midline collection of fluid is likely a hydrocolpos (a fluid-filled vagina). Answers A and B are incorrect. Differences in sexual development (DSD), along with congenital adrenal hyperplasia on examination, may take on a spectrum in appearance of the genitalia (Prader score); also, DSD are not associated with imperforate anus. Answer D is incorrect. An imperforate hymen is usually an isolated anatomic finding and may show a mucocolpos (mucous-filled vagina) in the infant on imaging. On examination, it appears as a bulging introitus below the urethral meatus. Imperforate hymen is not associated with imperforate anus.

CHAPTER 29

1. Correct Answer: D. The most common benign ovarian neoplasm of childhood is a benign dermoid. Common ultrasound findings include cystic components, the dot-dash pattern and presence of a Rokitansky nodule (solid nodule). Increased vascularity would be suggestive of a malignant lesion.

2. Correct Answer: C. A pre-pubertal child presenting with a solid-cystic mass with isosexual precocious puberty would raise suspicion for a granulosa cell tumor. Inhibit B is the associated tumor maker. HCG and LDH would be associated germ cell tumors, while Ca-125 would be most associated with an epithelial lesion.

3. Correct Answer: C. Increased vascularity and size >8 cm have been associated with malignancy. Similarly, patients aged 1 to 8 years have a threefold increase in the risk of malignancy compared to infants and adolescents. Associated abdominal pain does not predict benign versus malignant lesion.

CHAPTER 30

1. Correct Answer: D. All laparoscopic entry techniques have been described in pediatric and adolescent patients. A Cochrane review from 2015 suggested that the benefit of open over Veress or direct entry was a lower risk of failed entry, but no statistically significant increased risk of injury was associated with any of the entry techniques in adult laparoscopic surgery.

2. Correct Answer: A. Low-molecular-weight heparins (LMWHs) are the mainstay of chemical prophylaxis in adults and children. Answers B and C are incorrect. LMWHs are preferred to unfractionated heparin (UFH) and warfarin given more predictable pharmacokinetics, minimal need for serum monitoring, less alteration in the case of underlying disease, less interaction with concurrent medications, and greater ease of administration, as they are administered subcutaneously instead of intravenously. LMWHs also have less incidence of heparin-induced thrombocytopenia and osteoporosis as compared with UFH. Clinicians should be aware of the patient's kidney function before administration of LMWHs, as these medications are renally cleared. Answer D is incorrect.

3. Correct Answer: B. Loss of sensation to the upper thigh and inner leg and difficulty with knee extension are expected findings. Injury to the femoral nerve can present with paresthesia to the anteromedial aspect of the thigh and medial aspect of the calf. Additionally, if the motor fibers are involved, the patient may report difficulty with ambulation because of weakness with hip flexion, hip adduction, and knee extension, which classically present as falling when trying to get out of bed or difficulty walking up stairs. Care should be taken to appropriately position patients preoperatively. The hips should be positioned in a neutral position without sharp flexion, abduction, and external hip rotation to avoid femoral nerve injury from entrapment or compression of the nerve. The ankle, knee, and contralateral shoulder should be maintained in a relatively straight line, and the knees should not be flexed more than 90 degrees. It is important to ensure that the heels are properly seated in the heels of the boots and there are not pressure points on the calf. Answer A is incorrect. It describes a genitofemoral nerve injury. Answer C is incorrect. It describes an obturator nerve injury. Answer D is incorrect. It describes a lateral femoral cutaneous nerve injury.

MENSTRUAL SUPPRESSION

What Is Menstrual Suppression?
Menstrual suppression refers to using hormone medications to make periods lighter or, in some cases, to stop periods completely (amenorrhea).

Why Would I Choose Menstrual Suppression?
For some people, their periods can be heavy and painful. Some have irregular periods that are hard to control. Others are athletes, and their period gets in the way of sports. Some just choose not to have a period. There are many medical reasons to suppress periods!

Is It Safe to Lighten or Stop My Periods?
It is safe to control or stop your period using hormone medications. Using hormonal medications to stop your period is not harmful. However, different methods may have different side effects. You should discuss those with your health care provider.

How Long Will It Take for My Periods to Lighten or Stop?
Different methods take different amounts of time. For the first few months, you might have some unpredictable bleeding, but the bleeding will generally lighten or stop over time. Keeping a menstrual calendar (charting your bleeding and spotting) can be helpful both for you and your health care provider. If you are not achieving enough suppression of your period after 6 to 12 months, you can talk to your provider about other therapies.

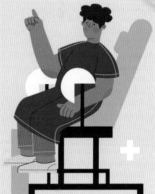

Methods	Pros	Cons	Amenorrhea at 1 Year
Combined hormonal contraceptives (patch/pill/ring)	Easy to start/stop	Contains estrogen, which for some patients is either contraindicated or not desired	Taking continuously (skipping period pills): **60%**
Progesterone-only pills	Easy to start/stop Can achieve reliable suppression at higher doses	Side effects at higher doses: weight gain, mood changes, acne	Dose dependent: **10%** with mini-pill, near **100%** with moderate to high doses
Depo-Provera	Not daily (every 3 months)	Side effects: weight gain, mood changes, acne Requires injection. Bone density changes (although no higher fracture risk).	**60%–70%**
Etonogestrel implant (Nexplanon)	Not daily (lasts 5 years)	Requires insertion procedure. Irregular bleeding is common.	**33%**
Progesterone IUD (Mirena/Liletta)	Not daily (lasts 8 years)	Requires insertion procedure.	**60%–70%**
GnRH analogues (Lupron)	Not daily (can be up to 3 months)	Requires injection. Menopausal effects. Potential impact on bone density.	**95%**

GnRH, Gonadotropin-releasing hormone; *IUD*, intrauterine device.
All data in this handout are taken from the following article: Altshuler AL, Adams Hillard PJ. Menstrual suppression for adolescents. *Curr Opin Obstet Gynecol.* 2014;26(5):323-331.

Courtesy Dr. Megan McCracken

INDEX

Note: Page numbers followed by '*f*' indicate figures '*t*' indicate tables and '*b*' indicate boxes.